Behavioral and Cognitive Neuroscience

Behavioral and Cognitive Neuroscience

Editor: Nell Croft

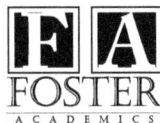

FOSTER
ACADEMICS

www.fosteracademics.com

www.fosteracademics.com

FA
FOSTER
ACADEMICS

Cataloging-in-Publication Data

Behavioral and cognitive neuroscience / edited by Nell Croft.
 p. cm.
Includes bibliographical references and index.
ISBN 978-1-63242-714-4
1. Neuropsychology. 2. Cognitive neuroscience. 3. Neurosciences. I. Croft, Nell.
RC341 .B44 2019
612.8--dc23

Foster Academics,
118-35 Queens Blvd., Suite 400,
Forest Hills, NY 11375, USA

ISBN 978-1-63242-714-4 (Hardback)

Contents

Preface IX

Chapter 1   **Neural correlates of interference resolution in the multi-source interference
task: a meta-analysis of functional neuroimaging studies** 1
Yuqin Deng, Xiaochun Wang, Yan Wang and Chenglin Zhou

Chapter 2   **Mothers' pupillary responses to infant facial expressions** 9
Santeri Yrttiaho, Dana Niehaus, Eileen Thomas and Jukka M. Leppänen

Chapter 3   **The effect of epilepsy on autistic symptom severity assessed by the social
responsiveness scale in children with autism spectrum disorder** 21
Chanyoung Ko, Namwook Kim, Eunjoo Kim, Dong Ho Song and
Keun-Ah Cheon

Chapter 4   **Age, environment, object recognition and morphological diversity of
GFAP-immunolabeled astrocytes** 30
Daniel Guerreiro Diniz, Marcus Augusto de Oliveira, Camila Mendes de Lima,
César Augusto Raiol Fôro, Marcia Consentino Kronka Sosthenes,
João Bento-Torres, Pedro Fernando da Costa Vasconcelos,
Daniel Clive Anthony and Cristovam Wanderley Picanço Diniz

Chapter 5   **Patterns of motor activity in spontaneously hypertensive rats compared to
Wistar Kyoto rats** 49
Ole Bernt Fasmer and Espen Borgå Johansen

Chapter 6   **Transplantation of bone marrow-derived mesenchymal stem
cells (BMSCs) improves brain ischemia-induced pulmonary injury in
rats associated to TNF-α expression** 61
Qin-qin He, Xiang He, Yan-ping Wang, Yu Zou, Qing-jie Xia, Liu-Lin Xiong,
Chao-zhi Luo, Xiao-song Hu, Jia Liu and Ting-hua Wang

Chapter 7   **The social brain network in 22q11.2 deletion syndrome: a diffusion
tensor imaging study** 75
Amy K. Olszewski, Zora Kikinis, Christie S. Gonzalez, Ioana L. Coman,
Nikolaos Makris, Xue Gong, Yogesh Rathi, Anni Zhu, Kevin M. Antshel,
Wanda Fremont, Marek R. Kubicki, Sylvain Bouix, Martha E. Shenton and
Wendy R. Kates

Chapter 8   **Venlafaxine ameliorates the depression-like behaviors and hippocampal
S100B expression in a rat depression model** 92
Chang-Hong Wang, Jing-Yang Gu, Xiao-Li Zhang, Jiao Dong, Jun Yang,
Ying-Li Zhang, Qiu-Fen Ning, Xiao-Wen Shan and Yan Li

Chapter 9   **Cognitive-enhancing and antioxidant activities of the aqueous extract from
Markhamia tomentosa (Benth.) K. Schum. stem bark in a rat model of
scopolamine** 102
Radu Ionita, Paula Alexandra Postu, Galba Jean Beppe, Marius Mihasan,
Brindusa Alina Petre, Monica Hancianu, Oana Cioanca and Lucian Hritcu

Chapter 10   **Transgenerational effects of paternal heroin addiction on anxiety and
aggression behavior in male offspring** 115
Mohd Zaki Farah Naquiah, Richard Johari James, Suraya Suratman,
Lian Shien Lee, Mohd Izhar Mohd Hafidz, Mohd Zaki Salleh and Lay Kek Teh

Chapter 11   **Acute immobilization stress following contextual fear conditioning reduces fear
memory: timing is essential** 125
Akemi Uwaya, Hyunjin Lee, Jonghyuk Park, Hosung Lee, Junko Muto,
Sanae Nakajima, Shigeo Ohta and Toshio Mikami

Chapter 12   **Sex differences in avoidance behaviour after perceiving potential
risk in mice** 138
Sayaka Yokota, Yusuke Suzuki, Keigo Hamami, Akiko Harada and
Shoji Komai

Chapter 13   **Visual food stimulus changes resting oscillatory brain activities related to
appetitive motive** 148
Takahiro Yoshikawa, Masaaki Tanaka, Akira Ishii, Yoko Yamano and
Yasuyoshi Watanabe

Chapter 14   **Involvement of hippocampal acetylcholinergic receptors in
electroacupuncture analgesia in neuropathic pain rats** 159
Shu Ping Chen, Yu Kan, Jian Liang Zhang, Jun Ying Wang, Yong Hui Gao,
Li Na Qiao, Xiu Mei Feng, Ya Xia Yan and Jun Ling Liu

Chapter 15   ***Scutellaria barbata* flavonoids alleviate memory deficits and
neuronal injuries induced by composited Aβ in rats** 169
Xiao G. Wu, Shu S. Wang, Hong Miao, Jian J. Cheng,
Shu F. Zhang and Ya Z. Shang

Chapter 16   ***BDNF* DNA methylation changes as a biomarker of psychiatric
disorders** 179
Galina Y. Zheleznyakova, Hao Cao and Helgi B. Schiöth

Chapter 17   **Interaction between cytochrome P450 2A6 and Catechol-*O*-Methyltransferase
genes and their association with smoking risk in young men** 193
Wei-Chih Ou, Yi-Chin Huang, Chih-Ling Huang, Min-Hsuan Lin,
Yi-Chun Chen, Yi-Ju Chen, Chen-Nu Liu, Mei-Chih Chen,
Ching-Shan Huang and Pei-Lain Chen

Chapter 18   **A novel approach to emotion recognition using local subset feature
selection and modified Dempster-Shafer theory** 202
Morteza Zangeneh Soroush, Keivan Maghooli,
Seyed Kamaledin Setarehdan and Ali Motie Nasrabadi

Chapter 19   **Interaction of basolateral amygdala, ventral hippocampus and**
medial prefrontal cortex regulates the consolidation and extinction of
social fear.. 217
Chu-Chu Qi, Qing-Jun Wang, Xue-zhu Ma, Hai-Chao Chen, Li-Ping Gao,
Jie Yin and Yu-Hong Jing

Chapter 20   **Assessing ADHD symptoms in children and adults: evaluating the role of**
objective measures 230
Theresa S. Emser, Blair A. Johnston, J. Douglas Steele, Sandra Kooij,
Lisa Thorell and Hanna Christiansen

Chapter 21   **Effects of social defeat stress on dopamine D2 receptor isoforms and proteins**
involved in intracellular trafficking... 243
Vishwanath Vasudev Prabhu, Thong Ba Nguyen, Yin Cui, Young-Eun Oh,
Keon-Hak Lee, Tarique R. Bagalkot and Young-Chul Chung

Chapter 22   **Frontal dysconnectivity in 22q11.2 deletion syndrome: an atlas-based**
functional connectivity analysis 260
Leah M. Mattiaccio, Ioana L. Coman, Carlie A. Thompson, Wanda P. Fremont,
Kevin M. Antshel and Wendy R. Kates

Permissions

List of Contributors

Index

Preface

Neuroscience is a multidisciplinary branch of biology that is concerned with the scientific study of the nervous system. It integrates principles of molecular biology, anatomy, developmental biology, cytology, physiology, etc. to develop an understanding of neurons and neural circuits. At the cognitive level, the understanding of psychological functions and their production by neural circuitry is addressed from the branch of cognitive neuroscience. Neuroimaging techniques like PET, SPECT, fMRI scans etc., human genetic analysis and electrophysiology are combined with advanced sophisticated experimental techniques to provide insights into human cognition and emotion. The complex questions pertaining to the interactions of the brain with its environment are dealt through an integration with social and behavioral sciences. The developmental, physiological and genetic mechanisms of behavior are studied in behavioral neuroscience. Research in behavioral neuroscience investigates changes relative to increase or decrease of neural function and enhanced neural activity. This can be measured using electroencephalography, fMRI, PET, various optical techniques, etc. This book covers in detail some existing theories and innovative concepts revolving around behavioral and cognitive neuroscience. It presents these complex subjects in the most comprehensible language. Researchers and students in these fields will be assisted by this book.

Various studies have approached the subject by analyzing it with a single perspective, but the present book provides diverse methodologies and techniques to address this field. This book contains theories and applications needed for understanding the subject from different perspectives. The aim is to keep the readers informed about the progresses in the field; therefore, the contributions were carefully examined to compile novel researches by specialists from across the globe.

Indeed, the job of the editor is the most crucial and challenging in compiling all chapters into a single book. In the end, I would extend my sincere thanks to the chapter authors for their profound work. I am also thankful for the support provided by my family and colleagues during the compilation of this book.

Editor

Neural correlates of interference resolution in the multi-source interference task: a meta-analysis of functional neuroimaging studies

Yuqin Deng[1] 📷, Xiaochun Wang[1], Yan Wang[2] and Chenglin Zhou[1*]

Abstract

Background: Interference resolution refers to cognitive control processes enabling one to focus on task-related information while filtering out unrelated information. But the exact neural areas, which underlie a specific cognitive task on interference resolution, are still equivocal. The multi-source interference task (MSIT), as a particular cognitive task, is a well-established experimental paradigm used to evaluate interference resolution. Studies combining the MSIT with functional magnetic resonance imaging (fMRI) have shown that the MSIT evokes the dorsal anterior cingulate cortex (dACC) and cingulate–frontal–parietal cognitive-attentional networks. However, these brain areas have not been evaluated quantitatively and these findings have not been replicated.

Methods: In the current study, we firstly report a voxel-based meta-analysis of functional brain activation associated with the MSIT so as to identify the localization of interference resolution in such a specific cognitive task. Articles on MSIT-related fMRI published between 2003 and July 2017 were eligible. The electronic databases searched included PubMed, Web of Knowledge, and Google Scholar. Differential BOLD activation patterns between the incongruent and congruent condition were meta-analyzed in anisotropic effect-size signed differential mapping software.

Results: Robustness meta-analysis indicated that two significant activation clusters were shown to have reliable functional activity in comparisons between incongruent and congruent conditions. The first reliable activation cluster, which included the dACC, medial prefrontal cortex, supplementary motor area, replicated the previous MSIT-related fMRI study results. Furthermore, we found another reliable activation cluster comprising areas of the right insula, right inferior frontal gyrus, and right lenticular nucleus-putamen, which were not typically discussed in previous MSIT-related fMRI studies.

Conclusions: The current meta-analysis study presents the reliable brain activation patterns on MSIT. These findings suggest that the cingulate-frontal-striatum network and right insula may allow control demands to resolve interference on MSIT. These results provide new insights into the neural mechanisms underlying interference resolution.

Keywords: Interference resolution, Multi-source interference task, Functional magnetic resonance imaging, Meta-analysis

*Correspondence: chenglin_600@126.com
[1] Department of Sport Psychology, School of Kinesiology, Shanghai University of Sport, 399 Chang Hai Road, Shanghai 200438, People's Republic of China
Full list of author information is available at the end of the article

Background

The interjection of goal-irrelevant information with goal-relevant information is referred to as cognitive interference. For instance, while trying to concentrate on your job, you may have to inhibit the habitual tendency to check your Facebook feed. Successful interference resolution depends on flexible cognitive control that suppresses goal-irrelevant inputs, while selecting and organizing goal-relevant inputs.

The multi-source interference task (MSIT) is a cognitively demanding well established paradigm for assessment of cognitive interference. In the MSIT, stimuli (e.g., the digits "1", "2", or "3", or a letter "X" or a digit "0") are organized into groups of three and participants are required to recognize a unique target among the three items under congruent and incongruent conditions [1, 2]. The spatial position of the unique target matches its correct button-press response in the **congruent condition** (e.g., "1XX" or "100", the unique targets were "1" and the button was responded at the 1st position) and is in conflict with its correct button-press response in the **incongruent condition** (e.g., "331", the unique targets were "1" but the button was responded at the 3nd position). In the MSIT, an interference effect is indexed by the difference in reaction time between incongruent and congruent conditions.

In an initial pilot imaging study of MSIT performance, Bush et al. reported that the dorsal anterior cingulate cortex (dACC) was reliably activated at either the individual- or group-level in the incongruent condition, compared with congruent condition, indicating that the dACC is important for interference processing [1]. Likewise, imaging studies with both youth and adults have shown increased activation in the dACC during MSIT performance and such dACC activity correlated with interference- and error-processing [3, 4]. Moreover, studies examining female twins [5] and subjects diagnosed with attention deficit hyperactivity disorder (ADHD) [6] have provided the evidence indicating that MSIT-related dACC activation may be attributable to genetic factors. Clinical studies have associated dACC dysfunctions with MSIT-related cognitive interference in patients with pediatric obsessive–compulsive disorder (OCD) [7], schizophrenia [8], and posttraumatic stress disorder (PTSD) [9, 10], suggesting that dACC abnormalities may contribute to cognitive difficulties.

Cingulate-frontal-parietal (CFP) cognitive-attentional networks have also been reported to be widely and significantly activated by MSIT [11, 12]. In a sample of younger and older adults, interference process on MSIT was associated with activation of the fronto-parietal and basal ganglia networks [13]. Patients with ADHD have been reported to show dysfunction of CFP cognitive-attention networks and abnormal ACC activity during interference processing [14, 15]. Also, relative to healthy controls, patients with chronic low back pain have been reported to have decreased MSIT-related activation in structures of the CFP network, including the dorsolateral prefrontal cortex, dACC, and superior parietal cortex [16]. Patients with OCD have been reported to exhibit functional abnormalities in the cingulate-frontal circuits, insular cortex and the putamen when performing the MSIT [17–19]. These findings could help to explain the inhibitory control deficits in OCD.

The MSIT interference effects on cortical activity in the aforementioned studies were variable, perhaps due to differences in study design and sample characteristics. Hence, a quantitative assessment of brain network activity in MSIT is needed. In the present study, we applied a meta-analytic approach to synthesize the published MSIT-fMRI studies with the aim of clarifying the locations of generators of interference processing during MSIT performance. We used effect-size signed differential mapping (ES-SDM) as the meta-analytic toolbox [20–22]. The ES-SDM is a reliable quantitative voxel-based meta-analytic method, which allow to integrate statistical parametric maps and peak coordinates. The meta-analytic method has to be superior to other coordinate-based meta-analytical methods owing to its ability to enable reconstruction of both positive and negative coordinate in the same map, leading to a signed differential map and keeping a special voxel from wrongly arising to be positive and negative at the same time [23]. It provides Jackknife sensitivity and heterogeneity analyses to further confirm the replicability of voxel-based meta-analytic findings. In this meta-analysis, we expected to demonstrate replicable brain activation patterns associated with MSIT interference processing within the dACC and in the CFP network.

Methods

Data sources and study selection

We conducted a systematic search of PubMed (http://www.pubmed.org), Web of Knowledge (http://apps.webofknowledge.com), and Google Scholar (http://scholar.google.com) for MSIT-related fMRI studies from 2003 to July 2017. The search term combinations used were: "multi-source interference task" and "functional magnetic resonance imaging". A total of 603 papers were found and assessed to determine if they met the following criteria: (1) an original article published in a peer-reviewed English-language journal; (2) a study employed MSIT during fMRI with a healthy control group; (3) the BOLD fMRI technique was used; (4) MSIT stimuli were numbers and MSIT trials included both incongruent and congruent conditions, as in Fig. 1; (5) the fMRI data were

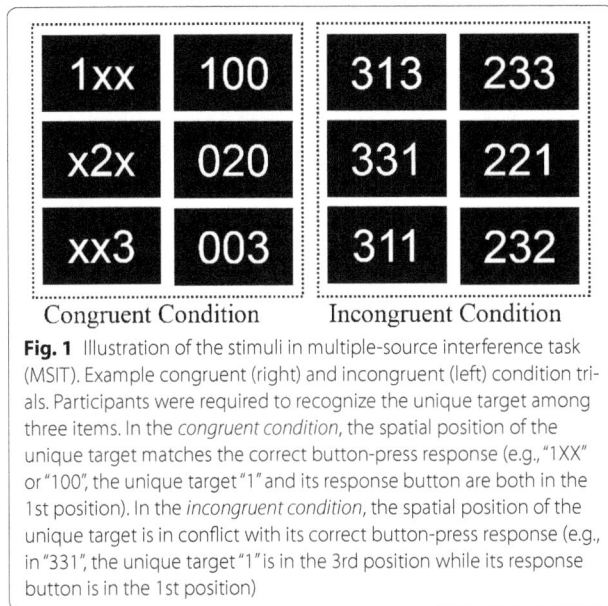

Fig. 1 Illustration of the stimuli in multiple-source interference task (MSIT). Example congruent (right) and incongruent (left) condition trials. Participants were required to recognize the unique target among three items. In the *congruent condition*, the spatial position of the unique target matches the correct button-press response (e.g., "1XX" or "100", the unique target "1" and its response button are both in the 1st position). In the *incongruent condition*, the spatial position of the unique target is in conflict with its correct button-press response (e.g., in "331", the unique target "1" is in the 3rd position while its response button is in the 1st position)

analyzed by contrasting of incongruent versus congruent conditions; (6) a whole-brain, voxel-wise analysis was applied in the fMRI data analysis; and (7) fMRI activation clusters were reported in Talairach or MNI coordinates.

Data analysis
Voxel-wise meta-analysis
Differential BOLD activation patterns between the incongruent and congruent condition were meta-analyzed in Anisotropic Effect-Size Signed Differential Mapping (ES-SDM) software, version 4.13 (http://www.sdmproject.com). ES-SDM, which is a voxel-based meta-analytic approach, is described in detail in the SDM tutorial and publications (http://www.sdmproject.com/software/tutorial.pdf) [20, 22, 23].

The meta-analysis procedure followed three steps. First, the peak coordinates of brain activation differences between incongruent and congruent conditions were retrieved from each study. Peak coordinates were recorded with their z-values, where z could be a positive z-statistic or a negative z-statistic. Second, effect-size and effect-size-variance maps were recreated for each study. Anisotropic kernels were used to optimize the accuracy of these maps [22]. Activation maps, both with contrast of incongruent > congruent conditions, and contrast of congruent > incongruent conditions were calculated by SDM [21]. Third, a voxel-wise random-effects meta-analysis that considered sample size, intra-study variance, and inter-study heterogeneity was conducted [20, 22]. The statistical significance was evaluated with a voxel-level (height) threshold of $p < 0.00001$ and a cluster-level (extent) threshold of k = 100 voxels [20].

Complementary analyses
To evaluate the robustness and replicability of meta-analytic results, whole-brain-voxel-based Jackknife sensitivity analysis was conducted, wherein the same meta-analysis is repeated nine times, each time with a different single study excluded. The principle of the procedure is that if the previous meta-analytic results remain significant, the results can be considered robust and reliable [20, 23]. Statistical significance was set based on the same thresholds applied in the voxel-wise meta-analytic results.

Employing a random effects model with Q statistics, we analyzed heterogeneity to determine whether the observed inter-study variance was larger than that resulting from sampling error alone [20, 23]. Such analyses can reveal any false-positive brain regions due to significant unexplained between-study variability. The default ES-SDM thresholds were set for the heterogeneous results based on a voxel-level threshold of $p < 0.005$ and a cluster-level threshold of k = 10 voxels [20].

A subgroup analysis of adult samples was conducted to examine if potential confounding effects of age contributed to the heterogeneity of the findings [20, 23]. To evaluate the replicability of meta-analytic results, the statistical significance of the subgroup analysis was also identified with the same thresholds applied in the voxel-wise meta-analytic results.

Results
Characteristics of the cohorts of the studies included for meta-analysis
In total, 20 studies met the inclusion criteria for our meta-analysis, of which 12 were excluded for overlapping or duplicating data, leaving eight studies eligible for the final meta-analysis. One of these involved two different healthy sample populations (an adult sample and a youth sample), and the interference effect results of each of the two samples were treated as an independent dataset in the meta-analysis [3]. Hence, our meta-analysis consisted of "nine" study datasets [1–3, 8, 24–27]. The detailed demographic and task-related variables of each study are presented in Table 1.

The characteristics of the analyzed MSIT-fMRI studies (nine datasets) are summarized in Table 1. Altogether, data from a total of 344 subjects (106 females), with a mean age of 29.22 years. Among them, there were 293 adults (80 females; mean age, 31.97 years) and 51 youths (26 females; mean age, 13.42 years).

Changes in regional brain responses to cognitive tasks in MSIT studies, complementary analyses
Voxel-wise meta-analysis showed that, compared to the congruent condition, the incongruent condition

Table 1 Summary of MSIT-fMRI studies (8 studies, 9 datasets) included in the meta-analysis

Study	Adults	Subjects, n (female, n)	Ages	Testa	Software	FWHM	Threshold	Interference condition	Control condition	Effect-size d
Bush et al. [1]	1	8 (4)	30.4±5.6	3	AFNI	NA	Corrected	787±129	479±92	2.75
Fitzgerald et al. [3] adult	1	21 (6)	39.8±9.4	3	SPM2	NA	Corrected	1044±193	803±197	1.24
Fitzgerald et al. [3] youth	0	23 (12)	13.2±3	3	SPM2	NA	Corrected	1062±338	754±212	1.09
Gianaros et al. [2]	1	97 (50)	40.1±6.2	3	SPM8	6	Corrected	905±199.6	540.4±108.9	2.27
Heckers et al. [8]	1	15 (0)	46.6±9.1	1.5	SPM99	8	Uncorrected	873±79	603±67	3.69
Kim et al. [24]	0	28 (14)	13.6±NA	3	SPM8	8	Corrected	969.8±NA	686.9±NA	NA
Shehzad et al. [25]	1	104 (0)	23.9±5.2	3	FSL	6	Corrected	977.57±135.41	632.81±84.79	3.05
Weissman et al. [26]	1	24 (9)	21±NA	3	SPM8	8	Corrected	858±NA	661±NA	NA
Yücel et al. [27]	1	24 (11)	29.58±6.45	3	FSL	5	Corrected	1190±172	861±162	1.97

Table 2 The main difference in activation between the incongruent and congruent conditions during multi-source inter-ference task

Region	Brodmann area	Maximum			Cluster		Jackknife sensitivity analysis
		MNI coordinates x, y, z	SDM value	p value	Number of voxels	Breakdown (number of voxels)	
dACC/MPFC/SMA	6/8/24/32	4, 14, 48	13.305	~0	2056	Supplementary motor area (911) Median cingulate/paracingulate gyri (734) Anterior cingulate/paracingulate gyri (105) Superior frontal gyrus, medial (141) Median network, cingulum (59) *Corpus callosum* (106)	9 out of 9
R insula/R IFG/R PUT	11/45/47/48	42, 20, −2	8.765	~0	902	R insula (366) R inferior frontal gyrus (207) R fronto-insular tract (26) R lenticular nucleus, putamen (136)	9 out of 9
L preCG/L IFG	6/44/48	−52, 2, 22	6.335	~0	279	L precentral gyrus (135) L inferior frontal gyrus (82) L middle frontal gyrus (16)	3 out of 9

L left; *R* right; *MNI* Montreal Neurological Institute; *SDM* signed differential mapping; *dACC* dorsal anterior cingulate cortex; *MPFC* medial prefrontal cortex; *SMA* supplementary motor area; *IFG* inferior frontal gyrus; *PUT* putamen; *preCG* precentral gyrus

produced significantly increased activity in three clusters, involving the dACC, medial prefrontal cortex (MPFC), supplementary motor area (SMA), right insula, right inferior frontal gyrus (IFG), right lenticular nucleus-putamen (PUT), left precentral gyrus, and left IFG (Table 2, Fig. 2). As reported in Table 2, whole-brain jackknife sensitivity analysis revealed two significant clusters involving the dACC, MPFC, SMA, right insula, right IFG, right PUT were highly replicable across all nine datasets. Only three datasets had significantly activated clusters in the left precentral gyrus and left IFG in common.

As reported in Table 3, our heterogeneity analysis detected a significant unexplained inter-study variance, focused mainly on the occipital lobe, parietal lobe, and right cerebellum. But the heterogeneity analysis did not reveal brain regions with significant incongruent versus congruent differences in voxel-wise meta-analysis results (Table 3). Significant clusters in the dACC, MPFC, SMA, right insula, right IFG, and right PUT, but not in the left precentral gyrus and left IFG, were retained in a sub-group analysis of adult subjects. Hence, significant clusters of activation in the voxel-wise meta-analysis results involving the dACC, MPFC, SMA, right insula, right IFG, and right PUT were reliable and robust.

Discussion

To our knowledge, this is the first report of a voxel-based meta-analysis that identified MSIT-associated functional brain activation. Robustness analyses confirmed that the significance of two major activation clusters involving the

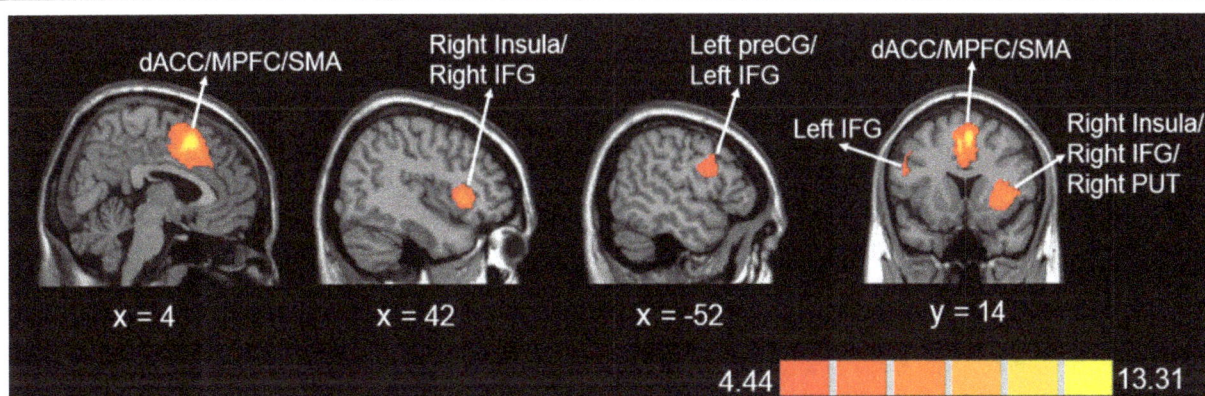

Fig. 2 Significant functional brain activation for incongruent condition > congruent condition determined by meta-analysis. Results with *p* < 0.00001 (cluster size ≥ 100 voxels) are shown. The color bar indicates the regional value of the signed differential mapping (SDM) statistic. *dACC* dorsal anterior cingulate cortex; *MPFC* medial prefrontal cortex; *SMA* supplementary motor area; *IFG* inferior frontal gyrus; *PUT* putamen; *preCG* precentral gyrus

Table 3 Heterogeneity analysis results

Regions	Brodmann area	Maximum MNI coordinates x, y, z	Voxels	SDM value	p value
R fusiform gyrus/R cerebellum	37	38, −50, −22	188	6.109	~0
R angular gyrus/R superior parietal gyrus/R superior occipital gyrus	7	26, −62, 48	105	6.564	~0
L middle frontal gyrus/L precentral gyrus	6	−28, −8, 50	78	6.29	~0
L middle occipital gyrus	18/19	−32, −88, 16	72	5.962	~0
L inferior occipital gyrus/L inferior temporal gyrus	19/37	−42, −66, −8	48	6.112	~0
R supramarginal gyrus/R inferior parietal gyri	2/40	44, −38, 44	47	5.907	~0
R inferior occipital gyrus	19	40, −78, −4	40	5.534	~0
L middle occipital gyrus/L superior occipital gyrus	19/7	−26, −68, 32	38	6.145	~0
L inferior occipital gyrus/L middle occipital gyrus	19	−34, −86, −6	37	5.962	~0
R middle occipital gyrus	19	34, −68, 30	23	5.920	~0
L anterior thalamic projections		−12, −16, 2	18	5.349	~0
L postcentral gyrus/L inferior parietal gyrus	2	−48, −34, 52	15	5.478	~0

L left; *R* right; *MNI* Montreal Neurological Institute; *SDM* signed differential mapping

dACC, MPFC, SMA, right insula, right IFG, and right PUT was reliable and robust during comparison between incongruent and congruent conditions.

Our findings are consistent with previous fMRI studies on MSIT indicating robust activation in the dACC, MPFC and SMA during interference processing when incongruent and congruent conditions are compared [1, 11, 28]. In the MSIT, subjects need to respond to the target while ignoring simultaneously presented unrelated information. Conflict is generated when the task-irrelevant information is incompatible with the target, thereby impeding the processing of task-relevant information. The dACC is recruited to monitor conflict. Higher dACC activity for incongruent trials has also been found in the flanker task [29, 30], Stroop task [30, 31], and Simon task [30, 32], providing further evidence for the supposition that the ACC is involved in detecting conflict in various interference tasks. Electrophysiological studies in both humans and monkeys have shown that dACC neurons firing rates increase during conflict processes and this increase is thought to promote ongoing behavioral adjustment [33–36]. Moreover, our findings are consistent with the conflict-monitoring hypothesis, which posits that increased ACC activity occurs when a high level of conflict is detected in incongruent trials, thereby recruiting top-down cognitive modulation to resolve the conflict and improve performance [37]. On the other hand, most imaging studies examining MSIT performance have found higher SMA activity in incongruent trials than in congruent ones and our meta-analysis results confirmed this conclusion. Anatomically, the SMA has ventral connections with the dACC [38]. Anatomically, the SMA has ventral connections with the dACC [38]. Thus, the SMA and dACC might work together to solve the interference

challenge in the MSIT. Functionally, the SMA participates in movement planning and in action initiation and inhibition [38–40]. In other conflict tasks, researchers have also found that the SMA played a leading role in guiding the process of action-monitoring [41]. In a recent review of neuroimaging, electrophysiological, and stimulation studies of the SMA, Coull et al. proposed that the SMA may be involved in the cognitive development of a sensory representation of time, in addition to its aforementioned roles [42]. Altogether, the SMA is implicated in the process of deciding when to initiate an action or not. This possibility is supported by a prior electrophysiological study showing that neuronal activity in the SMA is associated with proactive and reactive behavioral control in a stop-signal task [43]. The SMA plays a proactive role in controlling arm movements to regulate motor readiness, and is involved in inhibiting arm movements in response to an unexpected stop signal. Accordingly, in the MSIT, after conflict is detected by the dACC, the SMA might be activated to plan movements and to establish flexible adaptive behavior.

An unexpected finding in our meta-analysis was a significantly active cluster involving the right IFG, right insula, and right PUT in comparisons between incongruent and congruent conditions. But previous studies employing the MSIT have found that CFP cognitive-attentional networks are reliably activated under these conditions. Although the result was not predicted, it is in agreement with a previously proposed role of the right IFG [44]. In a systematic review of a decade of literature regarding right IFG functions, Aron et al. found that the right IFG, together with one or more fronto-basal-ganglia network regions (including the PUT), may play a critical role in outright action-stopping in response to external stop or salient signals or internal goals [44]. The authors of other reviews of empirical electrophysiological and neuroimaging data from various inhibition paradigms (e.g., Stroop, Simon, and flanker tasks) have proposed that right IFG/basal ganglia pathways may contribute to goal-directed and habitual inhibition [45–47]. However, Bari and Robbins, who contributed a systematic summary of inhibition and impulsivity studies, suggested that the right IFG appears to be involved not only in the processing of response inhibition but also in the updating of goal-related plans of action [48]. According to these reviews, incongruent MIST trials produce more interference and inhibitory control than congruent trials due to the need to suppress distracting stimuli. Thus, interference may be resolved by engagement of the right IFG and PUT.

The insula is a commonly activated region in the go/no-go task, flanker task, and stimulus–response compatibility task, and insula activation has been shown to be related to interference resolution in each task [49]. Cai et al. examined causal interactions within core frontal-cingulate-parietal regions in the stop-signal task and the flanker task [50]. The strength of causal interaction between the right anterior insula and dACC was found to be greater under high cognitive control conditions than under low ones, and to be significantly associated with cognitive control ability indices in both the stop-signal task and the flanker task, suggesting that both the right anterior insula and dACC may be involved in cognitive control in various interference tasks. On the other hand, the insula and dACC are constituents of "salient network", in which the right insula is thought to detect salient stimuli for recruitment of inhibitory control [51–56]. The salient feature is considered as a stimulus that is highlighted. The incongruent condition of MSIT, in which the target response is inconsistent with the target locations, has higher interference and stand out from the congruent one. Accordingly, in MSIT, the activation in right insula may involve in detecting interference and recruiting the interference-resolution.

Conclusion

In summary, our findings extend the results of prior MSIT studies, confirming that the dACC and prefrontal cortex are the main brain areas activated by MSIT performance. Our meta-analysis confirms cogently, for the first time, two robust activation clusters encompassing the dACC, MPFC, SMA, right IFG, right PUT, and right insula during MSIT performance. Compared to the congruent condition in the MSIT, the incongruent condition is characterized by more conflict and a greater need for cognitive control. On the basis of the functions of the aforementioned brain regions, we postulate that the right

insula may send saliently relevant (high interference) signals to the dACC to be used to induce conflict monitoring, and to the SMA, right IFG, and PUT to be used for movement planning and inhibitory control, enabling goal-related flexible, adaptive behavior to be established. Hence, our findings indicate that a cingulate-frontal-striatum network and the right insula may serve as a critical brain circuit in interference resolution.

Abbreviations
MSIT: multi-source interference task; fMRI: functional magnetic resonance imaging; dACC: dorsal anterior cingulate cortex; CFP: cingulate–frontal–parietal; ES-SDM: effect-size signed differential mapping; MPFC: medial prefrontal cortex; SMA: supplementary motor area; IFG: inferior frontal gyrus; PUT: putamen; preCG: precentral gyrus; ADHD: attention deficit hyperactivity disorder; OCD: obsessive–compulsive disorder; PTSD: posttraumatic stress disorder.

Authors' contributions
YD conceived the study. XW and YW acquired the data, which all authors analyzed and interpreted. YD wrote the article, which XW, YW and CZ reviewed. All authors read and approved the final manuscript.

Author details
[1] Department of Sport Psychology, School of Kinesiology, Shanghai University of Sport, 399 Chang Hai Road, Shanghai 200438, People's Republic of China. [2] Interdisciplinary Center for Social and Behavioral Studies, Dongbei University of Finance and Economics, Dalian 116025, Liaoning Province, People's Republic of China.

Acknowledgements
None.

Competing interests
The authors declare that they have no competing interests.

Funding
This work was supported by China Postdoctoral Science Foundation funded project (Grant Number 2017M610266) and the National Natural Science Foundation of China (Grant Number 31500911).

References
1. Bush G, Shin LM, Holmes J, Rosen BR, Vogt BA. The multi-source interference task: validation study with fMRI in individual subjects. Mol Psychiatry. 2003;8:60–70.
2. Gianaros PJ, Onyewuenyi IC, Sheu LK, Christie IC, Critchley HD. Brain systems for baroreflex suppression during stress in humans. Hum Brain Mapp. 2012;33:1700–16.
3. Fitzgerald KD, Perkins SC, Angstadt M, Johnson T, Stern ER, Welsh RC, Taylor SF. The development of performance-monitoring function in the posterior medial frontal cortex. Neuroimage. 2010;49:3463–73.
4. Liu Y, Angstadt M, Taylor SF, Fitzgerald KD. The typical development of posterior medial frontal cortex function and connectivity during task control demands in youth 8–19 years old. Neuroimage. 2016;137:97–106.
5. Matthews SC, Simmons AN, Strigo IA, Jang K, Stein MB, Paulus MP. Heritability of anterior cingulate response to conflict: an fMRI study in female twins. Neuroimage. 2007;38:223–7.
6. Brown A, Biederman J, Valera EM, Doyle AE, Bush G, Spencer T, Monuteaux MC, Mick E, Whitfield-Gabrieli S, Makris N, LaViolette PS, Oscar-Berman M, Faraone SV, Seidman LJ. Effect of dopamine transporter gene (SLC6A3) variation on dorsal anterior cingulate function in attention-deficit/hyperactivity disorder. Am J Med Genet B Neuropsychiatr Genet. 2010;153:365–75.
7. Fitzgerald KD, Stern ER, Angstadt M, Nicholson-Muth KC, Maynor MR, Welsh RC, Hanna GL, Taylor SF. Altered function and connectivity of the medial frontal cortex in pediatric obsessive–compulsive disorder. Biol Psychiatry. 2010;68:1039–47.

8. Heckers S, Weiss AP, Deckersbach T, Goff DC, Morecraft RJ, Bush G. Anterior cingulate cortex activation during cognitive interference in schizophrenia. Am J Psychiatry. 2004;161:707–15.

9. Shin LM, Bush G, Milad MR, Lasko NB, Brohawn KH, Hughes KC, Macklin ML, Gold AL, Karpf RD, Orr SP, Rauch SL, Pitman RK. Exaggerated activation of dorsal anterior cingulate cortex during cognitive interference: a monozygotic twin study of posttraumatic stress disorder. Am J Psychiatry. 2011;168:979–85.

10. Aupperle R, Stillman A, Francisco A, Bruce J, Martin L, McDowd J, Simmons A. Cognitive dysfunction in combat veterans is related to attenuated dorsal ACC activation during interference processing. Neuropsychopharmacology. 2014;39:S473–647.

11. Bush G, Shin LM. The multi-source interference task: an fMRI task that reliably activates the cingulo-fronto-parietal cognitive/attention network. Nat Protoc. 2006;1:308–13.

12. Bush G. Cingulate–frontal–parietal function in health and disease. In: Posner MI, editor. Cognitive neuroscience of attention. 2nd ed. New York: The Guilford Press; 2011. p. 374–87.

13. Salami A, Rieckmann A, Fischer H, Bäckman L. A multivariate analysis of age-related differences in functional networks supporting conflict resolution. Neuroimage. 2014;86:150–63.

14. Bush G, Holmes J, Shin LM, Surman C, Makris N, Mick E, Seidman LJ, Biederman J. Atomoxetine increases fronto-parietal functional MRI activation in attention-deficit/hyperactivity disorder: a pilot study. Psychiatry Res. 2013;211:88–91.

15. Stone W. Neural connectivity underlying cognitive control: Variations in ADHD participants. Degree of Bachelor of Science with Honors in Psychology. University of Michigan, 2010.

16. Mao CP, Zhang QL, Bao FX, Liao X, Yang XL, Zhang M. Decreased activation of cingulo-frontal-parietal cognitive/attention network during an attention-demanding task in patients with chronic low back pain. Neuroradiology. 2014;56:903–12.

17. Yücel M, Harrison BJ, Wood SJ, Fornito A, Wellard RM, Pujol J, Clarke K, Phillips ML, Kyrios M, Velakoulis D, Pantelis C. Functional and biochemical alterations of the medial frontal cortex in obsessive–compulsive disorder. Arch Gen Psychiatry. 2007;64:946–55.

18. Pathak Y, Schneck N, Nanda P, Gershkovich M, Simpson H, Sajda P, Sheth S. Identifying brain regions implicated in OCD using simultaneous EEG-fMRI. Stereotact Funct Neurosurg. 2017;95:16.

19. Fitzgerald KD, Liu Y, Welsh RC, Stern ER, Hanna GL, Monk CS, Phan KL, Taylor SF. Shared pathophysiology in the pediatric anxiety disorders: conflict-related hyperactivation of the anterior cingulate cortex. Neuropsychopharmacology. 2011;36:S75–197.

20. Radua J, Mataix-Cols D, Phillips ML, El-Hage W, Kronhaus DM, Cardoner N, Surguladze S. A new meta-analytic method for neuroimaging studies that combines reported peak coordinates and statistical parametric maps. Eur Psychiatry. 2012;27:605–11.

21. Radua J, Mataix-Cols D. Meta-analytic methods for neuroimaging data explained. Biol Mood Anxiety Disord. 2012;2:6.

22. Radua J, Rubia K, Canales-Rodríguez JE, Pomarol-Clotet E, Fusar-Poli P, Mataix-Cols D. Anisotropic kernels for coordinate-based meta-analyses of neuroimaging studies. Front Psychiatry. 2014;5:13.

23. Radua J, Mataixcols D. Voxel-wise meta-analysis of grey matter changes in obsessive–compulsive disorder. Br J Psychiatry. 2009;195:393–402.

24. Kim K, Carp J, Fitzgerald KD, Taylor SF, Weissman DH. Neural congruency effects in the multi-source interference task vanish in healthy youth after controlling for conditional differences in mean RT. PLoS ONE. 2013;8:e60710.

25. Shehzad Z, DeYoung CG, Kang Y, Grigorenko EL, Gray JR. Interaction of COMT val 158 met and externalizing behavior: relation to prefrontal brain activity and behavioral performance. Neuroimage. 2012;60:2158–68.

26. Weissman DH, Carp J. The congruency effect in the posterior medial frontal cortex is more consistent with time on task than with response conflict. PLoS ONE. 2013;8:e62405.

27. Yücel M, Lubman DI, Harrison BJ, Fornito A, Allen NB, Wellard RM, Roffel K, Clarke K, Wood SJ, Forman SD. A combined spectroscopic and functional MRI investigation of the dorsal anterior cingulate region in opiate addiction. Mol Psychiatry. 2007;12:691–702.

28. Ridderinkhof KR, Ullsperger M, Crone EA, Nieuwenhuis S. The role of the medial frontal cortex in cognitive control. Science. 2004;306:443–7.

29. Botvinick MM, Nystrom LE, Fissell K, Carter CS, Cohen JD. Conflict monitoring versus selection-for-action in anterior cingulate cortex. Nature. 1999;402:179–81.

30. Fan J, Flombaum JI, McCandliss BD, Thomas KM, Posner MI. Cognitive and brain consequences of conflict. Neuroimage. 2003;18:42–57.

31. Banich MT, Milham MP, Atchley RA, Cohen NJ, Webb AG, Wszalek T, Kramer AF, Liang Z, Wright A, Shenker JI. FMRI studies of Stroop tasks reveal unique roles of anterior and posterior brain systems in attentional selection. J Cogn Neurosci. 2000;12:988–1000.

32. Liu X, Banich MT, Jacobson BL, Tanabe JL. Common and distinct neural substrates of attentional control in an integrated Simon and spatial Stroop task as assessed by event-related fMRI. Neuroimage. 2004;22:1097–106.

33. Ebitz RB, Platt ML. Neuronal activity in primate dorsal anterior cingulate cortex signals task conflict and predicts adjustments in pupil-linked arousal. Neuron. 2015;85:628–40.

34. Michelet T, Bioulac B, Langbour N, Goillandeau M, Guehl D, Burbaud P. Electrophysiological correlates of a versatile executive control system in the monkey anterior cingulate cortex. Cereb Cortex. 2016;26:1684–97.

35. Sheth SA, Mian MK, Patel SR. Human dorsal anterior cingulate cortex neurons mediate ongoing behavioural adaptation. Nature. 2012;488:218–21.

36. Davis KD, Taylor KS, Hutchison WD, Dostrovsky JO, Mcandrews MP, Richter EO, Lozano AM. Human anterior cingulate cortex neurons encode cognitive and emotional demands. J Neurosci. 2005;25:8402–6.

37. Botvinick MM, Cohen JD, Carter CS. Conflict monitoring and anterior cingulate cortex: an update. Trends Cogn Sci. 2004;8:539–46.

38. Nachev P, Kennard C, Husain M. Functional role of the supplementary and pre-supplementary motor areas. Nat Rev Neurosci. 2008;9:856–69.

39. Chambers CD, Garavan H, Bellgrove MA. Insights into the neural basis of response inhibition from cognitive and clinical neuroscience. Neurosci Biobehav Rev. 2009;33:631–46.

40. Swick D, Ashley V, Turken U. Are the neural correlates of stopping and not going identical? Quantitative meta-analysis of two response inhibition tasks. Neuroimage. 2011;56:1655–65.

41. Bonini F, Burle B, Liegeoischauvel C, Regis J, Chauvel P, Vidal F. Action monitoring and medial frontal cortex: leading role of supplementary motor area. Science. 2014;343:888–91.

42. Coull JT, Vidal F, Burle B. When to act, or not to act: that's the SMA's question. Curr Opin Behav Sci. 2016;8:14–21.

43. Chen X, Scangos KW, Stuphorn V. Supplementary motor area exerts proactive and reactive control of arm movements. J Neurosci. 2010;30:14657–75.

44. Aron AR, Robbins TW, Poldrack RA. Inhibition and the right inferior frontal cortex: one decade on. Trends Cogn Sci. 2014;18:177–85.

45. Wiecki TV, Frank MJ. A computational model of inhibitory control in frontal cortex and basal ganglia. Psychol Rev. 2013;120:329–55.

46. Jahanshahi M, Obeso I, Rothwell JC, Obeso JA. A fronto-striato-subthalamic-pallidal network for goal-directed and habitual inhibition. Nat Rev Neurosci. 2015;16:719–32.

47. Aron AR, Herz DM, Brown P, Forstmann BU, Zaghloul KA. Fronto-subthalamic circuits for control of action and cognition. J Neurosci. 2016;36:11489–95.

48. Bari A, Robbins TW. Inhibition and impulsivity: behavioral and neural basis of response control. Prog Neurobiol. 2013;108:44–79.

49. Wager TD, Sylvester CC, Lacey SC, Nee DE, Franklin M, Jonides J. Common and unique components of response inhibition revealed by fMRI. Neuroimage. 2005;27:323–40.

50. Cai W, Chen T, Ryali S, Kochalka J, Li CR, Menon V. Causal interactions within a frontal-cingulate-parietal network during cognitive control: convergent evidence from a multisite–multitask investigation. Cereb Cortex. 2015;26:2140–53.

51. Cai W, Ryali S, Chen T, Li CR, Menon V. Dissociable roles of right inferior frontal cortex and anterior insula in inhibitory control: evidence from intrinsic and task-related functional parcellation, connectivity, and response profile analyses across multiple datasets. J Neurosci. 2014;34:14652–67.

Mothers' pupillary responses to infant facial expressions

Santeri Yrttiaho[1]*[iD], Dana Niehaus[2], Eileen Thomas[2] and Jukka M. Leppänen[1]

Abstract

Background: Human parental care relies heavily on the ability to monitor and respond to a child's affective states. The current study examined pupil diameter as a potential physiological index of mothers' affective response to infant facial expressions.

Methods: Pupillary time-series were measured from 86 mothers of young infants in response to an array of photographic infant faces falling into four emotive categories based on valence (positive vs. negative) and arousal (mild vs. strong).

Results: Pupil dilation was highly sensitive to the valence of facial expressions, being larger for negative vs. positive facial expressions. A separate control experiment with luminance-matched non-face stimuli indicated that the valence effect was specific to facial expressions and cannot be explained by luminance confounds. Pupil response was not sensitive to the arousal level of facial expressions.

Conclusions: The results show the feasibility of using pupil diameter as a marker of mothers' affective responses to ecologically valid infant stimuli and point to a particularly prompt maternal response to infant distress cues.

Keywords: Pupil, Emotion, Facial expressions, Attention, Mothers, Infant faces

Background

Parental care and parent-infant interaction relies heavily on the ability to receive and express nonverbal emotional signals through facial expressions [1]. There is increasing interest in the neurocognitive bases of these capacities in parents [2–4] and infants [5], and in the possibility that subtle variations in emotional signaling may have important influences on the quality of parent–child attachment [6]. In the current study, we extend these studies by examining whether mothers' pupil dilation is sensitive to children's affective cues and could, in future, serve as an accessible marker of interindividual variation in these responses. If the pupil is sensitive to mothers' affective responses, such as heightened vigilance towards infant signals of discomfort and distress [1], this index may prove useful in studying and understanding the mechanisms underlying maternal sensitivity or neglect.

To begin examining whether pupil diameter is a sensitive index of parents' physiological responses to children's affective cues, the present study focused on mothers' responses to infant facial expressions. Despite increasing involvement of fathers in childcare in many societies and the need for research on biological bases of paternal childcare, there are known intersex differences in the neural and hormonal bases for caregiving behaviors [3]. For this reason, we limited our current investigation on parental responsiveness to infant emotion to mothers rather than sampling parents of both sexes. The neural and physiological basis of mothering constitutes a distinct domain of research [7], with potentially important implications for maternal and infant mental health. Previous studies show differential patterns of brain and behavioral responses elicited by infant as opposed to adult faces [8–11], especially in women [11]. Further, mothers, compared to nulliparous women, show more marked early frontal (~100 ms) event-related potentials to infant facial expressions, as well as more pronounced modulation of posterior visual responses to infant faces

*Correspondence: santeri.yrttiaho@uta.fi
[1] Tampere Center for Child Health Research, School of Medicine, University of Tampere, Lääkärinkatu 1, 33520 Tampere, Finland
Full list of author information is available at the end of the article

displaying negative emotions [2, 12]. The current study extends the research on neurophysiological processes of mothering by examining the pupillary correlates of mothers' responses to infants' positive and negative facial expressions [12, 13].

Pupil size is largely determined by reflexive control over light entering the eye [14]. However, pupil diameter is also influenced by the activity of the sympathetic autonomic nervous system (ANS) during emotional arousal [15, 16]. The pupillary response to a visual stimulus can typically be characterized by two consecutive phases. First, in response to increased brightness, there is a constriction in pupil size around 600–1600 ms after stimulus onset [15]. Following the constriction, the pupil starts to dilate back to a baseline level over the course of several seconds. For example, an initial constriction of the pupil in response to visual stimuli is followed by a slow dilation that is augmented for emotionally positive and negative scenes [15, 17]. Pupil constriction and dilation per se are brought about by distinct branches of the nervous system, parasympathetic and sympathetic, innervating the constrictor and dilator muscles, respectively [16]. Pupil size at any time reflects the tone of both of these muscles. Therefore, both the constriction and the dilation phase are susceptible to emotional effects elicited by emotionally arousing scenes and facial expressions [15, 17–19]. Pupil response to emotional factors is thought to be mediated by the modulatory effects of the brain's noradrenergic system on neural circuitry controlling the muscles of the iris [20, 21]. Importantly, larger pupil dilation to emotional stimuli cannot be suppressed voluntarily [22], making it an accessible marker for studies examining human affective responses in a variety of contexts.

Because the dominant source of variability in pupil size comes simply from changes in stimulus luminance [20], pupillometry studies have traditionally required stringent control of luminance levels across experimental stimuli or, at minimum, equalization of mean luminance across different stimulus categories. While the luminance of many types of visual stimuli can, in principle, be easily adjusted to equal mean level, such equalization is not viable for all studies and small deviations from the mean levels will be unavoidable. This poses particular challenges for studies examining pupillary responses to ecologically valid stimuli such as infant facial expressions. The only available method to capture preverbal infants' facial expressions is to photograph them as they occur spontaneously in variable environments where strict control of luminance is difficult or may result in unnatural quality of the stimuli. Corresponding problems exists in other contexts such as studies using facial stimuli presented in live face-to-face or over-the-internet conditions, faces in variable background illumination, and faces of people with variable ethnicity or hair color. For this reason, an important challenge for pupillometric studies is to examine ways to disentangle unavoidable pupillary responses to luminance changes from those involved in affective processing.

The current study consisted of two experiments where pupil response was measured in response to infant facial stimuli. In Experiment 1, a large sample of mothers of young infants ($N = 86$) was recruited in order to examine whether pupil constriction and dilation are sensitive physiological measures of mothers' responses to mild and strong instances of infant positive and negative affect. Based on prior studies [15–20], we predicted relatively larger pupil diameter in response to high-arousal facial expressions (i.e., high intensity positive and negative expressions) in both the constriction and dilation phases. Our secondary aim was to disentangle affective pupillary responses to facial expressions from the response to unavoidable variations in stimulus luminance. To this end, we carried out Experiment 2, a control experiment, where participants were presented both with faces (face condition) and luminance-matched non-face stimuli (control condition). We hypothesized that an emotive pupil response, a greater pupil diameter during pupil dilation and constriction phases, would be manifested in the face condition but not in the control condition.

Experiment 1
Methods
Participants
The participants were mothers of young infants participating in an ongoing longitudinal study examining the mental health of mother-infant dyads in the Cape Town metropolitan area, South Africa. The participants had no mental health disorder as assessed by a psychiatrist through clinical assessment and the Mini International Neuropsychiatric Interview [23]. The eye-tracking assessment in mothers was conducted as a part of a scheduled immunization visit to a private well-baby clinic at the infant age of 6 weeks. All mothers recruited to this study and tested by the eye-tracking procedure by September 30th, 2015, were included in the current analyses. The final sample consisted of 86 mothers (Age: $M = 32.4$ years, SD $= 5.4$ years) of Caucasian ($N = 53$) and Black ($N = 33$) ethnicity. The Caucasian participants had higher socioeconomic status (SES) than the Black participants as indexed by monthly income [$X^2(3) = 57.91$, $p < .001$], level of education [$X^2(2) = 66.32$, $p < .001$] and employment [$X^2(3) = 66.89$, $p < .001$]. The number of pregnancies of the participants ranged from 1 to 5 with 68.7% of participants having more than one pregnancy.

Stimuli

The infant face stimuli were obtained from an existing stimulus set [13]. These 36 grayscale photographs were close-ups of infants with black uniform backgrounds, with infants producing four types of facial expressions (Fig. 1): mild positive (MP), strong positive (SP), mild negative (MN), and strong negative (SN). It is noteworthy that this classification is based on previous work showing that infants' emotional expressions during the first year of life are not readily categorized into discrete emotion categories, but instead, to primary dimensions of hedonic pleasure and arousal [13]. Nine instances of each category were used in the experiment. The selection was made to obtain sets of images that were matched for face-background ratio, models' head orientation, and models' age as closely as possible. As the original pool of images was taken from separate sources, some variations in above characteristics remained in each stimulus category. The infant's eyes were open in all positively-valenced (MP and SP) photographs but were closed in 67% of images with strong (SN) and in 22% of images with mild negative (MN) facial expressions. The infants had open eyes with direct gaze in 33, 56, 11, and in 33% of pictures classified as SP, MP, SN, and MN, respectively. All infants depicted in the stimuli were Caucasian.

The current infant stimuli were selected from an original pool of 208 images consistently rated (>75%) as reflecting one of the four emotions (i.e., MP, SP, MN, or SN) by human judges [12, 13]. However, the emotional content of the current face stimuli has been previously validated [12, 13] in a population which is geographically (Italy vs. South Africa), ethnically, and socioeconomically different from the current participants. Therefore, behavioral rating scores were obtained to ensure that the participants agreed with the emotional valence and arousal previously attributed to the stimuli. Participants were asked to judge the emotional valence of the face stimuli on a scale from 1 to 3, where 1 = positive (happy), 2 = neutral, and 3 = negative (sad) emotion. The rating scores varied according to the intended emotional category (i.e., SP, MP, MN, SN) of the stimuli [$F(1, 24) = 2405.73$, $p < .001$, $partial\ \eta^2 = .99$] in a subset of randomly selected 25 participants. The rating scores increased monotonically between SP, MP, and MN ($ps < .001$) and reached a plateau at MN vs. SN ($p = .37$). In effect, SP was rated as positive ($M = 1.0$, SD = .04), MP close to neutral ($M = 1.8$, SD = .1), and both MN and SN as negative ($Ms > 2.9$, SDs < .2).

In order to reduce the pupillary light reflex [15] elicited by the face stimuli, a visual non-face pattern was generated to be shown during the "pre-stimulus" interval before each face stimulus. This visual stimulus was produced by randomly permuting and then averaging the pixels derived from the entire set of face stimuli in order to match its grayscale intensity to that of the faces.

Procedure

The participants sat in a dimly lit room with no external light other than that laminating from the screen. Before data acquisition, eye-tracking calibration was performed for each participant by requiring the participant to fixate on five targets. In instances where the gaze was not found at these targets, the calibration-procedure was repeated. The calibration results from a subgroup of participants are shown in Additional file 1: Figure S2.

After calibration, participants were presented with a series of trials each consisting of (1) a short 1000-ms foreperiod with a black screen, (2) a 2000-ms pre-stimulus interval with a random visual pattern, (3) a 5000-ms face stimulus, and (4) a white rectangular border surrounding the face for 1000 ms to signal the end of the trial. A short sound signal, a "notification beep", was presented 2500 ms before each face stimulus. Illustration of the stimulus sequence is shown in Fig. 2. The face stimulus for a given trial was selected randomly, without replacement, from the set of 36 faces (9/category as explained above). The

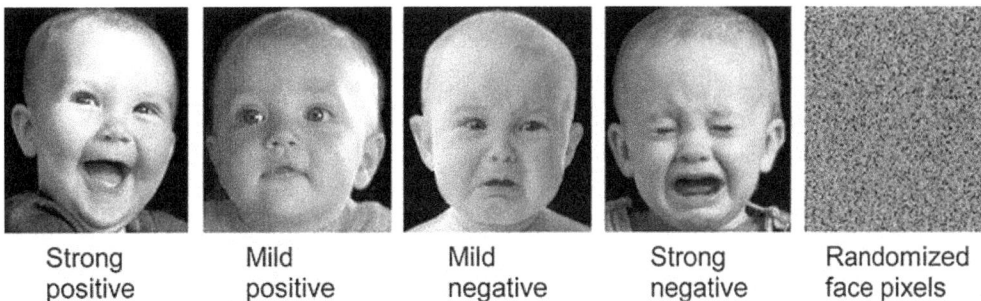

Fig. 1 Examples of infant face stimuli from each stimulus category defined by the intensity and valence of the facial expression of emotion. Randomized pixels (on the *right*), derived from all face stimuli were used as a pre-stimulus display. In the control experiment (Experiment 2) randomized face pixels, derived from each face stimulus individually, were used in place of the face stimuli in the "non-face" condition

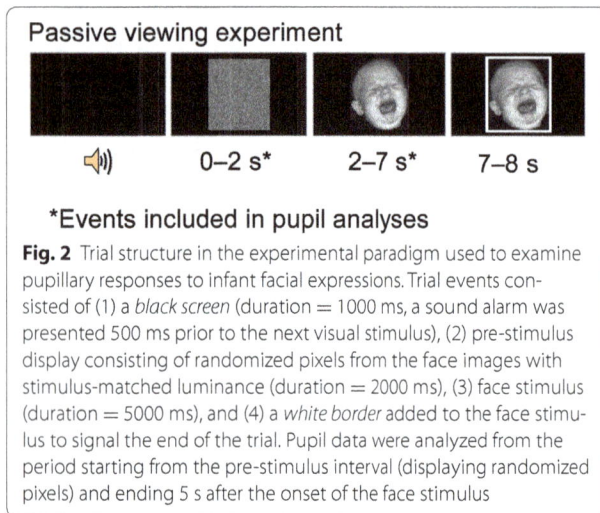

Passive viewing experiment

*Events included in pupil analyses

Fig. 2 Trial structure in the experimental paradigm used to examine pupillary responses to infant facial expressions. Trial events consisted of (1) a *black screen* (duration = 1000 ms, a sound alarm was presented 500 ms prior to the next visual stimulus), (2) pre-stimulus display consisting of randomized pixels from the face images with stimulus-matched luminance (duration = 2000 ms), (3) face stimulus (duration = 5000 ms), and (4) a *white border* added to the face stimulus to signal the end of the trial. Pupil data were analyzed from the period starting from the pre-stimulus interval (displaying randomized pixels) and ending 5 s after the onset of the face stimulus

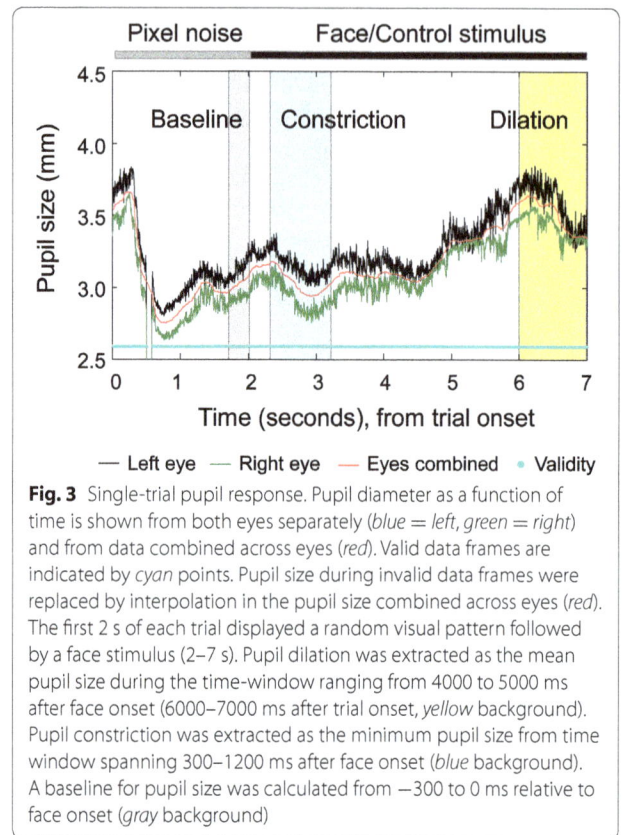

Fig. 3 Single-trial pupil response. Pupil diameter as a function of time is shown from both eyes separately (*blue = left, green = right*) and from data combined across eyes (*red*). Valid data frames are indicated by *cyan* points. Pupil size during invalid data frames were replaced by interpolation in the pupil size combined across eyes (*red*). The first 2 s of each trial displayed a random visual pattern followed by a face stimulus (2–7 s). Pupil dilation was extracted as the mean pupil size during the time-window ranging from 4000 to 5000 ms after face onset (6000–7000 ms after trial onset, *yellow* background). Pupil constriction was extracted as the minimum pupil size from time window spanning 300–1200 ms after face onset (*blue* background). A baseline for pupil size was calculated from −300 to 0 ms relative to face onset (*gray* background)

stimuli were presented on a black background. The participants were asked to simply view each stimulus presented without a specific requirement for a response. To collect subjective ratings, the experimenter presented the face pictures to participants as paper print-outs and collected verbal responses from participants onto separate sheets after the entire sequence of pupil data acquisition.

Acquisition and analysis of pupil diameter data
Pupil size was measured with a Tobii X-60 or X2-60 eye-tracker camera which measures corneal reflection of infrared light relative to the image of the pupil. The acquisition was controlled by custom-written MATLAB scripts, Psychtoolbox, and the Talk2Tobii toolbox, interfacing with a Tobii (Danderdyn, Sweden) eye-tracker.

Pupil size was measured from both eyes during the presentation of the face stimuli as well as during the pre-stimulus interval (with random visual pattern). The pupil data was acquired in conjunction with synchronous point-of-gaze (POG), eye-tracking validity (i.e., "valid" or "invalid"), and stimulus timing data at a sampling rate of 60 Hz. The data on pupil size was preprocessed using gazeAnalysisLib [24] to complete the following steps: averaging the diameter across the left and the right eye, replacing "invalid" frames of pupil size by the means of linear interpolation, median filtering, and baseline correction. The POG data was also combined across eyes and median filtered. The window size of the median filter was 7 frames (ca. 120 ms) for both POG and pupil data. A typical pupil response from a single trial is shown in Fig. 3.

Pupil response was baseline-corrected by subtracting the pupil size from a 300-ms pre-face time window. Based on visual inspection of the grand average pupil response, the minimum and maximum pupil diameters

were reached at 300–1200 and 4000–5000 ms after face onset, respectively (Fig. 4). These time intervals were thus selected for the extraction of pupil constriction

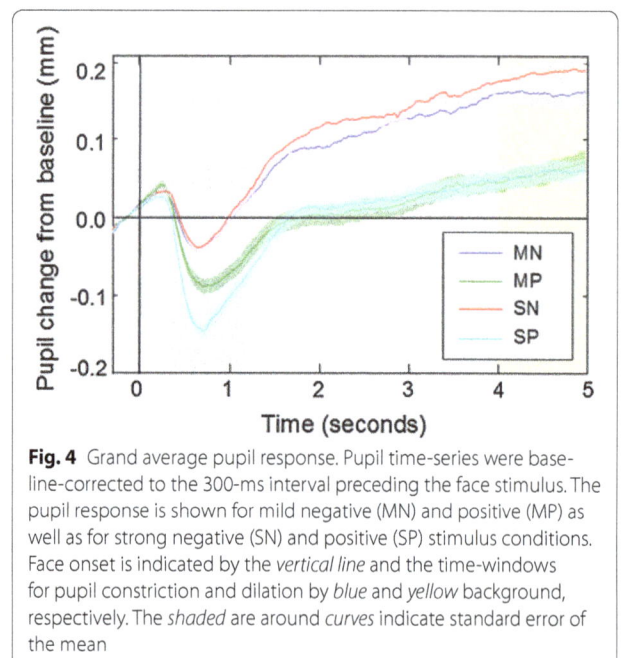

Fig. 4 Grand average pupil response. Pupil time-series were baseline-corrected to the 300-ms interval preceding the face stimulus. The pupil response is shown for mild negative (MN) and positive (MP) as well as for strong negative (SN) and positive (SP) stimulus conditions. Face onset is indicated by the *vertical line* and the time-windows for pupil constriction and dilation by *blue* and *yellow* background, respectively. The *shaded* are around *curves* indicate standard error of the mean

and dilation, respectively. While pupil constriction was determined as the minimum pupil size during the 300–1200 ms time window, pupil dilation was extracted as the mean pupil size during the latter 4000–5000 ms time-window.

Quality control (QC) of trial-by-trial pupil data was based on the following factors: (1) participant maintaining gaze within the face stimulus, (2) error-free pupil/eye-tracking, and (3) absence of outlier values. Quantitative indices of the participant gaze coordinates and error-free pupil tracking were acquired on a frame-by-frame basis together with pupil diameter. Using these metrics, trials where participant's gaze was directed at the location of the face stimulus less than 10% of time, either in the baseline or in the response interval, were rejected from analysis. Similarly, trials with excess of eye/pupil-tracking frames labeled as "invalid" by the acquisition software were discarded from the analyses. These trials were defined as those where the longest streaks of consecutive non-valid frames exceeded 250 ms within the baseline period, or 900 ms within the time-window used for extracting the pupil constriction or dilation response. In addition to these basic QC measures, we identified the first trial within each measurement as a systematic source of outlier data, and rejected these trials from further analyses as well (see Additional file 1 for further details about the rejection criteria used in the study). On the average 6.2 (SD = 6.1) trials were rejected (out of 35 available) from each participant (averaged across constriction and dilation). Two participants had less than 3 averaged trials available for the analysis of the effects of Arousal and Valence on pupil response, and were thus rejected from final statistical analyses.

The quality of the trials accepted for further analyses was then inspected by analyzing the average values of frame-by-frame pupil/eye-tracking data within these trials. The targeted metrics included the average percentage of valid frames for both eyes (during the response time-window), the duration of non-valid streaks during the baseline and response time-windows, and the percentage of gaze directed at the location of the face (minimum percentage across baseline and response time-windows). These statistics are shown in Table 1. In summary, mean valid eye-tracking reached 87–91%, and on the average, longest-non valid data streaks were shorter than 76–121 ms.

Statistical analyses

In order to determine whether significant pupil constriction and dilation were elicited by the current stimuli, baseline-corrected pupil diameter was contrasted to the zero-level (i.e., no response) with one sample

Table 1 Eye-tracking quality

	Constriction		Dilation	
	Mean	SD	Mean	SD
Valid eye-tracking (%)	90.5	17.6	87.0	19.8
Longest non-valid streak				
Baseline (ms)	28.5	61.0	27.9	60.5
Response (ms)	75.1	141.7	120.3	176.9
Inside AOI, valid frames (%)	96.1	21.6	95.4	23.5

t-tests. The emotive pupil response, in turn, was defined as a change in pupil size between conditions differing in emotive valence or arousal of the stimuli. Emotion-related differences in baseline-corrected pupil diameter across stimulus conditions and response time-windows were investigated with a Time-window (2) × Arousal (2) × Valence (2) repeated-measures Analysis of Variance (ANOVA). The factors comprised constriction vs. dilation phase (Time-window), strong vs. mild emotion (Arousal), and negative vs. positive emotion (Valence), respectively. Both main an interaction effects were analyzed. In case interaction effects were found in the initial ANOVA, further comparisons within pupil constriction and dilation data, separately, were conducted with Arousal × Valence ANOVAs. Any subsequent pairwise tests were conducted with pair-wise t-tests. Effect sizes are reported using Cohen's d for t-tests and *partial η^2* for ANOVA throughout the results.

Results

Following previous research [15–20], the presentation of faces was expected to elicit a typical visually induced pupil response consisting of an initial pupil constriction (decrease in pupil diameter Ø) and a subsequent dilation (increase in pupil diameter Ø). Further, as an increase in pupil size has been documented for pictures (not always including faces) with strong vs. mild emotive arousal [15, 17, 18], the pupil size was hypothesized to be larger both during the constriction and the dilation phase for strong vs. mild expressions. The corresponding effects were investigated also in response to negative vs. positive emotional valence of the facial expressions.

An ample pupil constriction, that is, a decrease in pupil diameter during 300–1200 ms after stimulus onset (Fig. 4) against baseline level, was found in response to all face stimuli [$|\Delta\varnothing| > .11$ mm, $|ts| > 13.18$, $ps < .001$, $|ds| > 1.43$]. Pupil constriction was followed by a subsequent pupil dilation (Fig. 4) and the pupil size increased significantly above the pre-stimulus baseline during the latter 4000–5000 ms time window [$.05 < \Delta\varnothing < .19$ mm, $ts > 3.96$, $ps < .001$, $.43 < |ds| < 1.44$].

Main effects of Time-window [constriction *vs.* dilation; $F(1, 83) = 532.40$, $p < .001$, *partial η^2* $= .87$], and Valence [$F(1, 83) = 157.03$, $p < .001$, *partial η^2* $= .65$] were found on baseline-corrected pupil size. These effects were due to greater pupil size during dilation ($\Delta\emptyset = .12$ mm) vs. constriction ($\Delta\emptyset = -.16$ mm) and greater pupil size in response to negatively-valenced vs. positively-valenced stimuli. Interaction effects on pupil size were found between Arousal and Valence [$F(1, 83) = 7.76$, $p < .01$], Time-window and Valence [$F(1, 83) = 15.03$, $p < .001$], as well as Time-window and Arousal [$F(1, 83) = 13.33$, $p < .001$]. Therefore, the effects of Arousal and Valence on pupil size were inspected separately for pupil constriction and dilation.

Main effects of Valence [$F(1, 84) = 83.60$, $p < .001$, *partial η^2* $= .50$] and Arousal [$F(1, 84) = 14.22$, $p < .001$, *partial η^2* $= .15$] were found on pupil constriction. Contrary to the hypothesis of increased pupil size in response to stimulus arousal, strong stimulus arousal was related to a decreased pupil size (i.e., increased constriction) within this early time window [strong < mild; $\Delta\emptyset = -.03$ mm]. Moreover, there was an interaction between Valence and Arousal on pupil constriction [$F(1, 84) = 11.64$, $p < .001$], reflecting a significant effect of arousal for the positively-valenced stimuli [$\Delta\emptyset = -.05$ mm, $t(84) = -4.77$, $p < .001$, $d = -.52$] but not for the negatively-valenced stimuli [$\Delta\emptyset = -.01$ mm, $t(84) = -.99$, $p = .33$, $d = -.11$]. While the hypothesized emotion-related increase in pupil diameter during constriction was not found for stimulus arousal, decreased pupil constriction (i.e., greater pupil diameter), was found for faces with negative *vs.* positive emotional valence across both levels of arousal [$\Delta\emptyset s > .05$ mm, $ts(84) > 6.10$, $ps < .001$, $|d|s > .66$].

A main effect of Valence [$F(1, 83) = 129.31$, $p < .001$, *partial η^2* $= .61$] was found on pupil dilation due to a .12-mm increase in pupil size to negatively-valenced ($\Delta\emptyset = .17$) vs. positively-valenced infant facial expressions ($\Delta\emptyset = .06$). Contrary to the hypothesized arousal-related pupil dilation, no effect of arousal on pupil dilation was found [$F(1, 83) = 1.41$, $p = .24$]. No interaction between Arousal and Valence [$F(1, 83) = 2.54$, $p = .12$] was found on pupil dilation either.

Experiment 2

Methods

Participants

The participants in Experiment 2 consisted of 15 volunteers (9 female, Age: $M = 28.9$ years, *range* $= 24$–50 years). None of the participants in Experiment 2 participated in Experiment 1 and parenthood was not required for the inclusion of participants into Experiment 2. The study was ethically approved by the institutional review board of the University of Stellenbosch

and written informed consent was obtained from all participants.

Stimuli

The stimuli in the original pool of infant facial expressions were matched for luminance [12], but as pupil diameter is highly sensitive to stimulus luminance, a further analysis of brightness was conducted for the purposes of the present study. Optical luminance data were unavailable (requires careful photometric measurements with appropriate equipment), but the possible differences in luminance were inspected from mean grayscale intensity (0–255) values of the bitmap files. A one-way ANOVA showed that, overall, there were no statistically significant differences between stimulus categories in grayscale intensity values, [$F(4,32) = 1.92$, $p = .13$, *partial η^2* $= .19$], but inspection of the bitmap intensity for individual images and direct pairwise comparisons showed noticeable variation within and across stimulus categories in intensity (Fig. 5). Furthermore, while the random visual pattern presented before each face stimulus had grayscale intensity equal to the mean intensity across *all faces* (horizontal line in Fig. 2), it differed somewhat in intensity from *each individual face* stimulus. Because such differences in stimulus luminance might bias the emotional effects on pupil response, we generated an array of control stimuli by randomly scrambling the bitmap matrices of the face images. The resultant control stimuli, thus, had exactly the same mean grayscale intensity as the face stimuli. These non-face stimuli were presented to a group of new participants ($N = 15$) who

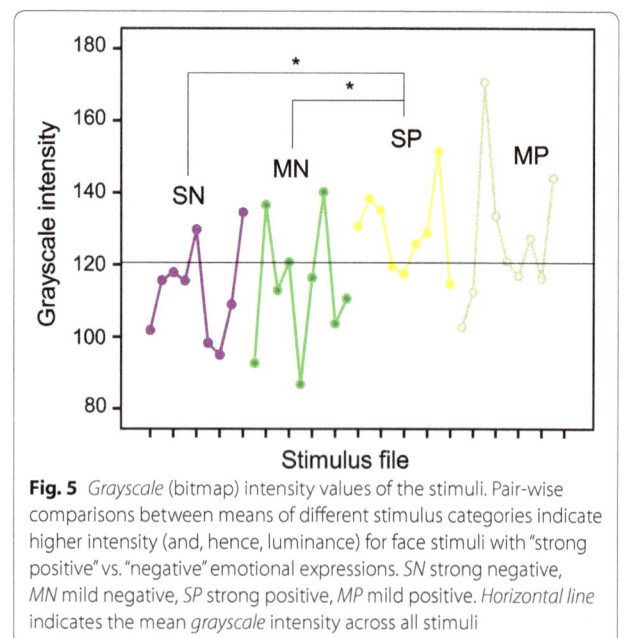

Fig. 5 *Grayscale* (bitmap) intensity values of the stimuli. Pair-wise comparisons between means of different stimulus categories indicate higher intensity (and, hence, luminance) for face stimuli with "strong positive" vs. "negative" emotional expressions. *SN* strong negative, *MN* mild negative, *SP* strong positive, *MP* mild positive. *Horizontal line* indicates the mean *grayscale* intensity across all stimuli

also viewed the original face pictures used in Experiment 1. The same visual pattern, consisting of randomly permuted pixels, was presented during the pre-stimulus interval as in Experiment 1.

Procedure

The stimulation paradigm was identical to that in Experiment 1 (Fig. 2). In particular, the sequence and timing of events within experimental trials was similar across the experiments. However, an additional experimental condition was included where the face stimuli were replaced by their pixel-scrambled counterparts. That is, in addition to face stimuli, random non-face patterns were presented in a separate experimental block preceding or following the face sequence in a counterbalanced order across participants.

Acquisition and analysis of pupil diameter data

The same equipment, software, and parameters were used in the acquisition of the pupil data as in Experiment 1. The pupil constriction and dilation were likewise extracted from the same time-windows spanning 300–1200 and 4000–5000 ms after face onset. An average of 6.0 (SD = 6.5) and 5.5 (SD = 7.6) trials were rejected per participant in the face and the control (pixel-scrambled face) condition, respectively. However, all participants had a sufficient number of averaged trials ($\geq$3) for the statistical analyses of the effects of Arousal and Valence. Thus data from all participants were included in the final statistical analyses from Experiment 2.

Statistical analyses

Pupil change from baseline (zero-level) in all stimulus conditions separately was first analyzed with one-sample t-tests. Then, emotion-related differences in baseline-corrected pupil diameter across stimulus conditions and response time-windows were compared with a Pixel randomization (2) × Time-window (2) × Arousal (2) × Valence (2) repeated-measures ANOVA. The repeated-measures factors comprised intact faces vs. scrambled non-faces (Pixel randomization), constriction vs. dilation phase (Time-window), strong vs. mild emotion (Arousal), and negative vs. positive emotion (Valence), respectively. Both main an interaction effects were analyzed. In case interaction effects were found in the initial ANOVA, further comparisons within pupil constriction and dilation data, separately, were conducted with Pixel randomization × Arousal × Valence ANOVAs. Finally, if an interaction was found between emotional pupil response (i.e., Arousal or Valence) and Pixel randomization, Arousal × Valence ANOVAs were conducted separately for the face and the-noise condition

to qualify the source of the interaction effect. Effect sizes are reported as *partial η^2*.

Results

Pupil constriction was elicited across all conditions ($|\Delta\varnothing| > .08$ mm, $|ts| > 4.19$, $ps < .001$, $|ds| > 1.08$) including both those with face stimuli and those with the non-face stimuli (randomly permuted pixels). However, significant pupil dilation above pre-stimulus baseline was observed only in the face condition ($\Delta\varnothing > .10$ mm, $2.24 < ts < 5.16$, $ps < .05$, $.58 < ds < 1.33$). Such pupil dilation was invariantly absent in the non-face condition ($\Delta\varnothing \leq .06$ mm, $-1.24 < ts < 2.01$, $ps > .06$, $-.32 < ds < .52$).

Main effects of Time-window [$F(1, 14) = 80.57$, $p < .001$, *partial η^2* = .85], Pixel randomization [$F(1, 14) = 13.05$, $p < .01$, *partial η^2* = .48], and Valence [$F(1, 14) = 51.22$, $p < .001$, *partial η^2* = .79] were found on pupil size across all conditions within Experiment 2. However, interaction effects on pupil size were found between Time-window and Pixel randomization [$F(1, 14) = 10.29$, $p < .01$] and between Valence, Time-window, and Pixel randomization [$F(1, 14) = 7.26$, $p < .05$]. Therefore, the effects of Valence on pupil size were inspected separately from the two different time-windows (constriction and dilation), and further, separately within the face and the non-face condition. The purpose of these further analyses was to determine whether the effect of Valence on pupil size differed between the face condition, with genuine emotional signals, and the non-face condition, without emotional content. No main or interaction effects of Emotional arousal on pupil size were found.

A main effect of emotional Valence was found on pupil constriction [$F(1, 14) = 41.93$, $p < .001$, *partial η^2* = .75]. A trend for interaction between Valence and Pixel randomization was further found on pupil constriction [$F(1, 14) = 3.07$, $p < .11$]. However, the effect of Valence was found both within the face condition [$F(1, 14) = 12.77$, $p < .001$, *partial η^2* = .48] and within the non-face condition [$F(1, 14) = 35.10$, $p < .001$, *partial η^2* = .72] in subsequent tests. As the effect of Valence on pupil constriction was found both in the face and in the non-face control condition, it cannot be considered to indicate an emotive pupil response (the non-face stimuli consisted of meaningless random patterns).

A main effect of emotional Valence was also found on pupil dilation [$F(1, 14) = 17.85$, $p < .001$, *partial η^2* = .56]. Furthermore, a trend level interaction [$F(1, 14) = 3.80$, $p < .08$] was found between Valence and Pixel randomization on pupil dilation (Fig. 6). This interaction was qualified by a significant effect of Valence on pupil dilation in the face condition [$F(1, 14) = 23.30$, $p < .001$,

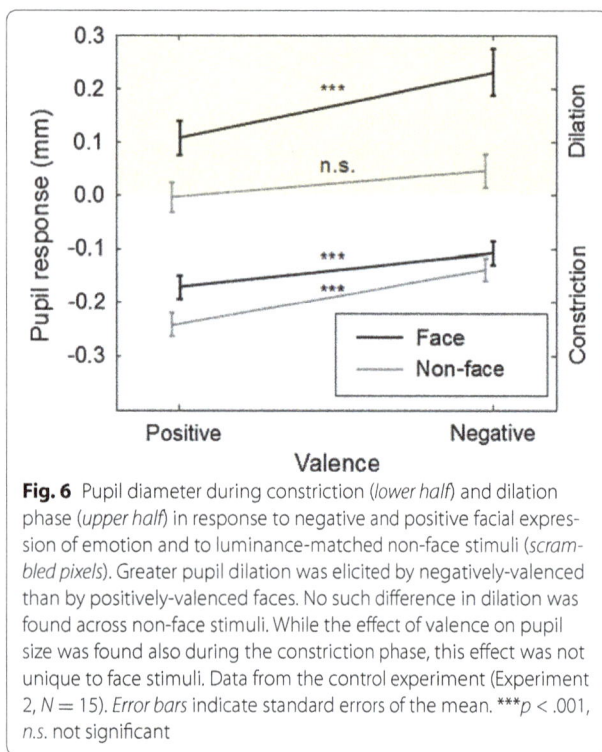

Fig. 6 Pupil diameter during constriction (*lower half*) and dilation phase (*upper half*) in response to negative and positive facial expression of emotion and to luminance-matched non-face stimuli (*scrambled pixels*). Greater pupil dilation was elicited by negatively-valenced than by positively-valenced faces. No such difference in dilation was found across non-face stimuli. While the effect of valence on pupil size was found also during the constriction phase, this effect was not unique to face stimuli. Data from the control experiment (Experiment 2, N = 15). *Error bars* indicate standard errors of the mean. ***p < .001, n.s. not significant

partial $\eta^2 = .63$] but not in the non-face condition [$F(1, 14) = 2.78$, $p < .12$, *partial* $\eta^2 = .17$]. In the face condition, greater pupil dilation was found for negatively-valenced ($\Delta\emptyset = .23$ mm) than for positively-valenced ($\Delta\emptyset = .11$ mm) infant face stimuli (difference = .12 mm).

As the non-face stimuli, consisting of random pixels, may be less motivating for participants to attend to than faces, it was necessary to ensure that the participants fixated equally on both stimulus types. Equal participant attentiveness and data quality in face and non-face condition was indicted by invariable number of acceptable trials across conditions [$F(1, 14) = .14$, $p = .72$, *partial* $\eta^2 = .01$]. Therefore, the difference between face and non-face condition reflect true effects of face and emotion processing as verified against conceivable data quality issues.

Discussion

Pupillary response, in particular pupil dilation, has been proposed as an indicator of variable psychophysiological states [14, 15, 20]. In the current study, we investigated whether the emotive pupil response could be used to index mothers' responsiveness to infant non-verbal communication. To this end, in Experiment 1, we measured pupillary responses in mothers while they viewed infant facial expressions. Larger pupil dilation was evoked by infant signals of distress or discomfort than by positively-valenced facial expressions. Emotive pupil dilation was

further replicated in comparison against a non-face control condition in Experiment 2, a separate control experiment. The control experiment further showed that the pupil dilation response triggered by infant distress was dissociable from a response to the brightness of stimuli in this category.

In child and adolescent participants, pupil dilation has been previously reported in response to face stimuli with direct as opposed to averted gaze, especially when depicting happy facial expressions [18]. In contrast, greater pupil dilation in response to angry vs. happy or fearful facial expressions has been reported in adult participants [31, 32]. Furthermore, the sensitivity of the pupil response to direct vs. averted gaze found in typically developing participants was absent in children diagnosed with autism spectrum disorders [18]. Therefore, the sensitivity of the pupil response to facial expressions of emotion seems to depend on participant population, stimulus material, or on their combination [18, 31, 32]. Consequently, previous literature on emotive pupil response is insufficient to describe the perception and physiological responsiveness to infant facial expressions in mothers or to describe how such processes are reflected in the pupil response. The current study (Experiment 1) is the first pupillometric study using specifically infant facial expressions of emotion as stimuli and mothers of young infants as participants. The current results characterize the pupil response in this particular context and indicate increased autonomic responsiveness in response to infant signals of discomfort and distress.

Adaptive infant-caregiver interaction rests on the ability of the interactants to receive and express emotional signals through facial expressions [1]. Mutually positive, optimally arousing social interaction involves the regulation of the activity of the autonomic nervous system as a component of emotion regulation [25] and correlates of maternal sensitivity have been found in both sympathetic and parasympathetic activity. Activation of the sympathetic nervous system is associated with emotional arousal and has been previously indicated in mothers' response to infant cry as indexed by electrodermal measures [26, 27]. Despite wide psychophysiological application [20, 28–30], relatively few studies have used pupillometry to investigate emotional processes evoked by the perception of facial expressions [18, 31, 32]. Such recent studies, using adult faces as stimuli, have indicated greater pupil dilation in response to angry vs. happy or fearful facial expressions in adult participants [31, 32]. In the current study, we investigated specifically whether the emotional responsiveness in mothers to infant facial expressions might be indexed with pupillometry. Our results were consistent with the previous studies on pupillary responses to facial expressions of emotion by indicating an increase in baseline-corrected pupil size in response to emotional face stimuli. Importantly, this effect was now replicated in the special case of infant stimuli viewed by mothers.

While autonomic responsiveness may be a prerequisite for adequate mother-infant interaction, overactive sympathetic arousal to infant or child cues has been linked with harsh parenting [26], lower maternal sensitivity [27], negative appraisal of children [33], and child abuse [34]. Also parasympathetic activity reflected in the respiratory sinus arrhythmia, in both baseline level [35] and in the regulation of the vagal tone [36], has been linked to maternal sensitivity. Moreover, the sympathetic and parasympathetic systems may act in concert in determining emotional response in mothers to infant crying and distress [27]. In the current study, emotive response to infant faces was established in pupil dilation which has been associated with sympathetic activity [16]. In this light, the current emotive pupil response is analogous to the increased skin conductance in mothers elicited by sounds of infant cry, which is also attributed to sympathetic arousal [26, 27]. This interpretation is further supported by covariance between emotive pupil dilation and skin conductance in response to affective pictures [15]. However, the pupil size during dilation may reflect the level of parasympathetic activity as well [16]. Based on findings from autonomic responses to infant cry [26, 27], the pupil response might index either sufficient or excessive autonomic arousal to infant negative affect for the maintenance of adaptive maternal sensitivity. In future studies, mapping the maternal pupil response to favorable level of autonomic responsiveness to infant cues might be achieved by relating the response to indices of caregiver behaviors and maternal sensitivity.

The norepinephrine attentional system of the brain originating in the locus coeruleus (i.e., the LC-NE system) has been suggested to underlie emotional pupil dilation [20, 37, 38]. Therefore, maternal pupil dilation in response to infant negative facial expressions is likely to share some common mechanisms with emotional pupil dilation in general which is elicited by a wide range of stimuli and conditions [20, 28–30]. Yet, there is evidence that effects of social signals of emotion on pupil size may reflect distinct social-cognitive processes. Firstly, interpersonal mimicry of gestures including mimicry of the pupil size [39] may specifically modulate the pupil response to faces. Secondly, previous studies suggest that there may be a dissociable neurocognitive system involved in monitoring infants' emotional cues which is important for supporting parental caregiving [2, 12, 13]. Thus, while probably mediated by the attentional LC-NE system, the current results may be viewed as indexing a specific subcategory of social cognition related to face-to-face interaction and caregiving behaviors.

Given inter-individual variability in the accuracy to interpret infant facial expressions [13], we used a behavioral rating task to assess recognition of infant emotional signals in the current participants. The results from the rating task indicated high accuracy in the recognition of infant facial expressions. In our pupillary analyses, a distinction between stimuli rated as indicating negative emotion produced a pupil dilation which was larger than that elicited by stimuli rated as positive or neutral. Thus, the pupil response was associated with the subjective identification of negative vs. positive affect in the infant pictures. In future studies, a comparable approach combining pupillometry and behavioral performance could be used in studies involving specific participant groups with variable social cognitive abilities especially related to infant signals of emotion (e.g., from families at-risk for maladaptive infant-caregiver interaction).

Previous research has demonstrated an effect of emotional arousal rather than that of valence on pupil dilation [15]. In contrast, in the current study we found an effect of emotional valence on pupil dilation but no effect of stimulus arousal. The difference between the findings may be related to the type of stimuli (face vs. IAPS, not limited to faces), the type of people depicted (infants vs. IAPS, not limited to infants), and the scale used in stimulus classification. Perceptual scaling of any stimulus is inherently arbitrary and heavily influenced by the reference stimulus or stimuli [40, 41]. In scaling emotional valence and arousal different sets of stimuli, and hence different reference(s), may have been used in the current stimulus set in comparison to IAPS pictures [42]. Thus, the arousal and valence categories used here may be different from those used in the IAPS. It further seems possible that the negatively-valenced stimuli in the current study depicting infant distress or discomfort may signal (and elicit) stronger emotional arousal than the positively-valenced faces used in the current study. That is, the dimensions of arousal and valence are not orthogonal as difference in valence between stimuli requires a sufficient level of arousal to emerge [42].

In principle, the onset and the time course of pupil dilation following an emotional stimulus could be estimated from the latencies of the LC-NE subsystems and their influence on pupil size [20]. To our knowledge, such estimates of the time course of the pupil response have not been established. In practice, the emotive pupil response has been investigated from different time-windows spanning 500–1300 ms [17], 600–1600 ms [18], 1000–1300 ms [43], 2–4 s [31, 32], or 2–6 s [15, 17] after stimulus onset. The early and late time-windows have been typically selected to cover the constriction and the dilation phase, respectively. In the current study, a relatively late time-window spanning 4–5 s after stimulus onset was chosen for the extraction of pupil dilation in order to minimize the contribution of the pupillary light response on the estimate. The current results indicate that the pupil dilation within this time-window was both sensitive to the emotive content of the stimuli and independent of stimulus brightness. In future studies using constant light conditions, a more detailed, frame-by-frame, analysis of the pupil response together with known latencies of the LC-NE system [20] might provide insight into the time course of LC activation in the context of emotional perception.

Pupillary response elicited by emotive face stimuli already around 600–1600 ms after stimulus onset in child participants [18], have been observed in previous studies. This latency overlaps with the pupil constriction reflex extracted in the current study. Furthermore, while a study [15] using pictures from the International Affective Picture System (IAPS), found no evidence for emotional effects in pupil constriction, a more recent study from the same authors indicated emotional suppression of this initial light reflex [17]. In the current study, modulations of pupil constriction in response to stimulus category were found across both experiments. However, the control experiment (Experiment 2) indicated that these effects were not specific to emotional content or to faces as they were found for the random non-face stimuli as well. The difference between the current results from those obtained with IAPS [17] may be related to the type of emotionally salient stimuli used to evoke the autonomic pupil response: in the IAPS study, the largest emotional suppression of pupil constriction was found for erotic and violent scenes which were not used in the current study but may elicit CNS [44] and ANS [45] activity distinct from other emotionally equally arousing stimuli. Further, the pupil constriction in the current study may have been partially suppressed by the presentation of the pre-stimulus visual pattern, which might also have suppressed emotional effects on this initial light reflex. Thus, further studies may be needed to clarify the modulations of pupil constriction by affective face processing, especially in the context of maternal responses to infant emotive cues.

Pupillary responses to emotional cues are relatively small and intermixed with the larger effects of stimulus or ambient luminance. In the current study, stimuli in different emotion categories were not significantly different with respect to their mean (bitmap) intensity values, but there was a clear trend for both within- and between-category variability. An ideal solution for avoiding these confounds in emotion research would be to use stimuli with invariable luminance levels as well as matched contrast and spatial frequency profile [46]. However, in many cases perfect matching between stimulus luminance and other low-level features may be difficult or result in unnatural stimulus qualities. In the current study, confounding effects of stimulus luminance (i.e., variable face luminance and the luminance variability between the stimulus and the pre-stimulus intervals) were controlled by contrasting pupil responses elicited by face stimuli to those elicited by pixel-scrambled version of the same face stimuli. In this control experiment (Experiment 2), the stimulus light intensity was exactly matched to the face condition while all facial and emotive cues were removed from the stimuli. If the difference in pupil size across stimulus conditions were to persist in the control condition, such effects could simply be attributed to differences in stimulus luminance. Conversely, if the effects are unique to the face condition, they most likely stem from genuine emotive processes related to face perception. While pupil constriction was affected by stimulus category in both face and control condition, pupil dilation and it's modulation by emotive stimulus category were confined to the face condition only. Thus, we may confidently interpret the current results as indicating emotive pupil dilation elicited by infant faces which is further intensified by negative emotional expressions.

Limitations of the study

(1) The participants were not perfectly matched across the main and the control experiment. For example, unlike in the main experiment, the participants in the control experiment were both male and female, and parenthood was not required as an inclusion criterion. However, participants in both experiments were healthy adults and manifested very similar pupil dilation in response to stimuli depicting infant distress or discomfort. (2) The infants depicted in face stimuli were Caucasian while the participants viewing the stimuli where both Black and Caucasian, with low and high SES, respectively. Therefore, own-race biases in face processing [47] and SES [48, 49] might have affected the emotive responses elicited by the stimuli. (3) The current study focused in testing intra-individual variation in pupil response across variable infant facial expressions. Therefore, measures of inter-individual variations in potentially related variables such as maternal sensitivity to infant cues were not presented. As such, positive effect of increased pupil size in response to pictures of infant negative affect was found within the current sample consisting of healthy mothers (main experiment) and adult controls (control experiment). Future studies are needed to indicate whether the

pupil response to infant faces is sensitive to inter-individual variations in general and in relation to motherhood in particular.

Conclusions

Our current results indicate that pupil diameter is a sensitive marker of emotional processes elicited by infant facial expressions in the targeted participant group of mothers of infant children. While the perception of infant signals of distress may constitute a specific case of face processing [2, 12, 13], the current approach may be applicable to other domains of social perception as well due to a common psychophysiological pathway, the LC-NE system. Consequently, it remains possible that comparable pupil response may be elicited by non-infant stimuli as well or in non-mother viewers exposed to affective facial stimuli. In order to address the specificity of the current emotive pupil response to infant cues, further studies with both adult and infant face stimuli as well as participants with sufficient inter-individual variability in responsiveness to facial expressions of emotion in both categories are needed. Nevertheless, the principle contribution of the current study is in indicating the feasibility of pupil diameter as an index of mothers' perception and responsiveness to infant non-verbal communication. As such, pupil diameter may provide a useful and accessible measure for studies of individual variations in mother-infant interaction [1].

Abbreviations
ANOVA: analysis of variance; ANS: autonomic nervous system; AOI: area of interest; CNS: central nervous system; GLM: general linear model; IAPS: International Affective Picture System; LC-NE: locus coeruleus-norepinephrine; MN: mild negative; MP: mild positive; POG: point of gaze; SES: socioeconomic status; SN: strong negative; SP: strong positive.

Authors' contributions
DN, ET, and JML conceived, designed, and coordinated the study. SY performed pupil and eye-tracking analyses, statistical analyses, and drafted the manuscript. JML and DN helped to draft the manuscript. All authors critically reviewed the manuscript and gave final approval for the version to be published. All authors read and approved the final manuscript.

Author details
[1] Tampere Center for Child Health Research, School of Medicine, University of Tampere, Lääkärinkatu 1, 33520 Tampere, Finland. [2] Department of Psychiatry, Faculty of Health Sciences, Stellenbosch University, Stellenbosch, South Africa.

Acknowledgements
The authors are grateful to Alice Mado Proverbio for the stimulus material, to Gerdia Harvey for assisting in data collection and to Jussi Kaatiala for the programming efforts (gazeAnalysisLib).

Competing interests
The authors declare that the research was conducted in the absence of any commercial, financial, or other relationships that could be construed as potential competing interests.

Funding
This research was supported by a joint project grant from the Academy of Finland and National Research Foundation, South Africa (# 2501271617). The funders had no role in study design, data collection and analysis, decision to publish, or preparation of the manuscript.

References
1. Strathearn L. Maternal neglect: oxytocin, dopamine and the neurobiology of attachment. J Neuroendocrinol. 2011;23(11):1054–65.
2. Peltola MJ, Yrttiaho S, Puura K, Proverbio AM, Mononen N, Lehtimäki T, et al. Motherhood and oxytocin receptor genetic variation are associated with selective changes in electrocortical responses to infant facial expressions. Emotion. 2014;14(3):469–77.
3. Rilling JK. The neural and hormonal bases of human parental care. Neuropsychologia. 2013;51(4):731–47.
4. Swain JE, Lorberbaum JP, Kose S, Strathearn L. Brain basis of early parent-infant interactions: psychology, physiology, and in vivo functional neuroimaging studies. J Child Psychol Psychiatry. 2007;48(3–4):262–87.
5. Yrttiaho S, Forssman L, Kaatiala J, Leppänen JM. Developmental precursors of social brain networks: the emergence of attentional and cortical sensitivity to facial expressions in 5 to 7 months old infants. PLoS ONE. 2014;9(6):e100811.
6. Peltola MJ, Forssman L, Puura K, van Ijzendoorn MH, Leppänen JM. Attention to faces expressing negative emotion at 7 months predicts attachment security at 14 months. Child Dev. 2015;86(5):1321–32.
7. Barrett J, Fleming AS. Annual research review: all mothers are not created equal: neural and psychobiological perspectives on mothering and the importance of individual differences. J Child Psychol Psychiatry. 2011;52(4):368–97.
8. Glocker ML, Langleben DD, Ruparel K, Loughead JW, Gur RC, Sachser N. Baby schema in infant faces induces cuteness perception and motivation for caretaking in adults. Ethology. 2009;115(3):257–63.
9. Glocker ML, Langleben DD, Ruparel K, Loughead JW, Valdez JN, Griffin MD, et al. Baby schema modulates the brain reward system in nulliparous women. Proc Natl Acad Sci USA. 2009;106(22):9115–9.
10. Kringelbach ML, Lehtonen A, Squire S, Harvey AG, Craske MG, Holliday IE, et al. A specific and rapid neural signature for parental instinct. PLoS ONE. 2008;3(2):e1664.
11. Proverbio AM, Riva F, Zani A, Martin E. Is it a baby? Perceived age affects brain processing of faces differently in women and men. J Cogn Neurosci. 2011;23(11):3197–208.
12. Proverbio AM, Brignone V, Matarazzo S, Del Zotto M, Zani A. Gender and parental status affect the visual cortical response to infant facial expression. Neuropsychologia. 2006;44(14):2987–99.
13. Proverbio AM, Matarazzo S, Brignone V, Del Zotto M, Zani A. Processing valence and intensity of infant expressions: the roles of expertise and gender. Scand J Psychol. 2007;48:477–85.
14. Beatty J, Lucero-Wagoner B. The Pupillary System. In: Cacioppo J, Tassinary LG, Berntson GG, editors. Handbook of psychophysiology. 3rd ed. New York: Cambridge University Press; 2007. p. 142–62.
15. Bradley MM, Miccoli L, Escrig MA, Lang PJ. The pupil as a measure of emotional arousal and autonomic activation. Psychophysiology. 2008;45(4):602–7.
16. Steinhauer SR, Siegle GJ, Condray R, Pless M. Sympathetic and parasympathetic innervation of pupillary dilation during sustained processing. Int J Psychophysiol. 2004;52(1):77–86.
17. Henderson RR, Bradley MM, Lang PJ. Modulation of the initial light reflex during affective picture viewing. Psychophysiology. 2014;51:815–8.

18. Sepeta L, Tsuchiya N, Davies MS, Sigman M, Bookheimer SY, Dapretto M. Abnormal social reward processing in autism as indexed by pupillary responses to happy faces. J Neurodev Disord. 2012;4(1):17.

19. Prehn K, Kazzer P, Lischke A, Heinrichs M, Herpertz SC, Domes G. Effects of intranasal oxytocin on pupil dilation indicate increased salience of socioaffective stimuli. Psychophysiology. 2013;50:528–37.

20. Laeng B, Sirois S, Gredebäck G. Pupillometry: a window to the preconscious? Perspect Psychol Sci. 2012;7(1):18–27.

21. Joshi S, Li Y, Kalwani RM, Gold JI. Relationships between pupil diameter and neuronal activity in the locus coeruleus, colliculi, and cingulate cortex. Neuron. 2016;89(1):221–34.

22. Loewenfeld I. The pupil: anatomy, physiology, and clinical applications. Detroit: Wayne State University Press; 1993.

23. Sheehan DV, Lecrubier Y, Sheehan KH, Amorim P, Janavs J, Weiller E, et al. The mini-international neuropsychiatric interview (M.I.N.I.): the development and validation of a structured diagnostic psychiatric interview for DSM-IV and ICD-10. J Clin Psychiatry. 1998;59:22–33.

24. Leppänen JM, Forssman L, Kaatiala J, Yrttiaho S, Wass S. Widely applicable MATLAB routines for automated analysis of saccadic reaction times. Behav Res Methods. 2015;47(2):538–48.

25. Koole SL. The psychology of emotion regulation: an integrative review. Cogn Emotion. 2009;23(1):4–41.

26. Joosen KJ, Mesman J, Bakermans-Kranenburg MJ, van Ijzendoorn MH. Maternal overreactive sympathetic nervous system responses to repeated infant crying predicts risk for impulsive harsh discipline of infants. Child Maltreat. 2013;18(4):252–63.

27. Leerkes EM, Supple AJ, O'Brien M, Calkins SD, Haltigan JD, Wong MS, et al. Antecedents of maternal sensitivity during distressing tasks: integrating attachment, social information processing, and psychobiological perspectives. Child Dev. 2015;86(1):94–111.

28. Laeng B, Orbo M, Holmlund T, Miozzo M. Pupillary Stroop effects. Cogn Process. 2011;12(1):13–21.

29. Dabbs JM Jr. Testosterone and pupillary response to auditory sexual stimuli. Physiol Behav. 1997;62(4):909–12.

30. Cassady JM, Farley GR, Weinberger NM, Kitzes LM. Pupillary activity measured by reflected infra-red light. Physiol Behav. 1982;28:851–4.

31. Kret ME, Roelofs K, Stekelenburg JJ, de Gelder B. Emotional signals from faces, bodies and scenes influence observers' face expressions, fixations and pupil-size. Front Hum Neurosci. 2013;7:810.

32. Kret ME, Stekelenburg JJ, Roelofs K, deGelder B. Perception of face and body expressions using electromyography, pupillometry and gaze measures. Front Psychol. 2013;4:28.

33. Lorber MF, O'Leary SG. Mediated paths to over-reactive discipline: mothers' experienced emotion, appraisals, and physiological responses. J Consult Clin Psychol. 2005;73(5):972–81.

34. Frodi AM, Lamb ME. Child abusers' responses to infant smiles and cries. Child Dev. 1980;51(1):238–41.

35. Musser ED, Ablow JC, Measelle JR. Predicting maternal sensitivity: the roles of postnatal depressive symptoms and parasympathetic dysregulation. Infant Ment Health J. 2012;33(4):350–9.

36. Moore GA, Hill-Soderlund AL, Propper CB, Calkins SD, Mills-Koonce WR, Cox MJ. Mother-infant vagal regulation in the face-to-face still-face paradigm is moderated by maternal sensitivity. Child Dev. 2009;80(1):209–23.

37. Aston-Jones G, Cohen JD. An integrative theory of locus coeruleus-norepinephrine function: adaptive gain and optimal performance. Annu Rev Neurosci. 2005;28:403–50.

38. Murphy PR, Robertson IH, Balsters JH, O'Connell RG. Pupillometry and P3 index the locus coeruleus-noradrenergic arousal function in humans. Psychophysiology. 2011;48:1532–43.

39. Kret ME, Tomonaga M, Matsuzawa T. Chimpanzees and humans mimic pupil-size of conspecifics. PLoS ONE. 2014;9(8):e104886.

40. Kreiman J, Gerratt BR, Ito M. When and why listeners disagree in voice quality assessment tasks. J Acoust Soc Am. 2007;122:2354–64.

41. Yrttiaho S, Alku P, May PJ, Tiitinen H. Representation of the vocal roughness of aperiodic speech sounds in the auditory cortex. J Acoust Soc Am. 2009;125(5):3177–85.

42. Bradley MM, Lang PJ. The international affective picture system (IAPS) in the study of emotion and attention. In: Coan JA, Allen JB, editors. The handbook of emotion elicitation and assessment. New York: Oxford University Press; 2007. p. 33.

43. Bradley MM, Lang PJ. Memory, emotion, and pupil diameter: repetition of natural scenes. Psychophysiology. 2015;52(9):1186–93.

44. Schupp H, Cuthbert B, Bradley M, Hillman C, Hamm A, Lang P. Brain processes in emotional perception: motivated attention. Cogn Emot. 2004;18(5):593–611.

45. Lang PJ, Bradley MM, Cuthbert BN. Motivated attention: Affect, activation, and action. In: Lang PJ, Simons RF, Balaban M, editors. Attention and orienting. Mahwah: Erlbaum; 1997. p. 97–135.

46. Link B, Junemann A, Rix R, Sembritzki O, Brenning A, Korth M, et al. Pupillographic measurements with pattern stimulation: the pupil's response in normal subjects and first measurements in glaucoma patients. Invest Ophthalmol Vis Sci. 2006;47(11):4947–55.

47. Ekman P, Friesen WV, O'Sullivan M, Chan A, Diacoyanni-Tarlatzis I, Heider K, et al. Universals and cultural differences in the judgments of facial expression of emotion. J Pers Soc Psychol. 1987;53:712–7.

48. Hackman DA, Gallop R, Evans GW, Farah MJ. Socioeconomic status and executive function: developmental trajectories and mediation. Dev Sci. 2015;18(5):686–702.

49. Kraus MW, Cote S, Keltner D. Social class, contextualism, and empathic accuracy. Psychol Sci. 2010;21(11):1716–23.

The effect of epilepsy on autistic symptom severity assessed by the social responsiveness scale in children with autism spectrum disorder

Chanyoung Ko[1], Namwook Kim[2,3], Eunjoo Kim[4], Dong Ho Song[2,3] and Keun-Ah Cheon[2,3*]

Abstract

Background: As the prevalence of autism spectrum disorders in people with epilepsy ranges from 15 to 47 % (Clarke et al. in Epilepsia 46:1970–1977, 2005), it is speculated that there is a special relationship between the two disorders, yet there has been a lack of systematic studies comparing the behavioral phenotype between autistic individuals and autistic individuals with epilepsy. This study aims to investigate how the co-occurrence of epilepsy and Autism Spectrum Disorder (ASD) affects autistic characteristics assessed by the Social Responsiveness Scale (SRS), which has been used as a measure of autism symptoms in previous studies. In this research we referred to all individuals with Autism or Autistic Disorder as individuals with ASD.

Methods: We reviewed the complete medical records of 182 participants who presented to a single tertiary care referral center from January 1, 2013 to July 28, 2015, and subsequently received complete child and adolescent psychiatric assessments. Of the 182 participants, 22 were diagnosed with Autism Spectrum Disorder and epilepsy. Types of epilepsy observed in these individuals included complex partial seizure, generalized tonic–clonic seizure, or infantile spasm. Using 'Propensity Score Matching' we selected 44 children, diagnosed with only Autism Spectrum Disorder, whose age, gender, and intelligence quotient (IQ) were closely matched with the 22 children diagnosed with Autism Spectrum Disorder and epilepsy. Social functioning of participants was assessed by the social responsiveness scale, which consists of five categories: social awareness, social cognition, social communication, social motivation, and autistic mannerisms. Bivariate analyses were conducted to compare the ASD participants with epilepsy group with the ASD-only group on demographic and clinical characteristics. Chi square and t test p values were calculated when appropriate.

Results: There was no significant difference in age (p = 0.172), gender (p > 0.999), IQ (FSIQ, p = 0.139; VIQ, p = 0.114; PIQ, p = 0.295) between the two groups. ASD participants with epilepsy were significantly more impaired than ASD participants on some measures of social functioning such as social awareness (p = 0.03) and social communication (p = 0.027). ASD participants with epilepsy also scored significantly higher on total SRS t-score than ASD participants (p = 0.023).

Conclusions: Understanding the relationship between ASD and epilepsy is critical for appropriate management (e.g. social skills training, seizure control) of ASD participants with co-occurring epilepsy. Results of this study suggest that mechanisms involved in producing epilepsy may play a role in producing or augmenting autistic features such as poor social functioning. Prospective study with larger sample sizes is warranted to further explore this association.

Keywords: Autism spectrum disorder, Epilepsy, Autistic symptom severity, Social responsiveness scale

*Correspondence: kacheon@yuhs.ac; psyreg88@gmail.com
[2] Division of Child and Adolescent Psychiatry, Department of Psychiatry, College of Medicine, Severance Hospital, Yonsei University, Seoul, South Korea
Full list of author information is available at the end of the article

Background

Autism spectrum disorder (ASD) is a childhood developmental disorder described by two core symptom dimensions—social communication and restricted, repetitive behavior (RRB) [2]. ASD encompasses a highly heterogeneous set of individuals with wide variations in clinical presentation, symptom severity, and cognitive ability [2]. Epilepsy is characterized by an enduring tendency to produce epileptic seizures and practically defined as having two un-triggered seizures occurring at least 24 h apart [3]. The co-occurrence of ASD and epilepsy is well recognized and has interested clinicians and researchers, yet the relationship between the two conditions has not been well established on a pathophysiologic level [4]. Prevalence estimates may vary, but between 11 and 39 % of individuals with ASD have been reported to develop epilepsy [4–6], which exceeds that of the general population (0.7–1 %) [7]. The prevalence of autism spectrum disorders in people with epilepsy ranges from 15 to 47 % [1].

Characteristics of individuals with both ASD and epilepsy have been explored in a handful of cross-sectional population-based studies [8–13]. Previous publications have reported findings about demographical variables such as age of onset, gender ratio, type of epilepsy, cognitive ability, and verbal ability. To date only one variable—lower cognitive ability—has consistently shown independent association with co-occurrence of epilepsy in individuals with ASD across all studies [8–13]. No specific epilepsy syndrome or seizure type has been associated, although focal or localization-related seizures are often reported [8]. While epilepsy onset in individuals without autism has been described to be highest in the first year of life [14, 15], in individuals with ASD, two peaks of seizure onset have been consistently reported, one in early childhood [16] and one in adolescence and continuing through adulthood [9, 17, 18]. Long-term follow-up cohort studies have shown higher prevalence of epilepsy in children with ASD of older age [8, 9, 13].

Only a few published studies have compared the clinical profiles of individuals who have both ASD and epilepsy with individuals who have only ASD [19–23]. Furthermore, little is known about the influence of epilepsy on the autistic symptoms in individuals with ASD. Clinical assessment of individuals with ASD and co-morbid epilepsy will give us an insight into how comorbid epilepsy affects the clinical features and natural history, certain cognitive-behavioral as well as psycho-pharmacological challenges associated with co-occurrence of ASD and epilepsy. One study showed a general trend towards greater developmental difficulties and stereotyped behaviors in children with epilepsy and ASD; their findings suggested that the presence of epilepsy may affect social

functioning and incite behavioral problems [20]. Tuchman and Cuccaro found an association between epilepsy and autistic mannerisms such as repetitive object use and unusual sensory interests [17]. These studies provided the initial evidence suggesting that individuals with ASD and co-morbid epilepsy have elevated autism symptoms. One way of determining the role of epilepsy in autistic characteristics is through the use of quantitative assessment that is known to measure ASD symptom severity.

The social responsiveness scale (SRS), developed by Constantino et al. is a brief screening questionnaire completed by a third party informant that is often used to evaluate ASD symptom severity [24]. Although the SRS refers to a measure of social deficiency, many SRS items describe other core features of ASD such as autistic mannerisms [24]. The SRS provides an overall quantitative score as well as treatment specific sub-scores pertaining to receptive, cognitive, expressive, and motivational aspects of social behavior. Recent studies evaluating the efficacy of the SRS have shown that the SRS scores are influenced by age, gender, IQ, and presence of psychiatric co-morbidities [25]. Therefore, results from trials that employ this metric must be interpreted in light of these possible confounding factors. For the purpose of comparison studies or large cohort studies, screening tools such as SRS may be more appropriate and practical than standard ASD diagnostic tools, which can take several hours to complete [24]. This scale permits rapid detection, hence early diagnosis, of ASD while providing a good index of the severity of autistic social impairment [26].

Two previous studies have employed the SRS to ascertain the relationship between epilepsy and autism symptoms [19, 27]. Viscidi et al. showed that ASD children with epilepsy had more severe autism symptoms than ASD children without epilepsy, which was mostly explained by the lower IQ of the epilepsy group. After statistically adjusting for the effect of IQ, SRS scores of children with and without epilepsy did not differ significantly [19]. Wakeford et al. utilized an abbreviated version of the SRS, social responsiveness scale—shortened (SRS-S), to study autistics characteristics in adults with epilepsy. They found that higher SRS-S scores were associated with having diagnosis of epilepsy and were perceived to increase during seizure activity [27].

To our knowledge, only two published studies have investigated the relationship between autism and epilepsy using the SRS. Whereas Wakeford et al. suggested that seizure activity itself might have an impact on social difficulties, Viscidi et al. implied that diagnosis of epilepsy might be associated with social impairment solely due to the effect of cognitive impairment. Based on these studies, it is unclear whether seizure activities or having diagnosis of epilepsy has a direct impact on autism symptoms. Therefore, the current study aimed to ascertain this possibility by utilizing the SRS, to observe any difference between individuals with ASD and co-morbid epilepsy and matched control sample (individuals with only ASD) that have similar distributions on covariates such as age, gender, and IQ. We hypothesized that in the group of individuals diagnosed with both disorders, there would be an increase of ASD characteristics represented by higher SRS scores.

Methods
Patients and controls
All participants were originally seen at a specialist outpatient clinic for children with autism at Severance Children's Hospital between January 1, 2013 and July 28, 2015. During this period, 182 patients had completed the SRS interview and routine developmental and cognitive assessments. Twenty seven of the 182 patients were reported to have shown epileptiform discharges on routine electroencephalogram (EEG); 22 of these 27 patients had been diagnosed with ASD and epilepsy (ASD + E). Forty-four ASD-only patients were selected from 155 patients with normal EEG using a statistical maneuver called *propensity score matching* [28]. *Propensity score matching* refers to a set of multivariate methods that estimate the effect of one factor by accounting for covariates known to affect the overall outcome [29]. This method allows the investigator to design and analyze an observational study mimicking certain characteristics of a randomized controlled trial [30]. For instance, conditional on the 'propensity score,' the distribution of observed baseline covariates will be similar between the participant and control group. A previous publication indicated that age, gender, and IQ influence scores on the SRS [25]. Accounting for these three covariates, one-to-two matching was performed, yielding 44 age-, gender-, and IQ- matched control ASD-only patients (Fig. 1). All study procedures were approved by the institutional review board at Severance Hospital, Yonsei University College of Medicine in Seoul, South Korea.

Clinical assessment
All study participants had had a previous clinical diagnosis of ASD. Diagnoses of childhood autism or atypical autism were established using the Childhood Autism Rating Scale (CARS), a behavior rating scale intended to help diagnose autism [31], or autism diagnostic interview-revised (ADI-R), the "gold" standard for ASD diagnosis [32]. Epilepsy had been diagnosed previously by a pediatric neurologist. For the purposes of this study, epilepsy was defined as 'two or more non-febrile seizures that were not confined to pre-school period (up to 5 years of

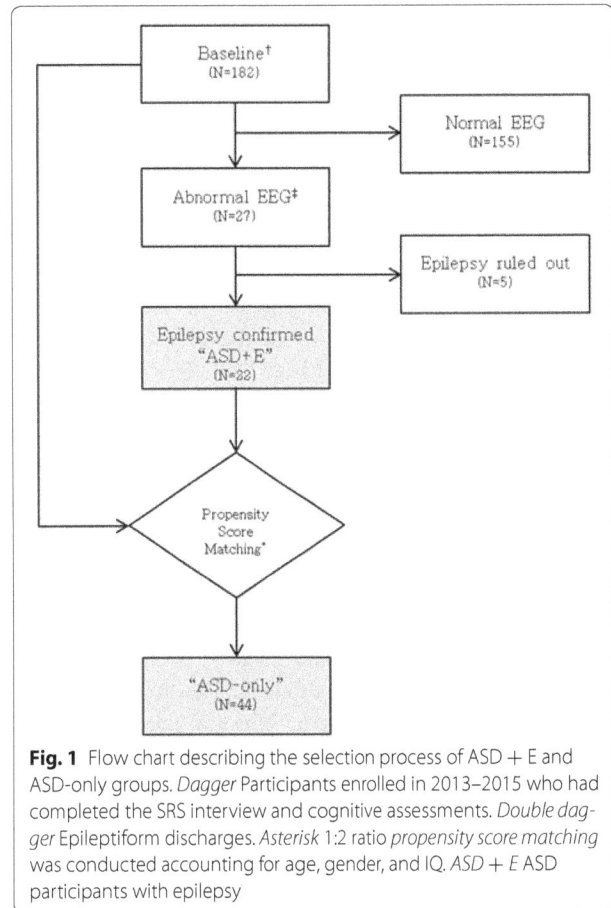

Fig. 1 Flow chart describing the selection process of ASD + E and ASD-only groups. *Dagger* Participants enrolled in 2013–2015 who had completed the SRS interview and cognitive assessments. *Double dagger* Epileptiform discharges. *Asterisk* 1:2 ratio *propensity score matching* was conducted accounting for age, gender, and IQ. *ASD + E* ASD participants with epilepsy

age).' The classification of seizure type followed the definitions of the International League against Epilepsy [3]. Individuals with neonatal seizures (i.e. seizures appearing before the age of 1 month which did not persist) were excluded from this study.

The medical records of all participants were retrospectively reviewed for demographic information, past medical history, medication history, main seizure type, age of seizure onset, and number of anti-epileptic drugs (AEDs) currently prescribed. Full Scale IQ (FSIQ), verbal IQ (VIQ), performance IQ (PIQ) were assessed with the Korean version [33] of the Wechsler Intelligence Scale for Children III [34], or the Korean version [35] of the Wechsler Adult Intelligence Scale III [36].

The SRS is a 65-item questionnaire that serves as a screening tool for ASD as well as a quantitative measure of ASD symptom severity in children aged 4 through 18. This scale was designed to be completed by an adult (parent or teacher) who is familiar with the child's current behavior and developmental history [37]. In this study, we used SRS scores based on the parent-completed questionnaire. The SRS assesses five domains, which include: social awareness, social information processing, expressive social communication, social anxiety/avoidance, and autistic preoccupations/mannerisms. Each item is scored on a scale ranging from 1 (not true) to 4 (almost always true). Raw scores are converted to T-scores (with mean of 50 and standard deviation of 10) for gender and rater type. T-score of ≥ 76 is considered severe and strongly associated with a clinical diagnosis of ASD. T-score of 60-75 falls in the mild to moderate range and considered typical for high functioning ASD, while a T-score of ≤ 59 suggests an absence of ASD symptoms [37]. The internal consistency of the SRS with a Cronbach's $\alpha > 0.90$ is considered high [24]. The SRS also has good inter-rater reliability of $r = 0.91$ [24, 38]. Studies have shown the SRS is capable of distinguishing individuals with pervasive developmental disorders such as ASD and other psychiatric disorders such as ADHD [24, 37]. Moderately strong associations were found between the SRS and the ADI-R, with correlation coefficients ≥ 0.52 across all subscales [24]. The SRS was translated into Korean language by Korean autism researchers and the Korean version of the SRS was back-translated into English by a bilingual child psychiatrist. The back-translated version was reconfirmed by a child and adolescent psychiatrist at the University of California San Francisco. Currently, the Korean version of the SRS has been well standardized and widely used (Cheon et al. under revision).

Statistical analysis

Statistical analyses were performed using Statistical Package for Social Sciences (SPSS PC, version 20.0). Statistical significance was defined at a level of $p < 0.05$, and a $p < 0.10$ was regarded as a statistical trend toward change. Bivariate analyses were conducted to compare ASD participants with epilepsy group with the ASD-only group on demographic and clinical characteristics. Chi square and t test p values were calculated when appropriate.

Results

Participant characteristics

The characteristics of all individuals in the study are summarized in Table 1. The ASD participants with epilepsy group had been matched with comparison group (ASD-only) based on age, gender, and IQ. Consequently there was no statistical difference in age ($p = 0.172$), gender ($p > 0.999$), IQ (FSIQ, $p = 0.139$; VIQ, $p = 0.114$; PIQ, $p = 0.295$) between the ASD participants with epilepsy group and the ASD-only group. There was no statistically significant difference in gestational age ($p = 0.386$), birth weight ($p = 0.072$), obstetric complications ($p = 0.485$), use of antipsychotic medication ($p = 0.191$) between the two groups.

Co-morbid conditions

Within the ASD participants with epilepsy group, 4 (18.2 %) reported to have ADHD; 2 (9.1 %) reported to have Tuberous sclerosis, 2 (9.1 %) reported to have depression; 1 (4.5 %) reported to have bipolar disorder; 3 (13.6 %) reported to have Tourette syndrome; 5 (22.7 %) reported to have additional diagnoses (Table 2). Within the ASD-only group, 16 (36.4 %) reported to have ADHD; 2 (4.5 %) reported to have depression; 2 (4.5 %) reported to have psychosis; 5 (11.4 %) reported to have bipolar disorder; 3 (6.8 %) reported to have anxiety disorder; 2 (4.5 %) reported to have additional diagnoses (Table 2). Additional diagnoses included neurofibromatosis type 1, fragile-X syndrome, subarachnoid hemorrhage, organic brain syndrome, cortical dysplasia, and childhood onset parkinsonism. ASD participants with epilepsy group and ASD-only group showed statistical difference in the percentage of Tourette syndrome ($p = 0.034$) and additional diagnoses ($p = 0.036$) (Table 2).

Epilepsy profile of ASD participants with co-occurring epilepsy

Epilepsy variables of the ASD participants with epilepsy ($N = 22$) are summarized in Table 3. The mean age at onset of confirmed epilepsy was 5.57 years (SD = 4.71). The number of AEDs prescribed at time of assessment were 1.45 (SD = 1.10), which means that the majority of them were receiving one or two anticonvulsants. Of the 22 participants with co-morbid epilepsy, two were diagnosed with infantile spasms, 14 reported to have complex partial seizures, and six reported to have generalized tonic–clonic seizures (Table 3).

Autistic symptom severity

Independent two sample t test was employed to compare the two samples in terms of their SRS ratings (Table 4). ASD participants with epilepsy scored generally higher than ASD-only participants across all SRS categories as represented by significantly higher SRS total t-score ($p = 0.023$). ASD participants with epilepsy showed significantly more marked severity in social awareness ($p = 0.03$) and social communication ($p = 0.027$). There was no statistical difference in social cognition ($p = 0.081$), social motivation ($p = 0.0505$), and autistic mannerisms ($p = 0.065$). However, the subscale scores for these three categories suggested a trend towards participants with ASD participants with epilepsy having greater severity in all three categories ($p < 0.1$).

Discussion

Among children diagnosed with ASD, we found significant difference in autistic characteristics between children with and without epilepsy. Even after adjusting

Table 1 Demographic characteristics of ASD + E and ASD-only participants

	ASD-only (N = 44)	ASD + E (N = 22)	p value
Age[a] (years)	8.273 ± 4.326	10.227 ± 5.814	0.172
Gender[b]			
Male	43 (97.7 %)	21 (95.5 %)	>0.999
Female	1 (2.3 %)	1 (4.5 %)	
FSIQ[a]	62.318 ± 17.095	55.455 ± 18.397	0.139
VIQ[a]	67.80 ± 22.130	58.68 ± 21.007	0.114
PIQ[a]	62.73 ± 15.813	58.27 ± 16.799	0.295
Intellectual disability based on FSIQ[b]			
Non-intellectual disability IQ >70	12 (27.3 %)	5 (22.7 %)	0.102
Mild intellectual disability IQ 50–70	20 (45.5 %)	6 (27.3 %)	
Moderate-severe intellectual disability IQ <50	12 (27.3 %)	11 (50.0 %)	
Gestation age (weeks)[b]			
≤31	1 (2.3 %)	0 (0 %)	0.386
32–36	8 (18.2 %)	2 (9.1 %)	
37–41	35 (79.5 %)	54 (81.8 %)	
≥42	0 (0 %)	1 (4.5 %)	
Birth weight (g)[b]			
1500–2499	2 (4.5 %)	1 (4.5 %)	0.072
2500–3999	41 (93.2 %)	17 (77.3 %)	
4000–4499	1 (2.3 %)	4 (18.2 %)	
Obstetrics complication[b]			
No	38 (86.4 %)	17 (77.3 %)	0.485
Yes	6 (13.6 %)	5 (22.7 %)	
Antipsychotic medication[b]			
No	25 (56.8 %)	8 (36.4 %)	0.191
Yes	19 (43.2 %)	14 (63.6 %)	

ASD + E ASD participants with epilepsy

[a] Independent two sample t test

[b] Chi square test

for baseline characteristics such as age, gender, and full scale IQ, ASD participants with epilepsy were found to be associated with higher scores on the SRS *total t-score*, *social awareness*, and *social communication*, indicating greater impairment. Based on our statistical model, there seemed to be a significant relationship between epilepsy and autistic characteristics in ASD children that is not explained by the association between epilepsy and low IQ. Participants diagnosed with both ASD and epilepsy appeared to be more socially impaired, especially in their capacity to pick up on social cues and organize expressive acts of social communication. In addition, ASD participants with epilepsy generally scored higher on other items that ascertain *social cognition* and *social motivation*.

Several studies have published in-depth reviews on the relationship between ASD and epilepsy [5, 8–10]. They have examined demographical variables such as the age of seizure onset, gender ratio, type of epilepsy, and intelligence level. Turk et al. was one of the first studies to compare the clinical profiles of matched groups of children with only ASD and children who were diagnosed with both ASD and epilepsy [20]. Utilizing the diagnostic interview for social and communication disorders (DISCO-11), they demonstrated that ASD participants with epilepsy were associated with greater motor difficulties, developmental delays, and challenging behavior in public places. Smith et al. study showed that individuals with intellectual disability (ID) combined with ASD and epilepsy were significantly more impaired than ID groups with a single co-morbid factor (ASD or epilepsy) on some measures of behavior problems including self-injury and disruptive behavior [21, 22]. No significant differences were found on stereotyped behaviors among all groups (ID-only vs. ASD-only vs. ASD and epilepsy vs. ID with ASD and epilepsy) [21]. Individuals with ID expressing co-morbid ASD and epilepsy had significantly more impaired social skills (e.g. sharing interests, playing,

Table 2 Reported co-morbid conditions in ASD + E and ASD-only participants

	ASD-only (N = 44) (%)	ASD + E (N = 22) (%)	p value
Attention deficit hyperactivity disorder (ADHD)			
No	28 (63.6)	18 (81.8)	0.163
Yes	16 (36.4)	4 (18.2)	
Tuberous sclerosis			
No	44 (100)	20 (90.9)	0.108
Yes	0 (0)	2 (9.1)	
Depression			
No	42 (95.5)	20 (90.9)	0.596
Yes	2 (4.5)	2 (9.1)	
Psychosis			
No	42 (95.5)	22 (100)	0.549
Yes	2 (4.5)	0 (0)	
Bipolar disorder			
No	39 (88.6)	21 (95.5)	0.655
Yes	5 (11.4)	1 (4.5)	
Anxiety disorder			
No	41 (93.2)	22 (100)	0.545
Yes	3 (6.8)	0 (0)	
Tourette disorder*			
No	44 (100)	19 (86.4)	0.034
Yes	0 (0)	3 (13.6)	
Other diagnoses[a],*			
No	42 (95.5)	17 (77.3)	0.036
Yes	2 (4.5)	5 (22.7)	

ASD + E ASD participants with epilepsy

[a] Other diagnoses: neurofibromatosis-type 1, fragile-x, subarachnoid hemorrhage, organic brain syndrome, cortical dysplasia, childhood-onset parkinsonism

* p < 0.05

Table 3 Epilepsy variables (seizure onset age, number of AEDs, type of epilepsy)

	ASD-only (N = 44)	ASD + E (N = 22)
Age at seizure onset, years	–	5.57 ± 4.71
Number of current AEDs	–	1.45 ± 1.10
Infantile spasms	–	2 (3.0 %)
Complex partial seizures	–	14 (21.2 %)
Generalized tonic–clonic seizures	–	6 (9.1 %)

AEDs anti-epileptic drugs; *ASD + E* ASD participants with epilepsy

smiling, and communicating using gestures) than groups containing a single factor (ID, ASD, or epilepsy only) [22]. Viscidi et al. underscored the large effect of IQ on the relationship between epilepsy and ASD as they failed to find a relationship between epilepsy and more severe autism symptoms after adjusting for IQ [19].

Table 4 Mean differences between groups on SRS total and subscale scores

	ASD-only (N = 44)	ASD + E (N = 22)	p value
Total**	82.14 ± 17.323	92.41 ± 16.141	0.023
Social awareness**	63.84 ± 15.749	73.14 ± 16.485	0.03
Social cognition*	71.98 ± 14.387	78.41 ± 12.812	0.081
Social communication**	82.89 ± 18.975	93.36 ± 15.041	0.027
Social motivation*	76.64 ± 19.569	86.18 ± 15.522	0.0505
Autistic mannerisms*	84.36 ± 17.062	93.68 ± 22.474	0.065

Independent two sample t test

ASD + E ASD participants with epilepsy

* p < 0.1

** p < 0.05

Findings from Smith et al. and Viscidi et al., therefore, implied that ASD children with epilepsy are at risk of having more severe autism symptoms due to the increased chance of these children having lower IQ. It is well established that cognitive impairment is an independent risk factor for developing epilepsy in individuals with ASD [12]. However, even the low rates of epilepsy reported in individuals with ASD without intellectual disability is higher than the general population rate; therefore, there is an increased risk of epilepsy in ASD even in the absence of intellectual disability [12]. In order to examine the effect of epilepsy on autistic symptom severity, without the influence of IQ, we designed a study that matched the 'ASD-only participants' with 'ASD participants with epilepsy' based on IQ measurements. As a result, there were no significant differences in FSIQ, VIQ, and PIQ between the two groups; consequently, any difference in SRS scores between the two groups would be due to the effect of epilepsy rather than lower cognitive ability.

Commensurate with previous studies [17, 20], our data indicated that individuals with ASD and epilepsy are more likely to be reported as having *autistic mannerisms*; however, statistical significance was not reached (p = 0.065). Our current data lack the statistical power to support the hypothesis that individuals with ASD and epilepsy are significantly more impaired than ASD-only participants on measures of RRBs; thus, it is not certain whether co-occurrence of epilepsy affects the development of autistic mannerisms. In previous studies, RRBs did not correlate with social communicatory difficulties in individuals with ASD, suggesting dissociation between the two symptom domains [39, 40]. One plausible hypothesis is that epilepsy plays a role in social functioning while having no effect on stereotypical behavior. Future direction for this research is to verify any correlation between RRBs and social-communicatory difficulties in ASD participants with epilepsy.

It is well established that epilepsy is more prevalent among individuals diagnosed with ASD than in the normal population [12, 15]. The vice versa is true as well [1]. However, very little do we know about the traits and characteristics of individuals with ASD and epilepsy and the common mechanisms linking the two types of disorders. While previous studies have highlighted the high co-morbidity between epilepsy and autism, there has been a lack of detailed examination of how certain hallmark features of autism such as impaired social functioning may be present in heterogeneous groups of individuals with epilepsy. One explanation might be that poor social skills are missed at the diagnostic-clinical level during assessment for epilepsy. Furthermore, studies of social cognition in epilepsy have been neglected, partly owing to findings from recent studies, which demonstrated a lack of association between epilepsy and social functioning after accounting for differences in IQ [18]. On the other hand, some studies have indicated that epilepsy can affect brain structures and neural networks associated with social cognition [41]; such findings allude to the possibility that pathogenesis of epilepsy may affect social functioning. Furthermore, social cognitive abilities in children may be associated with seizure frequency [42, 43]. To date, several studies attempted to establish the association between epilepsy and social cognitive abilities [19, 20, 23, 27, 44].

In contrast to findings from the Viscidi et al. study [19], our results demonstrated that there is a significant association between the two neurological conditions irrespective of difference in IQ. However, no further conclusion can be drawn in regard to whether co-occurrence of epilepsy causes elevated autism symptoms and disrupt social cognitive abilities since we do not understand the extent to which social functioning is shaped by neurobiological and psychological factors.

Nevertheless, findings of the present study point to several important clinical implications. First, individuals with ASD and epilepsy are more likely to have severe social impairments than those diagnosed solely with ASD. Secondly, individuals with ASD and epilepsy would benefit from an intensive social skills training, and aggressive treatment approaches for epilepsy may prevent decline in social functioning. Thirdly, the incidence of epilepsy may be higher for individuals with ASD who scored higher on the SRS; these individuals may benefit from thorough neurologic assessments and evaluation for epilepsy as part of their routine follow-up.

Limitations and strengths

A few limitations should be considered when interpreting the results of the current study. First, sample sizes of this study were relatively small; replication of the current findings with a larger sample is warranted. A large-sample birth cohort study as well as a study assessing the severity of autistic symptoms in relation to onset of epilepsy may further elucidate the cause-and-effect relationship between epilepsy and ASD. Second, much of the information was retrospectively gathered and based on parent report, so may have been participant to recall and other biases. Third, the study sample was selected from a clinic population following exclusion of individuals without a complete SRS measurement, which suggests exclusion of individuals with very severe intellectual disabilities who were unable to complete the interview. Thus, ASD with epilepsy sample included in this study is not necessarily representative of all children with epilepsy and autism. Fourth, *propensity score matching* is the observational study analog of randomization and that it can only balance the distribution of observed covariates, whereas randomization balances the distribution of observed as well as unobserved covariates. Fifth, despite successfully achieving group-matching using *propensity score matching*, the ASD-only group appeared to have a slight trend for higher FSIQ ($p = 0.102$). Although not statistically significant, ASD-only group may appear to have less intellectual disability than the ASD participants with epilepsy group. Sixth, although small in number, ASD participants with epilepsy group had more additional diagnoses such as neurofibromatosis type 1, fragile-x, organic brain syndrome, etc., which may also explain the significant difference in social functioning between the two groups. We were not able to control for these co-morbid conditions using the propensity score matching; hence, impaired social functioning in the ASD participants with epilepsy may not be a function of epilepsy alone. In spite of these limitations, there are also some positive aspects. Strengths of this study lie in the utility of the SRS as a measure of autistic symptom severity and the methodology in selecting a well-matched control group. Using the *propensity score matching*, we were able to construct ASD participants with epilepsy and matched control samples (ASD-only) that have similar distributions on covariates such as age, gender, and IQ. In contrast to Viscidi et al. study [19], which used the Poisson regression models and generalized linear models to adjust for the covariates in the later stages of data analysis, we employed a proven statistical technique that accounted for these covariates from the beginning. As a result, complicated multiple regression analyses and statistical errors associated with such analyses could be avoided. Previous studies on ASD were prone to preselect those having DSM-IV autistic disorder with little reference to the frequently associated cognitive impairment or co-morbidities such as epilepsy. Careful statistical measures were taken to account for several variables that were previously reported to confound any analysis of population studies of autism.

Conclusions

The co-occurrence of epilepsy and ASD is quite frequent and poses numerous challenges for the affected individuals including increased risk of worsened cognitive and behavioral profiles and overall worse prognosis. In the current study, individuals with ASD and co-morbid epilepsy appear to be at a higher risk for worsened social functioning. Large systematic studies employing strict ascertainment of samples, certain statistical tools to control for confounding factors such as IQ and other co-morbid conditions, as well as appropriate longitudinal follow-up are necessary to better shed light on the relationship between ASD and epilepsy. Early detection of social deficits as well as intensive social skills training should be considered as an integral part of their long-term care plans. Given that ASD and epilepsy affect one another's behavioral phenotype as well as response to psychopharmacological treatment, proper management for epilepsy may in turn reduce autistic symptom severity in these individuals with ASD and epilepsy.

Abbreviations

ASD: autism spectrum disorder; RRB: restricted, repetitive behavior; SRS: social responsiveness scale; IQ: intelligence quotient; FSIQ: full scale intelligence quotient; VIQ: verbal intelligence quotient; PIQ: performance intelligence quotient; AED: antiepileptic drug; EEG: electroencephalogram; ASD + E: ASD participants with epilepsy; CARS: childhood autism rating scale; ADI-R: autism diagnostic interview-revised; SPSS: statistical package for social sciences; ADHD: attention deficit hyperactivity disorder.

Authors' contributions

CK and KC created the design of the study and the experimental paradigm, managed the acquisition of the data. CK analyzed the data and KC and NK interpreted the data. CK wrote the first draft. NK, EK and DS have been involved in drafting and revising the manuscript, in the design regarding the interpreting the data. KC and NK supervised each step of the work, criticizing and improving the design, the statistical analyses, the drafts (revising), and the interpretations of the results. All authors read and approved the final manuscript.

Author details

[1] College of Medicine, Yonsei University, 50 Yonsei-ro, Seodaemun-Gu, Seoul 120-752, South Korea. [2] Division of Child and Adolescent Psychiatry, Department of Psychiatry, College of Medicine, Severance Hospital, Yonsei University, Seoul, South Korea. [3] Institute of Behavioral Science in Medicine, College of Medicine, Yonsei University, 50 Yonsei-ro, Seodaemun-Gu, Seoul 120-752, South Korea. [4] Department of Psychiatry, Institute of Behavioral Science in Medicine, College of Medicine, Gangnam Severance Hospital, Yonsei University, 211 Eonju-ro, Gangnam-gu, Seoul 06273, South Korea.

Acknowledgements

We are grateful to all of the study participants and their families. This research was supported by a Grant from the Korean Health Technology R&D Project, Ministry of Health and Welfare, Republic of Korea (HI12C0021-A120029).

Competing interests

The authors of this study declare that the research was conducted in the absence of any commercial, financial (or non-financial) relationships which could be construed as potential competing interests.

References

1. Clarke DF, Roberts W, Daraksan M, Dupuis A, McCabe J, Wood H, Snead OC 3rd, Weiss SK. The prevalence of autistic spectrum disorder in children surveyed in a tertiary care epilepsy clinic. Epilepsia. 2005;46:1970–7.
2. Association AP. Diagnostic and statistical manual of mental disorders (DSM-5®): American Psychiatric Pub. 2013.
3. Fisher RS, van Emde Boas W, Blume W, Elger C, Genton P, Lee P, Engel J Jr. Epileptic seizures and epilepsy: definitions proposed by the International League Against Epilepsy (ILAE) and the International Bureau for Epilepsy (IBE). Epilepsia. 2005;46:470–2.
4. Tuchman R, Rapin I. Epilepsy in autism. Lancet Neurol. 2002;1:352–8.
5. Olsson I, Steffenburg S, Gillberg C. Epilepsy in autism and autisticlike conditions. A population-based study. Arch Neurol. 1988;45:666–8.
6. Canitano R. Epilepsy in autism spectrum disorders. Eur Child Adolesc Psychiatry. 2007;16:61–6.
7. Forsgren L, Beghi E, Oun A, Sillanpaa M. The epidemiology of epilepsy in Europe—a systematic review. Eur J Neurol. 2005;12:245–53.
8. Bolton PF, Carcani-Rathwell I, Hutton J, Goode S, Howlin P, Rutter M. Epilepsy in autism: features and correlates. Br J Psychiatry. 2011;198:289–94.
9. Viscidi EW, Triche EW, Pescosolido MF, McLean RL, Joseph RM, Spence SJ, Morrow EM. Clinical characteristics of children with autism spectrum disorder and co-occurring epilepsy. PLoS One. 2013;8:e67797.
10. Jokiranta E, Sourander A, Suominen A, Timonen-Soivio L, Brown AS, Sillanpaa M. Epilepsy among children and adolescents with autism spectrum disorders: a population-based study. J Autism Dev Disord. 2014;44:2547–57.
11. Hara H. Autism and epilepsy: a retrospective follow-up study. Brain Dev. 2007;29:486–90.
12. Amiet C, Gourfinkel-An I, Bouzamondo A, Tordjman S, Baulac M, Lechat P, Mottron L, Cohen D. Epilepsy in autism is associated with intellectual disability and gender: evidence from a meta-analysis. Biol Psychiatry. 2008;64:577–82.
13. Danielsson S, Gillberg IC, Billstedt E, Gillberg C, Olsson I. Epilepsy in young adults with autism: a prospective population-based follow-up study of 120 individuals diagnosed in childhood. Epilepsia. 2005;46:918–23.
14. Ellenberg JH, Hirtz DG, Nelson KB. Age at onset of seizures in young children. Ann Neurol. 1984;15:127–34.
15. Hauser WA. The prevalence and incidence of convulsive disorders in children. Epilepsia. 1994;35(Suppl 2):S1–6.
16. Volkmar FR, Nelson DS. Seizure disorders in autism. J Am Acad Child Adolesc Psychiatry. 1990;29:127–9.
17. Tuchman R, Cuccaro M. Epilepsy and autism: neurodevelopmental perspective. Curr Neurol Neurosci Rep. 2011;11:428–34.
18. Cohen DJ, Volkmar FR. Handbook of autism and pervasive developmental disorders. 2nd ed. New York: Wiley; 1997.
19. Viscidi EW, Johnson AL, Spence SJ, Buka SL, Morrow EM, Triche EW. The association between epilepsy and autism symptoms and maladaptive behaviors in children with autism spectrum disorder. Autism. 2014;18:996–1006.
20. Turk J, Bax M, Williams C, Amin P, Eriksson M, Gillberg C. Autism spectrum disorder in children with and without epilepsy: impact on social functioning and communication. Acta Paediatr. 2009;98:675–81.
21. Smith KR, Matson JL. Psychopathology: differences among adults with intellectually disabled, comorbid autism spectrum disorders and epilepsy. Res Dev Disabil. 2010;31:743–9.
22. Smith KR, Matson JL. Behavior problems: differences among intellectually disabled adults with co-morbid autism spectrum disorders and epilepsy. Res Dev Disabil. 2010;31:1062–9.
23. Smith KR, Matson JL. Social skills: differences among adults with intellectual disabilities, co-morbid autism spectrum disorders and epilepsy. Res Dev Disabil. 2010;31:1366–72.
24. Constantino JN, Davis SA, Todd RD, Schindler MK, Gross MM, Brophy SL, Metzger LM, Shoushtari CS, Splinter R, Reich W. Validation of a brief quantitative measure of autistic traits: comparison of the social responsiveness scale with the autism diagnostic interview-revised. J Autism Dev Disord. 2003;33:427–33.
25. Hus V, Bishop S, Gotham K, Huerta M, Lord C. Factors influencing scores on the social responsiveness scale. J Child Psychol Psychiatry. 2013;54:216–24.
26. Charman T, Baird G, Simonoff E, Loucas T, Chandler S, Meldrum D, Pickles A. Efficacy of three screening instruments in the identification of autistic-spectrum disorders. Br J Psychiatry. 2007;191:554–9.

27. Wakeford S, Hinvest N, Ring H, Brosnan M. Autistic characteristics in adults with epilepsy and perceived seizure activity. Epilepsy Behav. 2015;52:244–50.

28. Rosenbaum PR, Rubin DB. The central role of the propensity score in observational studies for causal effects. Biometrika. 1983;70:41–55.

29. Austin PC. An introduction to propensity score methods for reducing the effects of confounding in observational studies. Multivariate Behav Res. 2011;46:399–424.

30. Ross ME, Kreider AR, Huang YS, Matone M, Rubin DM, Localio AR. Propensity score methods for analyzing observational data like randomized experiments: challenges and solutions for rare outcomes and exposures. Am J Epidemiol. 2015;181:989–95.

31. Schopler E, Reichler RJ, DeVellis RF, Daly K. Toward objective classification of childhood autism: childhood Autism Rating Scale (CARS). J Autism Dev Disord. 1980;10:91–103.

32. Rutter M, Le Couteur A, Lord C, Faggioli R. ADI-R: Autism diagnostic interview–revised: Manual. Florence: Giunti O. S. Organizzazioni Speciali; 2005.

33. Kwak K, Park H, Kim C. Korean Wechsler intelligence scale for children-III (K-WISC-III). Seoul: Seoul Special Education Publishing Co; 2001.

34. Wechsler D. WISC-III: Wechsler intelligence scale for children: Manual. Agra: Psychological Corporation; 1991.

35. Oh K, Yum T, Park Y, Kim C, Lee Y. Korean Wechsler adult intelligence scale (K-WAIS). Seoul: Guidance; 1992.

36. Wechsler D. WAIS-III: administration and scoring manual: Wechsler adult intelligence scale. Agra: Psychological Corporation; 1997.

37. Constantino JN, Gruber CP. The social responsiveness scale. Los Angeles: Western Psychological Services; 2002.

38. Constantino JN, Przybeck T, Friesen D, Todd RD. Reciprocal social behavior in children with and without pervasive developmental disorders. J Dev Behav Pediatr. 2000;21:2–11.

39. Harrop C, McConachie H, Emsley R, Leadbitter K, Green J, Consortium P. Restricted and repetitive behaviors in autism spectrum disorders and typical development: cross-sectional and longitudinal comparisons. J Autism Dev Disord. 2014;44:1207–19.

40. Hus V, Gotham K, Lord C. Standardizing ADOS domain scores: separating severity of social affect and restricted and repetitive behaviors. J Autism Dev Disord. 2014;44:2400–12.

41. Schacher M, Winkler R, Grunwald T, Kraemer G, Kurthen M, Reed V, Jokeit H. Mesial temporal lobe epilepsy impairs advanced social cognition. Epilepsia. 2006;47:2141–6.

42. Austin JK, Risinger MW, Beckett LA. Correlates of behavior problems in children with epilepsy. Epilepsia. 1992;33:1115–22.

43. Schachter SC, Holmes GL, Kasteleijn-Nolst Trenité DG. Behavioral aspects of epilepsy: principles and practice. New York: Demos Medical Publishing; 2008.

44. Wakeford S, Hinvest N, Ring H, Brosnan M. Autistic characteristics in adults with epilepsy. Epilepsy Behav. 2014;41:203–7.

Age, environment, object recognition and morphological diversity of GFAP-immunolabeled astrocytes

Daniel Guerreiro Diniz[1,3], Marcus Augusto de Oliveira[1], Camila Mendes de Lima[1], César Augusto Raiol Fôro[1], Marcia Consentino Kronka Sosthenes[1], João Bento-Torres[1], Pedro Fernando da Costa Vasconcelos[2], Daniel Clive Anthony[3] and Cristovam Wanderley Picanço Diniz[1,3]*

Abstract

Background: Few studies have explored the glial response to a standard environment and how the response may be associated with age-related cognitive decline in learning and memory. Here we investigated aging and environmental influences on hippocampal-dependent tasks and on the morphology of an unbiased selected population of astrocytes from the molecular layer of dentate gyrus, which is the main target of perforant pathway.

Results: Six and twenty-month-old female, albino Swiss mice were housed, from weaning, in a standard or enriched environment, including running wheels for exercise and tested for object recognition and contextual memories. Young adult and aged subjects, independent of environment, were able to distinguish familiar from novel objects. All experimental groups, except aged mice from standard environment, distinguish stationary from displaced objects. Young adult but not aged mice, independent of environment, were able to distinguish older from recent objects. Only young mice from an enriched environment were able to distinguish novel from familiar contexts. Unbiased selected astrocytes from the molecular layer of the dentate gyrus were reconstructed in three-dimensions and classified using hierarchical cluster analysis of bimodal or multimodal morphological features. We found two morphological phenotypes of astrocytes and we designated type I the astrocytes that exhibited significantly higher values of morphological complexity as compared with type II. Complexity = [Sum of the terminal orders + Number of terminals] × [Total branch length/Number of primary branches]. On average, type I morphological complexity seems to be much more sensitive to age and environmental influences than that of type II. Indeed, aging and environmental impoverishment interact and reduce the morphological complexity of type I astrocytes at a point that they could not be distinguished anymore from type II.

Conclusions: We suggest these two types of astrocytes may have different physiological roles and that the detrimental effects of aging on memory in mice from a standard environment may be associated with a reduction of astrocytes morphological diversity.

Keywords: Environment, Exercise, Aging, Astrocytes morphology, Dentate gyrus, Memory

*Correspondence: cwpdiniz@gmail.com
[1] Laboratório de Investigações Em Neurodegeneração e Infecção, Instituto de Ciências Biológicas, Universidade Federal do Pará, Hospital Universitário João de Barros Barreto, Rua dos Mundurucus 4487, Guamá, Belém, Pará CEP 66073-000, Brazil
Full list of author information is available at the end of the article

Background

Epidemiological studies have correlated physical and cognitive inactivity with a greater risk of age-related cognitive decline [1, 2]. In contrast, an active lifestyle may help prevent cognitive impairment in old age [3–5]; for recent reviews see [6–9]. Consistent with this view, the decline in memory that is associated with normal or pathological aging appears to be aggravated after institutionalization [10, 11]. Institutionalization is often associated with a standard-like environment with reduced sensory-motor and cognitive stimulation, social interactions, and physical activity, which contribute to a sedentary lifestyle [4, 5, 10, 12]. Similarly, it has been demonstrated that aged mice and rats, maintained in the standard environment of standard laboratory cages, perform worse in learning and memory tasks than those living in an enriched environment [13–24]. To perform spatial learning and memory tasks, the brain must accentuate the differences between old and new experiences, before coding occurs [25]. For that purpose, medial and lateral perforant pathways transmit to dentate gyrus, spatial and non-spatial information that would be necessary to recognize object placement (Where?), identity (What?) and timing (When?) [25].

Cellular and molecular analyses of these events demonstrate that the beneficial effects of environmental enrichment with voluntary exercise are associated with a variety of neuronal and neuroimmunological changes in both young and aged individuals [23, 26–35]. However, most of the documented changes in cell behavior relate to neuronal populations [36–40].

More recently significant contributions have explored possible roles of astrocytes in physiological and pathological brain aging [41]. Much of these outstanding work was done by Verkhratsky and Rodríguez-Arellano (see [104] for recent review), who showed that aging is associated with complex and region-dependent astrocyte remodeling, that may represent life-long adaptive responses [69] and that astrocytes participate in the morphological remodeling associated with synaptic plasticity [42]. However, astrocyte quantitative morphological studies under combined environmental and aging influences, in particular, is not yet largely explored [43–46].

A recent study showed that long-term potentiation and learning improved in chimeric mice generated by transplanting human astroglial progenitor cells into the forebrain [47]. In those chimeric mice, large regions of the CNS, including the hippocampus, consisted of mouse neurons (and oligodendrocytes) surrounded by human astrocytes and progenitor cells [48]. Both transplanted and control mice were then subject to a battery of learning and memory tasks and chimeric mice demonstrated enhanced performance on all tests. Those findings suggested that human astrocytes in particular, might contribute significantly, at least in part, to improved cognition [49, 50]. Morphologically, human astrocytes are larger and structurally more complex than mouse astrocytes [51]. Compared with mouse astrocytes, human astrocytes have soma diameters 2.6 mm longer, with tenfold more glial fibrillary acid protein (GFAP)-positive processes and fourfold faster calcium waves [52].

Taken together, these findings raise important questions related to the morphology of astrocytes and cognition. For example, is the performance of animals with more complexes immunolabeled astrocytes in the dentate gyrus, associated with better performances in object-identity tasks?

Thus, in the present report we described possible associations between environmental and age changes with alterations in the morphological complexity of GFAP immunolabeled astrocytes of the molecular layer of dentate gyrus, the main target of perforant pathway in mammals [53], and searched for potential associations between higher performances in the object recognition tests and higher morphological complexity of astrocytes.

Methods

Animals and experimental groups

More detailed experimental procedures have been previously described elsewhere [13]. Seventy-one Swiss female adult (6 months old—6 M) and aged (20 months old—20 M) mice were housed from 21st postnatal day either in enriched conditions (n = 42) or in standard conditions (n = 29). They remained as such until the sacrifice in each time window. These formed four experimental groups: enriched environment, young adults (EY, n = 12); standard environment, young adults (IY, n = 13); enriched environment, aged adults (EA, n = 30); and standard environment, aged adults (IA, n = 16). Enriched conditions comprised 2-level wire cages (100 × 50 × 100 cm) equipped with ropes, rod bridges, tunnels, running wheels, and toys. Toys were made of different forms of plastic, wood and metal of different colors, and were changed periodically. Each enriched cage housed 12-15 young and aged mice from housed from weaning in enriched conditions (EC, n = 27) or impoverished conditions (IC, n = 29). Water and food were delivered to the top and bottom levels, respectively. This obliged mouse to move from one compartment to another for drinking and eating. Standard conditions comprised plastic cages (32 × 39 × 100 cm) without equipment or toys. Each standard cage housed 12–13 young and aged mice. All mice had free access to water and food. In addition, 12-h dark and light cycles were maintained. Behavioral tests were administered during the light cycle.

Object recognition tasks

Behavioral procedures

Current learning analyses do not use dynamic estimation methods and require many trials across many animals to assess significant differences in learning. Moreover, they provide no consensus on how best to identify when learning was occurred [54]. In the present work we used single trial tests to assess object recognition [55].

The apparatus for the single trial object recognition test consisted of an open box (30 × 30 × 40 cm) made of painted white wood. The floor was painted with lines to form nine squares (10 × 10 cm) and the luminance at the center of the cage floor was 2.4 cd/m^2. Detailed protocols and reasons for test choices were discussed elsewhere [55, 56]; see also [57, 58] for reviews). In brief, behavioral essays were performed over 17 days: 7 days for handling, 3 days for open field habituation, 2 days for object habituation, and 5 days for testing: 1 day for each test. *Handling*: each day mice were placed in the center of the arena for 1 min and then removed to their cages. *Open field habituation*: each day mice were placed in the arena, free of objects, for 5 min to explore the open field. *Object habituation*: each day mice were exposed to two identical objects placed at the corners of the arena for 5 min, three times, with 50 min in between. These objects were not used on the test days. *Testing*: one-trial recognition tests were administered on five consecutive days: the object identity test, the object placement test, the object timing test, the context test, and the episodic-like memory test.

In order to minimize the influence of natural preferences for particular objects or materials, we chose objects of the same material but different geometries that could be easily discriminated and had similar possibilities for interaction [55]. All objects were plastic with different shapes, heights, and colors. Before each mouse entered the arena, the box and objects were cleaned with 75 % ethanol to minimize distinguishing olfactory cues.

One-trial object identity recognition consisted of a 5-min sample trial, during which subjects explored two identical objects in a familiar arena, followed by a 50-min intermission and then a second 5-min test trial, in which a "novel" object was presented together with one "familiar" object already explored during the sample trial. Objects differed in form, dimensions, color, and texture and had no ethological significance for mice.

One-trial object placement recognition followed the same procedure as above, except in the test trial, one of the two identical objects was shifted to a novel location ('displaced" object).

One-trial object timing recognition consisted of three trials: two 5-min sample trials during which subjects explored two different object pairs; each trial was followed by a 50-min intermission; then one 5-min test trial in which one "former" and one "recent" object were presented together.

One-trial object context recognition also consisted of three trials: two 5-min sample trials and one 5-min test trial, each separated by 50 min intermissions. During the sample trials objects were presented in different ambient contexts. In the first sample trial two identical objects were presented under a bright light with extra-arena visual cues. In the second sample trial two different identical objects were presented under a dim light with different extra-arena visual cues. In the test trial two objects, one from each sample trial, were presented simultaneously in the bright light context [59].

All tests were video recorded by web cam and most images were analyzed with a computer program to score the time spent interacting with objects and the water maze performances (ANYMAZE tracking system, Stöelting). Computer analysis was done off-line. Exploration of an object was assumed when a mouse approached an object, the head was directed towards it, and the head was placed within 0–3 cm from the object. This definition required that each object be fixed to the apparatus floor, thus we chose heavy objects for interaction. Diagrams of the object recognition memory tests used in the present report are shown in Fig. 2 and the performance on each test is defined as the percentage of time spent exploring one object. To account for individual variability in exploratory activity, the time spent with each object was normalized by the total exploration time for each individual.

Statistical analysis

Detailed statistical procedures for object recognition tests were described elsewhere [60]. Normality of the data distribution was tested and outliers were rarely removed from samples based on standard deviations. In brief, for object recognition tests, the basic measure obtained from video-images was the time a mouse spent exploring each object during the test trial, and scores were determined for recognition of identity (novel vs familiar), placement (displaced vs stationary), timing (recent vs former) and contextual (new context vs familiar context) memories. The data were analyzed by parametric statistics and the two-tailed t test for dependent groups was used to detect significant differences. The performance was the time of exploration for each object expressed as a proportion (percentage) of the total time of exploration, and possible significant differences were also detected with the two-tailed t test for dependent groups [59]. In all statistical tests the threshold for significance was set at p < 0.05.

Perfusion and histological procedures

At the end of behavioral tests, 5–9 animals from each experimental group were weighed and killed with an overdose of ketamine (100 mg/kg) and xylazine (10 mg/kg) (Konig Laboratories). They were then perfused transcardially with heparinized saline for 10 min, followed by an aldehyde fixative (4 % paraformaldehyde in 0.1 M phosphate buffer, pH 7.2–7.4) for 30 min. All other chemicals were purchased from Sigma (São Paulo, Brazil). After perfusion and craniotomy, the brains were removed and cut on a vibratome (70 μm thickness). One of each five sections was used to detect GFAP by free-floating immunohistochemistry. Free-floating sections were rinsed once in 0.1 M phosphate buffer, transferred to 0.2 M boric acid pH 9.0, heated to 65–70 °C for 1 h, and then washed 3 × 5 min in 5 % PBST. The sections were incubated under constant gentle shaking in a 1 % hydrogen peroxide solution in methanol for 10 min, then rinsed 2 × 2 min in 0.1 M PBS. The sections were blocked with immunoglobulin for 1 h using the Mouse-on-Mouse Immunodetection kit (M.O.M. kit, Vector Laboratories, USA) according to the manufacturer's instructions. Blocking was followed by washing for 3 × 2 min in PBS. Sections were incubated in a working solution of protein concentrate for 5 min, then incubated with monoclonal mouse anti-GFAP primary antibody (MAB360, CHEMICON Int., USA), diluted in protein concentrate solution (M.O.M. kit), at 4 °C for 3 days with continuous, gentle agitation. Next, the sections were washed 3 × 2 min in PBS and incubated for 20 h with biotinylated horse anti-mouse secondary antibody (M.O.M. kit), diluted 1:100 in PBS. After washing 3 × 2 min in PBS, sections were transferred to an avidin–biotin-peroxidase complex solution (ABC, Vector Laboratories, USA, 1:200) for 1.5 h, washed 3 × 2 min in 0.1 M PBS, and processed with the glucose oxidase-DAB-nickel method and peroxidase histochemistry [61].

The reaction was interrupted after fine astrocytic branches were detected under the microscope. Sections were rinsed 4 × 5 min in 0.1 M PBS, mounted on gelatinized slides, dehydrated in alcohol and xylene, and coverslipped with Enthelan (Merck). Five animals from each group with complete GFAP immunohistochemistry slide collections that contained conspicuous morphological details of astrocytes were used for 3-D reconstruction and morphometric analysis.

3-D astrocyte reconstruction and quantitative morphology

We selected five brains from each experimental group for GFAP immunolabeling and 3-D reconstruction. To analyze brain sections, we used a NIKON Eclipse 80i microscope (Nikon, Japan) equipped with a motorized stage (MAC6000, Ludl Electronic Products, Hawthorne, NY, USA). Astrocytes from the layer of interest were analyzed under oil immersion, with a high-resolution,

100 × oil immersion, plan fluoride objective (Nikon, NA 1.3, DF = 0.19 μm). Images were acquired with Neurolucida and analyzed with Neurolucida explorer software (MBF Bioscience Inc., Frederick, MD, USA). Although shrinkage in the z-axis is not a linear event, we corrected the shrinkage in the z-axis, based on previous evidence of 75 % shrinkage [62]. Without correction, this shrinkage would significantly distort the length measurements along this axis. Only cells with processes that were unequivocally complete were included for 3-D analysis; cells were discarded when branches appeared artificially cut or not fully immunolabeled. Terminal branches were typically thin.

Morphometric analysis and statistics

To accomplish the analysis, we used 20 animals, five from each experimental group (IY, n = 5; EY, n = 5; EA, n = 5; IA, n = 5). From these four groups, we digitally reconstructed 309 astrocytes in three-dimensions from the molecular layer (EY = 79, IY = 75, EA = 76, IA = 79) of the dentate gyrus. Astrocytes for 3-D reconstructions were selected in an unbiased, randomized, and systematic way (Fig. 1). We used architectonic differences in the neuropil region, readily visible in immunolabeled sections, to define the limits of the dentate gyrus layers of the hippocampus. Systematic and random samples were taken from a series of sections containing dorsal and ventral dentate gyrus to guarantee that all regions had the same probability of being included among the analyzed samples. Each box inside the outlined dentate gyrus layers indicates a site from which we selected a single astrocyte for 3-D reconstruction (Fig. 1).

We first investigated the presence of morphological features shared by the astrocytes observed in each layer of interest in our sample, inside each experimental group. We selected all morphometric quantitative variables with multimodality indices (MMI) higher than 0.55, to an initial cluster analysis (Ward's hierarchical clustering method), which included all animals from each group. To estimate the multimodality index (MI) based on skewness and kurtosis of our sample for each morphometric variable as previously defined elsewhere: $MI = [M3^2 + 1]/[M4 + 3(n-1)^2/(n-2)(n-3)]$, where M3 is skewness and M4 is kurtosis and n is sample size [63, 64]. Kurtosis and skewness describe the shape of the data distribution and enable to distinguish between unimodal, bimodal or multimodal curves. Multimodal data sets are essential for separating a population of cells into cell types [63]. The multimodal index of each variable was estimate based on the measurements of 30 morphometric features of astrocytes, 10 related to the soma and 20 to the branches, as follows: 1. Soma area (μm^2); 2. Soma perimeter; 3. Feret

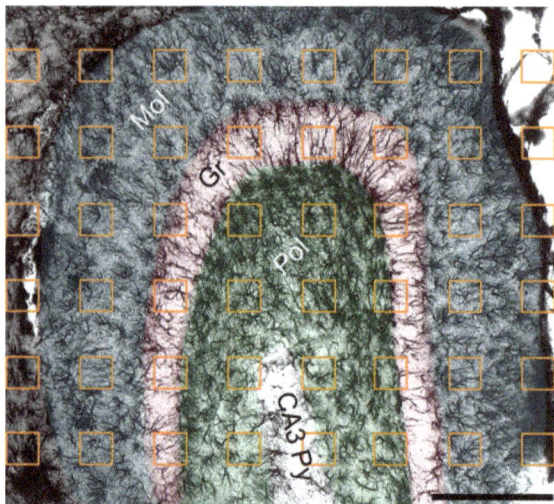

Fig. 1 Low-power photomicrograph of mouse dentate gyrus from a section immunolabeled with anti-GFAP antibody to reveal the laminar distribution of astrocytes and to define the layers and limits of the dentate gyrus. Note the boundaries of the granular layer (Gr, *pink*) are demarcated by adjacent molecular (Mol, *blue*) and polymorphic (Pol, *green*) layers. Reduced GFAP immunostaining in the CA3 pyramidal layer (CA3Py) clearly delineates the boundary between the polymorphic layer and the pyramidal layer. The grid (straight *green lines* parallel to the *x*- and *y-axes*) establishes the intervals between the *orange square boxes* and illustrates the random and systematic sampling approach. The *number of boxes* in each section is proportional to the area covered by the dentate gyrus. A single astrocyte located inside every *box* was selected for three-dimensional reconstruction. *Scale bar* 250 μm

generated by cluster analysis. From hierarchical cluster analysis we categorized astrocytes into two groups designated types I and II.

We applied this multivariate statistical procedure to our sample of astrocytes in order to search for potential astroglial morphological classes inside of each experimental group. The classification of astrocytes suggested by cluster analysis was assessed using a forward stepwise discriminant function analysis performed with Statistica 12.0 (Statsoft, Tulsa, OK). Discriminant function analysis was used to determine which variables discriminate between two or more naturally occurring groups. The purpose of this procedure is to determine whether the groups differ with regard to the mean of a variable, and then to use that variable to predict group membership. In the present study, we used this software to perform comparisons between matrices of total variances and co-variances. These matrices were compared using multivariate F tests to determine whether there were any significant between-group differences (with regard to all variables). In the step-forward discriminant function analysis, the program builds a model of discrimination step-by-step. In this model, at each step, all variables are reviewed and evaluated to determine which variable contributes most to the discrimination between groups. We applied this procedure to determine morphometric variables that provided the best separation between the astroglial classes suggested by the cluster analysis. In addition, we calculated the arithmetic mean and standard deviation for the variables chosen as the best predictors for the astroglial groups. Parametric statistical analyses with t tests were applied to compare groups of astrocytes inside each experimental group and to detect possible morphological differences between average astrocytes from molecular layer of each experimental group. In the selected sections, the margins of the polymorphic, granular, and molecular layers were clearly distinguished with Nissl counterstaining.

All astrocytes from each layer of interest were measured multiple times, and dedicated software (Neurolucida explorer, MicroBright Field Inc.) was used to process data obtained with Neurolucida.

minimum diameter; 4. Feret Mouse maximum diameter (maximum diameter in a shape); 5. Compactness; 6. Form factor; 7. Solidity; 8. Roundness; 9. Aspect ratio; 10. Convexity; 11. Branch length (μm); 12. Total tree length (μm) 13. Surface area (μm^2); 14. Branch volume (μm^3); 15. Segments/mm; 16. Tortuosity; 17. Fractal dimensions (k-dim); 18. Base diameter of the primary branch (μm); 19. Total number of segments; 20. Number of varicosities; 21. Planar angle; 22. Number of trees; 23. Complexity; 24. Convex hull volume; 25. Convex hull surface; 26. Convex hull area; 27. Convex hull perimeter; 28. Vertex Va; 29. Vertex Vb; 30. Vertex Vc. Table 1 contains descriptions of all morphometric variables used.

We found that a few microglial morphological features showed a multimodality index greater than 0.55 and this index value indicates that the distribution is at least bimodal and may be multimodal, and these particular features were selected for cluster analysis as previously described [63]. We used the Ward's method with standardized variables, square Euclidian distances and a tree diagram (dendrogram) to illustrate the classification

Results
Behavioral outcomes
Results of the object recognition tests are shown in Fig. 2. All experimental groups were able to distinguish familiar from new objects (identity—What?). All other tasks were significantly influenced by age, environment, or both as follow:

Table 1 Morphometric features definitions

Branched structure analysis

Segment	Any portion of microglial branched structure with endings that are either nodes or terminations with no intermediate nodes
Segments/mm	Number of segments/total length of the segments expressed in millimeters
No of trees	Number of trees in the astrocytes
Total no of segments	Refer to the total number of segments in the tree
Branch length	Total length of the line segments used to trace the branch of interest.
Total branch length	Total length for all branches in the tree Mean = [length]/[number of branches]
Tortuosity	=[Actual length of the segment]/[distance between the endpoints of the segment]. The smallest value is 1; this represents a straight segment. Tortuosity allows segments of different lengths to be compared in terms of the complexity of the paths they take
Surface area	Computed by modeling each branch as a frustum (truncated right circular cone)
Tree surface area	
Branch volume	Computed by modeling each piece of each branch as a frustum.
Total branch volume	Total volume for all branches in the tree
Base diameter of primary branch	Diameter at the start of the 1st segment
Planar Angle	Computed based on the endpoints of the segments. It refers to the change in direction of a segment relative to the previous segment
Fractal dimension	The "k-dim" of the fractal analysis, describes how the structure of interest fills space. Significant statistical differences in k-dim suggest morphological dissimilarities
Convex hull-perimeter	Convex hull measures the size of the branching field by interpreting a branched structure as a solid object controlling a given amount of physical space. The amount of physical space is defined in terms of convex-hull volume, surface area, area, and or perimeter
Vertex analysis	Describes the overall structure of a branched object based on topological and metrical properties. Root (or origin) point: For neurons, microglia or astrocytes, the origin is the point at which the structure is attached to the soma. Main types of vertices: V_d (bifurcation) or V_t (trifurcation): Nodal (or branching) points. V_p: Terminal (or pendant) vertices. V_a: primary vertices connecting 2 pendant vertices; V_b: secondary vertices connecting 1 pendant vertex (V_p) to 1 bifurcation (V_d) or 1 trifurcation (V_t); V_c: tertiary vertices connecting either 2 bifurcations (V_d), 2 trifurcations (V_t), or 1 bifurcation (V_d) and 1 trifurcation (V_t). In the present report we measure the number of vertices Va, Vb and Vc
Complexity	Complexity = [sum of the terminal orders + number of terminals] × [total branch length/number of primary branches]

Cell body

Area	Refers to the 2-dimensional cross-sectional area contained within the boundary of the cell body
Perimeter	Length of the contour representing the cell body
Feret max/min	Largest and smallest dimensions of the cell body as if a caliper was used to measure across the contour. The two measurements are independent of one another and not necessarily at right angles to each other
Aspect ratio	Aspect ratio = [min diameter]/[max diameter] Indicates the degree of flatness of the cell body Range of values is 0–1 A circle has an aspect ratio of 1
Compactness	$$Compactness = \frac{\sqrt{\left(\frac{4}{\pi}\right) \times Area}}{MaxDiam}$$ The range of values is 0–1 A circle is the most compact shape (compactness = 1)
Convexity	Convexity = [convex perimeter]/[perimeter] A completely convex object does not have indentations, and has a convexity value of 1 (e.g., circles, ellipses, and squares) Concave objects have convexity values less than 1 Contours with low convexity have a large boundary between inside and outside areas
Form factor	$$Formfactor = 4\pi \times \frac{Area}{perimeter^2}$$ As the contour shape approaches that of a perfect circle, this value approaches a maximum of 1.0 As the contour shape flattens out, this value approaches 0
Roundness	Roundness = [compactness]^2 Use to differentiate objects that have small compactness values

Table 1 continued

Solidity	Solidity = [area]/[convex Area]
	The area enclosed by a 'rubber band' stretched around a contour is called the convex area
	Circles, squares, and ellipses have a solidity of 1
	Indentations in the contour take area away from the convex area, decreasing the actual area within the contour

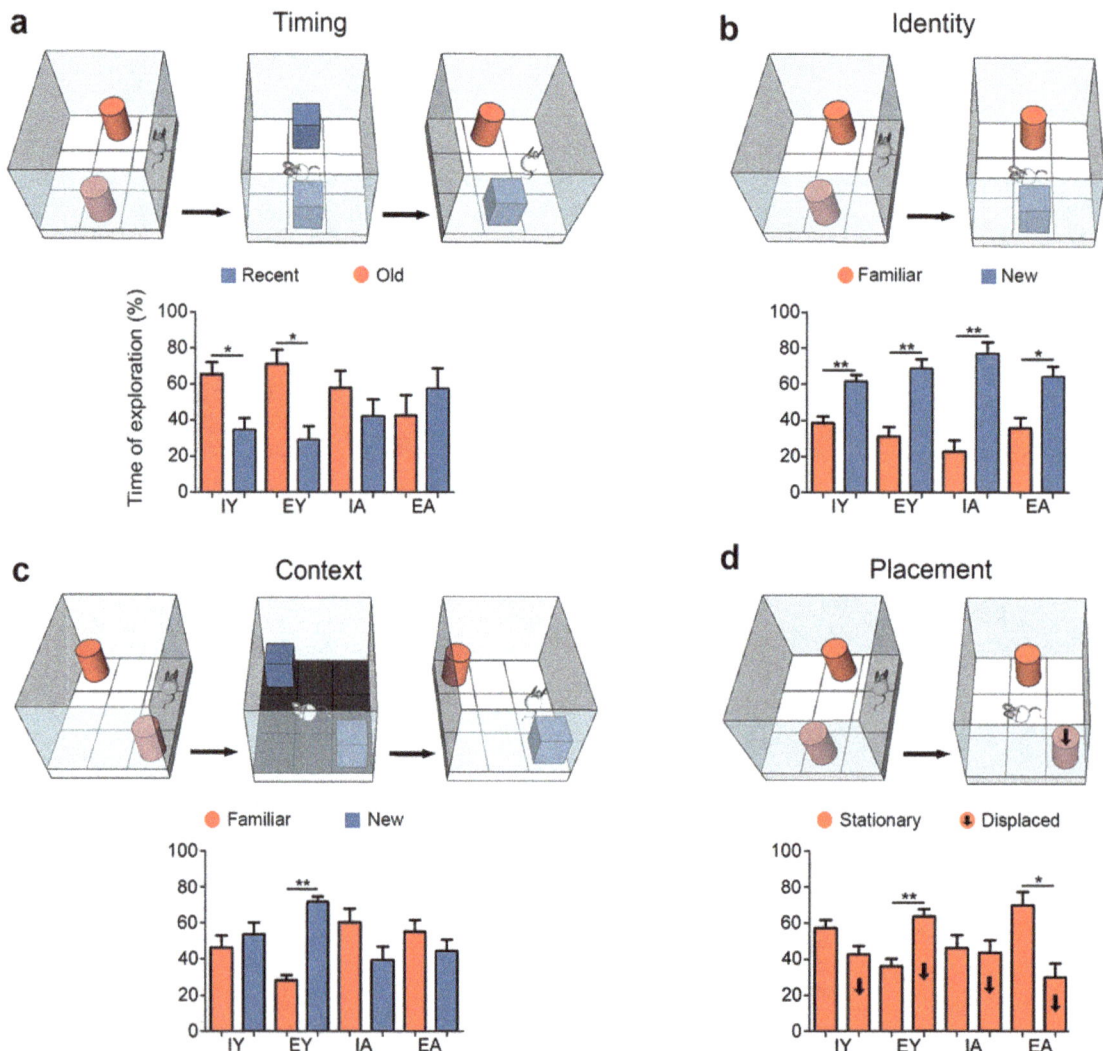

Fig. 2 Object recognition and contextual memories. **a** Timing; **b** Identity; **c** Context; **d** Placement. *Bars* indicate average values of the exploration time ± s.e. for each group. *Red* and *blue filled bars* represent differences between objects (displaced vs. stationary, old vs. recent, familiar vs. new). Two-tailed t test for dependent samples; *p < 0.05; **p < 0.001. *A SE* aged mice from standard environment; *A EE* aged mice from enriched environment; *Y SE* young mice from standard environment; *Y EE* young mice from enriched environment

One trial object timing recognition

Young adult mice, independent of environment, were able to distinguish older from recent objects (When?) (Y SE: t = 2.38, p = 0.0411; Y EE: t = 2.72, p = 0.0235). In contrast, aged mice independent of environment were unable to make this distinction (A SE: t = 0.83, p = 0.426; A EE: t = 0.66, p = 0.526).

One-trial object identity recognition

Young adult and aged subjects, independent of environment, were able to distinguish familiar from novel objects. Y SE: t = 4.49, p = 0.0015; Y EE: t = 3.60, p = 0.0058; A SE: t = 4.30, p = 0.0020; A EE: t = 2.45, p = 0.0364.

One trial object context recognition

Only young mice from an enriched environment were able to distinguish novel from familiar contexts. Y SE: t = 0.033, p = 0.973; Y EE: t = 7.56, p < 0.0001; A SE: t = 1.39, p = 0.201; A EE: t = 0.87, p = 0.406.

One trial object placement recognition

Aged mice from standard conditions were unable to distinguish stationary from displaced objects (A SE: t = 0.274, p = 0.789), however young mice, raised in similar conditions were able to do so (Y SE: t = 2258, p = 0.0503). In contrast, animals from enriched environments, independent of age, were able to distinguish stationary from displaced objects (Where?) with different preferences: young mice spent more time with displaced objects and aged mice with stationary objects (Y EE: t = 3.38, p = 0.0081; A EE: t = 2.62, p = 0.0305). Additional file 1: Table S1 shows absolute values of time of exploration on each hippocampal-dependent task for all experimental groups.

Morphological phenotypes of astrocytes in the molecular layer of dentate gyrus

We used microscopic 3-D reconstructions and an unbiased, systematic, randomized sampling approach to select astrocytes from the molecular layers of the dentate gyrus. Cluster and discriminant analysis illustrate these findings, together with 3-D reconstructions of astrocytes with morphological features close to the "mean astrocyte" of each experimental group. These findings are shown in Figs. 3, 4, 5, 6.

Based on morphometric features and hierarchical cluster analysis using multimodal parameters, we proposed to designate type I and type II as a function of their morphological complexities. As compared to type II, type I was the group of astrocytes with significant higher mean values of complexity. Table 2 summarizes discriminant analysis results and reveals that a few morphological measurements are enough to distinguish Type I from Type II astrocytes in the molecular layer of different experimental groups. Among them, morphological complexity was the morphological feature that contributed most to cluster formation. Complexity is a combination of different morphological features of astrocytes trees. Longer and more ramified astrocytes show higher values of complexity. Based on this parameter we measured the influence of aging and environment on dentate gyrus astrocytes morphology.

Figure 3a represents the hierarchical cluster analysis of the molecular layer astrocytes morphological features from young mice raised in enriched environment. As previously mentioned, this analysis was done using the morphological parameters with MMI >0.55 as

follow: branch volume, aspect ratio, convexity, form factor, complexity, convex hull volume, convex hull surface, convex hull area. Two main clusters of astrocytes were distinguished in the molecular layer of this group and the variables that most contributed to their formation were complexity ($p < 0.29 \times 10^{-9}$) and convex hull volume ($p < 0.12 \times 10^{-4}$). The astrocyte features corresponding to clusters I (Fig. 3b) and II (Fig. 3D) where the presence of significant differences in complexity and convex hull volumes. Figure 3c is a graphic representation of the discriminant analysis to illustrate the distribution of astrocytes in X–Y plot. Note that type I astrocytes dots are more dispersed than type II and the spatial distribution of type I and II dots are quite distinct. Similar analysis was applied to the astrocytes from young adult raised in standard cages (Fig. 4a–d), and to the astrocytes from aged mice raised in enriched (Fig. 5a–d) or in standard cages (not illustrated). Except for the aged mice group from standard environment, showing a single morphological phenotype, all other cases showed two distinct astrocyte morphologies, with notable differences in the mean values of complexity. Indeed, because molecular layer astrocytes from aged mice raised in standard environment were morphologically homogeneous with small Euclidian distances, we could not distinguish type I from type II astrocytes in this group (not illustrated). Surprisingly, in relative terms, the reduction of morphological complexity in both type I and II astrocytes was higher in aged mice maintained in enriched environment than in aged mice from standard environment (Fig. 6). We found no difference between type I and II astrocytes in the molecular layer of aged mice from a standard environment and this was associated with spatial memory impaired performance. In contrast, we still detected significant differences between type I and II astrocytes in aged animals from enriched environment and this was associated with intact spatial memory suggesting that the morphological diversity of astrocytes may be important to maintain spatial memory integrity.

Influences of environment and age on the morphological complexity of astrocytes in the dentate gyrus

Complexity has been defined previously [65] using the following equation:

$$\text{Complexity} = [\text{Sum of the terminal orders} + \text{Number of terminals}]$$
$$\times [\text{Total branch length/Number of primary branches}].$$

See http://www.mbfbioscience.com/help/nx11/Default. htm#Analyses/BranchedStructure/neuronSumm.htm for details.

As previously mentioned, more ramified and longer astrocytes are given higher values of complexity. Based on cluster and discriminant analysis we categorized astrocytes into two groups with respect to complexity, and designated

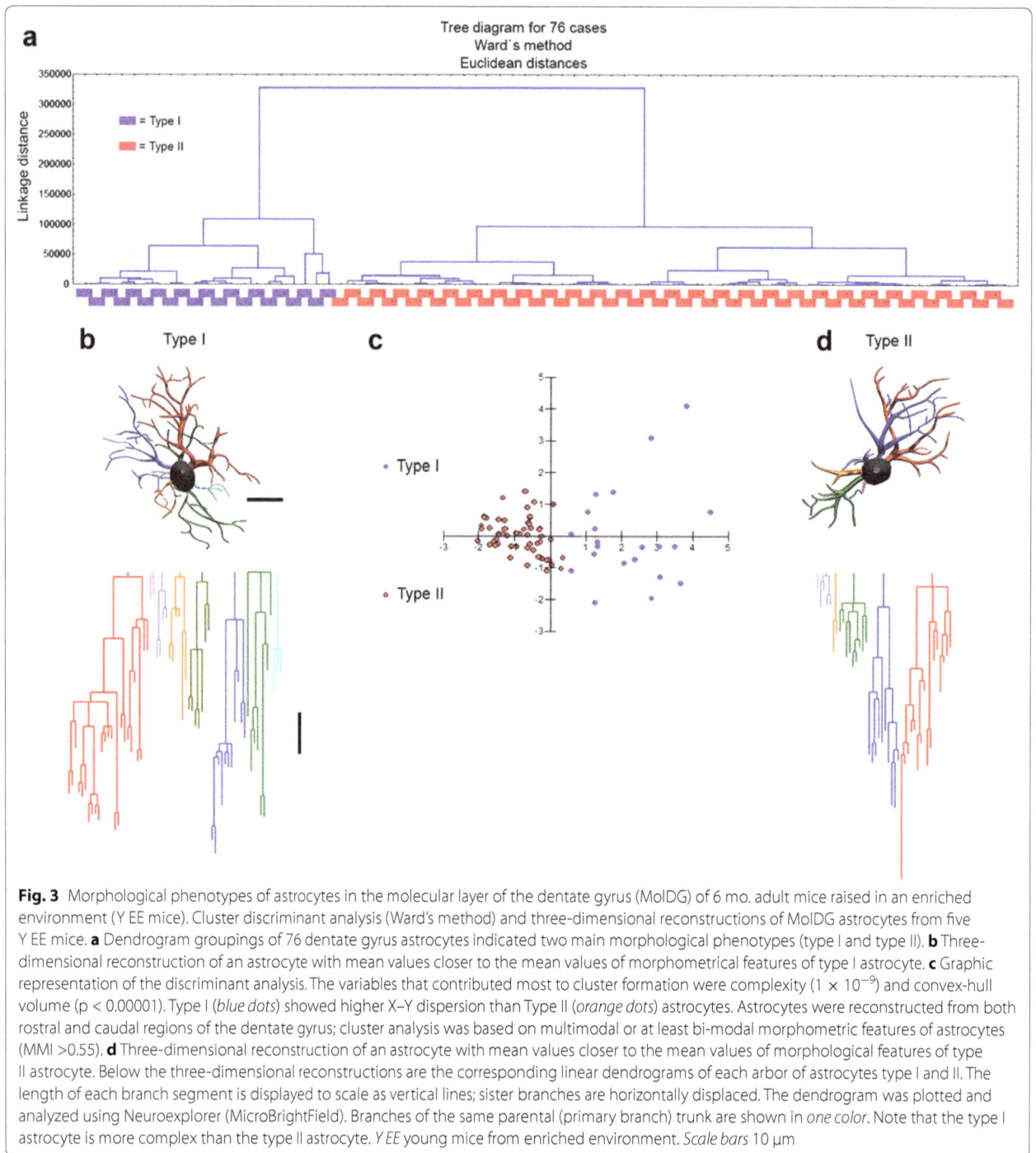

Fig. 3 Morphological phenotypes of astrocytes in the molecular layer of the dentate gyrus (MolDG) of 6 mo. adult mice raised in an enriched environment (Y EE mice). Cluster discriminant analysis (Ward's method) and three-dimensional reconstructions of MolDG astrocytes from five Y EE mice. **a** Dendrogram groupings of 76 dentate gyrus astrocytes indicated two main morphological phenotypes (type I and type II). **b** Three-dimensional reconstruction of an astrocyte with mean values closer to the mean values of morphometrical features of type I astrocyte. **c** Graphic representation of the discriminant analysis. The variables that contributed most to cluster formation were complexity (1×10^{-9}) and convex-hull volume ($p < 0.00001$). Type I (*blue dots*) showed higher X–Y dispersion than Type II (*orange dots*) astrocytes. Astrocytes were reconstructed from both rostral and caudal regions of the dentate gyrus; cluster analysis was based on multimodal or at least bi-modal morphometric features of astrocytes (MMI >0.55). **d** Three-dimensional reconstruction of an astrocyte with mean values closer to the mean values of morphological features of type II astrocyte. Below the three-dimensional reconstructions are the corresponding linear dendrograms of each arbor of astrocytes type I and II. The length of each branch segment is displayed to scale as vertical lines; sister branches are horizontally displaced. The dendrogram was plotted and analyzed using Neuroexplorer (MicroBrightField). Branches of the same parental (primary branch) trunk are shown in *one color*. Note that the type I astrocyte is more complex than the type II astrocyte. *Y EE* young mice from enriched environment. *Scale bars* 10 μm

as type I the astrocytes that exhibited significantly higher values of complexity in comparison with type II.

Figure 6 and Tables 3 and 4 demonstrate the influences of age and environmental effects on the complexity of type I and II astrocytes (A–C) and on the "mean astrocyte' (D–F). In the last case complexity represents the mean of complexity of all astrocytes (without distinction between type I and II). Two-way ANOVA applied to the "mean astrocyte' complexity values revealed that aging and environmental impoverishment, acting together, reduces astrocytes complexity (Table 3). However, the analysis of aging and environment influences on complexity of type I and II astrocytes separately (Fig. 6), revealed that the long term effects of aging and environment seems

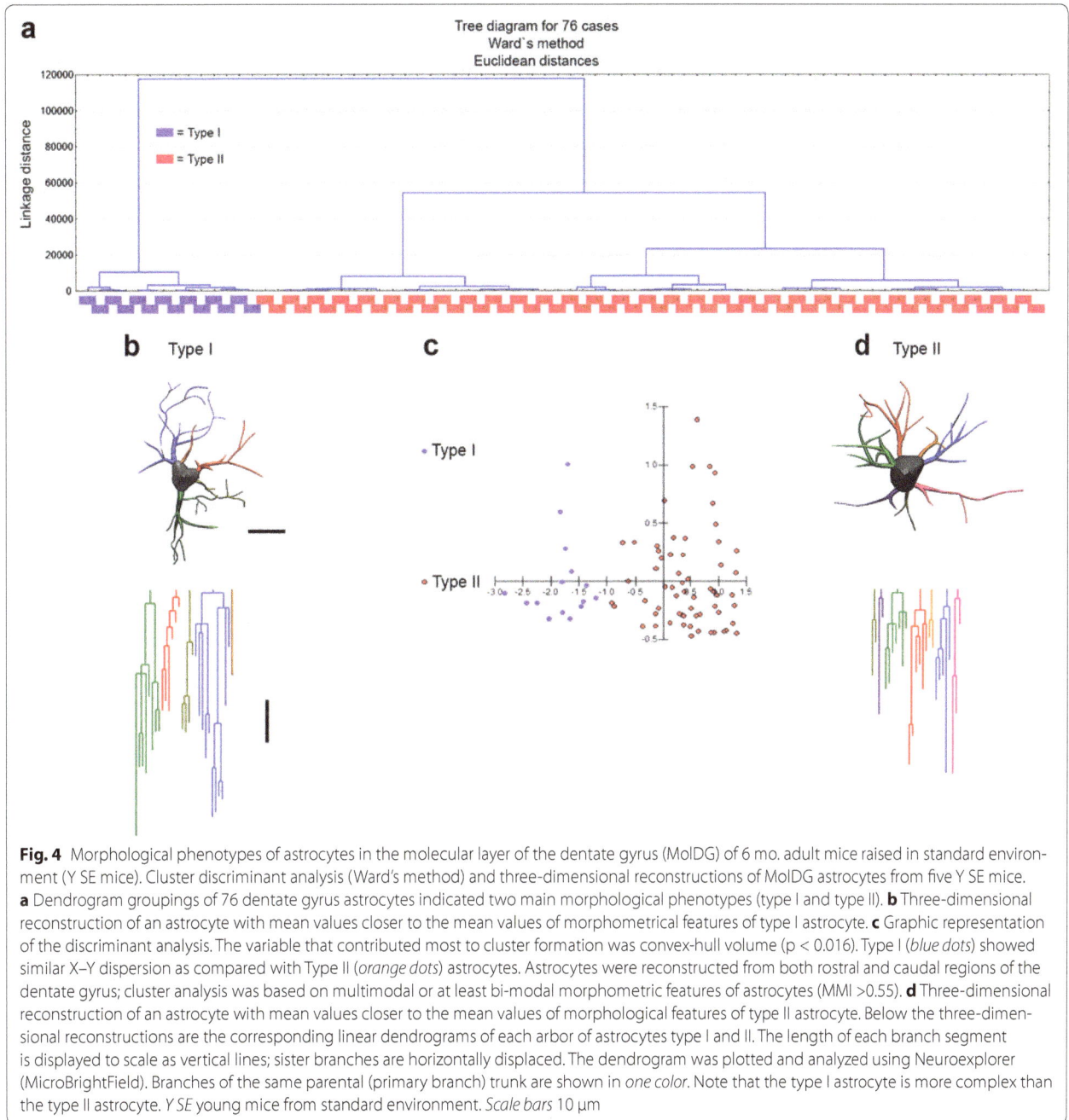

Fig. 4 Morphological phenotypes of astrocytes in the molecular layer of the dentate gyrus (MolDG) of 6 mo. adult mice raised in standard environment (Y SE mice). Cluster discriminant analysis (Ward's method) and three-dimensional reconstructions of MolDG astrocytes from five Y SE mice. **a** Dendrogram groupings of 76 dentate gyrus astrocytes indicated two main morphological phenotypes (type I and type II). **b** Three-dimensional reconstruction of an astrocyte with mean values closer to the mean values of morphometrical features of type I astrocyte. **c** Graphic representation of the discriminant analysis. The variable that contributed most to cluster formation was convex-hull volume (p < 0.016). Type I (*blue dots*) showed similar X–Y dispersion as compared with Type II (*orange dots*) astrocytes. Astrocytes were reconstructed from both rostral and caudal regions of the dentate gyrus; cluster analysis was based on multimodal or at least bi-modal morphometric features of astrocytes (MMI >0.55). **d** Three-dimensional reconstruction of an astrocyte with mean values closer to the mean values of morphological features of type II astrocyte. Below the three-dimensional reconstructions are the corresponding linear dendrograms of each arbor of astrocytes type I and II. The length of each branch segment is displayed to scale as vertical lines; sister branches are horizontally displaced. The dendrogram was plotted and analyzed using Neuroexplorer (MicroBrightField). Branches of the same parental (primary branch) trunk are shown in *one color*. Note that the type I astrocyte is more complex than the type II astrocyte. *Y SE* young mice from standard environment. *Scale bars* 10 μm

to affect type I and type II astrocytes from aged mice raised in enriched environment to a greater extent than astrocytes from aged mice maintained in standard environment (Table 4). Indeed, in the molecular layer, except for the A-SE group, which was submitted to impoverishment environment throughout life, type I cells were preserved quite distinct from type II in terms of complexity in all groups. Type I astrocytes were more complex in young adults than in aged groups and more complex in aged mice raised in enriched environment than in standard environment. However, type I astrocytes complexity mean values were not different from type II values in aged mice raised in standard environment.

No simple correlations were detected between identity, placement or timing test results and the morphological complexity (Fig. 7). Similar analysis applied separately to type I or II astrocytes complexities and behavioral performances (not illustrated) showed similar negative results suggesting that cognition and morphological complexity of dentate gyrus astrocytes may not be linearly related.

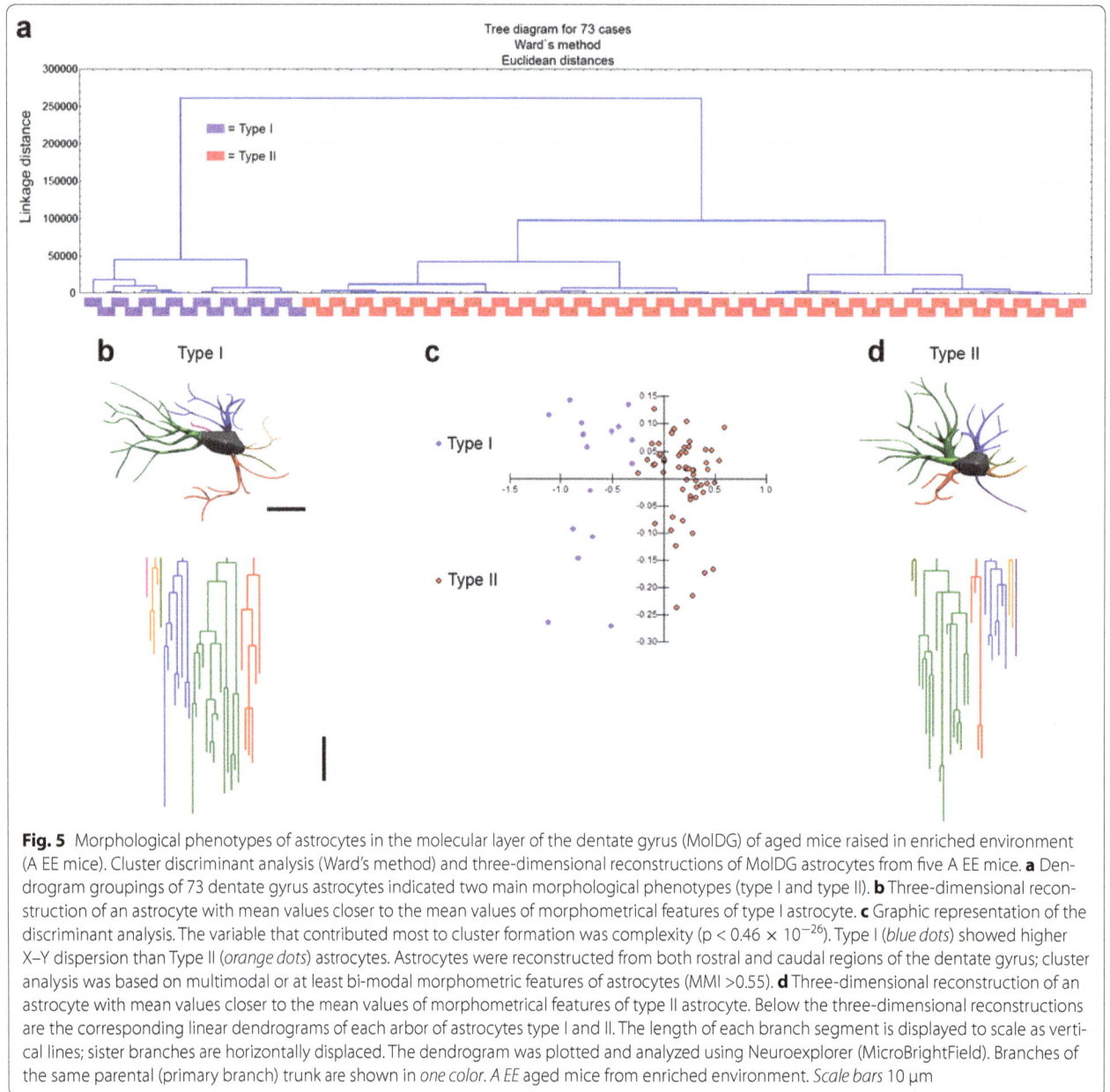

Fig. 5 Morphological phenotypes of astrocytes in the molecular layer of the dentate gyrus (MolDG) of aged mice raised in enriched environment (A EE mice). Cluster discriminant analysis (Ward's method) and three-dimensional reconstructions of MolDG astrocytes from five A EE mice. **a** Dendrogram groupings of 73 dentate gyrus astrocytes indicated two main morphological phenotypes (type I and type II). **b** Three-dimensional reconstruction of an astrocyte with mean values closer to the mean values of morphometrical features of type I astrocyte. **c** Graphic representation of the discriminant analysis. The variable that contributed most to cluster formation was complexity (p < 0.46 × 10^{-26}). Type I (*blue dots*) showed higher X–Y dispersion than Type II (*orange dots*) astrocytes. Astrocytes were reconstructed from both rostral and caudal regions of the dentate gyrus; cluster analysis was based on multimodal or at least bi-modal morphometric features of astrocytes (MMI >0.55). **d** Three-dimensional reconstruction of an astrocyte with mean values closer to the mean values of morphometrical features of type II astrocyte. Below the three-dimensional reconstructions are the corresponding linear dendrograms of each arbor of astrocytes type I and II. The length of each branch segment is displayed to scale as vertical lines; sister branches are horizontally displaced. The dendrogram was plotted and analyzed using Neuroexplorer (MicroBrightField). Branches of the same parental (primary branch) trunk are shown in *one color*. A EE aged mice from enriched environment. *Scale bars* 10 μm

Discussion

We used stereological random and systematic sampling [66], combined with 3-D reconstruction of astrocytes to show that astrocyte morphological complexity is experience-dependent. We also demonstrated that young mice with more complex astrocyte structures showed, on average, better performance in object recognition tests. To our knowledge, there are no previous findings that result from applying an unbiased sample approach with 3-D microscopic reconstruction to the assessment of an astrocytes' morphological phenotype in the mouse dentate gyrus. This approach was chosen to guarantee

that all regions from the area of interest would have the same probability of inclusion in the (systematic and randomized) sample, and that fine anatomical details (from 3-D reconstructed astrocytes) could be quantified in all experimental groups using unbiased methods. From this sampling approach, associated with cluster and discriminant analysis of the morphometric features, we have found that, with the exception of the aged mice raised in the standard environment, which showed great homogeneity in the morphology of astrocytes, two main morphological phenotypes occupy the molecular layer of the dentate gyrus in adult and aged female albino Swiss mice.

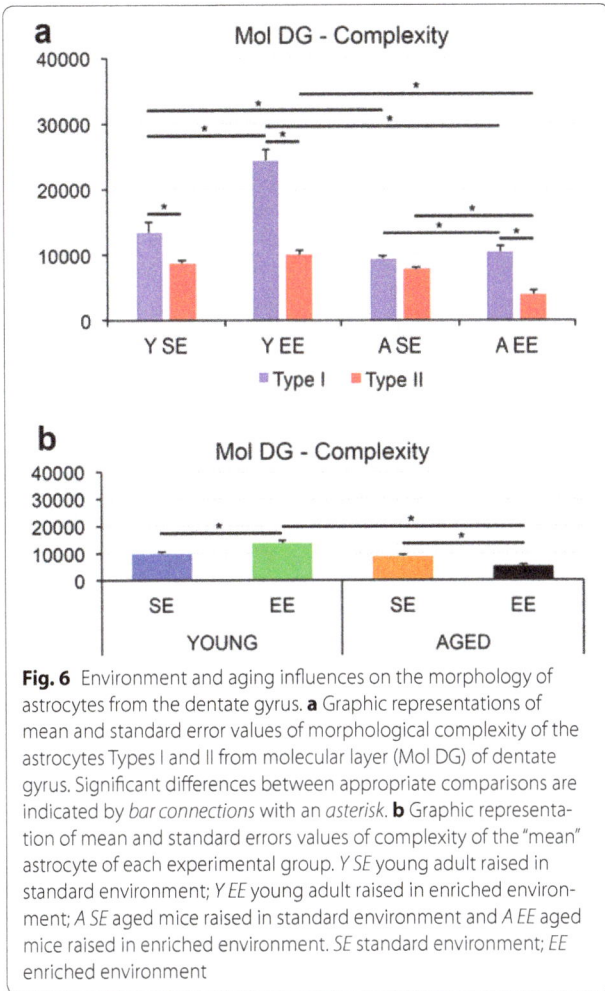

Fig. 6 Environment and aging influences on the morphology of astrocytes from the dentate gyrus. **a** Graphic representations of mean and standard error values of morphological complexity of the astrocytes Types I and II from molecular layer (Mol DG) of dentate gyrus. Significant differences between appropriate comparisons are indicated by *bar connections* with an *asterisk*. **b** Graphic representation of mean and standard errors values of complexity of the "mean" astrocyte of each experimental group. *Y SE* young adult raised in standard environment; *Y EE* young adult raised in enriched environment; *A SE* aged mice raised in standard environment and *A EE* aged mice raised in enriched environment. *SE* standard environment; *EE* enriched environment

We also discovered that relatively few morphological parameters are sufficient to distinguish the morphological changes in astrocytes associated with environment and age in our sample. Because complexity was the morphological feature that best exemplifies such morphological changes, we will discuss it as a basis for the classification of astrocytes, as well as possible functional implications.

Aging, astrocytes' morphological complexity and object recognition

Emerging evidence indicates that the number of cells that express biomarkers of cellular senescence increases with aging and astrocytes in the aging brain express characteristics of senescence-associated secretory phenotype. Indeed, aged astrocytes exhibit increased intermediate GFAP- and vimentin-positive filaments, increased expression of several cytokines (TNFα, IL-1β, and IL-6) in the rat brain [67], and increased accumulation of proteotoxic aggregates [68]. Indeed, aged astrocytes exhibit increased intermediate GFAP- and vimentin-positive filaments, increased expression of several cytokines (TNFα, IL-1β, and IL-6) in the rat brain [67], and increased accumulation of proteotoxic aggregates [68]. However, the increase in GFAP-positive filaments in the aging brain is not a consensus. As reported elsewhere, changes in astroglia in ageing and neurodegeneration seem to be highly heterogeneous and region-specific [69] and this include significant differences between white and grey matter astrocytic and microglial activation as ageing progresses [70]. In addition, hippocampal astrocyte cultures from adult and aged rats seem to reproduce changes in glial functionality observed in the aging brain and this seem to include a reduction in GFAP expression that may reflect astroglial degeneration at early stages followed by an increase of GFAP at late stages [71]. Independent of the reasons associated to these contradictory findings an important question that remain to be investigated is how these changes affect astrocytic glutamate exocytosis at the entorhinal-to-dentate granular cells (perforant pathway), because through this mechanism, astrocytes

Table 2 Discriminant analysis summary to indicate the morphological variables that most contribute to cluster formation of types I and II astrocytes from the molecular layer of dentate gyrus of each experimental group

	Wilks'	Partial	F-remove	p level	Toler.	1-Toler.
Molecular layer						
Y EE						
Complexity	0.449649	0.574029	53.429	0.0000000003	0.809881	0.19012
Convex hull volume (μm³)	0.337713	0.764293	22.205	0.0000116304	0.826130	0.17387
Y SE						
Convex hull volume (μm³)	0.550693	0.4469105	84.15575	0.00000000000016	0.952663	0.04734
A EE						
Complexity	0.9949113	0.2732307	194.1735	2.946224E^{-22}	0.9189208	0.08108

Because astrocytes from the molecular layer of aged mice from standard environment (A SE) were morphologically quite homogeneous (very short Euclidian distances), data is not included here

Y EE young mice from enriched environment; *Y SE* young mice from standard environment; *A EE* aged mice from enriched environment

Table 3 Influences of age and environment on the morphological complexity of the "mean astrocyte" from molecular layer of dentate gyrus

Molecular layer of dentate gyrus	F	P		
Age	49.529	0.000		
Environment	0.091	0.763		
Age and environment	32.231	0.000		
Two-tail t test	*Y EE x Y SE*	*Y EE x A EE*	*Y SE x A SE*	*A EE x A SE*
t=	34,475	85,256	10,210	−53,432
p=	0.001	<0.0001	0.309	<0.0001

Two-way ANOVA with correspondent F and p values and two-tail t tests with correspondent t and p values

Y EE young mice from enriched environment; *Y SE* young mice from standard environment; *A EE* aged mice from enriched environment; *A SE* aged mice from standard environment

Table 4 Influences of age and environment on the morphological complexity of Type I and Type II astrocytes from molecular layer of dentate gyrus (Mol-DG)

Mol-DG type I x II	Y SE	Y EE	A SE	A EE
t=	30,689	82,001	−14,087	129,240
p=	0.003	<0.0001	0.1629	<0.0001
Type I	*Y EE X Y SE*	*Y EE X A EE*	*Y SE X A SE*	*A EE X A SE*
t=	45,419	82,187	32,042	27,412
p=	<0.0001	<0.0001	0.003	0.010
Type II	*Y EE X Y SE*	*Y EE X A EE*	*Y SE X A SE*	*A EE X A SE*
t=	15,521	101,537	−0.8054	−70,682
p=	0.1234	<0.0001	0.4224	<0.0001

Two-tail t tests with correspondent t and p values

Y EE young mice from enriched environment; *Y SE* young mice from standard environment; *A EE* aged mice from enriched environment; *A SE* aged mice from standard environment

participate in synaptic tuning in circuits involved in cognitive processing and the control of mossy fiber-to-CA3 synaptic input [72]. In addition, even in the absence of

neurological disease, a more reactive astrocyte phenotype is expressed during aging as part of an increased and maintained pro-inflammatory profile that may be associated with cognitive dysfunction [73]. A decrease in the ability of aged rats to sustain long-term potentiation in the perforant pathway of the dentate gyrus also appears to be associated with microglial activation [74]. Taking these observations together, it would be reasonable to suggest that the number of astrocytes with senescence-associated secretory phenotype may be increased in animals raised in standard conditions (reducing astrocytic complexity) compared with aged mice housed in enriched conditions [74]. Although this was not the case of the "mean astrocyte" of the molecular layer from aged mice of enriched environment, when we analyzed type I and type II separately, type I astrocytes were significantly more complex than type II in this mice group. In contrast, only one morphological phenotype was found in aged mice raised in standard environment and this was morphologically similar to type II astrocytes.

Object recognition enables the unambiguous distinction between new and familiar objects; see [75, 76] for recent reviews. To cope with memory tasks, the brain must accentuate the differences between old and new experiences before coding occurs [25]. For that purpose, medial and lateral perforant pathways transmit spatial and non-spatial information to the dentate gyrus, which is necessary for recognizing object placement (Where?), identity (What?), and timing (When?). Lateral portions of the entorhinal cortex project to the caudal levels of the dentate gyrus and hippocampus, and medial portions of the entorhinal cortex project to the rostral levels [77, 78]. We have learned from earlier experiments that only 6 mo. adult and aged mice from the enriched environment were able to integrate object recognition into a spatial–temporal context [13]. Mice from standard environments were unable to make the appropriate distinctions. In the spatial memory component of episodic-like memory (Where?),

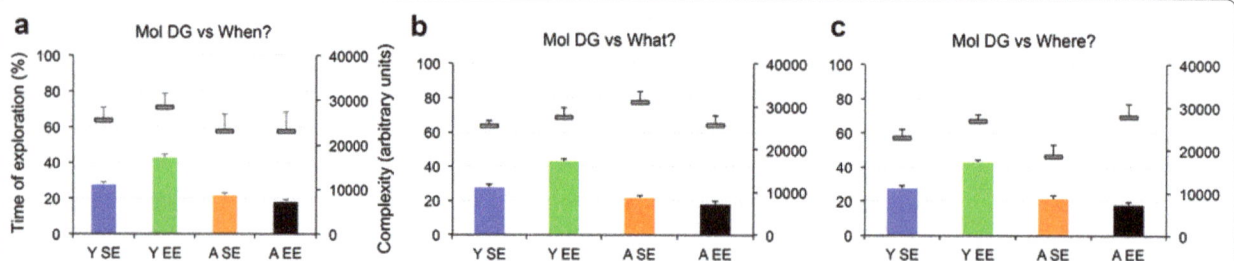

Fig. 7 Object identity recognition (What?), timing (When?), spatial memory (Where?), and astrocytes complexity. Object discrimination index is expressed as percentage values on the left *Y-axis* and astrocyte morphological complexity is indicated as arbitrary values on the right *Y-axis*. Discrimination index of 60 % or higher was set to indicate that mice distinguished between the objects (familiar vs new; stationary vs displaced; old vs recent) whereas indices below 60 % indicate no object recognition. *Mol DG* molecular layer of dentate gyrus, *Y SE* young mice from standard environment, *Y EE* young mice from enriched environment, *A SE* aged mice from standard environment, *A EE* aged mice from enriched environment. **a** Object timing recognition and astrocytes morphological complexity. **b** Object identity recognition and astrocytes morphological complexity. **c** Object placement recognition and astrocytes morphological complexity

young and aged animals housed in enriched conditions spent significantly more time in the displaced than stationary objects. In the identity and temporal memory components (What? and When?), young and aged animals housed in enriched conditions spent significantly more time in the old than recent objects [13]. Coherently, subsequent analysis of the behavior of aged mice found similar results in tasks that engaged episodic-like memory [79, 80] and working and recognition memories [81]. In the present report using object identity recognition, similar results were found. Indeed, all experimental groups recognized the identity of the objects, only mice from enriched environment (both young and aged) succeeded in the placement task, only young mice both from standard and enriched environments succeeded in the timing task but only young mice from enriched environment distinguished the context where the objects were displaced.

Enriched environment, neurogenesis, spatial memory improvement and glial cells

Neuronal progenitor cells in the subgranular zone continuously proliferate, migrate into de granular cell layer and differentiate into granule cells [82]. These new neurons, which have been implicated in pattern separation [83], are continually generated in the dentate gyrus in the adult hippocampus [35, 84]. Molecular layer perforant path-associated cells contribute to feed-forward inhibition of these granular cells in the adult dentate gyrus [85] and the integrity of these projections seems to be essential to maintain granular dendritic arbors [86] and spatial learning and memory [87]. Medial and lateral perforant pathways transmit to dentate gyrus, spatial and non-spatial information that would be necessary to learn and recognize object placement (Where?), identity (What?) and timing (When?) [88]. The newborn neurons targeted by perforant pathway, seem to increase significantly in the dentate gyrus of rodents raised in an enriched environment, and this has been associated with spatial memory improvements [89, 90]. In line with these observations our findings demonstrated that spatial memory is influenced by both age and environment and that object recognition memory seems to be resistant to both normal aging and impoverished environment of standard cages

During our previous stereological analysis of the dentate gyrus of aged mice raised in standard environment, we observed hyperplasia of astrocytes in the molecular layer compared with equivalent sections from young adults raised in the same conditions. Interestingly, aged mice from enriched but not from standard exhibited the ability to form integrated memories in the spatial–temporal context [13] However, environment and aging affected the molecular layer of the dentate gyrus

in an additive way; thus, we speculated that astrocytosis induced by environmental enrichment might have a different functional role from that induced by aging [13]. Paradoxically, our preliminary morphometric analysis in the molecular layer of the dentate gyrus, using a random but not systematic sampling approach, [45] confirmed earlier descriptions in aged rats [44], that hippocampal astrocytes from aged mice, maintained in an enriched environment, were smaller than those from aged mice maintained in an standard environment. In the present report, we confirmed our preliminary report on the "mean astrocyte" molecular layer. However, hierarchical cluster and discriminant analysis revealed two different morphological phenotypes that had their morphologies distinctly influenced by environment and age.

Although the molecular basis of those changes remains to be investigated, it is important to discuss possible implications associated with the influences of aging and the environment on the morphology of astrocytes in the dentate gyrus.

Possible physiological implications of an increase in astrocytic complexity

It is interesting to discuss possible connections between the quantitative astrocyte morphological response and the cognitive protection observed after environmental enrichment. In the rodent brain, a single astrocyte is the third element of hundreds of thousands of synapses [91–93]. This ramified complex morphological substrate provides the structural basis for functional interactions with neurons, other glial cell processes, and blood vessels [94]. Studies of neuronal stimulation and astrocyte morphology have taught us that astrocytes react to neuronal stimulation by changing their morphology, and ultrastructural analysis of targeted projections from the stimulated region have demonstrated that neural stimulation causes a significant increase in the astrocytic envelopment of excitatory synapses on dendritic spines [95].

Our findings showed that mice living all life on an impoverished environment lose astrocytic morphological diversity. In contrast, individuals maintained for the same time extent in an enriched environment, did not lose astrocytic diversity. Indeed, 6 months of enriched environment increase 113 % the number of higher complexity astrocytes, and the absolute number of these type I astrocytes are not reduced later in life. aged mice from enriched environment showed the same number of type I astrocytes. Although type II is less influenced by environmental changes (26 % increase in Y EE vs Y SE), it seems that this morphological phenotype is responsible for significant increase in the total number of astrocytes on aged mice from enriched environment (Fig. 8).

Because environmental enrichment is associated with a greater degree of long-term somatosensory/motor and visuospatial stimulation, and in the present report, we observed better performance of an object recognition placement and context tasks in young mice from the enriched environment, with more complex astrocytes, we suggest that at least part of this improvement in hippocampal-dependent tasks performances in young mice, might be associated with astrocytic plasticity. These findings are in line with recent report which demonstrate that housing complexity alters GFAP-immunoreactive astrocyte morphology in the rat dentate gyrus [41]. It is important to highlight that our analysis was done in the molecular layer of dentate gyrus, the main target of the perforant pathway and type I astrocytes were more ramified and longer than type II. Thus, it is reasonable to propose they will affect a higher number of synapses in that layer than type II.

Because type I morphology is affected in higher proportion by aging and environmental impoverishment than type II and aged mice raised in enriched environment had better performances in hippocampal-dependent tasks than aged mice from standard environment it is reasonable to propose different physiological roles for these two phenotypes.

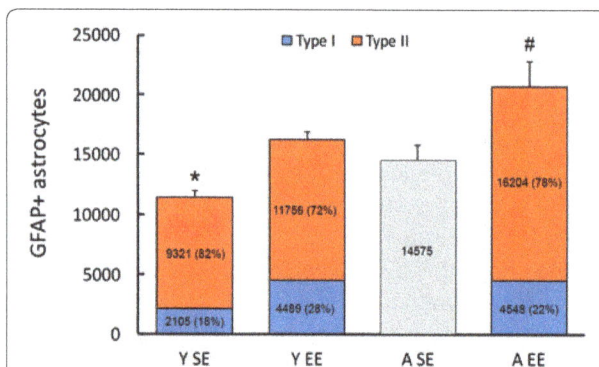

Fig. 8 Environment and aging influences on the number and morphology of astrocytes from the molecular layer of dentate gyrus. Relative number of astrocytes morphological phenotypes Type I and Type II as a function of the total number of GFAP immunolabeled astrocytes (GFAP + astrocytes). To estimate these numbers, we used percentage values of type I and type II reconstructed astrocytes in combination with previous stereological data described elsewhere [106]. Note that young mice independent of environment, and aged mice from enriched environment show Type I and II morphological phenotypes, whereas aged mice from standard environment did not. *Y SE* young adult raised in standard environment; *Y EE* young adult raised in enriched environment; *A SE* aged mice raised in standard environment and *A EE* aged mice raised in enriched environment. *SE* standard environment; *EE* enriched environment. (*) and (#) indicate significant differences between the number of total astrocytes from different experimental groups (Y EE vs Y SE; Y EE vs A EE; Y SE vs A SE; A EE vs A SE)

Hormones and astrocytes

When male Swiss mice were group housed in the laboratory, aggressive interactions between cage mates caused severe injury and stress in the animals. These findings previously described elsewhere, may hamper the validity of experimental results, for review see [96]. To minimize the level of aggression in the cages, female mice were chosen to compose the experimental groups. This choice however, may have included estrogenic changes late in life induced by aging, that may contribute to age-related cognitive impairments and to associated astrocytic morphological changes. Indeed, apart from aging and environment, sexual hormones may change the number [97–99] and morphology [98, 100] of neuroglial cells. In the dentate gyrus, aged C57Bl6J female mice presented 35 % more astrocytes than age-matched males [97] and estrogen and raloxifene changed both the number and morphology of astrocytes of aged female mice [101]. In the present report, aged females may have been depleted of estrogenic protection; thus, we suggest that at least part of the morphological changes detected in aged female mice from both enriched and impoverished environments might be related to estropause. In agreement, ovariectomized female mice given an estrogenic replacement showed significant changes in both the number and morphology of astrocytes in the dentate gyrus compared to an ovariectomized placebo group [101].

Finally, it is important to consider that manipulation-induced stress during behavioral tasks might have altered plasma corticosteroid levels, with implications on astrocytic plasticity [102]. Although we cannot exclude the possibility that different levels of corticosteroids might explain the results the behavioral tests were applied to all animals of all experimental groups which minimizes the possibility that manipulation-induced stress might explain the results.

Limitations of the experimental design and technical approaches

Comparative analysis of different astrocytes immunomarkers demonstrated that anti-GFAP immunolabeling offers complementary information to anti-S-100ß or anti-glutamine synthetase [103]. Indeed, morphometric analysis of astrocytes, labeled with these three distinct markers revealed region-specific changes in the astroglial morphological phenotypes.

Although the number of GFAP immunolabeled astrocytes may not represent the total number of astrocytes, we and others using GFAP immunolabeling and unbiased stereological methods demonstrated that age [13, 97] and environmental changes [13] were associated with significant changes in the number of the subpopulation of GFAP immunolabeled astrocytes in dentate gyrus.

In addition, the environmental enrichment stimulated neurogenenesis and gliogenesis [104], increaseed the GFAP immunolabeled cellular network [105], showing astrocytes with longer branches and higher number of branching points [43, 46]. We [45] and others [32, 44, 46, 103] also demonstrated that as compared to aged mice raised in standard environment, long-life environmental enrichment is associated with shorter GFAP astrocytes branches, lower number of nodes and reduction in the tree surface areas and complexity.

Finally, the influences of environmental enrichment and age on astrocytes' morphological changes and memory investigated previously in mice and rats using different approaches, models, and techniques [13, 43, 44, 105, 106] were sometimes contradictory. Because different methods, different animal lineages, variations in histological procedures, different stereological protocols, and ambiguities in the definition of the objects and areas of interest were applied, it is reasonable to suppose that at least part of these contradictions might be explained by these differences. To minimize possible sources of variations all samples were obtained with the same tissue processing protocols (perfusion, immunoreaction, dehydration, counterstaining, and clearing) and all data were collected and analyzed with the same unbiased methodology. We also confirmed the results by having different investigators reconstructing the same cells, using the same monoclonal anti-GFAP antibody as a selective marker for astrocytes. Thus, it is expected that non-biological sources were reduced to acceptable levels in the present report [97, 107]. Microscopic, 3-D reconstructions might be affected by non-uniform shrinkage in the z-axis of sections [108]. It was recently demonstrated that sections that the final thickness in the Z-axis is approximately 25 % of the cut thickness after dehydration and clearing [62]. We used this percentage value to implement corrections on all astrocyte reconstructions, assuming 75 % shrinkage of thickness along the z-axis and because the tissue size did not change along X–Y axes after histological dehydration and clearing no corrections were applied to the x/y dimensions.

Conclusions

Using a combination of stereological sampling approach and three-dimensional reconstruction we found two morphological phenotypes on the molecular layer of dentate gyrus. On average, type I morphological complexity seems to be much more sensitive to age and environmental influences than that of type II. Indeed, aging and environmental impoverishment interact and reduce the morphological complexity of type I astrocytes at a point that they could not be distinguished anymore from type II. Our findings confirm previous reports that the morphological complexity of astrocytes is experience-dependent and suggest at least

in young mice that astrocytes of higher complexity may be associated with better performances in object recognition hippocampal-dependent tasks. Although aged mice from enriched environment preserved object recognition, their astrocytes revealed significant degree of shrinkage.

Abbreviations
A EE: aged mice raised in enriched environment; Y EE: young mice raised in enriched environment; A SE: aged mice raised in standard environment; Y SE: young mice raised in standard environment; GFAP: glial fibrillary acid protein; GrDG: granular layer of the dentate gyrus; MolDG: molecular layer of the dentate gyrus; PolDG: polymorphic layer of the dentate gyrus; 3-D: three-dimensional.

Authors' contributions
Study concept and design: CWPD, DGD, PFCV and JBT. Acquisition of data: CARF, MAO, CML, DGD. Analysis and interpretation of data: JBT, DCA, DGD, CWPD, MCKS. Drafting of the manuscript: CWPD, DCA, JBT and DGD. Critical revision of the manuscript for important intellectual content: DCA, CWPD, JBT, DGD. Statistical analysis: JBT, DGD, CWPD. Obtained funding: CWPD, PFCV. Administrative, technical and material support: CARF, MCKS, CML, MAO. Study supervision: CWPD. All authors read and approved the final manuscript.

Author details
[1] Laboratório de Investigações Em Neurodegeneração e Infecção, Instituto de Ciências Biológicas, Universidade Federal do Pará, Hospital Universitário João de Barros Barreto, Rua dos Mundurucus 4487, Guamá, Belém, Pará CEP 66073-000, Brazil. [2] Departamento de Arbovirologia e Febres Hemorrágicas, Instituto Evandro Chagas, Ananindeua, Pará, Brazil. [3] Laboratory of Experimental Neuropathology, Department of Pharmacology, University of Oxford, Oxford, England, UK.

Acknowledgements
Not applicable.

Competing interests
The authors declare that they have no competing interests.

Funding
This study received financial support from Conselho Nacional de Pesquisa—CNPq (Grant Numbers: 300203/2010-1, 471077/2007-0 and 441007/2014-7) for CWPD; Coordenação de Aperfeiçoamento de Pessoal de Nível Superior—CAPES (Process Number: 99999.001533/2014-02) for CWPD; Universidade Federal do Pará—Edital PROPESP/FADESP—PIAPA 2015.

References
1. Tyndall AV, Davenport MH, Wilson BJ, Burek GM, Arsenault-Lapierre G, Haley E, Eskes GA, Friedenreich CM, Hill MD, Hogan DB, et al. The brain-in-motion study: effect of a 6-month aerobic exercise intervention on cerebrovascular regulation and cognitive function in older adults. BMC Geriatr. 2013;13:21.

2. Erickson KI, Weinstein AM, Lopez OL. Physical activity, brain plasticity, and Alzheimer's disease. Arch Med Res. 2012;43:615–21.

3. Small BJ, Dixon RA, McArdle JJ, Grimm KJ. Do changes in lifestyle engagement moderate cognitive decline in normal aging? Evidence from the Victoria Longitudinal Study. Neuropsychology. 2012;26:144–55.

4. Fernández-Mayoralas G, Rojo-Pérez F, Martínez-Martín P, Prieto-Flores ME, Rodríguez-Blázquez C, Martín-García S, Rojo-Abuín JM, Forjaz MJ. Active ageing and quality of life: factors associated with participation in leisure activities among institutionalized older adults, with and without dementia. Aging Ment Health. 2015;19:1031–41.

5. Pedrero-Chamizo R, Albers U, Tobaruela JL, Meléndez A, Castillo MJ, González-Gross M. Physical strength is associated with Mini-Mental State Examination scores in Spanish institutionalized elderly. Geriatr Gerontol Int. 2013;13:1026–34.

6. Lovden M, Xu W, Wang HX. Lifestyle change and the prevention of cognitive decline and dementia: what is the evidence? Curr Opin Psychiatry. 2013;26:239–43.

7. Zhao E, Tranovich MJ, Wright VJ. The role of mobility as a protective factor of cognitive functioning in aging adults: a review. Sports Health. 2014;6:63–9.

8. Stranahan AM, Mattson MP. Metabolic reserve as a determinant of cognitive aging. J Alzheimers Dis. 2012;30(Suppl 2):S5–13.

9. Mangialasche F, Kivipelto M, Solomon A, Fratiglioni L. Dementia prevention: current epidemiological evidence and future perspective. Alzheimers Res Ther. 2012;4:6.

10. Volkers KM, Scherder EJ. Impoverished environment, cognition, aging and dementia. Rev Neurosci. 2011;22:259–66.

11. Zalik E, Zalar B. Differences in mood between elderly persons living in different residential environments in Slovenia. Psychiatr Danub. 2013;25:40–8.

12. Maseda A, Balo A, Lorenzo-López L, Lodeiro-Fernández L, Rodríguez-Villamil JL, Millán-Calenti JC. Cognitive and affective assessment in day care versus institutionalized elderly patients: a 1-year longitudinal study. Clin Interv Aging. 2014;9:887–94.

13. Diniz D, Foro CA, Rego C, Gloria DA, de Oliveira FR, Paes JM, de Sousa AA, Tokuhashi TP, Trindade LS, Turiel MC, et al. Environmental impoverishment and aging alter object recognition, spatial learning, and dentate gyrus astrocytes. Eur J Neurosci. 2010;32:509–19.

14. Teather LA, Wurtman RJ. Chronic administration of UMP ameliorates the impairment of hippocampal-dependent memory in impoverished rats. J Nutr. 2006;136:2834–7.

15. Teather LA, Wurtman RJ. Dietary CDP-choline supplementation prevents memory impairment caused by impoverished environmental conditions in rats. Learn Mem. 2005;12:39–43.

16. Gregory ML, Szumlinski KK. Impoverished rearing impairs working memory and metabotropic glutamate receptor 5 expression. NeuroReport. 2008;19:239–43.

17. Mendes Fde C, de Almeida MN, Felício AP, Fadel AC, Silva Dde J, Borralho TG, da Silva RP, Bento-Torres J, Vasconcelos PF, Perry VH, et al. Enriched environment and masticatory activity rehabilitation recover spatial memory decline in aged mice. BMC Neurosci. 2013;14:63.

18. Winocur G. Environmental influences on cognitive decline in aged rats. Neurobiol Aging. 1998;19:589–97.

19. Bell JA, Livesey PJ, Meyer JF. Environmental enrichment influences survival rate and enhances exploration and learning but produces variable responses to the radial maze in old rats. Dev Psychobiol. 2009;51:564–78.

20. Kumar A, Rani A, Tchigranova O, Lee WH, Foster TC. Influence of late-life exposure to environmental enrichment or exercise on hippocampal function and CA1 senescent physiology. Neurobiol Aging. 2012;33:828 **(e821–817)**.

21. Speisman RB, Kumar A, Rani A, Pastoriza JM, Severance JE, Foster TC, Ormerod BK. Environmental enrichment restores neurogenesis and rapid acquisition in aged rats. Neurobiol Aging. 2012;34:263–74.

22. Speisman RB, Kumar A, Rani A, Pastoriza JM, Severance JE, Foster TC, Ormerod BK. Environmental enrichment restores neurogenesis and rapid acquisition in aged rats. Neurobiol Aging. 2013;34:263–74.

23. Speisman RB, Kumar A, Rani A, Foster TC, Ormerod BK. Daily exercise improves memory, stimulates hippocampal neurogenesis and

modulates immune and neuroimmune cytokines in aging rats. Brain Behav Immun. 2013;28:25–43.

24. Yuan Z, Wang M, Yan B, Gu P, Jiang X, Yang X, Cui D. An enriched environment improves cognitive performance in mice from the senescence-accelerated prone mouse 8 strain: role of upregulated neurotrophic factor expression in the hippocampus. Neural Regen Res. 2012;7:1797–804.

25. Schmidt B, Marrone DF, Markus EJ. Disambiguating the similar: the dentate gyrus and pattern separation. Behav Brain Res. 2012;226:56–65.

26. Cheng L, Wang SH, Jia N, Xie M, Liao XM. Environmental stimulation influence the cognition of developing mice by inducing changes in oxidative and apoptosis status. Brain Dev. 2014;36:51–6.

27. Leger M, Quiedeville A, Paizanis E, Natkunarajah S, Freret T, Boulouard M, Schumann-Bard P. Environmental enrichment enhances episodic-like memory in association with a modified neuronal activation profile in adult mice. PLoS One. 2012;7:e48043.

28. Suzuki H, Kanagawa D, Nakazawa H, Tawara-Hirata Y, Kogure Y, Shimizu-Okabe C, Takayama C, Ishikawa Y, Shiosaka S. Role of neuropsin in parvalbumin immunoreactivity changes in hippocampal basket terminals of mice reared in various environments. Front Cell Neurosci. 2014;8:420.

29. Bureš Z, Bartošová J, Lindovský J, Chumak T, Popelář J, Syka J. Acoustical enrichment during early postnatal development changes response properties of inferior colliculus neurons in rats. Eur J Neurosci. 2014;40:3674–83.

30. Vallès A, Granic I, De Weerd P, Martens GJ. Molecular correlates of cortical network modulation by long-term sensory experience in the adult rat barrel cortex. Learn Mem. 2014;21:305–10.

31. Hosseiny S, Pietri M, PetitPaitel A, Zarif H, Heurteaux C, Chabry J, Guyon A. Differential neuronal plasticity in mouse hippocampus associated with various periods of enriched environment during postnatal development. Brain Struct Funct. 2014;220:3435–48.

32. Sampedro-Piquero P, Begega A, Arias JL. Increase of glucocorticoid receptor expression after environmental enrichment: relations to spatial memory, exploration and anxiety-related behaviors. Physiol Behav. 2014;129:118–29.

33. Kobilo T, Liu QR, Gandhi K, Mughal M, Shaham Y, van Praag H. Running is the neurogenic and neurotrophic stimulus in environmental enrichment. Learn Mem. 2011;18:605–9.

34. van Praag H, Shubert T, Zhao C, Gage FH. Exercise enhances learning and hippocampal neurogenesis in aged mice. J Neurosci. 2005;25:8680–5.

35. Kempermann G, Kuhn HG, Gage FH. More hippocampal neurons in adult mice living in an enriched environment. Nature. 1997;386:493–5.

36. Ramírez-Rodríguez G, Ocaña-Fernández MA, Vega-Rivera NM, Torres-Pérez OM, Gómez-Sánchez A, Estrada-Camarena E, Ortiz-López L. Environmental enrichment induces neuroplastic changes in middle age female Balb/c mice and increases the hippocampal levels of BDNF, p-Akt and p-MAPK1/2. Neuroscience. 2014;260:158–70.

37. Merkley CM, Jian C, Mosa A, Tan YF, Wojtowicz JM. Homeostatic regulation of adult hippocampal neurogenesis in aging rats: long-term effects of early exercise. Front Neurosci. 2014;8:174.

38. Bergami M, Masserdotti G, Temprana SG, Motori E, Eriksson TM, Göbel J, Yang SM, Conzelmann KK, Schinder AF, Götz M, Berninger B. A critical period for experience-dependent remodeling of adult-born neuron connectivity. Neuron. 2015;85:710–7.

39. Donato F, Chowdhury A, Lahr M, Caroni P. Early- and late-born parvalbumin basket cell subpopulations exhibiting distinct regulation and roles in learning. Neuron. 2015;85:770–86.

40. Huang W, Ming GL, Song H. Experience matters: enrichment remodels synaptic inputs to adult-born neurons. Neuron. 2015;85:659–61.

41. Salois G, Smith JS. Housing complexity alters GFAP-immunoreactive astrocyte morphology in the rat dentate gyrus. Neural Plast. 2016;2016:3928726.

42. Zorec R, Horvat A, Vardjan N, Verkhratsky A. Memory Formation Shaped by Astroglia. Front Integr Neurosci. 2015;9:56. doi:10.3389/fnint.2015.00056.

43. Sampedro-Piquero P, De Bartolo P, Petrosini L, Zancada-Menendez C, Arias JL, Begega A. Astrocytic plasticity as a possible mediator of the cognitive improvements after environmental enrichment in aged rats. Neurobiol Learn Mem. 2014;114:16–25.

44. Soffie M, Hahn K, Terao E, Eclancher F. Behavioural and glial changes in old rats following environmental enrichment. Behav Brain Res. 1999;101:37–49.

45. Diniz D, Foro C, Bento-Torres J, Vasconcelos P, Diniz CW. Aging, environmental enrichment, object recognition and astrocyte plasticity in dentate gyrus. In: Gonzalez-Perez O, editor. Astrocytes: structure, functions and role in disease. 1st ed. Hauppauge, New York: Nova Science Publisher Inc; 2012. p. 91–108.

46. Viola GG, Rodrigues L, Americo JC, Hansel G, Vargas RS, Biasibetti R, Swarowsky A, Goncalves CA, Xavier LL, Achaval M, et al. Morphological changes in hippocampal astrocytes induced by environmental enrichment in mice. Brain Res. 2009;1274:47–54.

47. Han X, Chen M, Wang F, Windrem M, Wang S, Shanz S, Xu Q, Oberheim NA, Bekar L, Betstadt S, et al. Forebrain engraftment by human glial progenitor cells enhances synaptic plasticity and learning in adult mice. Cell Stem Cell. 2013;12:342–53.

48. Windrem MS, Schanz SJ, Guo M, Tian GF, Washco V, Stanwood N, Rasband M, Roy NS, Nedergaard M, Havton LA, et al. Neonatal chimerization with human glial progenitor cells can both remyelinate and rescue the otherwise lethally hypomyelinated shiverer mouse. Cell Stem Cell. 2008;2:553–65.

49. Zhang Y, Barres BA. A smarter mouse with human astrocytes. Bioessays. 2013;35:876–80.

50. Franklin RJ, Bussey TJ. Do your glial cells make you clever? Cell Stem Cell. 2013;12:265–6.

51. Oberheim NA, Wang X, Goldman S, Nedergaard M. Astrocytic complexity distinguishes the human brain. Trends Neurosci. 2006;29:547–53.

52. Oberheim NA, Takano T, Han X, He W, Lin JH, Wang F, Xu Q, Wyatt JD, Pilcher W, Ojemann JG, et al. Uniquely hominid features of adult human astrocytes. J Neurosci. 2009;29:3276–87.

53. Witter MP. The perforant path: projections from the entorhinal cortex to the dentate gyrus. Prog Brain Res. 2007;163:43–61.

54. Smith AC, Frank LM, Wirth S, Yanike M, Hu D, Kubota Y, Graybiel AM, Suzuki WA, Brown EN. Dynamic analysis of learning in behavioral experiments. J Neurosci. 2004;24:447–61.

55. Dere E, Huston JP, De Souza Silva MA. Episodic-like memory in mice: simultaneous assessment of object, place and temporal order memory. Brain Res Brain Res Protoc. 2005;16:10–9.

56. Dere E, Huston JP, De Souza Silva MA. Integrated memory for objects, places, and temporal order: evidence for episodic-like memory in mice. Neurobiol Learn Mem. 2005;84:214–21.

57. Dere E, Huston JP, De Souza Silva MA. The pharmacology, neuroanatomy and neurogenetics of one-trial object recognition in rodents. Neurosci Biobehav Rev. 2007;31:673–704.

58. Tulving E. Episodic memory and common sense: how far apart? Philos Trans R Soc Lond B Biol Sci. 2001;356:1505–15.

59. Dix SL, Aggleton JP. Extending the spontaneous preference test of recognition: evidence of object-location and object-context recognition. Behav Brain Res. 1999;99:191–200.

60. Dere M, Huston JP, Silva MAS. Episodic-like memory in mice: simultaneous assessment of object, place and temporal order memory. Brain Res. 2005;16:10–9.

61. Shu S, Ju G, Fan L. The glucose oxidase-DAB-nickel method in peroxidase histochemistry of the nervous system. Neurosci Lett. 1988;85:169–71.

62. Carlo CN, Stevens CF. Analysis of differential shrinkage in frozen brain sections and its implications for the use of guard zones in stereology. J Comp Neurol. 2011;519:2803–10.

63. Schweitzer L, Renehan WE. The use of cluster analysis for cell typing. Brain Res Brain Res Protoc. 1997;1:100–8.

64. Kolb H, Fernandez E, Schouten J, Ahnelt P, Linberg KA, Fisher SK. Are there three types of horizontal cell in the human retina? J Comp Neurol. 1994;343:370–86.

65. Pillai AG, de Jong D, Kanatsou S, Krugers H, Knapman A, Heinzmann JM, Holsboer F, Landgraf R, Joëls M, Touma C. Dendritic morphology of hippocampal and amygdalar neurons in adolescent mice is resilient to genetic differences in stress reactivity. PLoS One. 2012;7:e38971.

66. West MJ. Stereological methods for estimating the total number of neurons and synapses: issues of precision and bias. Trends Neurosci. 1999;22(2):51–61.

67. Campuzano O, Castillo-Ruiz MM, Acarin L, Castellano B, Gonzalez B. Increased levels of proinflammatory cytokines in the aged rat brain attenuate injury-induced cytokine response after excitotoxic damage. J Neurosci Res. 2009;87:2484–97.

68. Salminen A, Ojala J, Kaarniranta K, Haapasalo A, Hiltunen M, Soininen H. Astrocytes in the aging brain express characteristics of senescence-associated secretory phenotype. Eur J Neurosci. 2011;34:3–11.

69. Rodríguez-Arellano JJ, Parpura V, Zorec R, Verkhratsky A. Astrocytes in physiological aging and Alzheimer's disease. Neuroscience. 2016;323:170–82.

70. Robillard KN, Lee KM, Chiu KB, MacLean AG. Glial cell morphological and density changes through the lifespan of rhesus macaques. Brain Behav Immun. 2016;55:60–9.

71. Bellaver B, Souza DG, Souza DO, Quincozes-Santos A. Hippocampal astrocyte cultures from adult and aged rats reproduce changes in glial functionality observed in the aging brain. Mol Neurobiol. 2016:1–17. doi:10.1007/s12035-016-9880-8.

72. Jourdain P, Bergersen LH, Bhaukaurally K, Bezzi P, Santello M, Domercq M, Matute C, Tonello F, Gundersen V, Volterra A. Glutamate exocytosis from astrocytes controls synaptic strength. Nat Neurosci. 2007;10:331–9.

73. Godbout JP, Johnson RW. Age and neuroinflammation: a lifetime of psychoneuroimmune consequences. Immunol Allerg Clin North Am. 2009;29:321–37.

74. Lynch MA. Age-related neuroinflammatory changes negatively impact on neuronal function. Front Aging Neurosci. 2010;1:6.

75. Pause BM, Zlomuzica A, Kinugawa K, Mariani J, Pietrowsky R, Dere E. Perspectives on episodic-like and episodic memory. Front Behav Neurosci. 2013;7:33.

76. Eichenbaum H, Sauvage M, Fortin N, Komorowski R, Lipton P. Towards a functional organization of episodic memory in the medial temporal lobe. Neurosci Biobehav Rev. 2012;36:1597–608.

77. Witter MP, Van Hoesen GW, Amaral DG. Topographical organization of the entorhinal projection to the dentate gyrus of the monkey. J Neurosci. 1989;9(1):216–28.

78. Witter MP, Amaral DG. Entorhinal cortex of the monkey: V. Projections to the dentate gyrus, hippocampus, and subicular complex. J Comp Neurol. 1991;307(3):437–59.

79. Davis KE, Eacott MJ, Easton A, Gigg J. Episodic-like memory is sensitive to both Alzheimer's-like pathological accumulation and normal ageing processes in mice. Behav Brain Res. 2013;254:73–82.

80. Tronche C, Lestage P, Louis C, Carrie I, Béracochéa D. Pharmacological modulation of contextual "episodic-like" memory in aged mice. Behav Brain Res. 2010;215:255–60.

81. Da Silva Costa-Aze V, Dauphin F, Boulouard M. Serotonin 5-HT6 receptor blockade reverses the age-related deficits of recognition memory and working memory in mice. Behav Brain Res. 2011;222:134–40.

82. Cameron HA, Woolley CS, McEwen BS, Gould E. Differentiation of newly born neurons and glia in the dentate gyrus of the adult rat. Neuroscience. 1993;56:337–44.

83. Nakashiba T, Cushman JD, Pelkey KA, Renaudineau S, Buhl DL, McHugh TJ, Rodriguez Barrera V, Chittajallu R, Iwamoto KS, McBain CJ, et al. Young dentate granule cells mediate pattern separation, whereas old granule cells facilitate pattern completion. Cell. 2012;149:188–201.

84. Zhao C, Deng W, Gage FH. Mechanisms and functional implications of adult neurogenesis. Cell. 2008;132:645–60.

85. Li Y, Stam FJ, Aimone JB, Goulding M, Callaway EM, Gage FH. Molecular layer perforant path-associated cells contribute to feed-forward inhibition in the adult dentate gyrus. Proc Natl Acad Sci USA. 2013;110:9106–11.

86. Vuksic M, Del Turco D, Vlachos A, Schuldt G, Müller CM, Schneider G, Deller T. Unilateral entorhinal denervation leads to long-lasting dendritic alterations of mouse hippocampal granule cells. Exp Neurol. 2011;230:176–85.

87. Moorthi P, Premkumar P, Priyanka R, Jayachandran KS, Anusuyadevi M. Pathological changes in hippocampal neuronal circuits underlie age-associated neurodegeneration and memory loss: positive clue toward SAD. Neuroscience. 2015;301:90–105.

88. Kesner RP, Rolls ET. A computational theory of hippocampal function, and tests of the theory: new developments. Neurosci Biobehav Rev. 2015;48:92–147.

89. Nilsson M, Perfilieva E, Johansson U, Orwar O, Eriksson PS. Enriched environment increases neurogenesis in the adult rat dentate gyrus and improves spatial memory. J Neurobiol. 1999;39:569–78.

90. Bruel-Jungerman E, Laroche S, Rampon C. New neurons in the dentate gyrus are involved in the expression of enhanced long-term memory following environmental enrichment. Eur J Neurosci. 2005;21:513–21.

91. Halassa MM, Haydon PG. Integrated brain circuits: astrocytic networks modulate neuronal activity and behavior. Annu Rev Physiol. 2010;72:335–55.

92. Halassa MM, Fellin T, Haydon PG. Tripartite synapses: roles for astrocytic purines in the control of synaptic physiology and behavior. Neuropharmacology. 2009;57:343–6.

93. Halassa MM, Fellin T, Takano H, Dong JH, Haydon PG. Synaptic islands defined by the territory of a single astrocyte. J Neurosci. 2007;27:6473–7.

94. Reichenbach A, Derouiche A, Kirchhoff F. Morphology and dynamics of perisynaptic glia. Brain Res Rev. 2010;63:11–25.

95. Genoud C, Quairiaux C, Steiner P, Hirling H, Welker E, Knott GW. Plasticity of astrocytic coverage and glutamate transporter expression in adult mouse cortex. PLoS Biol. 2006;4:e343.

96. Van Loo PL, Van Zutphen LF, Baumans V. Male management: Coping with aggression problems in male laboratory mice. Lab Anim. 2003;37(4):300–13.

97. Mouton PR, Long JM, Lei DL, Howard V, Jucker M, Calhoun ME, Ingram DK. Age and gender effects on microglia and astrocyte numbers in brains of mice. Brain Res. 2002;956:30–5.

98. Johnson RT, Breedlove SM, Jordan CL. Sex differences and laterality in astrocyte number and complexity in the adult rat medial amygdala. J Comp Neurol. 2008;511:599–609.

99. Luquin S, Naftolin F, Garcia-Segura LM. Natural fluctuation and gonadal hormone regulation of astrocyte immunoreactivity in dentate gyrus. J Neurobiol. 1993;24:913–24.

100. Johnson RT, Schneider A, DonCarlos LL, Breedlove SM, Jordan CL. Astrocytes in the rat medial amygdala are responsive to adult androgens. J Comp Neurol. 2012;520:2531–44.

101. Lei DL, Long JM, Hengemihle J, O'Neill J, Manaye KF, Ingram DK, Mouton PR. Effects of estrogen and raloxifene on neuroglia number and morphology in the hippocampus of aged female mice. Neuroscience. 2003;121:659–66.

102. Liu WL, Lee YH, Tsai SY, Hsu CY, Sun YY, Yang LY, Tsai SH, Yang WC. Methylprednisolone inhibits the expression of glial fibrillary acidic protein and chondroitin sulfate proteoglycans in reactivated astrocytes. Glia. 2008;56:1390–400.

103. Rodríguez JJ, Yeh CY, Terzieva S, Olabarria M, Kulijewicz-Nawrot M, Verkhratsky A. Complex and region-specific changes in astroglial markers in the aging brain. Neurobiol Aging. 2014;35:15–23. doi:10.1016/j.neurobiolaging.2013.07.002.

104. van Praag H, Kempermann G, Gage FH. Running increases cell proliferation and neurogenesis in the adult mouse dentate gyrus. Nat Neurosci. 1999;2:266–70.

105. Williamson LL, Chao A, Bilbo SD. Environmental enrichment alters glial antigen expression and neuroimmune function in the adult rat hippocampus. Brain Behav Immun. 2012;26:500–10.

106. Diniz DG, Foro CAR, Rego CMD, Gloria DA, de Oliveira FRR, Paes JMP, de Sousa AA, Tokuhashi TP, Trindade LS, Turiel MCP, et al. Environmental impoverishment and aging alter object recognition, spatial learning, and dentate gyrus astrocytes. Eur J Neurosci. 2010;32:509–19.

107. Slomianka L, West MJ. Estimators of the precision of stereological estimates: an example based on the CA1 pyramidal cell layer of rats. Neuroscience. 2005;136(3):757–67.

108. Hosseini-Sharifabad M, Nyengaard JR. Design-based estimation of neuronal number and individual neuronal volume in the rat hippocampus. J Neurosci Methods. 2007;162:206–14.

5

Patterns of motor activity in spontaneously hypertensive rats compared to Wistar Kyoto rats

Ole Bernt Fasmer[1,2,3] and Espen Borgå Johansen[4*]

Abstract

Background: Increased motor activity is a defining characteristic of patients with ADHD, and spontaneously hypertensive rats have been suggested to be an animal model of this disorder. In the present study, we wanted to use linear and non-linear methods to explore differences in motor activity patterns in SHR/NCrl rats compared to Wistar Kyoto (WKY/NHsd) rats.

Methods: A total number of 42 rats (23 SHR/NCrl and 19 WKY/NHsd, male and female) were tested. At PND 51, the animals' movements were video-recorded during an operant test procedure that lasted 90 min. Total activity level and velocity (mean and maximum), standard deviation (SD) and root mean square successive differences (RMSSD) were calculated. In addition, we used Fourier analysis, autocorrelations and two measures of complexity to characterize the time series; sample entropy and symbolic dynamics.

Results: The SHR/NCrl rats showed increased total activity levels in addition to increased mean and maximum velocity of movements. The variability measures, SD and RMSSD, were markedly lower in the SHR/NCrl compared to the WKY/NHsd rats. At the same time, the SHR/NCrl rats displayed a higher complexity of the time series, particularly with regard to the total activity level as evidenced by analyses of sample entropy and symbolic dynamics. Autocorrelation analyses also showed differences between the two strains. In the Fourier analysis, the SHR/NCrl rats had an increased variance in the high frequency part of the spectrum, corresponding to the time period of 9–17 s.

Conclusion: The findings show that in addition to increased total activity and velocity of movement, the organization of behavior is different in SHR/NCrl relative to WKY/NHsd controls. Compared to controls, behavioral variability is reduced in SHR/NCrl at an aggregate level, and, concomitantly, more complex and unpredictable from moment-to-moment. These finding emphasize the importance of the measures and methods used when characterizing behavioral variability. If valid for ADHD, the results indicate that decreased behavioral variability can co-exist with increased behavioral complexity, thus representing a challenge to current theories of variability in ADHD.

Keywords: ADHD, SHR, WKY, Behavioral variability, Motor activity, Video-analyses

Background

Increased motor activity is a defining characteristic of patients with attention-deficit/hyperactivity disorder (ADHD), combined and hyperactive subgroups. This is based on observations of children with ADHD and on objective registrations with actigraphs [1]. Studies of reaction times, as well as other behavioral measures in patients with ADHD, have repeatedly shown increased intraindividual variability (IIV) as a characteristic feature of ADHD [2–18].

Spontaneously hypertensive (SHR/NCrl) rats have been suggested to be an animal model of ADHD [19], and in several test paradigms display behavior similar to that seen in patients with ADHD, including increased motor activity, impulsivity, and inattention. Another similar feature observed in the behavior of SHR/NCrl is increased IIV

---

*Correspondence: espenborga.johansen@hioa.no
[4] Oslo and Akershus University College, Stensberggata 26, 0170 Oslo, Norway
Full list of author information is available at the end of the article

[20–24]. However, there are divergent views on SHR/NCrl as a valid model of ADHD [25] which may possibly be related to the control strain used in the experiments [26].

A characteristic feature of different disorders or disease processes may be increased order and regularity of behavior, i.e. reduced complexity [27, 28]. Biological systems can seldom be fully characterized by simple linear processes, and additional mathematical methods are required obtained from the field of non-linear system, complexity theory and chaos theory [29]. At a molar, aggregated level, behavioral variability is quantitatively described by measures such as standard deviation and root mean square of successive differences. However, such measures do not capture behavior variability at a local, molecular, moment-to-moment level [30]. Therefore, non-linear methods, such as different measures of complexity and entropy, have in recent years been employed to analyze biological time series. Such methods may give additional information to that obtained by traditional linear methods, and can be used to identify the underlying neural mechanisms of the system being studied.

In the present report, we have analyzed video-recorded motor behavior of SHR/NCrl rats in order to look for differences in behavioral organization between this strain and control rats of the WKY/NHsd strain. In addition to total activity levels and velocity of movement, we have used both linear and non-linear methods to analyze movement patterns. We have used standard deviation (SD) and root mean square successive differences (RMSSD) to indicate the molar, overall level of variability. These measures have been used in the study of reaction time variability in ADHD patients [31] and also in the study of motor activity of psychiatric patients assessed with actigraphs [32–34]. For analyses of molecular behavioral variability, we included analyses of autocorrelations, which have been used to assess response variability in children with ADHD [2, 3]. Additionally, to investigate variability in different frequency domains, we have employed Fourier analyses, which is a well-established method in many different fields, and which have been used together with SD and RMSSD in studies of motor activity [32–34]. To obtain a measure of complexity we have used sample entropy and symbolic dynamics which are two methods that tolerate a reasonable degree of noise (as usually is the case with biological systems). Both methods were used in the actigraph-studies mentioned above [32–34] and also in the study of reaction time variability in ADHD patients where increased variability and reduced complexity were found [31].

Reduced behavioral complexity is suggested to be a characteristic of different disorders or disease processes, and several studies show that intraindividual variability is increased in ADHD as well as in SHR/NCrl. Thus, our hypothesis when conducting this study was that the behavior of SHR/NCrl rats would be characterized by increased variability and reduced complexity compared to WKY/NHsd rats, both with regard to total activity and velocity of movement.

Methods
Subjects
A total number of 42 animals, 23 SHR/NCrl rats (11 females and 12 males) and 19 WKY/NHsd rats (11 females and 8 males) participated in the present experiment. The rats were primarily employed as controls in a behavioral study on the effects of polychlorinated biphenyl 153 in a rat model of ADHD, and had been orally administered corn oil at postnatal days (PND) 8, 14, and 20 [35]. Data from PND 51 were used in the present analyses. The study was approved by the Norwegian Animal Research Authority (NARA) (project id. no. 590), and conducted in accordance with the laws and regulations controlling experiments on live animals in Norway.

Apparatus and behavioral procedure
Details of the apparatus and experimental procedure are described in [35, 36]. In brief, 16 Campden Instruments operant chambers enclosed in sound-resistant outer housings were used in the current study. The animal's working space was 25 × 25 × 25 (height) in half of the chambers, and 25 × 25 × 20 (height) in the other half. Each chamber was equipped with two levers, one positioned on each side of a small, recessed cubicle where reinforcers (water) were delivered contingent on lever-pressing.

A variable interval 180 s schedule of reinforcement was in effect for the session analyzed in the present study and for the 17 prior sessions. A cue light was located above each lever, and only presses on the lever signaled by light produced reinforcers. Then, the cue light above the other lever was off, and pressing this lever had no consequences. Following each reinforcer delivery, the reinforcer-producing lever randomly switched side. The behavioral procedure has been described as a simultaneous visual discrimination task [36].

Behavior was recorded by a video camera manufactured by Tracer Technology Co., Ltd, Taiwan (Mini Color Hidden Cameras, 420TVL, 0,1 lux) mounted in the upper rear corner of the ceiling. The camera was controlled by the VR Live Capture computer program (Novus Security, Warsaw, Poland) saving video-files (15 frames/s) for analyses.

Video recordings
The animals were video-recorded during the whole 90-min session, and frame-to-frame analyses of changes

in pixels were performed using a computer program developed by Jensenius [37]. Changes in pixels occurred whenever the animal moved, and the total number of pixel-changes was used to quantitate the animal's locomotion [38]: Total motor activity was calculated as the sum of all pixels that changed from frame to frame divided by the total number of pixels in the video image. The center of the active pixels was used to estimate the animal's position and calculate velocity (i.e. velocity = change in position/time). For the present analyzes, seven recordings per second were used to calculate total amount of movement and velocity (mean and maximum).

Data analysis

The first 84 min of each session were used for the analysis of motor activity, either analyzed as one continuous period or divided into three separate periods of 28 min each. Data were analyzed using SPSS 18. Differences between SHR/NCrl and WKY/NHsd rats were compared using t tests except for the autocorrelations that were analyzed by way of ANOVA using Statistica 12.

Several different measures of variability were calculated and analyzed in order to characterize behavioral variability at a molar level as well as at a local level. For analyses of behavioral variability at a molar level, mean values, SD, and the RMSSD were used. Additionally, we used four other measures to characterize these motor patterns at a local, fine-grained level; sample entropy, symbolic dynamics, Fourier analysis and autocorrelations.

Standard deviation and root mean square successive differences

Each of the three 28-min periods obtained when dividing the first 84 min of the test session in three equal parts contained 130 data points. Each of these points thus encompasses data from a time period of 12.9 s, and represent respectively the total amount of motion, the average (mean) velocity or the maximum velocity during this time period. Standard deviation (SD) and RMSSD were both expressed as percent of the mean.

Sample entropy

Sample entropy (http://www.physionet.org) is a non-linear measure developed to compute the regularity of heart rate and other time series [32, 39–41]. Sample entropy is the negative natural logarithm of an estimate of the conditional probability that two sequences that are similar for m points, within a tolerance, remain similar at the next point. Data were normalized before analysis. According to Richman and Moorman [41], we chose the following parameters: $m = 2$ and $r = 0.2$. Time periods of 12.9 s were used for the sample entropy analyses. Sample entropy was calculated using a program downloaded

from the web-site PhysioNet, a resource site for the analysis of physiological signals (http://www.physionet.org). This program calculates the sample entropy of time series given in a text format input-file.

Symbolic dynamics

The same time series as used for the sample entropy analyses were employed to analyze symbolic dynamics (time periods of 12.9 s). The time series were transformed into series of symbols according to the method described by [42, 43]. For each sequence analyzed, the difference between the maximum and minimum value was divided into 6 equal portions (1–6) and each value of the series was assigned a number from 1 to 6, such that the transformed time series consisted of a string of numbers from 1 to 6. The series were then divided into overlapping sequences of three consecutive numbers. Each sequence was assigned one of four symbols according to the following rule: (1) 0 V—a pattern with no variation (e.g. pattern 333 or 555), (2) 1 V—a pattern with only one variation where two consecutive symbols are equal and the remaining symbol is different (e.g. 522 or 331), (3) 2LV—a pattern with two like variations, such that the 3 symbols ascend or descend (e.g., 641 or 235), and, (4) 2UV—a pattern with two unlike variations (both ascending and descending, e.g., 312 or 451). The occurrence of these four patterns (0, 1 V, 2LV, 2UV) were counted and the results presented as the percentage of the total number of sequences analyzed (n = 129). The symbolic dynamic analyses give an indication of the complexity of the time series.

Fourier analysis

For the Fourier analyses (http://www.physionet.org), the first 84 min of the test session were divided into three equal parts, each containing 390 data points, and the middle 256 points from these time series were used. Each data point thus represents a time period of 4.3 s. The reason for using 256 data points is that the Fourier analysis requires series with a length that represents a power of 2 (64, 128, 256). Data were normalized before analysis and no windows were applied. Results are presented as the relation between variance in the high frequency part of the spectrum, 0.116–0.0581 Hz, corresponding to the period 9–17 s, and the low frequency part, 0.0581–0.00091 Hz, corresponding to 17–1100 s.

Autocorrelations

The first 84 min of the session were divided into three 28-min sequences, and serial correlations (autocorrelations) of movement and velocity were calculated for each of the three sequences thus expressing the predictability or variability of behavior within a sequence of observations. A total of 42 lags were calculated, where the correlation between e.g. movement at time t and movement at time t + 1 represents lag 1, the correlation between movement at time t and movement at time t + 2 represents lag 2, and so forth. The autocorrelations were calculated for seven recordings of movement or velocity per second. Thus, the 42 lags represent a time period of approximately 6 s.

Results

Total motor activity

The SHR/NCrl rats showed substantially higher total motor activity than the WKY/NHsd rats during all three sequences of the test session; 437, 542 and 426% of the activity of the WKY/NHsd rats (Table 1).

At a molar level, both the SD and the RMSSD measures showed reduced behavioral variability in the SHR/NCrl rats. In the three sequences, the SDs in SHR/NCrl were 52, 53 and 53% and the RMSSDs were 55, 51 and 53% of the corresponding values for the WKY/NHsd. Calculating variability for total motor activity without correcting for mean values (using absolute SD values) showed higher variability for SHR/NCrl compared to WKY/NHsd rats, with values that were 214, 284 and 275% of the corresponding values for the WKY/NHsd rats in the three sequences. For RMSSD, the absolute values were also higher for SHR/NCrl compared to WKY/NHsd rats. The values were 226, 279 and 271% of the corresponding values for the WKY/NHsd rats in the three sequences (Table 4).

At a molecular level, the Fourier analysis showed that the SHR/NCrl rats had an increased ratio of variance in the high frequency range compared to the low frequency range (16, 13 and 22% higher than the WKY/NHsd rats),

but these differences were not significant. The sample entropy was for the SHR/NCrl rats increased to 150, 151 and 164% of the corresponding values for the WKY/NHsd rats in the three sequences. The symbolic dynamic analyses showed that the SHR/NCrl rats had lower values for the 0 and 1 V measures, particularly in the second and third sequences, and correspondingly higher values for 2LV and 2UV. Analyses of motor activity autocorrelations (Fig. 1) showed no statistically significant main effects of strain for the three sequences analyzed. However, statistically significant strain x lag interaction effects were found in all three sequences (0–28, 28–56 and 56–84 min): $F_{(41, 1640)} = 3.59$; $p < 0.0001$, $F_{(41, 1640)} = 6.68$; $p < 0.0001$, and $F_{(41, 1640)} = 7.94$; $p < 0.0001$, respectively. Newman-Keuls post hoc analyses of these significant effects showed that the autocorrelation for lag 1 was higher in SHR/NCrl than in WKY/NHsd controls in all the three sequences, were lower for lags 3–5 in the second sequence, and higher for lags 3–4 in the third sequence ($ps < 0.05$).

Velocity

The mean velocities of the SHR/NCrl were also significantly higher than in the WKY/NHsd rats, but the differences were smaller than for the motor activity. Mean velocity for the SHR/NCrl rats were 164, 195 and 185% of the corresponding values for the WKY/NHsd rats in the three test sequences (Table 2). This difference is illustrated in Fig. 2 showing mean velocity over time during the third sequence for one SHR/NCrl and one WKY/NHsd rat.

At a molar level, and similar to the findings for the motor activity, both the SD and the RMSSD measures showed lower variability in the SHR/NCrl rats. In the

Table 1 Total amount of motor activity

	WKY	SHR	WKY	SHR	WKY	SHR
	0–28 min		28–56 min		56–84 min	
Mean	671 ± 256	2935 ± 919***	424 ± 205	2298 ± 818***	482 ± 259	2054 ± 658***
SD	136 ± 72	71 ± 33**	125 ± 33	66 ± 19***	124 ± 31	66 ± 11***
RMSSD	159 ± 91	87 ± 43**	163 ± 41	83 ± 26***	162 ± 40	86 ± 16***
Sample entropy	1.25 ± 0.65	1.87 ± 0.53**	1.32 ± 0.40	1.99 ± 0.40***	1.27 ± 0.46	2.08 ± 0.36**
Fourier analysis	0.56 ± 0.19	0.65 ± 0.17	0.62 ± 0.18	0.70 ± 0.21	0.63 ± 0.22	0.77 ± 0.26
Symbolic dynamics						
0 V	0.6 ± 1.8	0.0 ± 0.0	3.0 ± 3.4	0.0 ± 0.0**	3.7 ± 4.8	0.0 ± 0.2**
1 V	3.7 ± 3.0	0.1 ± 0.4***	10.1 ± 6.0	0.2 ± 0.5***	9.9 ± 6.1	0.6 ± 1.0***
2LV	33.8 ± 3.4	35.5 ± 3.6	28.6 ± 4.8	36.0 ± 4.7***	30.0 ± 5.0	34.4 ± 5.7*
2UV	61.9 ± 3.7	64.4 ± 3.6*	58.3 ± 7.6	63.8 ± 4.5**	56.5 ± 8.0	64.9 ± 5.4***

Activity was analyzed using time periods of 12.9 s. SD and RMSSD are given as % of the mean. For the Fourier analysis results are presented as variance in the high frequency range divided by the variance in the low frequency range. All data are given as mean ± SD

t tests: * p < 0.05, ** p < 0.01, *** p < 0.001

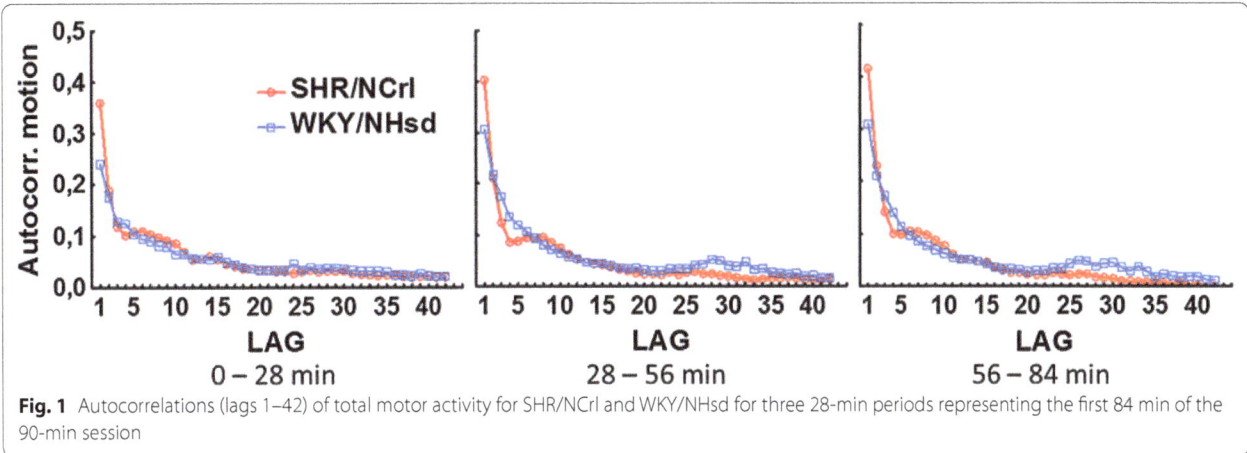

Fig. 1 Autocorrelations (lags 1–42) of total motor activity for SHR/NCrl and WKY/NHsd for three 28-min periods representing the first 84 min of the 90-min session

Table 2 Mean velocity

	WKY	SHR	WKY	SHR	WKY	SHR
	0–28 min		28–56 min		56–84 min	
Mean	146 ± 20	240 ± 37***	110 ± 24	214 ± 36***	107 ± 25	198 ± 32***
SD	51 ± 9	32 ± 4***	65 ± 10	35 ± 4***	66 ± 13	37 ± 7***
RMSSD	59 ± 10	39 ± 5***	80 ± 16	45 ± 7***	81 ± 16	49 ± 10***
Sample entropy	2.01 ± 0.24	2.20 ± 0.36	2.14 ± 0.33	2.15 ± 0.25	2.05 ± 0.4	2.25 ± 0.28
Fourier analysis	0.52 ± 0.10	0.68 ± 0.20**	0.42 ± 0.09	0.71 ± 0.16***	0.43 ± 0.10	0.76 ± 0.22***
Symbolic dynamics						
0 V	0.1 ± 0.3	0.0 ± 0.0	0.3 ± 0.8	0.0 ± 0.0	1.3 ± 3.5	0.0 ± 0.0
1 V	2.3 ± 2.1	1.0 ± 1.2*	3.0 ± 3.1	1.3 ± 1.0*	3.9 ± 4.6	2.1 ± 1.6
2LV	33.6 ± 4.0	34.9 ± 4.7	34.2 ± 5.1	34.9 ± 4.1	35.0 ± 4.6	32.8 ± 3.9
2UV	64.1 ± 4.1	63.8 ± 4.1	62.5 ± 5.0	63.8 ± 4.3	59.8 ± 6.2	65.1 ± 3.8**

Mean velocity was analyzed using time periods of 12.9 s. SD and RMSSD are given as % of the mean. For the Fourier analysis results are presented as variance in the high frequency range divided by the variance in the low frequency range. All data are given as mean ± SD

t tests: * $p < 0.05$, ** $p < 0.01$, *** $p < 0.001$

three test sequences, the SDs of the SHR/NCrl rats were 63, 54 and 56% of the values for the WKY/NHsd rats, and 66, 56 and 60% for the RMSSDs. Calculating variability without correcting for mean values (using absolute SD values) showed higher variability for SHR/NCrl compared to WKY/NHsd rats, with SDs that were 103, 106 and 104% of the corresponding values for the WKY/NHsd rats in the three sequences. For RMSSD, the absolute values were also higher for SHR/NCrl compared to WKY/NHsd rats with values that were 108, 111 and 113% of the corresponding values for the WKY/NHsd rats in the three sequences (Table 4).

At a molecular level, the Fourier analysis showed that the SHR/NCrl rats had a significantly increased ratio of variance in the high frequency range compared to the low frequency range. In SHR/NCrl, this ratio was found to be 31, 69 and 77% higher than for the WKY/NHsd rats

in the three sequences. As an illustration, Fig. 3 shows the Fourier analysis results during the third sequence for the same animals as in Fig. 2. Contrary to the findings for motor activity, the sample entropy values did not differ between the SHR/NCrl and the WKY/NHsd rats. The symbolic dynamic analyses showed lower values in SHR/NCrl for the 0 and 1 V measures, but only significantly different from WKY/NHsd for 1 V in the first and second sequences, and significantly higher values in SHR/NCrl for 2UV in the third sequence. Further, the analyses showed that autocorrelations of velocity (Fig. 4) were lower in SHR/NCrl than in WKY/NHsd controls in all three sequences (0–28, 28–56 and 56–84 min): $F_{(1, 40)} = 5.69$; $p < 0.05$, $F_{(1, 40)} = 17.11$; $p < 0.001$, and $F_{(1, 40)} = 8.97$; $p < 0.01$, respectively. The analyses also showed a statistically significant strain × lag interaction effect during the third sequence, $F_{(41, 1640)} = 1.84$;

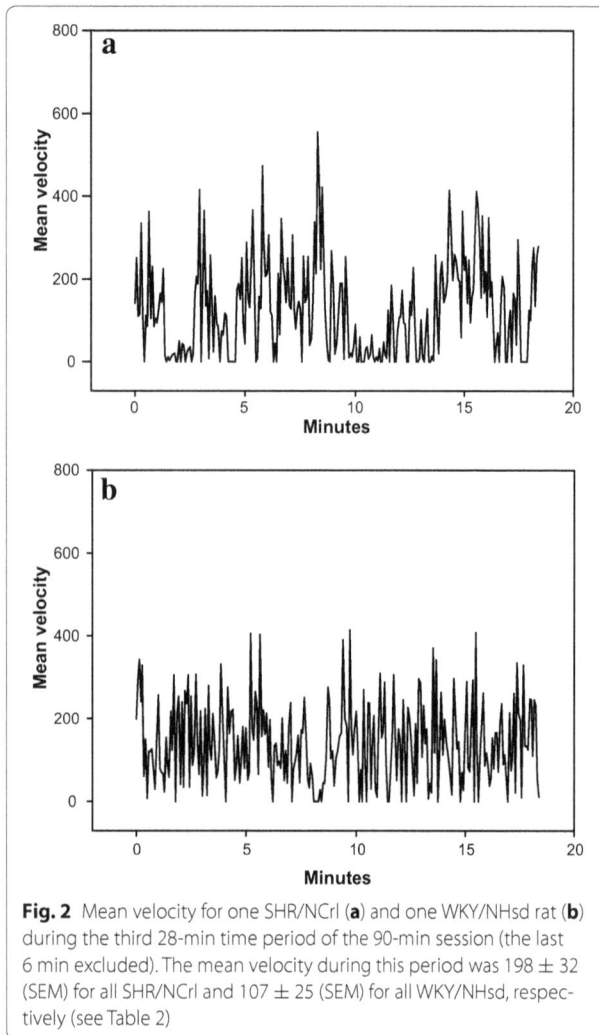

Fig. 2 Mean velocity for one SHR/NCrl (**a**) and one WKY/NHsd rat (**b**) during the third 28-min time period of the 90-min session (the last 6 min excluded). The mean velocity during this period was 198 ± 32 (SEM) for all SHR/NCrl and 107 ± 25 (SEM) for all WKY/NHsd, respectively (see Table 2)

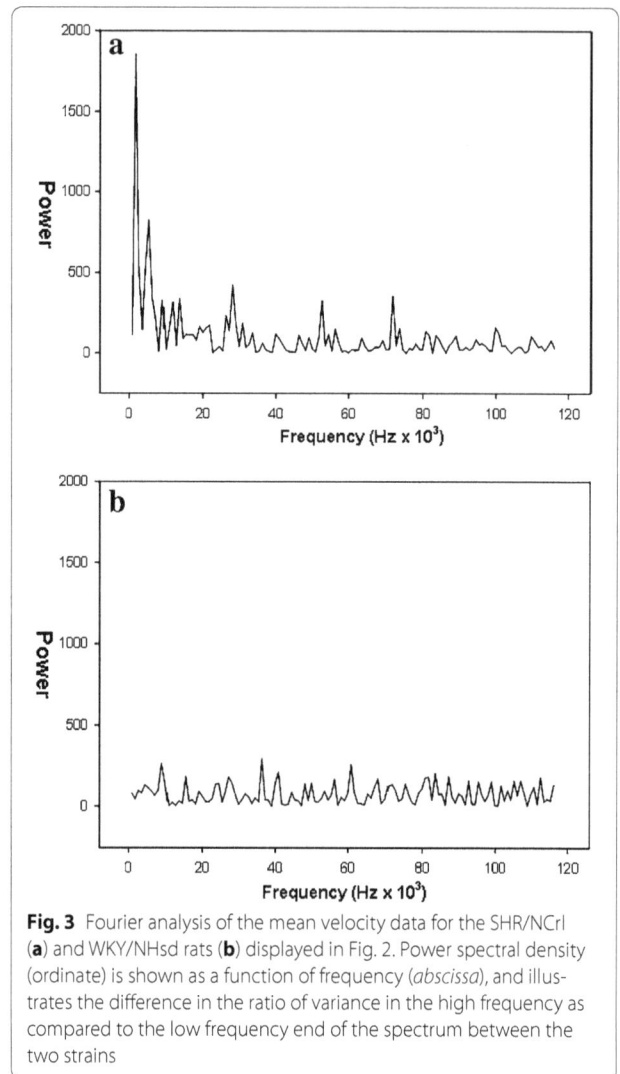

Fig. 3 Fourier analysis of the mean velocity data for the SHR/NCrl (**a**) and WKY/NHsd rats (**b**) displayed in Fig. 2. Power spectral density (ordinate) is shown as a function of frequency (*abscissa*), and illustrates the difference in the ratio of variance in the high frequency as compared to the low frequency end of the spectrum between the two strains

$p < 0.001$. Newman-Keuls post hoc tests showed that autocorrelations were lower in SHR/NCrl than in WKY/NHsd for lags 2–5 (*ps* < 0.05).

The maximum velocities of the SHR/NCrl rats were significantly higher than those of the WKY/NHsd rats, but the differences were smaller than for the mean velocity. The values for the SHR/NCrl rats were 12, 23 and 22% higher than the corresponding values for the WKY/NHsd rats in the three test sequences (Table 3). Similar to the findings for the motor activity and the mean velocity, both the SD and the RMSSD measures showed lower variability in the SHR/NCrl rats. In the three test sequences, the SDs for the SHR/NCrl rats were 67, 55 and 59% of the values for the WKY/NHsd rats, whereas the corresponding values for the RMSSDs were 69, 61 and 63%. Calculating variability without correcting for mean values (using absolute SD values) showed lower variability for SHR/NCrl compared to WKY/NHsd rats for maximum velocity, with values that were 76, 69 and 73% of the corresponding values for the WKY/NHsd rats in the three sequences. For RMSSD, the absolute values were also lower for SHR/NCrl compared to WKY/NHsd rats, with values that were 78, 75 and 77% of the corresponding values for the WKY/NHsd rats in the three sequences (Table 4).

Again, and similar to the findings for the mean velocity, the Fourier analysis showed that the SHR/NCrl rats had an increased ratio of variance in the high frequency range compared to the low frequency range. In SHR/NCrl, these were found to be 24, 44 and 38% higher than for the WKY/NHsd rats. The sample entropy values did not differ between the SHR/NCrl and the WKY/NHsd rats. The symbolic dynamic analyses showed that the SHR/NCrl rats had significantly lower values for the 1 V measure in all three sequences, and correspondingly higher values for 2UV in the second and third sequence.

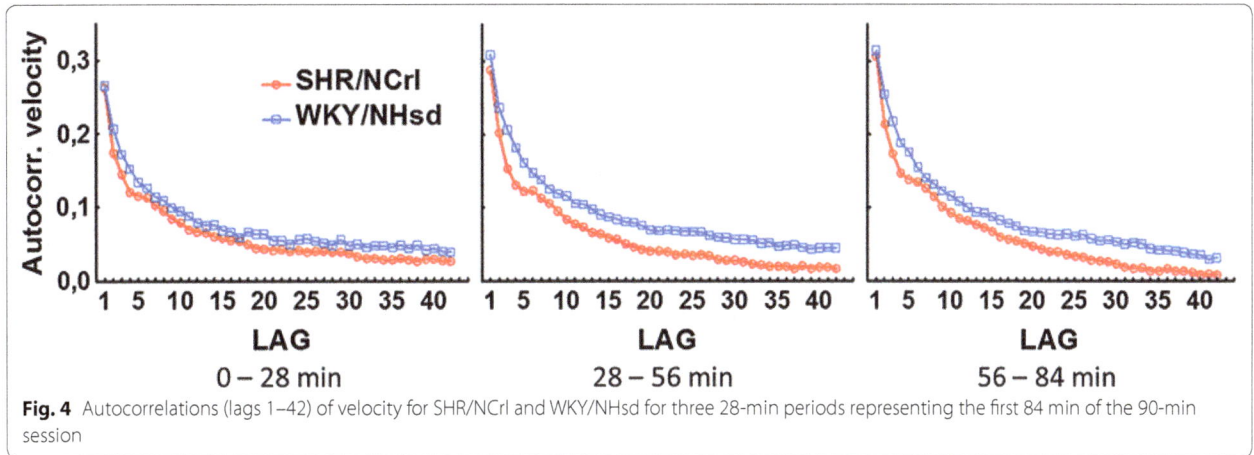

Fig. 4 Autocorrelations (lags 1–42) of velocity for SHR/NCrl and WKY/NHsd for three 28-min periods representing the first 84 min of the 90-min session

Table 3 Maximum velocity

	WKY	SHR	WKY	SHR	WKY	SHR
	0–28 min		28–56 min		56–84 min	
Mean	1302 ± 185	1455 ± 174**	1133 ± 206	1391 ± 166***	1137 ± 203	1388 ± 194***
SD	49 ± 8	33 ± 7***	56 ± 9	31 ± 5***	56 ± 12	33 ± 4***
RMSSD	62 ± 8	43 ± 8***	71 ± 11	43 ± 8***	72 ± 15	45 ± 7***
Sample entropy	1.94 ± 0.24	1.90 ± 0.21	2.01 ± 0.19	2.02 ± 0.19	1.96 ± 0.49	2.13 ± 0.27
Fourier analysis	0.66 ± 0.16	0.82 ± 0.18**	0.52 ± 0.09	0.75 ± 0.15***	0.55 ± 0.13	0.76 ± 0.22**
Symbolic dynamics						
0 V	0.1 ± 0.4	0.0 ± 0.0	0.3 ± 0.8	0.0 ± 0.0	1.2 ± 3.5	0.0 ± 0.0
1 V	1.8 ± 1.8	0.7 ± 0.9*	2.3 ± 3.0	0.8 ± 1.2*	3.7 ± 4.3	0.9 ± 1.0*
2LV	33.6 ± 2.9	34.2 ± 3.4	34.4 ± 3.3	32.3 ± 3.9	35.1 ± 4.7	33.7 ± 2.4
2UV	64.6 ± 3.4	65.1 ± 3.6	63.0 ± 3.4	66.9 ± 4.1**	60.0 ± 6.3	65.5 ± 2.5**

Maximum velocity was analyzed using time periods of 12.9 s. SD and RMSSD are given as % of the mean. For the Fourier analysis results are presented as variance in the high frequency range divided by the variance in the low frequency range. All data are given as mean ± SD

t tests: * $p < 0.05$, ** $p < 0.01$, *** $p < 0.001$

Table 4 Results from analysis of variability without correcting for mean values, but using absolute values for SD and RMSSD

	Motor activity			Mean velocity			Maximum velocity		
	WKY	SHR	p	WKY	SHR	p	WKY	SHR	p
SD									
0–28 min	880	1882	0.001	73	75	0.591	633	484	0.001
28–56 min	506	1438	0.001	70	74	0.452	631	435	0.001
56–84 min	481	1325	0.001	69	72	0.353	630	461	0.001
RMSSD									
0–28 min	2308	1021	0.001	86	93	0.095	813	634	0.001
28–56 min	1788	641	0.001	85	94	0.042	801	602	0.001
56–84 min	1702	629	0.001	84	95	0.016	809	624	0.001

In Table 5 are presented correlations between mean values of motor activity, mean velocity, maximum velocity and the different variability measures we have used in Tables 1, 2 and 3. These correlations are given for each strain separately and together. Analysis of sex differences did not reveal any consistent pattern with regard to differences between SHR/NCrl and WKY/NHsd rats, test sequences or the different parameters used, and are therefore not reported.

Discussion

The present study examined organization of video-recorded motor behavior in SHR/NCrl and WKY/NHsd controls using linear and non-linear methods. The main finding of the present study is that the motor activity of SHR/NCrl rats is different from WKY/NHsd rats in a number of ways, not only at the level of activity. The SHR/NCrl rats display increased mean and maximum velocity of their movements in addition to a pronounced increased total activity level. Concurrently, the organization of behavior is different in SHR/NCrl and WKY/NHsd controls. At a molar level of analysis, the variability of the time series, the SD and RMSSD, is markedly lower in SHR/NCrl compared to the WKY/NHsd rats when

these measures are expressed as percent of the mean. At a molecular level of analysis, in contrast, the Fourier analysis shows that in the SHR/NCrl rats there is an increased variance in the high frequency part of the spectrum, corresponding to a time period of 9–17 s. When analyzing the time series with symbolic dynamics, the SHR/NCrl rats appear to have a higher behavioral complexity, particularly with regard to the total activity level. Similarly, using sample entropy, the complexity of the time series of total activity is higher in the SHR/NCrl rats than in the WKY/NHsd rats, and the lower autocorrelations of velocity in SHR/NCrl than in WKY/NHsd controls show that behavior is less systematic and less predictable from one occurrence to the next in the SHR/NCrl.

The increased total activity level of SHR/NCrl rats compared to the WKY/NHsd strain is in accordance with previous studies and in agreement with SHR/NCrl rats as a model of ADHD [20–24, 44, 45]. Increased activity is a defining feature of ADHD and has been confirmed using objective registrations of motor activity in patients [1, 46].

In SHR/NCrl, increased IIV has been found across a variety of behaviors including maze performance, lever pressing and nose poking [20–24, 44, 45]. The markedly

Table 5 Correlations between motor activity, mean velocity, maximum velocity and measures of variability in WKY and SHR rats in sequence 2 (28–56 min), each strain analyzed separately (A) and together (B)

	Motor activity		Mean velocity		Maximum velocity	
	WKY	SHR	WKY	SHR	WKY	SHR
A						
SD	−0.391	−0.523*	−0.691**	−0.114	−0.009	0.253
RMSSD	−0.611**	−0.596**	−0.821***	−0.443*	−0.091	0.171
Sample entropy	0.195	0.428*	−0.086	−0.382	0.653**	0.030
Fourier analysis	0.092	−0.328	0.250	−0.417*	0.315	−0.165
Symbolic dynamics						
0V	−0.439	–	−0.207	–	0.115	–
1V	−0.678**	−0.401	−0.211	−0.169	0.015	−0.417**
2LV	0.471*	0.016	0.278	0.018	−0.178	−0.112
2UV	0.437	0.026	−0.121	0.021	0.141	0.217

	Motor activity	Mean velocity	Maximum velocity
B			
SD	−0.760***	−0.859***	−0.466**
RMSSD	−0.802***	−0.875***	−0.472**
Sample entropy	0.686***	−0.107	0.307*
Fourier analysis	0.041	0.559***	0.407**
Symbolic dynamics			
0V	−0.505**	−0.283	−0.088
1V	−0.719***	−0.388*	−0.266
2LV	0.559***	0.132	−0.272
2UV	0.397**	0.102	0.396**

reduced molar IIV in SHR/NCrl, as measured with SD and RMSSD, found in the present study is therefore at first glance surprising and inconsistent with the findings of Perry et al. [24] who used an identical experimental procedure to the one used in the present study, where total test-time was divided into 5 segments, and IIV for operant lever-pressing was expressed as the absolute difference between behavior in each segment and the total test-time mean. One important difference between the studies is that Perry et al. analyzed reinforcer-controlled lever pressing only, whereas the video-recorded behavior analyzed in the present study included reinforcer-controlled movements (lever approach, presses, tray visits, and reinforcer consummation) as well as other movements not controlled by the scheduled reinforcers (e.g. grooming, exploration and motor control). The impact of each of these processes on the observed changes in IIV in SHR/NCrl cannot be disentangled in the present study, but may have contributed to the inconsistent findings. A second important difference between the two studies is that Perry et al. used variability measures corrected for mean whereas SD and RMSSD mean corrections were used in the present study. Although uncorrected SDs and RMSSDs in the present study were higher in SHR/NCrl than in controls for total activity, the means were also much higher in SHR/NCrl than in controls. Thus, the mean-corrections produced lower SDs and RMSSDs in SHR/NCrl than in controls, and it has been argued that this procedure may be overly conservative and over-correct for SHR/NCrl phenotype [24]. In the analysis of mean velocity, uncorrected SDs and RMSSDs were also higher in SHR/NCrl than in controls, but the differences were smaller, whereas uncorrected SDs and RMSSDs for maximum velocity were lower in SHR/NCrl than in controls. Comparing total activity, mean and maximum velocity using uncorrected SD and RMSSD would therefore give inconsistent results, while correcting for mean gives a consistent picture, with lower SD and RMSSD for SHR/NCrl compared to controls in the range of 51–69%.

Mean corrections have been discussed within the ADHD literature for measures of reaction time (RT) and reaction time variability. In these studies, intraindividual variability has commonly been measured as the standard deviation of RTs without mean correction. Studies have shown that although correlated, RT mean and RT standard deviation have independent components of variance [47]. Additionally, increased mean RT and RT variability may have shared etiology in ADHD [48]. Thus, by correcting for mean, there is a risk of controlling for what one intends to study [49].

The question of dependence between the mean and measures of variability is highly relevant in the present study because the increased mean activity level and variability measures in SHR/NCrl could be expressions of one underlying factor. When looking at data from both rat strains, there are strong correlations between the variability measures and mean values for motor activity, velocity and maximum velocity, and these correlations parallel the differences in variability measures between the strains. However, when examining each strain separately there are fewer correlations and the pattern is clearly different for the two strains. We think this shows that the differences seen between the two strains do not simply reflect differences in total motor activity or velocity of movement, and that studying variability measures give added information concerning the organization of motor activity.

Overall, the analyses of video-recorded behavior during the operant task suggest that behavior is organized differently in SHR/NCrl as compared to WKY/NHsd controls: At a molar level, SHR/NCrl behavior is less variable whereas behavior at a molecular level is more complex than in controls. Increased molecular behavioral complexity in SHR/NCrl compared to WKY/NHsd was found in the Fourier analyses for both mean velocity and maximum velocity of movement, and is consistent with the symbolic dynamics analyses, and the autocorrelations analyses for velocity of movement.

Studying movement patterns, Paulus et al. [50] found differences between Fischer, Lewis, and Sprague–Dawley rats using a spatial scaling exponent quantifying the degree of linear movement versus movement within a circumscribed area (low versus high scaling exponent, respectively), that may in some respect resemble the complexity test we have used. They suggested that a lower scaling exponent in Sprague–Dawley rats compared to Fischer and Lewis rats was related to differences in central serotonergic systems. In a study of SHR and WKY rats, Li and Huang [51] found that the scaling exponent was higher in SHR rats, in accordance with our finding of a higher complexity of total motor activity in these rats. Previous studies have shown a range of neurological changes in SHR. We are in our study unable to separate the possible role of dopaminergic and serotonergic systems in the regulation of movement patterns, and there are differences between SHR and WKY rats in both these systems. Additionally, changes in noradrenergic, glutaminergic neurotransmission and several other systems have been shown in SHR [19, 26, 52–55].

The present finding may partly reflect basic motor processes and point to important differences in the neuronal organization of basic motor activity in SHR/NCrl compared to WKY/NHsd rats. This may indicate similar differences in motor activity regulation in patients with ADHD vs. controls. In a study of reaction times during the CPT-II test, higher variability (using SD and RMSSD) was found in adult ADHD patients compared to clinical controls, but at the same time lower complexity as measured with sample entropy and symbolic dynamic analysis was found in the ADHD group [31]. This finding, an inverse relation between measures of variability and complexity, mirrors the relation between the same measures in the present study. We have seen this same inverse relationship also in a study of motor activity in depressed and schizophrenic patients [32].

Reduced complexity of physiological systems has been postulated to be associated with disease and aging [28], but this may depend on the dynamics of the system under study. Vaillancourt and Newell [56] have suggested that in systems with intrinsic oscillations the opposite may occur, namely that disease processes are accompanied by increased complexity. This has been found in the motor activity of schizophrenic patients [32], and the present findings may fit the same pattern.

Another way to conceptualize the present findings on intraindividual variability is to compare them with human studies showing that variability patterns are different when comparing measures of brain function and behavior. Garrett et al. [57] found in an imaging study that blood oxygen level-dependent signal variability (brain variability) was lower in older compared to younger persons, while reaction time speed variability on different cognitive tasks was higher. Similarly, McIntosh et al. [58] found, when comparing children and young adults, that maturation was accompanied by increased variability of EEG-signals and reduced variability of response times on a facial recognition task.

Studies of behavioral variability in ADHD have produced a complex set of findings. Studying children with ADHD using autocorrelations, predictability of responses was found to be lower in ADHD (i.e. responding was more variable), consistent with the current findings [2]. Additionally, the autocorrelations in ADHD were found to be sensitive to the reinforcement contingencies [3], which has also been found for response time variability [59]. In a study of reaction times in children with ADHD, Castellanos et al. [6] found evidence of multisecond oscillations, with a cycle length of approximately 20 s, and they suggested that this might be due to deficiencies in dopaminergic regulations in the patients. This is intriguingly similar to the findings with Fourier analysis in the present study. Using Fourier analyses, Karalunas et al. found more low-frequency variability and higher faster-frequency variability in ADHD, with non-significant differences between frequency bands [60]. In a study of children with ADHD, Wood et al. [46] found, in addition to increased motor activity, also increased intraindividual variability of the intensity of movements. On the

other hand [61], a study of adult ADHD patients found that the patients had both increased activity levels and reduced daytime variability patterns compared to controls. In another study in adults, ADHD patients did not show increased activity levels compared to controls, and variability measures (SD and RMSSD) were not altered, but Fourier analyses revealed higher power in the high frequency range, corresponding to the period from 2 to 8 min [31].

Several mechanisms underlying the increased IIV observed in ADHD have been proposed, including deficient astrocyte energy supply to active neurons, state regulation and working memory problems, arousal-attention regulation, and altered learning processes (see [11, 49] for reviews of etiological models of reaction time variability). The complexity of findings is a challenge to current theories of IIV in ADHD, and obviously underscore the need for further studies that compare measures used to characterize variability, examine possible discrepancies between molar and molecular analyses of variability, and explore variability patterns in both patients and animal models.

The current findings add to this complexity by suggesting the presence of both increased molecular as well as decreased molar behavioral variability in SHR. If valid for ADHD, this finding is a new and interesting contribution to the research on IIV, and suggests that IIV in ADHD is not unitary and explained by one common principle, but may have several underlying mechanism depending on the task used and the behavior analyzed, and may be changed in opposite directions depending on the variability measures used.

There are some important limitations to the present study that must be considered. First, it is not clear what the video-recorded behavior during the operant task reflect (i.e. reinforcer-effects, grooming, exploration, basic motor organization, or other processes) or how the behavioral changes relate to underlying mechanisms. Nevertheless, several changes in IIV in SHR/NCrl were found suggesting that analyses of video-recorded behavior may be a valuable supplement to traditional behavioral measures used in studies of IIV. Second, the decreased molar IIV found in SHR/NCrl relative to controls is based on analyses of SD and RMSSD correcting for mean. However, the use of mean correction has been debated in the ADHD literature, and has been argued to overcorrect for phenotype in studies of SHR/NCrl [24]. The present analyses using mean corrections produced more consistent results, with variability changes in opposite directions, compared to analyses using mean corrections, underscoring the importance of mean corrections in analyses of variability.

Conclusion

This study shows that SHR/NCrl rats, a postulated animal model of ADHD, are different form WKY/NHsd rats in a number of measures related to motor activity. In addition to increased activity levels, the most pronounced findings are increased mean and maximum velocity of movements, and reduced variability for all these measures when assessed with SD and RMSSD corrected for mean. There is also an increased complexity of movement patterns in the SHR/NCrl rats. These results point to differences in the neuronal organization of movements that may be related to the known differences in neurotransmitter systems between these two rat strains. Even though these findings have no immediate implications for the diagnosis or treatment of ADHD patients, they may be used to explore further the mechanisms of motor activity regulation in general, and alterations in neurodevelopmental disorders such as ADHD.

Abbreviations
ADHD: attention-deficit/hyperactivity disorder; ANOVA: analysis of variance; EEG: electroencephalogram; IIV: intra-individual variability; PND: post-natal day; RMSSD: root mean square successive difference (the square root of the mean of the squares of the differences between adjacent time periods); SD: standard deviation; SHR/NCrl: spontaneously hypertensive rats bred by Charles River (an animal model of ADHD); WKY/NHsd: Wistar Kyoto rats bred by Harlan (a control animal for the SHR); 0V: symbolic dynamic measure representing a pattern with no variation (e.g. pattern 333 or 555); 1V: symbolic dynamic measure representing a pattern with only one variation (two consecutive symbols are equal and the remaining symbol is different, e.g. 522 or 331); 2LV: symbolic dynamic measure representing a pattern with two like variations (the 3 symbols ascend or descend, e.g., 641 or 235); 2UV: symbolic dynamic measure representing a patterns with two unlike variations (both ascending and descending, e.g., 312 or 451).

Authors' contributions
OBF had the main responsibility for analyzing the data and for drafting the manuscript. EBJ participated in designing the PCB-study from which the data are collected, performed the autocorrelation analyses, and helped drafting the manuscript. Both authors read and approved the final manuscript.

Author details
[1] Department of Clinical Medicine, Section for Psychiatry, Faculty of Medicine and Dentistry, University of Bergen, Bergen, Norway. [2] Division of Psychiatry, Haukeland University Hospital, Bergen, Norway. [3] K.G. Jebsen Centre for Research on Neuropsychiatric Disorders, Bergen, Norway. [4] Oslo and Akershus University College, Stensberggata 26, 0170 Oslo, Norway.

Acknowledgements
We thank Erlend Fasmer for making available to us the program for the symbolic dynamical analyses. We also wish to thank Alexander Refsum Jensenius and Kristian Nymoen for assistance in setting up the video equipment and providing video-analyses software, and Grete Wøien who performed the daily behavioral testing. Finally, we would like to express our sincere gratitude to Terje Sagvolden who founded *Behavioral and Brain Functions* a decade ago, was an important contributor to ADHD and SHR research, and with great enthusiasm and collaborative skills inspired and initiated studies on SHR including the present one.

Competing interests
The authors declare that they have no competing interests.

Funding
The present study was supported by grants from the Research Council of Norway (NFR 175096 and 173046), and by the European Commission (Food-CT-2006-022923-ATHON).

References
1. Teicher MH. Actigraphy and motion analysis: new tools for psychiatry. Harv Rev Psychiatry. 1995;3(1):18–35.
2. Aase H, Meyer A, Sagvolden T. Moment-to-moment dynamics of ADHD behaviour in South African children. Behav Brain Funct. 2006;2:11.
3. Aase H, Sagvolden T. Moment-to-moment dynamics of ADHD behaviour. Behav Brain Funct. 2005;1:12.
4. Adamo N, Huo L, Adelsberg S, Petkova E, Castellanos FX, Di Martino A. Response time intra-subject variability: commonalities between children with autism spectrum disorders and children with ADHD. Eur Child Adolesc Psychiatry. 2014;23(2):69–79.
5. Castellanos FX, Kelly C, Milham MP. The restless brain: attention-deficit hyperactivity disorder, resting-state functional connectivity, and intrasubject variability. Can J Psychiatry. 2009;54(10):665–72.
6. Castellanos FX, Sonuga-Barke EJ, Scheres A, Di Martino A, Hyde C, Walters JR. Varieties of attention-deficit/hyperactivity disorder-related intra-individual variability. Biol Psychiatry. 2005;57(11):1416–23.
7. Di Martino A, Ghaffari M, Curchack J, Reiss P, Hyde C, Vannucci M, Petkova E, Klein DF, Castellanos FX. Decomposing intra-subject variability in children with attention-deficit/hyperactivity disorder. Biol Psychiatry. 2008;64(7):607–14.
8. Johnson KA, Kelly SP, Bellgrove MA, Barry E, Cox M, Gill M, Robertson IH. Response variability in attention deficit hyperactivity disorder: evidence for neuropsychological heterogeneity. Neuropsychologia. 2007;45(4):630–8.
9. Karalunas SL, Geurts HM, Konrad K, Bender S, Nigg JT. Annual research review: reaction time variability in ADHD and autism spectrum disorders: measurement and mechanisms of a proposed trans-diagnostic phenotype. J Child Psychol Psychiatry. 2014;55(6):685–710.
10. Klein C, Wendling K, Huettner P, Ruder H, Peper M. Intra-subject variability in attention-deficit hyperactivity disorder. Biol Psychiatry. 2006;60(10):1088–97.
11. Kofler MJ, Rapport MD, Sarver DE, Raiker JS, Orban SA, Friedman LM, Kolomeyer EG. Reaction time variability in ADHD: a meta-analytic review of 319 studies. Clin Psychol Rev. 2013;33(6):795–811.
12. Luman M, Papanikolau A, Oosterlaan J. The unique and combined effects of reinforcement and methylphenidate on temporal information processing in attention-deficit/hyperactivity disorder. J Clin Psychopharmacol. 2015;35(4):414–21.
13. Russell VA, Oades RD, Tannock R, Killeen PR, Auerbach JG, Johansen EB, Sagvolden T. Response variability in attention-deficit/hyperactivity disorder: a neuronal and glial energetics hypothesis. Behav Brain Funct. 2006;2:30.
14. Sagvolden T, Aase H, Zeiner P, Berger D. Altered reinforcement mechanisms in attention-deficit/hyperactivity disorder. Behav Brain Res. 1998;94(1):61–71.
15. Shiels Rosch K, Dirlikov B, Mostofsky SH. Increased intrasubject variability in boys with ADHD across tests of motor and cognitive control. J Abnorm Child Psychol. 2013;41(3):485–95.
16. Tamm L, Narad ME, Antonini TN, O'Brien KM, Hawk LW Jr, Epstein JN. Reaction time variability in ADHD: a review. Neurotherapeutics. 2012;9(3):500–8.
17. van Belle J, van Hulst BM, Durston S. Developmental differences in intra-individual variability in children with ADHD and ASD. J Child Psychol Psychiatry. 2015;56(12):1316–26.
18. Williams BR, Strauss EH, Hultsch DF, Hunter MA, Tannock R. Reaction time performance in adolescents with attention deficit/hyperactivity disorder: evidence of inconsistency in the fast and slow portions of the RT distribution. J Clin Exp Neuropsychol. 2007;29(3):277–89.
19. Sagvolden T, Johansen EB. Rat models of ADHD. Curr Top Behav Neurosci. 2012;9:301–15.

20. Hunziker MH, Saldana RL, Neuringer A. Behavioral variability in SHR and WKY rats as a function of rearing environment and reinforcement contingency. J Exp Anal Behav. 1996;65(1):129–44.

21. Johansen EB, Killeen PR, Sagvolden T. Behavioral variability, elimination of responses, and delay-of-reinforcement gradients in SHR and WKY rats. Behav Brain Funct. 2007;3:60.

22. Mook DM, Jeffrey J, Neuringer A. Spontaneously hypertensive rats (SHR) readily learn to vary but not repeat instrumental responses. Behav Neural Biol. 1993;59(2):126–35.

23. Perry GM, Sagvolden T, Faraone SV. Intra-individual variability in genetic and environmental models of attention-deficit/hyperactivity disorder. Am J Med Genet B Neuropsychiatr Genet. 2010;153B(5):1094–101.

24. Perry GM, Sagvolden T, Faraone SV. Intraindividual variability (IIV) in an animal model of ADHD– the spontaneously hypertensive Rat. Behav Brain Funct. 2010;6:56.

25. van den Bergh FS, Bloemarts E, Chan JS, Groenink L, Olivier B, Oosting RS. Spontaneously hypertensive rats do not predict symptoms of attention-deficit hyperactivity disorder. Pharmacol Biochem Behav. 2006;83(3):380–90.

26. Sagvolden T, Johansen EB, Woien G, Walaas SI, Storm-Mathisen J, Bergersen LH, Hvalby O, Jensen V, Aase H, Russell VA, et al. The spontaneously hypertensive rat model of ADHD—the importance of selecting the appropriate reference strain. Neuropharmacology. 2009;57(7–8):619–26.

27. Goldberger AL. Non-linear dynamics for clinicians: chaos theory, fractals, and complexity at the bedside. Lancet. 1996;347(9011):1312–4.

28. Goldberger AL. Fractal variability versus pathologic periodicity: complexity loss and stereotypy in disease. Perspect Biol Med. 1997;40(4):543–61.

29. Tang L, Lv H, Yang F, Yu L. Complexity testing techniques for time series data: a comprehensive literature review. Chaos Solitons Fractals. 2015;81:117–35.

30. Shimp CP. What means in molecular, molar, and unified analyses. Int J Comp Psychol. 2014;27(2):224–7.

31. Fasmer OB, Mjeldheim K, Forland W, Hansen AL, Syrstad VE, Oedegaard KJ, Berle JO. Linear and non-linear analyses of Conner's continuous performance test-II discriminate adult patients with attention deficit hyperactivity disorder from patients with mood and anxiety disorders. BMC Psychiatry. 2016;16(1):284.

32. Hauge ER, Berle JO, Oedegaard KJ, Holsten F, Fasmer OB. Nonlinear analysis of motor activity shows differences between schizophrenia and depression: a study using Fourier analysis and sample entropy. PLoS ONE. 2011;6(1):e16291.

33. Krane-Gartiser K, Henriksen TE, Morken G, Vaaler A, Fasmer OB. Actigraphic assessment of motor activity in acutely admitted inpatients with bipolar disorder. PLoS ONE. 2014;9(2):e89574.

34. Fasmer OB, Hauge E, Berle JO, Dilsaver S, Oedegaard KJ. Distribution of active and resting periods in the motor activity of patients with depression and Schizophrenia. Psychiatry Investig. 2016;13(1):112–20.

35. Johansen EB, Fonnum F, Lausund PL, Walaas SI, Baerland NE, Woien G, Sagvolden T. Behavioral changes following PCB 153 exposure in the spontaneously hypertensive rat-an animal model of attention-deficit/hyperactivity disorder. Behav Brain Funct. 2014;10:1.

36. Sagvolden T, Xu T. l-Amphetamine improves poor sustained attention while d-amphetamine reduces overactivity and impulsiveness as well as improves sustained attention in an animal model of attention-deficit/hyperactivity disorder (ADHD). Behav Brain Funct. 2008;4:3.

37. Jensenius AR, Godøy RI, Wanderley MM. Developing tools for studying musical gestures within the Max/MSP/Jitter environment. In: Proceedings of the International Computer Music Conference. 2005: 282–5.

38. Jensenius AR. Action-sound: developing methods and tools to study music-related body movement. Oslo: University of Oslo; 2007.

39. Fasmer OB, Liao H, Huang Y, Berle JO, Wu J, Oedegaard KJ, Wik G, Zhang Z. A naturalistic study of the effect of acupuncture on heart-rate variability. J Acupunct Meridian Stud. 2012;5(1):15–20.

40. Goldberger AL, Amaral LA, Glass L, Hausdorff JM, Ivanov PC, Mark RG, Mietus JE, Moody GB, Peng CK, Stanley HE. PhysioBank, PhysioToolkit, and PhysioNet: components of a new research resource for complex physiologic signals. Circulation. 2000;101(23):E215–20.

41. Richman JS, Moorman JR. Physiological time-series analysis using approximate entropy and sample entropy. Am J Physiol Heart Circ Physiol. 2000;278(6):H2039–49.

42. Guzzetti S, Borroni E, Garbelli PE, Ceriani E, Della Bella P, Montano N, Cogliati C, Somers VK, Malliani A, Porta A. Symbolic dynamics of heart rate variability: a probe to investigate cardiac autonomic modulation. Circulation. 2005;112(4):465–70.

43. Porta A, Tobaldini E, Guzzetti S, Furlan R, Montano N, Gnecchi-Ruscone T. Assessment of cardiac autonomic modulation during graded head-up tilt by symbolic analysis of heart rate variability. Am J Physiol Heart Circ Physiol. 2007;293(1):H702–8.

44. Low WC, Whitehorn D, Hendley ED. Genetically related rats with differences in hippocampal uptake of norepinephrine and maze performance. Brain Res Bull. 1984;12(6):703–9.

45. Mook DM, Neuringer A. Different effects of amphetamine on reinforced variations versus repetitions in spontaneously hypertensive rats (SHR). Physiol Behav. 1994;56(5):939–44.

46. Wood AC, Asherson P, Rijsdijk F, Kuntsi J. Is overactivity a core feature in ADHD? Familial and receiver operating characteristic curve analysis of mechanically assessed activity level. J Am Acad Child Adolesc Psychiatry. 2009;48(10):1023–30.

47. Jensen AR. The importance of intraindividual variation in reaction time. Personal Individ Differ. 1992;13(8):869–81.

48. McLoughlin G, Palmer JA, Rijsdijk F, Makeig S. Genetic overlap between evoked frontocentral theta-band phase variability, reaction time variability, and attention-deficit/hyperactivity disorder symptoms in a twin study. Biol Psychiatry. 2014;75(3):238–47.

49. Kuntsi J, Klein C. Intraindividual variability in ADHD and its implications for research of causal links. In: Behavioral neuroscience of attention deficit hyperactivity disorder and its treatment. Berlin: Springer; 2011. p. 67–91.

50. Paulus MP, Geyer MA, Sternberg E. Differential movement patterns but not amount of activity in unconditioned motor behavior of Fischer, Lewis, and Sprague-Dawley rats. Physiol Behav. 1998;65(3):601–6.

51. Li JS, Huang YC. Early androgen treatment influences the pattern and amount of locomotion activity differently and sexually differentially in an animal model of ADHD. Behav Brain Res. 2006;175(1):176–82.

52. Dervola KS, Roberg BA, Woien G, Bogen IL, Sandvik TH, Sagvolden T, Drevon CA, Johansen EB, Walaas SI. Marine Omicron-3 polyunsaturated fatty acids induce sex-specific changes in reinforcer-controlled behaviour and neurotransmitter metabolism in a spontaneously hypertensive rat model of ADHD. Behav Brain Funct. 2012;8:56.

53. Russell VA. Dopamine hypofunction possibly results from a defect in glutamate-stimulated release of dopamine in the nucleus accumbens shell of a rat model for attention deficit hyperactivity disorder—the spontaneously hypertensive rat. Neurosci Biobehav Rev. 2003;27(7):671–82.

54. Russell VA, Sagvolden T, Johansen EB. Animal models of attention-deficit hyperactivity disorder. Behav Brain Funct. 2005;1:9.

55. Sagvolden T, Russell VA, Aase H, Johansen EB, Farshbaf M. Rodent models of attention-deficit/hyperactivity disorder. Biol Psychiatry. 2005;57(11):1239–47.

56. Vaillancourt DE, Newell KM. Changing complexity in human behavior and physiology through aging and disease. Neurobiol Aging. 2002;23(1):1–11.

57. Garrett DD, Kovacevic N, McIntosh AR, Grady CL. The importance of being variable. J Neurosci. 2011;31(12):4496–503.

58. McIntosh AR, Kovacevic N, Itier RJ. Increased brain signal variability accompanies lower behavioral variability in development. PLoS Comput Biol. 2008;4(7):e1000106.

59. Tye C, Johnson KA, Kelly SP, Asherson P, Kuntsi J, Ashwood KL, Azadi B, Bolton P, McLoughlin G. Response time variability under slow and fast-incentive conditions in children with ASD, ADHD and ASD+ADHD. J Child Psychol Psychiatry. 2016;57(12):1414–23.

60. Karalunas SL, Huang-Pollock CL, Nigg JT. Is reaction time variability in ADHD mainly at low frequencies? J Child Psychol Psychiatry. 2013;54(5):536–44.

61. Boonstra AM, Kooij JJ, Oosterlaan J, Sergeant JA, Buitelaar JK, Van Someren EJ. Hyperactive night and day? Actigraphy studies in adult ADHD: a baseline comparison and the effect of methylphenidate. Sleep. 2007;30(4):433–42.

6

Transplantation of bone marrow-derived mesenchymal stem cells (BMSCs) improves brain ischemia-induced pulmonary injury in rats associated to TNF-α expression

Qin-qin He[1†], Xiang He[1†], Yan-ping Wang[2], Yu Zou[1], Qing-jie Xia[1], Liu-Lin Xiong[1], Chao-zhi Luo[1], Xiao-song Hu[3], Jia Liu[2*] and Ting-hua Wang[1,2*]

Abstract

Background: Bone marrow mesenchymal stem cell (BMSCs)-based therapy seems to be a promising treatment for acute lung injury, but the therapeutic effects of BMSCs transplantation on acute lung injury induced by brain ischemia and the mechanisms have not been totally elucidated. This study explores the effects of transplantation of BMSCs on acute lung injury induced by focal cerebral ischemia and investigates the underlying mechanism.

Methods: Acute lung injury model was induced by middle cerebral artery occlusion (MCAO). BMSCs (with concentration of 1×10^6/ml) were transplanted into host through tail vein 1 day after MCAO. Then, the survival, proliferation and migration of BMSCs in lung were observed at 4 days after transplantation, and histology observation and lung function were assessed for 7 days. Meanwhile, in situ hybridization (ISH), qRT-PCR and western blotting were employed to detect the expression of TNF-α in lung.

Results: Neurobehavioral deficits and acute lung injury could be seen in brain ischemia rats. Implanted BMSCs could survive in the lung, and relieve pulmonary edema, improve lung function, as well as down regulate TNF-α expression.

Conclusions: The grafted BMSCs can survive and migrate widespread in lung and ameliorate lung injury induced by focal cerebral ischemia in the MCAO rat models. The underlying molecular mechanism, at least partially, is related to the suppression of TNF-α.

Keywords: Brain ischemia, Acute lung injury, Bone marrow mesenchymal stem cells, TNF-α

Background

Over the past decades in the United States, the relative rate of stroke death has fallen and the actual number of stroke deaths has declined from the third to the fourth leading cause of death in population suffered stroke [1]. However, in low- and middle- income countries, the incidence and mortality of stroke were still disproportionately high [2], in which, about 95,000 people still experience new or recurrent stroke (ischemic or hemorrhagic). After stroke, several complications are still great challenges to physicians. Among them, not only is the presence of pulmonary dysfunction after stroke well recognized, but also brain lung crosstalk as a complex interaction, has been recognized [3–7]. Severe pulmonary injuries occurred not only in stroke condition, but also induced in brain injuries, such as severe traumatic brain injury (TBI) or subarachnoid hemorrhage (SAH) [8–11]. As pulmonary dysfunction, such as pulmonary edema (NPE) [6, 12], pneumonia [7], acute lung injury and the acute respiratory distress syndrome (ALI/ARDS) [9], is

*Correspondence: liujiaaixuexi@163.com; tinghua_neuron@263.net
†Qin-qin He and Xiang He contributed equally to this work
[1] Department of Anesthesia and Critical Care Medicine Translational Neuroscience Center, West China Hospital, Sichuan University, Chengdu 610041, Sichuan, China
[2] Institute of Neuroscience and Experiment Animal Center, Kunming Medical University, Kunming 650031, China
Full list of author information is available at the end of the article

severe and often result in the increase of mortality, or lead to the poor neurological outcome and longer intensive care unit (ICU) and longer length of hospital stay after stroke [8, 9, 13]. Therefore, it is very important to find the effective method for the treatment of lung injury, and investigate the molecular mechanism for find the intervention strategy.

Currently, the pathophysiology of lung dysfunction after stroke is still in debate, with several theories proposed. Theodore and Robin et al. first defined the "blast theory" of neurogenic pulmonary edema (NPE). In the blast theory, transient increase of intravascular pressure, caused by an acute increase in intracranial pressure (ICP), damages the capillary-alveolar membranes which may cause a leak of protein-rich plasma [14]. However, continuous hemodynamic monitoring indicated that NPE may be irrelevant with hemodynamic instability [15, 16]. Some researchers proposed that NPE may be resulted, in part, from select pulmonary venoconstriction after massive sympathetic discharge following brain injury. Videlicet, pulmonary venues may be α- and β-adrenergic hypersensitive after brain injury. This could increase ICP and pulmonary pressures, and then induce direct myocyte injuries with wall motion abnormalities [17]. These suggested that vasomotor centers by autonomic nervous system were over-estimated, which could to be an explanation to the association of the edema with central nervous system [18]. However, it could not explain the presence of red blood cells and protein in the alveolar fluid [19, 20]. In 2009, Mascia et al. [21] described the "double hit" model, in which, they observed that systemic inflammatory reaction could induce alteration in blood–brain barrier permeability and promote infiltration of activated neutrophils and macrophages to lung, thus cause direct damage to lung. Cascade of inflammatory response can cause extravasation of intravascular fluid and the damage of blood vessel walls, which can cause intra-alveolar hemorrhage [21, 22]. These observations suggested that a new therapeutic intervention for lung dysfunction is necessary after stroke.

Bone marrow mesenchymal stem cell (BMSCs), as multiple differentiation progenitor cells, are noted to be able to influence native immunomodulatory function [23], suppress local inflammatory response [24] and attenuate sepsis by means of maintaining the normal pulmonary endothelial, establishing epithelial interactions and promoting epithelial function [25, 26]. Therefore, it may be considered as a potential strategy for the treatment of lung injury, and the underlying mechanism needs to be investigated.

In this study, we firstly explored whether BMSCs transplantation could alleviate inflammatory activities and improve functional consequence in lung injury induced by brain ischemia, then investigated the possible molecular mechanism involving in the expression of TNF-α.

Methods
Animal and grouping
Forty-five adult male Sprague–Dawley (SD) rats (weighing 180–220 g) were provided by the Center of Experimental Animals, Sichuan University. All animal care, breeding, and testing procedures conform to the principle of *Guidance Suggestions for the Care and Use of Laboratory Animals* promulgated by Ministry of Science and Technology of the People's Republic of China in 2006, and was approved by the Animal Care and Use Committee, Sichuan, University, Chengdu, China. All animals were housed in individual cages in a room with a temperature of 21–25 °C and a humidity of 45–50 % with a 12 h light/dark cycle and ad libitum access to pellet chow and water. Three groups, 15 rats in each group, were randomly designated as sham group, brain ischemia group (BI) and BMSCs transplantation group (BMSCs), as shown in Fig. 1.

Induction of focal cerebral ischemia
Permanent focal cerebral infarction was introduced by bipolar coagulation of the left middle cerebral artery (MCA) as described previously [10]. After 3.6 % chloral hydrate (1 ml/100 g) intraperitoneally injection, left common, internal and external carotid arteries were exposed through a midline neck incision and were carefully

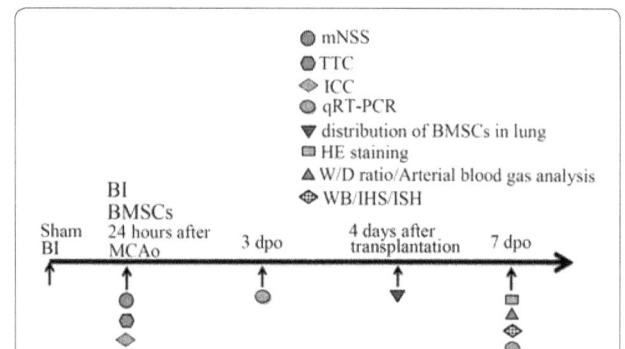

Fig. 1 Experiment design for transplantation of BMSCs in rat with brain ischemia-induced pulmonary injury. *mNSS* modified neurological severity score for measuring neural function after brain ischemia. *TTC staining* 2, 3, 5-Triphenyltetrazolium chloride for measuring the viability of brain tissue. *ICC* immunocytochemistry staining to identify the BMSCs. *qRT-PCR* quantitative real-time polymerase chain reaction for detecting the mRNA expression of TNF-α. *HE staining* hematoxylin-eosin staining. *W/D ratio* wet-to-dry weight ratio of lung. *WB* western blot analysis for quantifying the protein level of TNF-α. *IHS* immunohistochemistry staining for analyzing the expression of TNFα. *ISH* in situ hybridization for determining the location of TNF-α in lung with cerebral ischemia. *BI* brain ischemia. *BMSCs* brain ischemia with BMSCs transplantation

dissected from the surrounding tissues with help of an operating microscope. After electrocoagulation of the external and common carotid arteries, a 3-0 silicon rubber-coated monofilament (Shadong Biotech, Beijing, China) was inserted through the common carotid artery into the internal carotid artery 18–20 mm beyond the carotid bifurcation to the base of the middle cerebral artery, while 10 mm for sham group. The pterygopalatine branch of the internal carotid artery was exposed before the insertion in order to avoid the filament turning into it. Rectal temperature was maintained at 36.5–37 °C using a heat lamp during the operation and for 2 h after MCAO, and breath and heart rate were monitored all the time.

Assessment of neurological function

Each rat was subjected to a series of behavioral tests by using modified neurological severity score (mNSS) [27] 24 h after MCAO to identify the model reliability. The mNSS (0–18) is determined by motor (muscle status, abnormal movement), sensory (visual, tactile, proprioceptive), reflex, and balance tests. In the severity score of injury, one score point is awarded for the inability to perform the test or for the lack of a tested reflex; thus, the higher the score is, the more severe the injury is. All rats were given enough time to become familiar with the testing environment before inflicting the brain injury. This test was completed by three trained and qualified observers who were blinded to the groups of animals.

Isolation of bone marrow mesenchymal stem cell (BMSCs)

BMSCs from SD rats (4 weeks, 60–80 g) were isolated and harvested as described previously [11]. In brief, bone marrow tissues were acquired from the cavities of femurs and tibias with a syringe and 22-gauge needle and injected into the culture medium (Dulbecco's modified Eagle's medium, Gibco, Carlsbad, CA, USA; 10 % fetal bovine serum, Hyclone, Logan, UT, USA; 2 mM L-glutamine; 10,000 U/L penicillin, and 10 mg/L streptomycin, Gibco BRL, Life Technologies, Paisley, United Kingdom). All the flushing fluid was turned into the single-cell suspension and seeded into 15 ml culture flasks with culture medium. Cells were cultured at 37 °C in a humidified environment with 5 % CO_2. Non adherent cells were removed 24 h later, and adherent cell colonies were washed three times with phosphate-buffered saline solution (PBS, Life Technologies). Fresh complete medium was added and changed every 3–4 days. Cells were subcultured 1:2 or 1:4 when they reached 80–90 % confluence. Cells used in this experiment were all harvested from the third passage. Cell surface markers CD29, CD44 and CD45 were detected by immunocytochemistry staining to identify BMSCs.

Immunocytochemistry staining

Monolayer and single colony-derived adherent cells (at the third passage in culture) were analyzed by immunocytochemistry. Cytospin preparations and growing cells in 6-well culture plate were fixed in 4 % paraformaldehyde for 20 min at 4 °C, washed three times with PBS, and then incubated with 3 % hydrogen-peroxide (H_2O_2; Sigma-Aldrich) at room temperature for 30 min. The cells were permeabilized and pre-incubated with blocking solution (containing 2 % goat serum, 0.3 % Triton X-100, and 0.1 %BSA in PBS) for 30 min at room temperature, and then blocked with 5 % normal goat serum at room temperature for 30 min. Washed slides were separately incubated with anti-CD44 (1:50, Abcam, USA), anti-CD29 (1:50, Abcam, USA) and anti-CD45 (1:50, Abcam, USA) primary antibody at 4 °C overnight. After washing with PBS, Alexa Fluor 488 anti-goat IgG (1:200; Molecular Probes, Carlsbad, CA, USA) was incubated for 1 h at 37 °C. Nuclear staining was performed by treatment with 4′, 6-diamidino-2-phenylindole (DAPI, 1:20,000; Molecular Probes, Carlsbad, CA, USA) for 5 min. Slices were then mounted and observed with a florescent microscope (Leica, Solms, Germany).

BMSCs death assessments of Trypan Blue staining in vitro

Before transplantation, the cell mortality of BMSCs was evaluated by Trypan blue assay (Sigma-Aldrich, St. Louis, MO, USA). BMSCs suspension was balanced in PBS. 500 μL of 0.4 % Trypan Blue solution (w/v) was transferred to a test tube. Then 300 μL of PBS and 200 μL BMSCs suspension (dilution factor = 5) were added and mix thoroughly. Cells were counted using a countess automated cell counter (Invitrogen Life Technologies, Grand Island, NY Life Technologies, Grand Island, NY, USA) after 3 min staining at room temperature. The dead cells were stained with blue color. Count cells on top and left touching middle line of the perimeter of each square. And cells touching the middle line at bottom and right sides were not count. Cell inhibitory ratio was calculated by the following formula: cell mortality (%) = (the dead cell number/the total number) × 100 %.

BMSCs transplantation procedures

BMSCs from SD rats were prepared and transplanted into SD rats. Two days before and after BMSCs transplantation, SD rats were injected Cyclosporin A (10 mg/kg) for three consecutive days. To trace the BMSCs after transplantation, they were labeled with Hoechst33342 with a final concentration of 10 μM in the culture medium and were incubated for 2 h. BMSCs were washed three times with PBS to remove unbound Hoechst dye, digested with 0.25 % (w/v) trypsin (Gibco), and then suspended in complete medium. After centrifuged and washed with PBS for several times, cells were suspended in a serum-free medium at 1×10^6 cells per 1 ml. In BMSCs group, the rats were given an intravenous (through tail vein) injection of 2 ml of BMSCs suspension with 2×10^6 cells for 10 min one day after MCAO. Penicillin (20 U/rat/day) was injected intraperitoneally for three consecutive days after BMSCs transplantation to prevent infection. The route, dose and timing of administration have been used in a previous study [28–30].

Tissue preparation

Animals were re-anaesthetized with 3.6 % chloral hydrate (1 ml/100 g). The chest cavity was opened and the hilum of left lung was ligatured. The right lung was perfused with normal saline for 10 min and then slowly fixed with 4 % paraformaldehyde for 30 min. The brain and right lung were obtained and post fixed in 4 % paraformaldehyde (solution in 0.1 mol/L phosphate buffer, pH 7.4) overnight at 4 °C. The sample was then dehydrated in 20 % sucrose solution in 4 % paraformaldehyde, and then with 30 % sucrose solution in 0.1 mol/L phosphate buffer. Subsequently, samples were embedded in paraffin and sectioned (5 μm in thickness). The left lung without fixing was harvested and stored at −80 °C for west blotting. In addition, 3 days after MCAO, lung tissue was also harvested for qRT-PCR. Sections obtained 4 days after BMSCs transplantation were also employed to observe the distribution of Hochest33342 labeled BMSCs lung tissue under fluorescence microscope.

2, 3, 5-Triphenyltetrazolium chlorides(TTC) staining and evaluation of infarction volume after MCAO

Viability of brain ischemia was evaluated using TTC (Sigma-Aldrich, St. Louis, Missouri, USA) 24 h after MCAO. Rat brains were rapidly removed, frozen at −80 °C for 5 min and then sliced coronal into serial 2-mm-thick slices at the level of the bregma. Sets of five serial slices from each brain were incubated for 30 min at 37 °C in 2 % TTC (Sigma Co., St Louis, MO, USA) in the dark washed in PBS, and then fixed by 4 % formaldehyde in PBS. Images of sections from the exact center of the forebrain were captured using digital camera system (Leica, Solms, Germany). The infarction area and hemisphere area of each section were traced and measured using Image Pro plus 6.0 software (Media Cybernetics, Inc., MD, USA). To eliminate the interference of brain edema, the infarct volume was corrected by standard methods (contralateral hemisphere volume–volume of non-ischemic ipsilateral hemisphere). Infracted volume was expressed as a percentage of the contralateral hemisphere, as described previously [31, 32].

Lung function assessment and edema measurement

Arterial blood gas analysis and wet-to-dry weight (W/D) ratio of lung were used to represent the severity of lung edema. Seven days after MCAO, rats were re-anaesthetized with 3.6 % chloral hydrate (2 ml/100 g) intraperitoneally. Arterial blood samples (100 μl) of rats were extracted into a heparinized syringe by left ventricular sampling, and then blood gas analysis was immediately performed with blood-gas analyzer (RADUOMETER ABL800). In addition, after equivalent lung tissue in bilateral was separated from the thoracic cavity, the lungs were weighed and then dried to constant weight at 80 °C for 24 h. The ratio of wet-to-dry was finally calculated using the formula of (dry weight/wet weight) × 100 %.

Hematoxylin–eosin staining and immunohistochemical assay

Brains and lung were removed and placed in 10 % paraformaldehyde in phosphate-buffer overnight, dehydrated, and embedded in paraffin. 5 μm-thick serial sections of the right lung and brain were stained with hematoxylin-eosin (HE). For immunohistochemical assay, the paraffin embedded sections were routinely de-paraffinized and rehydrated. After non-specific antigen site blocking, the slices of lung tissue were incubated with monoclonal mouse anti-TNF-α (dilution 1:50, Abcam, Cambridge, UK), and then the slices were performed at room temperature for 1 h and then incubated overnight at 4 °C. The sections were incubated in biotin-conjugated secondary antibody for 30 min at 37 °C and then incubated with horseradish peroxidase conjugated streptavidin avidin for 20 min at 37 °C. Washing was performed with PBS (pH 7.4) for three times (5 min for each time) between any two adjacent procedures, except for blocking in serum. Then, visualization was done with diaminobenzidine (DAB), followed by dehydration, transparentization and mounting. Counterstaining of sections by hematoxylin was also performed. Negative controls were stained similarly. However, PBS was used, instead of a primary antibody. Images were taken with a laser scanning confocal microscope (Nikon, Tokyo, Japan). Quantification of the immunolabeled lung sections was performed separately. For each slice, ×200 magnification photomicrographs were taken to measure the density of TNF-α. The mean density was presented as IOD over the area of interest using Image-Pro plus 6.0 software (Media Cybernetics, Silver Spring, MD, USA), which was described previously [18]. Data are presented as mean ± SEM. Observers were blinded to group identity.

In situ hybridization

Slides, prepared as described, were used for ISH. Briefly, sections were de-waxed in xylene, rehydrated in gradedalcohols, and placed in diethyl pyrocarbonate (DEPC) H$_2$O. Endogenous peroxidase was inactivated by incubation in 3 % H$_2$O$_2$ for 15 min at room temperature. Sections were then digested in proteinase K (20 µg/ml) for 20 min, rinsed in NaCl/Tris, and then fixed in 4 % PFA for 10 min. Following this, slides were rinsed with PBS twice for 5 min. Slices were blocked at room temperature for 2 h in hybridization buffer (50 % formamide, 25 % 5× saline sodium citrate (SSC), 10 % 5× Denhardt's and 15 % DEPC-H$_2$O (containing 200 ng/ml yeast RNA, 500 g/ml salmon sperm DNA and 20 mg/ml Roche blocking reagent)), hybridized with 30 nmol of locked nucleic acid (LNA)-modified oligonucleotide probe (Exiqon, Woburn, MA, USA) complementary to TNF-α, and then labeled with digoxigenin (DIG) at 52 °C overnight. After hybridization, the slides were washed in 2× SSC twice at 37 °C for 15 min after washing with 0.5× SSC (15 min at 37 °C) and 0.2× SSC (15 min at 37 °C). The slides were then incubated with HRP conjugated anti-DIG antibody. Sections were rinsed in PBS three times for 5 min. Peroxidase staining was visualized with DAB for 3 min.

Detection of BMSCs cells and phenotypic analysis in vivo

Four days after transplantation, the phenotype of BMSCs in vivo was detected. Lungs of the deeply-anesthetized rats were removed, fixed in 4 % paraformaldehyde in phosphate-buffer, dehydrated with 30 % sucrose in 0.1 M PBS for overnight, and frozen in powdered dry ice. Cryostat sections (10 µm) were processed. Phenotypic analysis of the transplanted cells in vivo was carried out using fluorescence microscope (Leica, Solms, Germany).

Quantitative real-time polymerase chain reaction (qRT-PCR)

Three and seven days after MCAO, the mRNA expressions of TNF-α and β-actin in the lung were detected by qRT-PCR. In brief, the left upper lung tissues were kept at −80 °C, then the total RNA was isolated from lung homogenates with Trizol reagent (Takara Bio Inc., Otsu, Japan) and reverse transcribed using PrimerScript® RT reagent Kit with cDNA eraser (Takara Bio Inc., Otsu, Japan). Each PCR was performed with a iQ™5Multicolor RealTime PCR Detection System (Bio-Rad Laboratories, Inc., USA) and a SYBR Green PCR kit (Takara Bio Inc., Otsu, Japan) in a final volume of 20 µL, containing 1.6 µL cDNA template, forward and backward primers 0.8 µL each, 10 µL SYBR® Premix Ex Taq™II and 6.8 µL dH2O. The primers and Taqman probes were designed using Primer Premier (PREMIER Biosoft International, Canada). The premier sequences were as follows: TNF-α (forward) 5′-AATGACCCAGATTAT GTTTGAGAC-C-3′ and (reverse) 5′-TCCAGAGTCCA GCACAATACCAG-3′; β-actin (forward) 5′-GATTA CTGCTCTGGCTCCTAGC-3′ and (reverse) 5′-ACT CATCGTACTCCTGCTTGCT-3′. The mouse β-actin housekeeping gene was used as an internal control. The fluorescence emitted by the reporter dye was detected in real time, and the threshold cycle (Ct) of each sample was recorded as a quantitative measure of the amount of PCR product in the sample. The target signal was normalized against the relative quantity of β-actin and expressed as $\Delta Ct = Ct_{target} - Ct_{\beta\text{-actin}}$. The changes in target signal relative to the total amount of genomic DNA were expressed as $\Delta\Delta Ct = \Delta Ct_{treatment} - \Delta Ct_{control}$. Relative changes in metastasis were then calculated as $2^{-\Delta\Delta Ct}$ [13].

Western blot analysis

Seven days after MCAO, the protein expression of TNF-α was determined by western blot. The left middle lung tissues were kept at −80 °C and homogenized in PBS containing the protease inhibitor cocktail with the aid of a tissue grinder. The homogenates were centrifuged for 15 min at 12,000 rpm and 4 °C. Supernatants were collected, and the protein concentration of each sample was measured with Bradford protein assay kit (BioRad Laboratories, Inc., USA) using bovine serum albumin (BSA) as the standard. An equal amount of protein from each sample (25 µg) was resolved in 15 % SDS-polyacryamide gel (SDS-PAGE). After electrophoresis, the separated protein bands were wet transferred to the polyvinylidenedifluoride (PVDF) membrane (Millipore, Bedford, MA, USA). Nonspecific binding to membrane was blocked with 5 % skim milk (Sigma, USA) in TBST (10 mmol/L Tris, pH 8.0,150 mmol/L NaCl, 0.05 % Tween 20) for 1 h at room temperature. The membranes were incubated for 24 h at 4 °C with primary anti-TNF-α IgG (1:1000, Abcam, Cambridge, UK),and anti-β-actin antibody(1:2500, Santa Cruz Biotechnology, Inc., USA) respectively. The secondary antibody (horseradish peroxidase-conjugated goat anti-mouse IgG in 5 % skim milk-TBS-T) was added at 1:20,000 dilutions and incubated for 2 h at room temperature. Immunodetected proteins were visualized using ECL assay kit (Millipore, Bedford, MA, USA) with glyco doc imaging system (Bio-Rad Laboratories, Inc., USA) and analyzed by Quantity One software. The relative protein level was normalized to β-actin.

Statistic analysis

Sigma plot software SPSS version 17.0 (SPSS Inc., Chicago, USA) was used to perform data analysis. All data were expressed as mean ± standard deviation (SD). Differences between control and experimental group were compared by One-Way analysis of variance (ANOVA) and $P < 0.05$ was considered to be statistically significant.

Results

Cerebral ischemia induced acute lung injury

MCAO has a high mortality, about 60–70 %, in our study. After brain ischemia, the pyramidal cells in the cortex were exhibited acellular edema (Fig. 2a, b). Neurologic function evaluation showed that mNSS score was higher in the brain ischemia group 24 h after MCAO, as compared with the Sham group (P < 0.05) (Fig. 2c). Normal lung tissue structures and clear alveoli existed in rats of Sham group, and there are few inflammatory cells in the lung tissue (Fig. 2d). Comparatively, in brain ischemia group, many cells with nuclei were large and deep dyed were observed, and these cells were considered as macrophages (Fig. 2e). The alveolar walls are thickened; capillaries in the alveolar walls are congested with many red blood cells, local hemorrhage, interstitial edema, alveoli exudation and inflammatory cells were observed in lungs in brain ischemia group. Some inflammatory cells were passing through the vascular wall to the pulmonary interstitial. Various pathological changes were observed in the same pulmonary lobe (Fig. 2e). In the brain ischemia group, the counts of red cells in lung were significant increased, as compared with the Sham group (Fig. 2f). Moreover, 7 days after MCAO, wet-to-dry weight (W/D) ratio of lung in brain ischemia group elevated, as compared with the Sham group (P < 0.05, Fig. 2g). TTC staining showed the volume of infarct in the brain of MCAO is apparent as compared with Sham one (Fig. 2h). Ischemic infarcts include ipsilateral frontal lobe, parietal lobe and the front of the temporal lobe after MCAO (Fig. 2h), and the average infarct percentage is approximately 21 %.

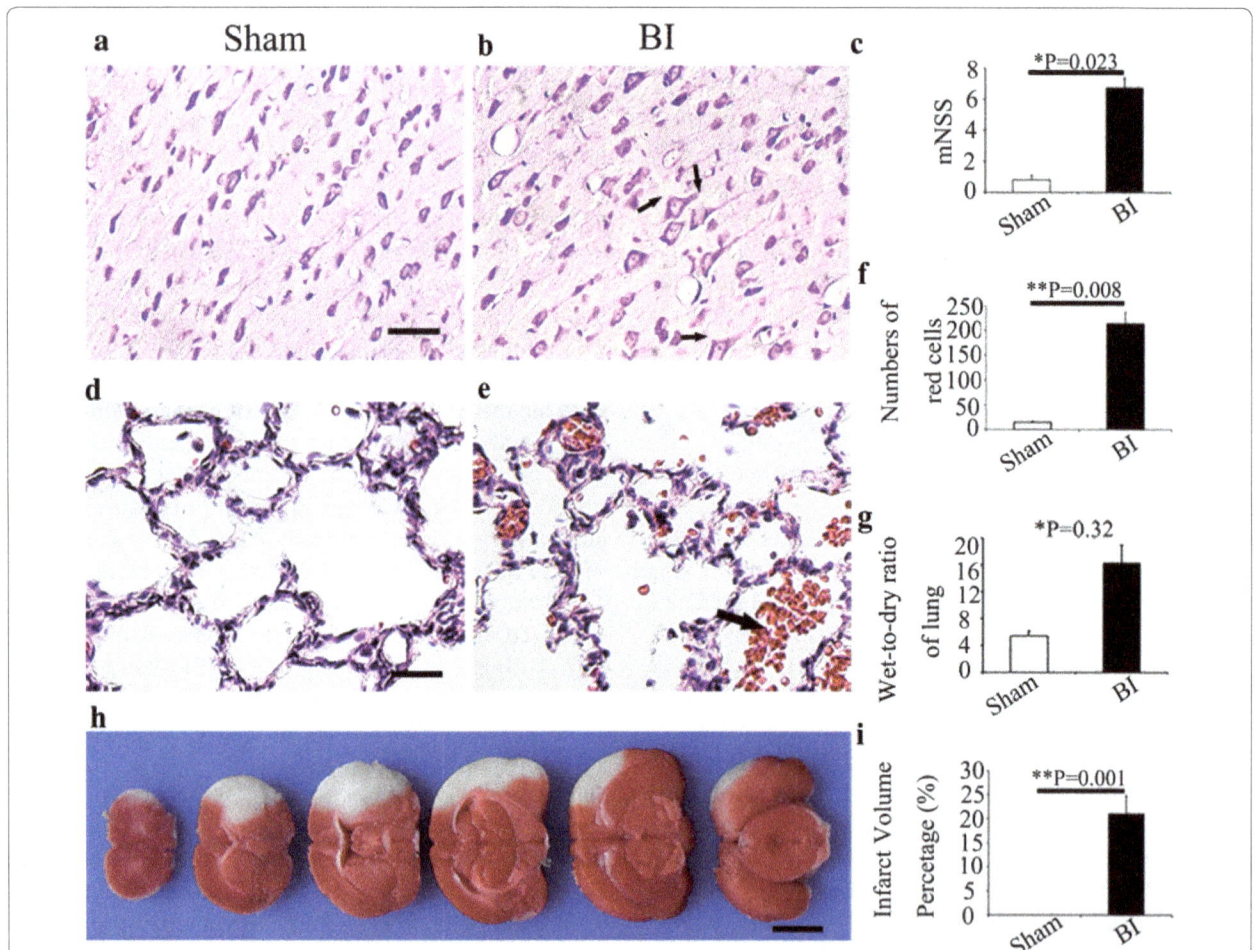

Fig. 2 Cerebral ischemia induced by MCAO produces lung injury in rat. **a, b** Morphological examination of the cerebral cortex neurons by H&E staining. **a** Sham group; **b** BI group. **a** In Sham group, there were abundant pyramidal cells. **b** After brain ischemia, the nuclei of pyramidal cells (*bold arrow*) were shrunken and surrounded with acidophilic cytoplasm. **c** mNSS score in the Sham group and BI group at 24 h after MCAO. **d, e** H&E staining of the lung tissue in Sham group (**d**) and BI group (**e**). Red blood cells (*bold arrow*) were observed in the pulmonary alveoli (**e**). **f** *Bar graph* of the numbers of red cells in the lung in Sham group and BI group was shown. **g** Wet-to-dry weight (W/D) ratio of lung in Sham group and BI group was shown. **h** Viability of brain tissue was shown by TTC staining in rats suffered MCAO. **i** *Bar graph* of the infarct volume percentage in Sham group and BI group were shown. *P < 0.05;**P < 0.01, n = 5 in each group. *Scale bars* **a,b, d, e**, 25 μm; **h**, 200 μm

Analysis of lung function and TNF-α expression after brain ischemia

Blood gas analysis confirmed that PaO_2 decreased and $PaCO_2$ increased after brain ischemia, compared with the Sham group(both $P < 0.05$, Fig. 3a, b). Either mRNA (Fig. 3c, d) or protein (Fig. 3e) expression of TNF-α in lung significantly increased after MCAO, compared with the Sham group ($P < 0.05$).

Expression and localization of TNF-α in lung after brain ischemia

Immunohistochemistry showed that in Sham group, TNF-α staining was junior in alveolar type I and type II epithelial cell, and few macrophagocytes was stained by TNF-α recognition (Fig. 4a). While in brain ischemia group, intensity of staining in typeI and II epithelial cells were both increased, a stronger dyeing of TNF-α was observed in alveolar type I and type II epithelial cells (Fig. 4b). What's more important, more

macrophagocytes with TNF-α strong positive staining were observed in lung after MCAO (Fig. 4b). ISH indicated that TNF-α was mainly located in macrophagocytes, which were significantly increased in the brain ischemia group (Fig. 4c, d).

Morphological and surface antigen characteristics of primary BMSCs

Primary BMSCs cultured as plastic adherent cells. They turned to confluency one week after culture and were expanded by serial subcultivation just prior to confluency. Figure 5a showed the morphological features of BMSCs at 0 h. At the 3rd day, their clonal-rosette derived round shape became elongated or spindle-shaped (Fig. 5b). At the 3rd passage, the form of primary BMSCs adherent cells was uniform with polygons-shaped appearance (Fig. 5c). To characterize primary BMSCs phenotype, we examined the cell surface markers CD29, CD44, and CD45 by means of immunocytochemistry staining. The

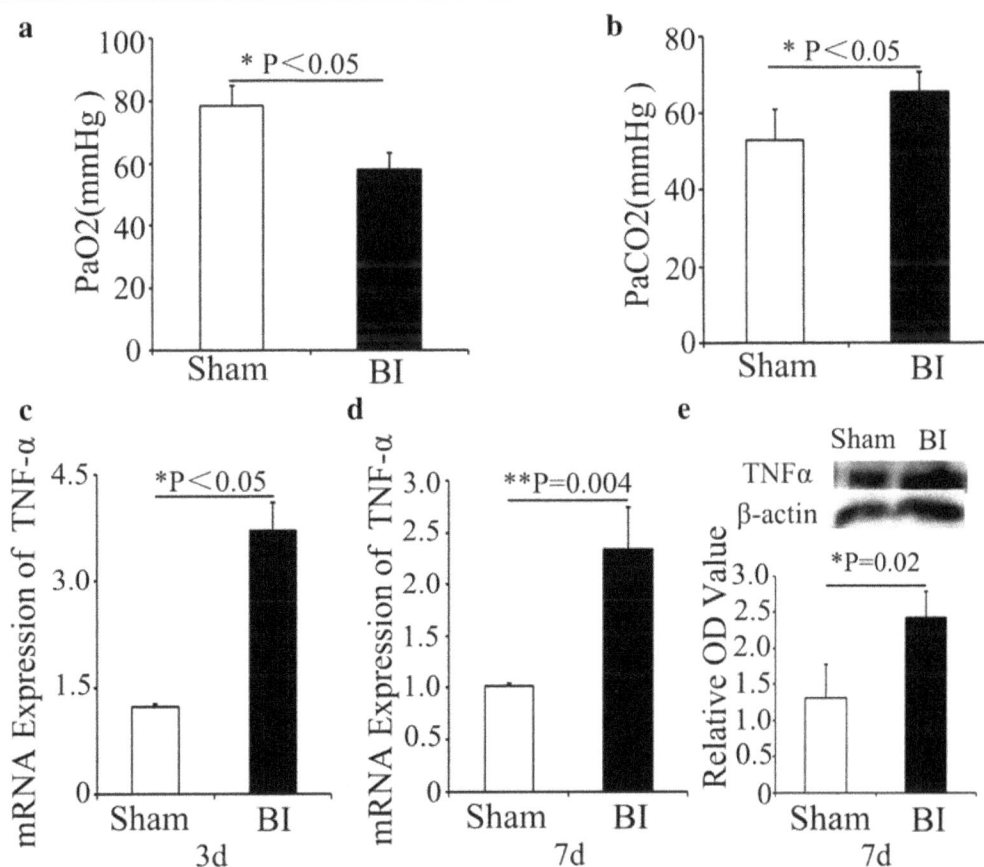

Fig. 3 Lung function was deteriorated and the expression of TNF-α in lung was increased after MCAO. **a, b** Blood gas analysis of the Sham group and BI group. PaO2 (**a**); PaCO2 (**b**). **c, d** qRT-PCR assessment of the mRNA expression of TNF-α in the Sham group and BI group at 3(**c**) and 7(**d**) days after MCAO. **e** Western blot assessment of the protein expression of TNF-α in lung tissues in the Sham group and BI group. A semi-quantitative analysis was used to represent the total protein level of TNF-α. Data are expressed as mean ± SD. *P < 0.05, **P < 0.01 compared to the Sham group, n = 5 in each group

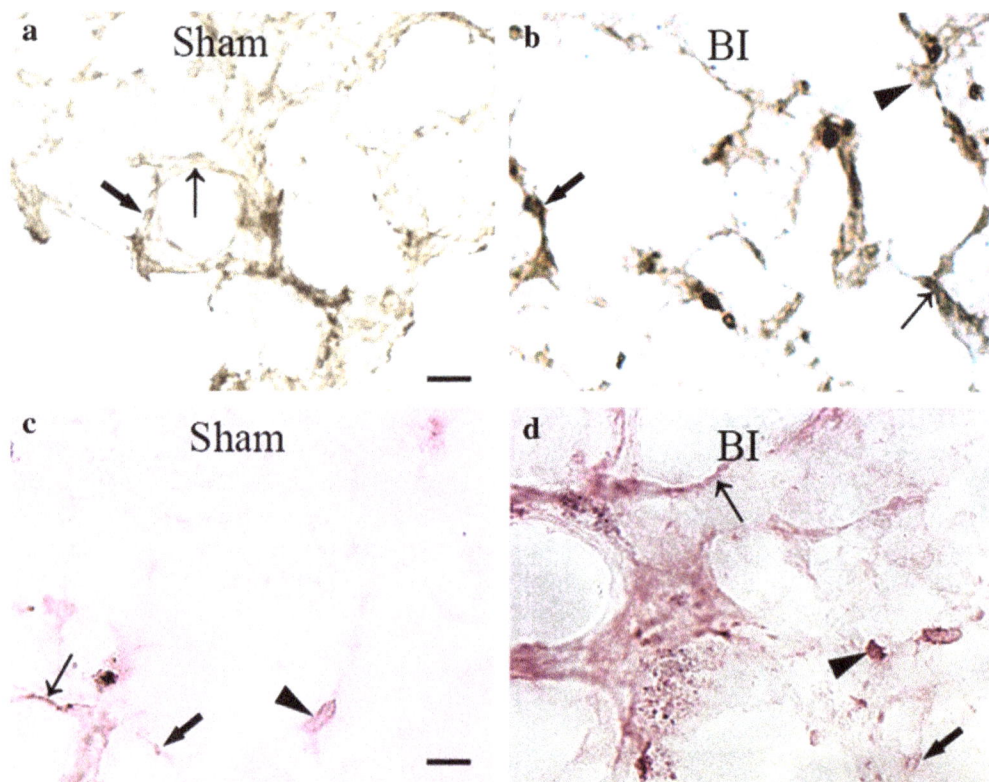

Fig. 4 Representative histopathological finding of TNF-α in the injured lung after brain ischemia. **a, b** Immunohistochemistry staining of TNF-α in type I (*brown signal, bold arrow*), II lung epithelial cells (*brown signal, thin arrow*) and macrophagocytes (*brown signal, arrow head*) in the Sham group (**a**) and BI group (**b**). **c, d** ISH of TNF-α (*red signals*) was detected in the typeI (ISH, *red signals, bold arrow*), II lung epithelial cells (ISH, *red signals, thin arrow*) and macrophagocytes (ISH, *red signals, arrow head*) in the Sham group (**c**) and BI group (**d**). *Scale bars* **a–d**, 25 μm

BMSCs were positive for CD29 (Fig. 5d–f) and CD44 (Fig. 5g–i), but negative for CD45 (Fig. 5j–l). This indicates that the cells were highly expressed markers of mesenchymal stem cells and were negative for endothelial and hematopoietic cell markers.

BMSCs engrafts improved lung morphology and alleviated TNF-α expression

Trypan Blue staining indicated that the viability of BMSCs is about 96 %, before transplantation. Brain ischemia induced prominent lesions in lung and increased the inflammatory exudations in alveolar and inflammatory cells (Fig. 6a, c). In contrast, inflammatory exudations in alveolar and inflammatory cells were partly ameliorated by BMSCs treatment (Fig. 6b, d). Within the lung tissue, the transplanted BMSCs could be easily identified under fluorescent microscopy, and their nucleic appearances were exactly the same as that before the transplantation (Fig. 6e). Cells derived from BMSCs were round-to-oval with irregular dark brown nuclei and thin cytoplasm by Hoechst33342 staining (Fig. 6e). Moreover, both the mean density of TNF-α (Fig. 6f) and the number of the inflammation cells (Fig. 6g) were significantly

decreased in BMSCs transplantation group (vs brain ischemia group, P < 0.05).

Analysis of lung function and TNF-α expression after treatment of BMSCs in brain ischemia rats

Seven days after BMSC transplantation, wet-to-dry weight(W/D) ratio of lung in BMSCs group decreased, as compared with rats subjected to only brain ischemia (P < 0.05, Fig. 7a). Blood gas analysis indicated that PaO_2 increased (P < 0.05, Fig. 7b) and $PaCO_2$ decreased (P < 0.05) (Fig. 7c) after BMSCs treatment, as compared with the brain ischemia group. Furthermore, there was a significantly decrease in the level of TNF-α (Fig. 7d, e) mRNA or protein expression (Fig. 7f) both 3 and 7 days after BMSCs transplantation, as compared with the brain ischemia group (both P < 0.05).

Discussion

The major findings of these experiments can be summarized as follows: (1) brain ischemia could induce lung injury, a kind of inflammatory lung damage; (2) intravenous injection of BMSCs could home to the lung and survive in brain ischemia induced lung injury model; (3)

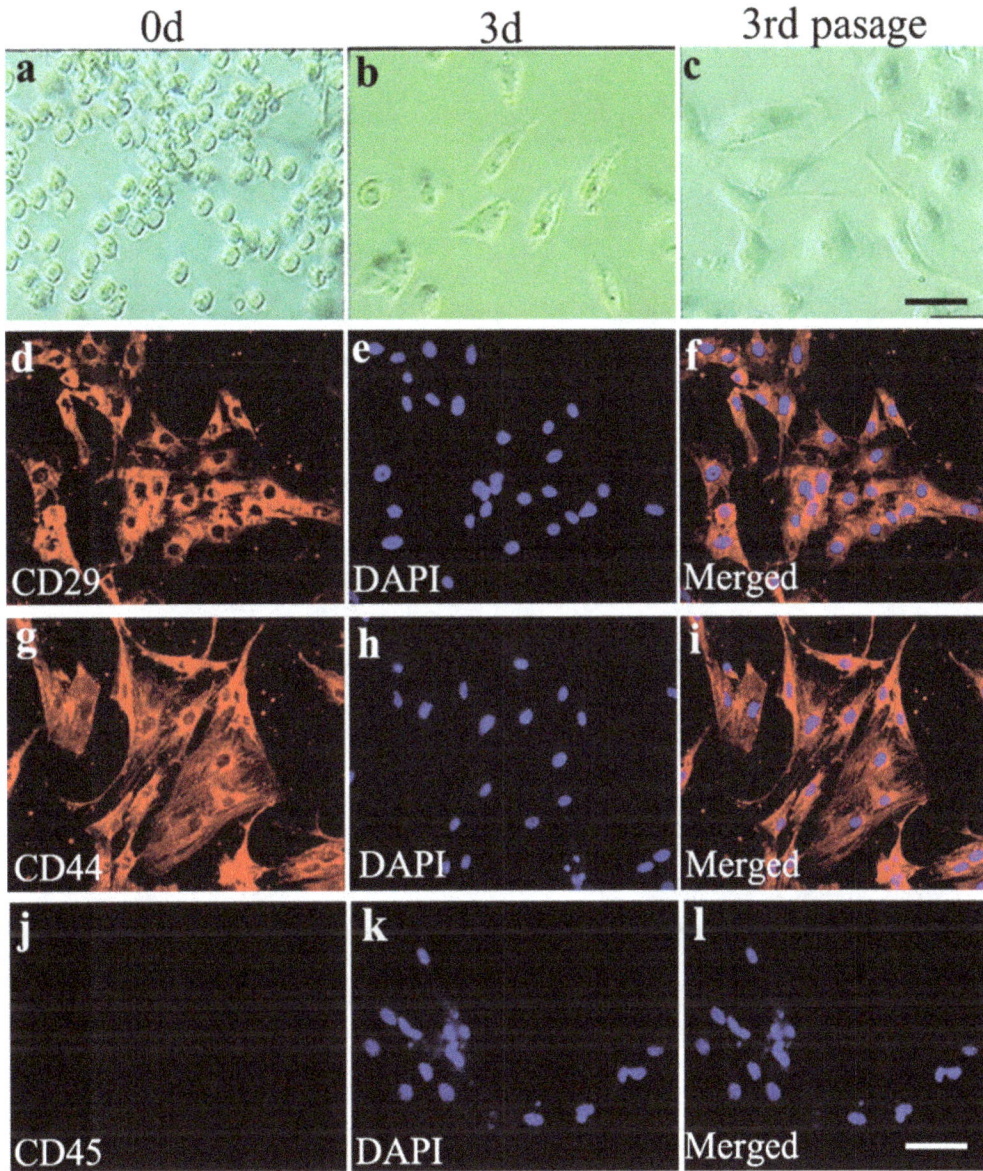

Fig. 5 Isolation and identification of BMSCs. **a, b, c** Cellular morphology of BMSCs at 0 h (**a**) 3-day (**b**) and the 3rd passage (**c**) in primary culture which were observed under inverted phase contrast microscope CD29, CD44 and CD45 immunostaining of the 3rd passage of BMSCs were performed. Immunostaining of CD29 (**d**, *red*), CD44 (**g**, *red*) and CD45 (**j**) with nucleus stained DAPI (**e, h, k** respectively, *blue*) and the merge graphs (**f, i, l**) were showed. *Scale bars* **a, b, c**, 100 μm; **d–l**, 25 μm

treatment with BMSCs could reduce pulmonary edema, improve lung function after brain ischemia; (4) BMSCs exhibited a positive role in suppressing inflammation mediators like TNF-α in lung after brain ischemia.

In this study, we found that permanent MCAO induced pulmonary injury in SD rats. Pulmonary dysfunction is an important independent factor that affects mortality in patients suffering brain injury and deteriorates the long-term neurologic outcome [13, 32–34]. Ségolène Mrozek et al. suggested that brain lung crosstalk is a

complex interaction from the brain to the lung but also from the lung to the brain. Several studies described the occurrence of severe pulmonary injuries after experiencing a brain injury, such as severe traumatic brain injury, subarachnoid hemorrhage, stroke or hypoxic-ischemic brain damage [8, 10, 33–35]. The pathophysiology of brain-lung interaction is complex and several hypotheses have been proposed with a particular described "double hit" model [21]. After brain ischemia, there was local hemorrhage, interstitial edema, alveoli exudation and

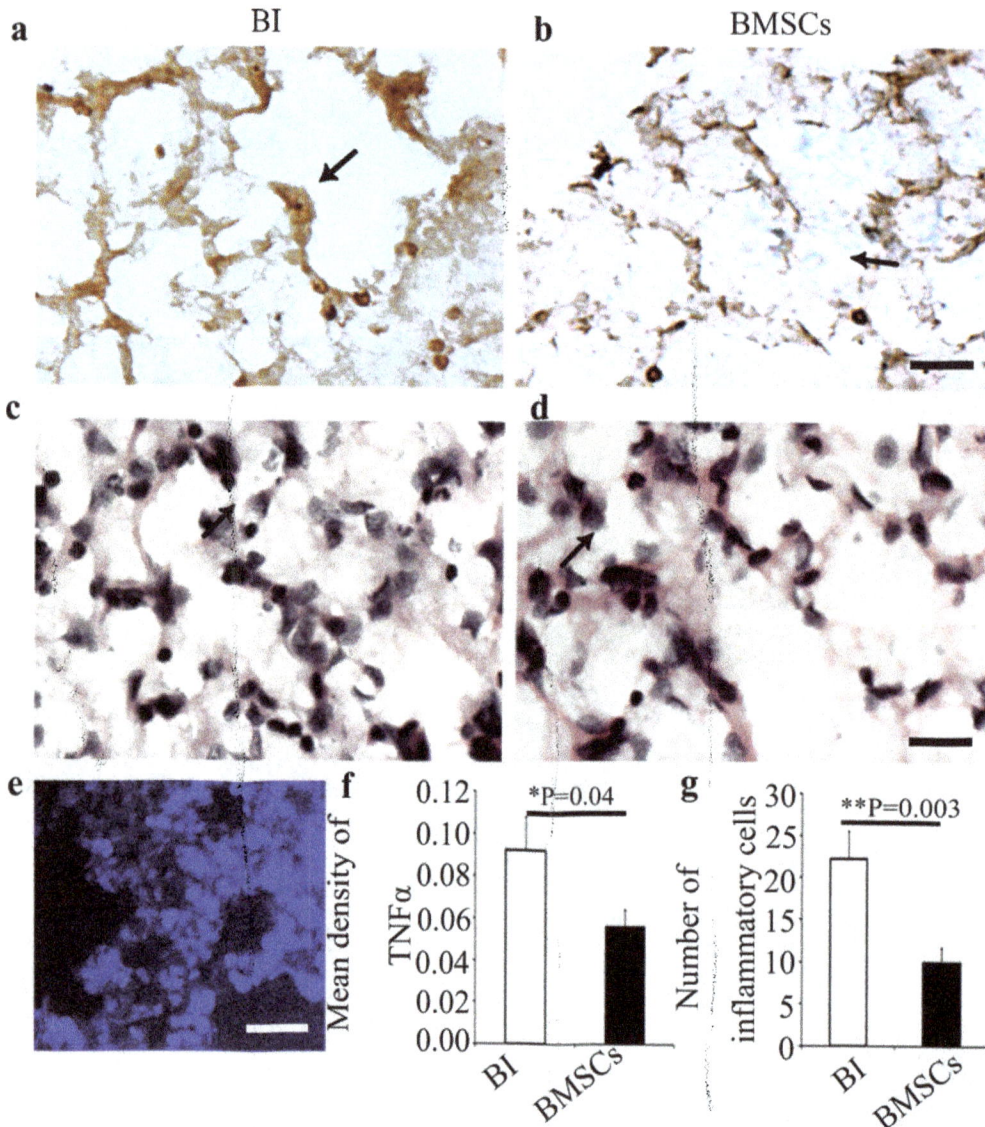

Fig. 6 BMSCs transplantation decreased the expression of TNF-α and the numbers of inflammatory cells in lungs of rats after MCAO. **a**, **b** The intracellular TNF-α in lung (*brown signal, thin arrow*) was detected by immunohistochemistry. The photos represented the intracellular TNF-α content of lung in BI group (**a**) and BMSCs group (**b**). **c**, **d** Inflammatory cells in lung of rats in BI group (**c**) and BMSCs group (**d**) were detected by HE staining. **e** Hochest33342 labeled cells (*blue*) in lung under fluorescence microscope. **f** *Bar graph* of mean density of TNF-α in the lung in BI group and BMSCs group. **g** Numbers of inflammatory cells were calculated in BI group and BMSCs group. (*P < 0.05, n = 5 in each group). **a–d**, 25 μm; **e**, 100 μm

inflammatory infiltrates in lung. This injury presents as a kind of inflammatory lung damage characterized by histology study and increased tissue TNF-α concentration in the lung.

Intravenous injection of BMSCs could home to the lung and survive after brain ischemia. The ability to self-renew and multi-directional differentiation make BMSCs attractive as a potential treatment for acute lung injury. Four days after BMSCs treatment, migration towards and adhesion of BMSCs with Hochest33342 labeled were observed in the rat lung tissue under fluorescence

microscope Muhammad Aslam et al. [23] did observe that a higher number of donor BMSCs can be detected in the injured lung compared with the normal lung at 10 days post injection. This elucidated that the intravenous transplanted BMSCs could partially maintain themselves in the injured lung. Although we cannot propose that BMSCs extensively replace injured lung cells to effectively improve lung architecture because of the minimal BMSC engraftment after transplantation, this may be the basis for functional and morphological improvement [23, 36].

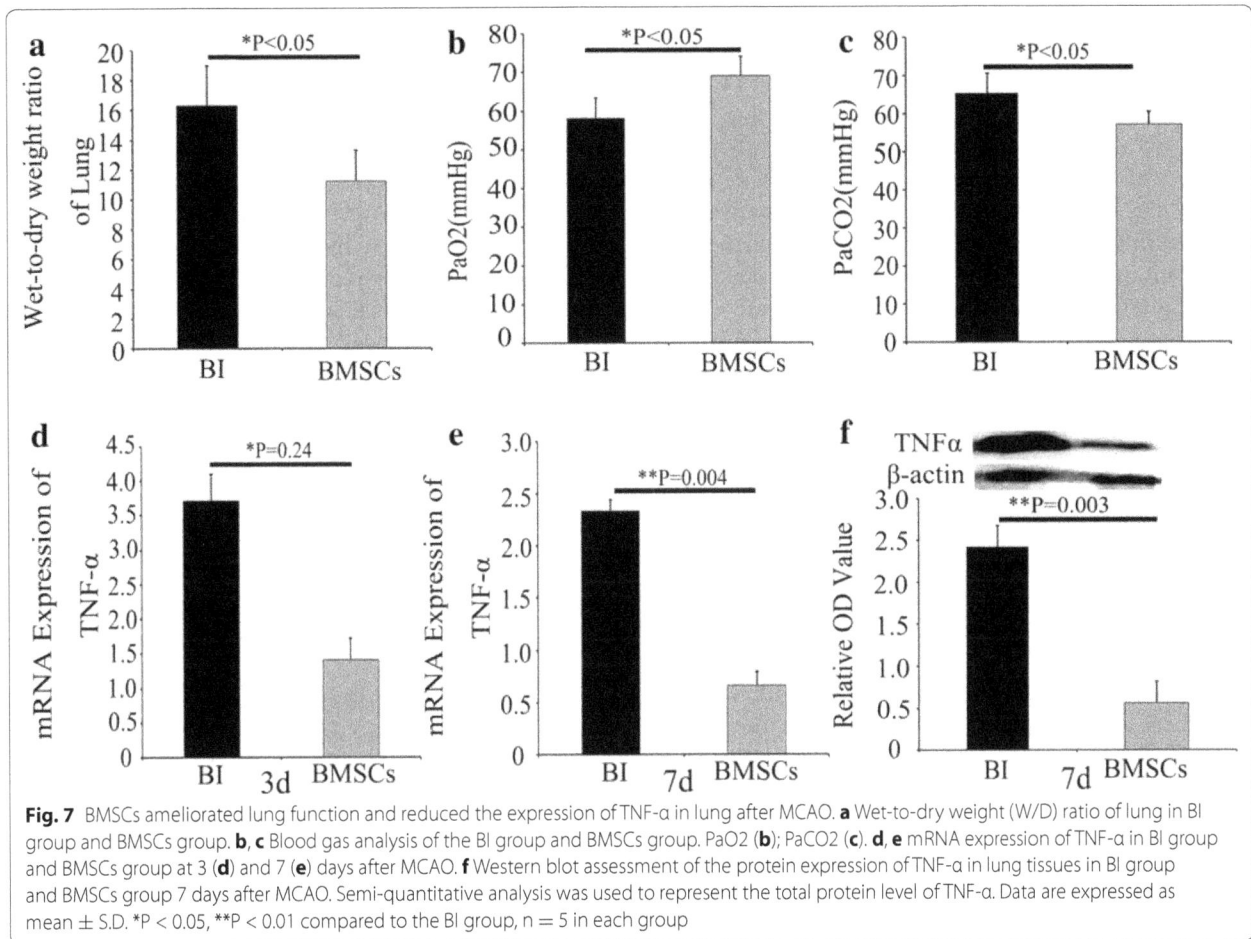

Fig. 7 BMSCs ameliorated lung function and reduced the expression of TNF-α in lung after MCAO. **a** Wet-to-dry weight (W/D) ratio of lung in BI group and BMSCs group. **b, c** Blood gas analysis of the BI group and BMSCs group. PaO2 (**b**); PaCO2 (**c**). **d, e** mRNA expression of TNF-α in BI group and BMSCs group at 3 (**d**) and 7 (**e**) days after MCAO. **f** Western blot assessment of the protein expression of TNF-α in lung tissues in BI group and BMSCs group 7 days after MCAO. Semi-quantitative analysis was used to represent the total protein level of TNF-α. Data are expressed as mean ± S.D. *P < 0.05, **P < 0.01 compared to the BI group, n = 5 in each group

In the present study, we have shown that BMSCs enhance the recovery of lung structure and function after brain ischemia. Specifically, BMSCs treatment improved lung architecture, restored static lung compliance, and ameliorate alveolar fluid exudation in lung, as evidenced by reduced lung wet- to- dry weight ratio, histological evidence of reduced alveolar tissue edema and the improved blood gas analysis. These findings support previous findings that BMSCs normalize lung fluid balance and alveolar fluid clearance through therapeutic effects on the lung endothelium [37]. The integrity of the lung microvascular endothelium is essential to prevent the influx of protein-rich fluid from the plasma as well as inflammatory cells which may further aggravate the ability of the lung epithelium to remove alveolar edema.

BMSCs suppress inflammation responses in lung after brain ischemia. BMSCs were demonstrated by prior studies to have anti-inflammatory effects on lung injury. Gupta et al. [11] found that intrapulmonary delivery of BMSCs in mice mediated a down-regulation of pro-inflammatory responses to endotoxin by reducing TNF-α and macrophage inflammatory protein-2,

while increasing the anti-inflammatory cytokine IL-10. BMSCs therapy can attenuate paraquat-induced ALI in rats through decreases plasma TNF-α and MDA levels. BMSCs have demonstrated benefit in oleic acid induced acute lung injury in rats by decreased TNF-α expression and increased IL-10 content [38]. BMSCs decreased lung inflammation ventilator-induced lung injury rat, by reduced TNF-α and upregulated IL-10 [39].

In our study, we found a significantly increase of TNF-α concentration in the lung tissue after brain ischemia. Inflammatory cytokines may key mediator for pulmonary alveoli injury. TNF-α could distract vascular endothelial cells, leading to the increase of capillary permeability and the development of lung inflammation response [40]. TNF-α induced NF-κB signaling activation in whole lung has been proven to be associated with inflammation damage in pulmonary complication [41, 42].

On the other hand, it's generally accepted that the beneficial effects of stem and progenitor cells in animal disease models are the result of immunomodulatory and trophic support properties delivered by the transplanted cells acting in a paracrine manner. BMSCs might produce a number of potent cytokines and growth factors, such as platelet-derived growth factor (PDGF) and transforming growth factor β (TGF-β1) to repair the process of lung injury [43, 44].

We performed the cell transplantation at 24 h after stroke, which needs to be justified. It was reported that BMSC transplantation acutely after stroke was deteriorating to the ischemic brain. The high level of VEGF in these cells may cause brain edema. However, the relationship between VEGF and brain edema has been debated, also. Some literatures demonstrated that the up-regulated VEGF after ischemic stroke may significantly increase the brain water content [45–47] and induce vasogenic brain edema [48, 49]. VEGF has the potency to increase vascular permeability [50, 51]. After brain ischemia, VEGF could significantly increase BBB leakage [52]. VEGF disrupts the organization of interendothelial junctions (IEJ) and the integrin-extracellular matrix (ECM) complexes, thereby opening the junctional barrier. Nicholas van Bruggen et al. [53] established that sequesters murine VEGF could significantly reduce the acute appearance of cortical edema after focal cerebral ischemia [53]. However, the role of VEGF in the pathogenesis of the formation of ischemic brain edema is unclear with contradictory experimental observations. For example, Hayashi et al. reported that VEGF itself, when applied topically to the surface of a reperfused rat brain after transient cerebral artery occlusion, reduced ischemic brain damage, infarct volume, and edema formation. Harrigan MR et al. [54] demonstrated that intracerebroventricular infusion of VEGF decreases infarct volume and brain edema after temporary MCAO. Betz et al. [55] suggested that ischemic brain edema formation in the relatively early phase is mainly caused by cytotoxic edema rather than vasogenic edema [56]. On the other hand, VEGF may protect the blood–brain barrier rather than destroy it after brain ischemia because Criscuolo et al. suggested that VEGF application through the carotid artery did not cause albumin extravasation. The amelioration of blood–brain barrier injury may be attributable to the protective effect of VEGF on endothelial cells [57]. One possible mechanism of VEGF in the reduction of ischemic brain edema is that VEGF could reduce the infarct volume by protection of endothelial cells, and thus reduce water content, without exacerbating vasogenic edema. Chen Bo et al. [54] suggested that VEGF gene modified BMSCs adenovirus could reduce reactive gliosis, ameliorate neurological deficit, diminish the percentage of cerebral infarction volume in rats, and facilitate angiogenesis [58]. In addition, BMSCs transplantation could ameliorate neurological deficit and increase neurogenesis as the result of VEGF-mediated angiogenesis without brain ischemia [59]. Therefore, it seems that BMSCs combined with VEGF may play a more significant role in protecting brain ischemia.

Together, our results give vital evidences that BMSCs treatment may be a potential effective therapy for pulmonary complication after brain ischemia derived brain ischemia. Moreover, BMSCs may regulate TNF-α expression in brain ischemia induced lung injury. Therefore, BMSCs treatment can reduce lung injury, in which, the possible mechanism may link to the inhibition of TNF-α in brain ischemia induced lung injured rats. Our findings is first time to show the protective effects of BMSCs in brain ischemia induced lung injury, which is linked to the inhibition of TNF-α expression.

Conclusions

We concluded that the intravenous transplantation of BMSCs originated from the bone marrow could partially ameliorate lung injury induced by brain ischemia, and inhibited the mobilization of inflammatory cells and reduce the TNF-α protein expression in lung. The present data indicate that BMSCs may serve as the basis of a novel therapeutic approach for patients suffering from pulmonary complications after brain injury, based on the TNF-α inhibition, in future clinic practice.

Authors' contributions
THW and JL conceived of the study and participated in its design and coordination and helped to revise the manuscript. QQH prepared the animal model and cultured the BMSCs cells. YPW and YZ performed the immunoassays. QJX performed the PCR. CZL revised the final the manuscript and gave valuable suggestions in the process of experiment. XH prepared the animal model in the revision work. LLX cultured the BMSCs cells in the revision work. XSH drafted the revision manuscript and replied the points of reviewers. All the authors read and approved the final manuscript.

Author details
[1] Department of Anesthesia and Critical Care Medicine Translational Neuroscience Center, West China Hospital, Sichuan University, Chengdu 610041, Sichuan, China. [2] Institute of Neuroscience and Experiment Animal Center, Kunming Medical University, Kunming 650031, China. [3] Center for Experimental Technology for Preclinical Medicine, Chengdu Medical College, Chengdu 610083, Sichuan, China.

Acknowledgements
We acknowledge contribution of Fei-fei Shang towards the article by making substantial contributions to analysis and interpretation of data. And acknowledge Dr. Visar for close editing of the language of the revision manuscript.

Competing interests
The authors declare that have no competing interests.

References
1. Mozaffarian D, et al. Heart disease and stroke statistics–2015 update: a report from the American Heart Association. Circulation. 2015;131(4):e29–322.

2. Krishnamurthi RV, et al. Global and regional burden of first-ever ischaemic and haemorrhagic stroke during 1990–2010: findings from the Global Burden of Disease Study 2010. Lancet Glob Health. 2013;1(5):e259–81.

3. Kim AS, Johnston SC. Global variation in the relative burden of stroke and ischemic heart disease. Circulation. 2011;124(3):314–23.

4. Lozano R, et al. Global and regional mortality from 235 causes of death for 20 age groups in 1990 and 2010: a systematic analysis for the Global Burden of Disease Study 2010. Lancet. 2012;380(9859):2095–128.

5. Lakshminarayan K, et al. Trends in 10-year survival of patients with stroke hospitalized between 1980 and 2000: the minnesota stroke survey. Stroke. 2014;45(9):2575–81.

6. Busl KM, Bleck TP. Neurogenic pulmonary edema. Crit Care Med. 2015;43(8):1710–5.

7. Hannawi Y, et al. Stroke-associated pneumonia: major advances and obstacles. Cerebrovasc Dis. 2013;35(5):430–43.

8. Rincon F, et al. The prevalence and impact of mortality of the acute respiratory distress syndrome on admissions of patients with ischemic stroke in the United States. J Intensive Care Med. 2014;29(6):357–64.

9. Rincon F, et al. Impact of acute lung injury and acute respiratory distress syndrome after traumatic brain injury in the United States. Neurosurgery. 2012;71(4):795–803.

10. Veeravagu A, et al. Acute lung injury in patients with subarachnoid hemorrhage: a nationwide inpatient sample study. World Neurosurg. 2014;82(1–2):e235–41.

11. Kahn JM, et al. Acute lung injury in patients with subarachnoid hemorrhage: incidence, risk factors, and outcome. Crit Care Med. 2006;34(1):196–202.

12. Otero HJ, Pollock AN. Neurogenic pulmonary edema. Pediatr Emerg Care. 2014;30(11):845–6.

13. Mrozek S, Constantin JM, Geeraerts T. Brain-lung crosstalk: implications for neurocritical care patients. World J Crit Care Med. 2015;4(3):163–78.

14. Bredin CP. Speculations on neurogenic pulmonary edema (NPE). Am Rev Respir Dis. 1976;114(4):814–5.

15. Keegan MT, Lanier WL. Pulmonary edema after resection of a fourth ventricle tumor: possible evidence for a medulla-mediated mechanism. Mayo Clin Proc. 1999;74(3):264–8.

16. Fein A, et al. The value of edema fluid protein measurement in patients with pulmonary edema. Am J Med. 1979;67(1):32–8.

17. Zaroff JG, et al. Regional patterns of left ventricular systolic dysfunction after subarachnoid hemorrhage: evidence for neurally mediated cardiac injury. J Am Soc Echocardiogr. 2000;13(8):774–9.

18. Baumann A, et al. Neurogenic pulmonary edema. Acta Anaesthesiol Scand. 2007;51(4):447–55.

19. Dongaonkar RM, et al. Balance point characterization of interstitial fluid volume regulation. Am J Physiol Regul Integr Comp Physiol. 2009;297(1):R6–16.

20. van der Zee H, et al. Lung fluid and protein exchange during intracranial hypertension and role of sympathetic mechanisms. J Appl Physiol Respir Environ Exerc Physiol. 1980;48(2):273–80.

21. Mascia L. Acute lung injury in patients with severe brain injury: a double hit model. Neurocrit Care. 2009;11(3):417–26.

22. Kalsotra A, et al. Brain trauma leads to enhanced lung inflammation and injury: evidence for role of P4504Fs in resolution. J Cereb Blood Flow Metab. 2007;27(5):963–74.

23. Aslam M, et al. Bone marrow stromal cells attenuate lung injury in a murine model of neonatal chronic lung disease. Am J Respir Crit Care Med. 2009;180(11):1122–30.

24. Liu QP, et al. Bone marrow mesenchymal stem cells ameliorates seawater-exposure-induced acute lung injury by inhibiting autophagy in lung tissue. Patholog Res Int. 2014;2014:104962.

25. Zhang ZH, et al. Effect of bone marrow mesenchymal stem cells on experimental pulmonary arterial hypertension. Exp Ther Med. 2012;4(5):839–43.

26. Islam MN, et al. Mitochondrial transfer from bone-marrow-derived stromal cells to pulmonary alveoli protects against acute lung injury. Nat Med. 2012;18(5):759–65.

27. Chen J, et al. Therapeutic benefit of intravenous administration of bone marrow stromal cells after cerebral ischemia in rats. Stroke. 2001;32(4):1005–11.

28. Gutierrez-Fernandez M, et al. Effects of intravenous administration of allogenic bone marrow- and adipose tissue-derived mesenchymal stem cells on functional recovery and brain repair markers in experimental ischemic stroke. Stem Cell Res Ther. 2013;4(1):11.

29. Gutierrez-Fernandez M, et al. Functional recovery after hematic administration of allogenic mesenchymal stem cells in acute ischemic stroke in rats. Neuroscience. 2011;175:394–405.

30. Li N, et al. Effect of bone marrow stromal cell transplantation on neurologic function and expression of VEGF in rats with focal cerebral ischemia. Mol Med Rep. 2014;10(5):2299–305.

31. Hu Q, et al. Therapeutic application of gene silencing MMP-9 in a middle cerebral artery occlusion-induced focal ischemia rat model. Exp Neurol. 2009;216(1):35–46.

32. Holland MC, et al. The development of acute lung injury is associated with worse neurologic outcome in patients with severe traumatic brain injury. J Trauma. 2003;55(1):106–11.

33. O'Phelan KH, et al. Therapeutic temperature modulation is associated with pulmonary complications in patients with severe traumatic brain injury. World J Crit Care Med. 2015;4(4):296–301.

34. Rodriguez-Gonzalez R, et al. Endotoxin-induced lung alveolar cell injury causes brain cell damage. Exp Biol Med (Maywood). 2015;240(1):135–42.

35. Arruza L et al. Hypoxic-ischemic brain damage induces distant inflammatory lung injury in newborn piglets. Pediatr Res. 2015.

36. Togel F, et al. Administered mesenchymal stem cells protect against ischemic acute renal failure through differentiation-independent mechanisms. Am J Physiol Renal Physiol. 2005;289(1):F31–42.

37. Lee JW, et al. Allogeneic human mesenchymal stem cells for treatment of E. coli endotoxin-induced acute lung injury in the ex vivo perfused human lung. Proc Natl Acad Sci USA. 2009;106(38):16357–62.

38. Xu YL, et al. Intravenous transplantation of mesenchymal stem cells attenuates oleic acid induced acute lung injury in rats. Chin Med J (Engl). 2012;125(11):2012–8.

39. Curley GF, et al. Mesenchymal stem cells enhance recovery and repair following ventilator-induced lung injury in the rat. Thorax. 2012;67(6):496–501.

40. Cobelens PM, et al. Interferon-beta attenuates lung inflammation following experimental subarachnoid hemorrhage. Crit Care. 2010;14(4):R157.

41. Lentsch AB, et al. Essential role of alveolar macrophages in intrapulmonary activation of NF-kappaB. Am J Respir Cell Mol Biol. 1999;20(4):692–8.

42. Morgan MJ, Liu ZG. Crosstalk of reactive oxygen species and NF-kappaB signaling. Cell Res. 2011;21(1):103–15.

43. Brody AR, Salazar KD, Lankford SM. Mesenchymal stem cells modulate lung injury. Proc Am Thorac Soc. 2010;7(2):130–3.

44. Uccelli A, Moretta L, Pistoia V. Immunoregulatory function of mesenchymal stem cells. Eur J Immunol. 2006;36(10):2566–73.

45. Nag S, Takahashi JL, Kilty DW. Role of vascular endothelial growth factor in blood–brain barrier breakdown and angiogenesis in brain trauma. J Neuropathol Exp Neurol. 1997;56(8):912–21.

46. Issa R, et al. Vascular endothelial growth factor and its receptor, KDR, in human brain tissue after ischemic stroke. Lab Invest. 1999;79(4):417–25.

47. Lennmyr F, et al. Vascular endothelial growth factor gene expression in middle cerebral artery occlusion in the rat. Acta Anaesthesiol Scand. 2005;49(4):488–93.

48. Yao X, et al. Protective effect of albumin on VEGF and brain edema in acute ischemia in rats. Neurosci Lett. 2010;472(3):179–83.

49. Schoch HJ, Fischer S, Marti HH. Hypoxia-induced vascular endothelial growth factor expression causes vascular leakage in the brain. Brain. 2002;125(Pt 11):2549–57.

50. Hayashi T, et al. Rapid induction of vascular endothelial growth factor gene expression after transient middle cerebral artery occlusion in rats. Stroke. 1997;28(10):2039–44.

51. Dvorak HF, et al. Vascular permeability factor/vascular endothelial growth factor and the significance of microvascular hyperpermeability in angiogenesis. Curr Top Microbiol Immunol. 1999;237:97–132.

52. Zhang ZG, et al. VEGF enhances angiogenesis and promotes blood-brain barrier leakage in the ischemic brain. J Clin Invest. 2000;106(7):829–38.

53. van Bruggen N, et al. VEGF antagonism reduces edema formation and tissue damage after ischemia/reperfusion injury in the mouse brain. J Clin Invest. 1999;104(11):1613–20.

54. Hayashi T, Abe K, Itoyama Y. Reduction of ischemic damage by application of vascular endothelial growth factor in rat brain after transient ischemia. J Cereb Blood Flow Metab. 1998;18(8):887–95.

55. Harrigan MR, et al. Effects of intraventricular infusion of vascular endothelial growth factor on cerebral blood flow, edema, and infarct volume. Acta Neurochir (Wien). 2003;145(1):49–53.

56. Betz AL, Coester HC. Effect of steroids on edema and sodium uptake of the brain during focal ischemia in rats. Stroke. 1990;21(8):1199–204.

57. Criscuolo GR, Merrill MJ, Oldfield EH. Characterization of a protein product of human malignant glial tumors that induces microvascular permeability. Adv Neurol. 1990;52:469–74.

58. Chen B, et al. Protective effect of Ad-VEGF-bone mesenchymal stem cells on cerebral infarction. Turk Neurosurg. 2016;26(1):8–15.

59. Yang Z, et al. Bone marrow stromal cell transplantation through tail vein injection promotes angiogenesis and vascular endothelial growth factor expression in cerebral infarct area in rats. Cytotherapy. 2015;17(9):1200–12.

The social brain network in 22q11.2 deletion syndrome: a diffusion tensor imaging study

Amy K. Olszewski[1], Zora Kikinis[2], Christie S. Gonzalez[3], Ioana L. Coman[1], Nikolaos Makris[2,4], Xue Gong[2], Yogesh Rathi[2], Anni Zhu[2], Kevin M. Antshel[3], Wanda Fremont[1], Marek R. Kubicki[2,5], Sylvain Bouix[2], Martha E. Shenton[5,6] and Wendy R. Kates[1]*

Abstract

Background: Chromosome 22q11.2 deletion syndrome (22q11.2DS) is a neurogenetic disorder that is associated with a 25-fold increase in schizophrenia. Both individuals with 22q11.2DS and those with schizophrenia present with social cognitive deficits, which are putatively subserved by a network of brain regions that are involved in the processing of social cognitive information. This study used two-tensor tractography to examine the white matter tracts believed to underlie the social brain network in a group of 57 young adults with 22q11.2DS compared to 30 unaffected controls.

Results: Results indicated that relative to controls, participants with 22q11.2DS showed significant differences in several DTI metrics within the inferior fronto-occipital fasciculus, cingulum bundle, thalamo-frontal tract, and inferior longitudinal fasciculus. In addition, participants with 22q11.2DS showed significant differences in scores on measures of social cognition, including the Social Responsiveness Scale and Trait Emotional Intelligence Questionnaire. Further analyses among individuals with 22q11.2DS demonstrated an association between DTI metrics and positive and negative symptoms of psychosis, as well as differentiation between individuals with 22q11.2DS and overt psychosis, relative to those with positive prodromal symptoms or no psychosis.

Conclusions: Findings suggest that white matter disruption, specifically disrupted axonal coherence in the right inferior fronto-occipital fasciculus, may be a biomarker for social cognitive difficulties and psychosis in individuals with 22q11.2DS.

Keywords: 22q11.2 deletion syndrome, Social brain network, Social cognition, Two-tensor tractography, White matter tracts

Background

Chromosome 22q11.2 deletion syndrome (22q11.2DS), also known as velo-cardio-facial syndrome (VCFS), or DiGeorge syndrome, is a genetic neurodevelopmental disorder that occurs as a result of an interstitial deletion of 40–50 genes on the long arm of chromosome 22 [1]. The most recent estimate of the syndrome's incidence is 1:992 live births [2]. The deletion is associated with a myriad of physical features, including distinctive facial characteristics, palatal abnormalities, and cardiac anomalies [3]. In addition to these physical characteristics, individuals with 22q11.2DS often possess a distinct neuropsychological profile, consisting of a full scale IQ in the borderline range, as well as deficits in executive function, working memory, and visuospatial abilities [4–6]. 22q11.2DS is also associated with multiple psychiatric comorbidities, including mood disorders [7–10], anxiety disorders [3, 9, 11–13], attention-deficit/hyperactivity disorder (ADHD; [9–11, 13]), autism spectrum disorder (ASD; [5, 14, 15]), and, in up to 30–40% of adults,

*Correspondence: katesw@upstate.edu
[1] Department of Psychiatry, SUNY Upstate Medical University, 750 E. Adams St., Syracuse, NY 13210, USA
Full list of author information is available at the end of the article

psychotic disorders such as schizophrenia [16, 17]. In fact, aside from having a monozygotic twin with schizophrenia, 22q11.2DS is the next highest risk for developing schizophrenia [16].

Social processing and the social brain

Many individuals with 22q11.2DS also experience social difficulties, including shyness, withdrawal, social immaturity, and deficits in social cognition [18–21]. Social cognition refers to the mental processes that subserve social interactions [22] and includes theory of mind, i.e., being able to see things from another's perspective, also referred to as "mentalizing skills," attributional style, social perception, and emotional processing abilities [22, 23]. Importantly, social cognitive impairments have also been identified in individuals with schizophrenia [24] and autism spectrum disorders [25].

Of further note, functional brain imaging studies have identified two major social networks that are involved in social cognition tasks: a mirror network, which is involved in reading another individual's body language, and a mentalizing network that allows for social mentalizing, or taking another's perspective [26–28]. These networks involve several brain regions in the prefrontal (i.e., dorsolateral-ventrolateral-medial prefrontal and premotor cortices), pregenual and dorsal anterior cingulate regions, the insula, the amygdala, inferior parietal lobule and precuneus as well as the temporopolar and the temporo-parieto-occipital junction areas [24, 29, 30]. Insofar as studies have shown associations between aberrant connectivity within the mentalizing network and social cognitive difficulties among individuals with schizophrenia [31–34], ASD [35–38], and 22q11.2DS [39, 40], our primary interest was to examine the white matter tracts underlying social cognition in 22q11.2DS.

Structural imaging: diffusion tensor imaging

Recent advances in imaging, including diffusion tensor imaging (DTI) and fiber tractography post-processing analyses, have enabled the use of noninvasive methods to measure structural white matter tract integrity in vivo by examining the diffusion of water molecules in the brain. DTI metrics, including fractional anisotropy (FA), a measure of white matter integrity, radial diffusivity (RD), a purported measure of myelin integrity, and axial diffusivity (AD), a purported measure of axonal integrity, make it possible to quantify differences in these metrics across groups. Studies in individuals with 22q11.2DS show altered white matter microstructure in long-range and limbic connections (see review by [41]), including fronto-parietal, fronto-temporal, and parieto-occipital networks, as well as in cingulum bundle (CB), anterior limb of the internal capsule (ALIC), anterior thalamic

radiation and uncinate fasciculus (UF), all areas known to show abnormalities in individuals with schizophrenia [41–46].

DTI tracts related to social functioning

Several white matter tracts are believed to play important roles in the transmission of social information. For example, the CB is an associative bundle of fibers running through the cingulate gyrus around the corpus callosum. Longer fibers run from the anterior temporal gyrus to the orbitofrontal cortex, while shorter fibers connect the four lobar regions of the brain and the cingulate cortex [47]. The location of the CB within the limbic system suggests that it plays an important role in emotional information processing. The UF is also part of the limbic system, and connects the amygdala to the anterior temporal lobe and orbitofrontal cortex [47]. Thus, the UF is also believed to play a role in emotion processing.

The superior longitudinal fasciculus (SLF) is composed of four separate components, SLF I—SLF III and the arcuate fasciculus. The SLF II composes the central core of white matter above the insula, and is believed to be the major link between the parietal lobe and prefrontal cortex, thereby implicating a role in the perception of visual space [48]. The inferior fronto-occipital fasciculus (IFOF) connects the ventral occipital lobe to the orbitofrontal cortex, and is involved in visual processing/facial emotion recognition [47]. A study by DeRosse and colleagues [49] found that lower FA in the IFOF is related to higher levels of schizotypy, indicating a possible role for IFOF in experience/affect sharing [49]. The inferior longitudinal fasciculus (ILF) connects the occipital and temporal lobes. While not much is known regarding the ILF's functionality, it is believed to be involved in face recognition and visual object perception [47, 50, 51]. Finally, the anterior thalamic radiation (ATR) connects the anterior nuclear and midline nuclear groups of the thalamus with the frontal lobe [52]. The ATR is located in the thalamolimbic area, and hypoconnectivity of the ATR has been demonstrated in males with ASD, a disorder associated with social cognitive impairment [53]. Studies have also shown that functional connectivity (i.e., fMRI) reflects structural connectivity (i.e., DTI) in the mentalizing network [54, 55].

The aim of the current project was to explore structural DTI tracts hypothesized to be involved in the social brain, as well as to investigate associations with measures of social and emotional processing. We predicted that there would be significant differences between individuals with 22q11.2DS and controls in DTI metrics, including FA, RD, AD, and the number of streamlines (an estimate of fiber bundles). Following the expected reductions in DTI metrics, we also hypothesized: (1) FA in IFOF, SLF, the thalamo-frontal tract, and CB would be correlated with a measure of social responsiveness; (2) FA in ILF and IFOF would be associated with a measure of experience and affect sharing; and (3) FA in UF and IFOF would be associated with emotion regulation and cognitive reappraisal. Finally, we predicted that alterations in DTI metrics in 22q11.2DS would be associated with a dimensional measure of both positive and negative symptoms of prodromal/overt psychosis.

Methods

Participants

The imaging and psychiatric data presented in this study were derived from a subsample of participants enrolled in a longitudinal study of risk factors for psychosis in 22q11.2DS [56]. This subsample consists of 57 participants with 22q11.2DS, 12 unaffected siblings, and 18 community controls who returned for the fourth time point of the study. Participants were recruited from the International Center for Evaluation, Treatment, and Study of Velo-Cardio-Facial Syndrome at SUNY Upstate Medical University, parent support groups, and the surrounding community. Presence of the 22q11.2 deletion was confirmed with fluorescence in situ hybridization (FISH). Informed consent was obtained under protocols approved by the medical center's institutional review board. Initial statistical analyses comparing sibling and community controls did not differ for any of the measures utilized in this study (see Additional file 1). Therefore, we combined the sibling and community controls into one control group for the remainder of the analyses. Demographic information is provided in Table 1.

Several papers examining white matter microstructure have been published on this cohort based on assessment at the third time point of the study (when they were between the ages of 15 and 21) [43, 45, 46]. However, this is the first paper to examine white matter microstructure based on participants' assessments at the 4th timepoint of the study, when they were between the ages of 18 and 24 years, representing the age window at which this cohort is at highest risk for developing psychotic symptoms. Moreover, whereas previous papers have been based on imaging data acquired from a 1.5 Tesla scanner, the current study is based on data acquired from a 3 Tesla scanner, utilizing state-of-the-art two-tensor tractography to measure white matter microstructure.

Exclusion criteria for all participants included: presence of a seizure disorder, fetal exposure to alcohol or drugs, parent-reported elevated lead levels, birthweight under 2500 g, history of loss of consciousness lasting longer than 15 min, paramagnetic implants, or orthodontic braces. Potential community control participants were also excluded if there was a personal or family history of

Table 1 Participant demographics

Demographic variable	22q11.2DS (N = 57)	Control (N = 30)
Age [Mean (SD)]	20.87 (2.29)	20.97 (1.46)
Gender [N (%)]		
Male	31 (54.4)	17 (56.7)
Female	26 (45.6)	13 (43.3)
FSIQ [Mean (SD)]	74.54 (11.82)***	109.47 (16.02)
Race [N (%)]		
Native American	0	1 (3.3)
Asian	1 (1.8)	2 (6.7)
African American	0	1 (3.3)
Caucasian	51 (89.5)	24 (80.0)
More than one	2 (3.5)	1 (3.3)
Unknown	3 (5.3)	1 (3.3)
Psychiatric diagnosis [N (%)]		
Mood disorder	7 (12.3)	1 (3.3)
Anxiety disorder	16 (28.1)	5 (16.7)
ASD	7 (12.3)	0
ADHD	9 (15.8)	5 (16.7)
Psychotic disorder	4 (7.0)	0
Other	3 (5.2)	0
Any psychiatric diagnosis	27 (47.4)	7 (23.3)

22q11.2DS, 22q11.2 deletion syndrome; FSIQ, full scale IQ; ASD, autism spectrum disorder; ADHD, attention-deficit/hyperactivity disorder

*** $p < .0001$

schizophrenia or bipolar disorder [57]. All participants were screened for psychiatric disorders using the structured clinical interview for DSM-IV-TR (SCID).

Procedures

As described in previous studies [7, 11, 14, 58], each participant and parent/caregiver completed measures of cognitive and/or social, emotional, and behavioral functioning. All diagnostic interviews were completed by a licensed psychiatrist or psychologist, and all neuropsychological measures were administered by an experienced doctoral-level examiner. Due to the facial features characteristic of 22q11.2DS, evaluator blindness to group assignment was not possible. A licensed psychologist or trained student assistant familiar with the measures double scored all protocols to ensure scoring accuracy. Caregivers completed behavior rating scales and background information while the children and adolescents were completing neuropsychological measures.

Measures

Wechsler Adult Intelligence Scale, third edition (WAIS-III)
The WAIS-III [59] is a test of cognitive ability that provides intelligence quotient (IQ) scores, including a full scale IQ (FSIQ), verbal IQ (VIQ), and performance

IQ (PIQ) for individuals 16 years of age and older. The WAIS-III consists of several subtests (mean = 10, SD = 3), which measure various domains. The WAIS-III has outstanding reliability, with internal consistency reliability coefficients at or above .93 for the WAIS-III FSIQ, VIQ, and PIQ [60].

Social Responsiveness Scale (SRS)

The SRS is a 65-item parent report questionnaire designed to assess the different dimensions of interpersonal behavior, communication, and repetitive/stereotypic behaviors that are characteristic of autism spectrum disorders [61]. Psychometric properties of the SRS are excellent, with total score alpha coefficients above .90 for both males and females in both clinical and normative sample [61]. In this study, we used the adult research version of the SRS to assess for social deficits, with higher total raw scores indicative of more severe social impairment [62].

Junior Schizotypy Scale (JSS)

The JSS is a 50-item self-report questionnaire used to measure schizotypal personality traits in adolescents, which are believed to indicate a predisposition to schizophrenia in adulthood. The JSS provides scores for five subscales, each of which reflect a particular aspect of schizotypy: cognitive, perceptual, social, impulsive nonconformity, and physical anhedonia [63]. Higher scores on each scale indicate higher levels of schizotypy.

Trait Emotional Intelligence Questionnaire (TEIQue)

The TEIQue [64] is a 153-item questionnaire based on trait emotion intelligence theory. The TEIQue uses a 7-point Likert response scale (1: disagree completely; 7: agree completely) to measure the level of various facets of emotional intelligence. Higher scores on each facet represent better levels of perceived abilities and dispositions [64]. This study used the parent version of the TEIQue, in which the parent or caregiver rated the participant's emotional intelligence. For the current study, we were particularly interested in the four facets that relate to social cognition; therefore, our analyses focused on emotion regulation (the degree to which an individual has control over his or her emotions), empathy (the ability to take another's perspective), social awareness (social skills and the ability to adapt to and interact in various social situations), and emotion perception (the ability to perceive one's own and others' emotions).

Structured interview for prodromal syndromes (SIPS)

The SIPS [65] is a scale that measures the severity and change of individuals who are experiencing pre-psychotic symptoms. The SIPS consists of five positive symptom items, six negative symptom items, four items related to disorganized symptoms, and four general symptom items, each of which are rated on a severity scale ranging from 0 (never or absent) to 6 (severe and psychotic, or extreme). The SIPS was administered to all study participants and separately to their parents. The positive symptoms (SIPS PS) and negative symptoms (SIPS NS) scores were used for the purpose of determining prodromal/psychotic symptoms.

MRI acquisition/DTI processing
Scan acquisitions

For the time point examined in this study (Time Four), images were acquired using a 3T Siemens Magnetom Tim Trio scanner (Siemens Medical Solutions, Erlangen, Germany).The high resolution anatomic scan consisted of an ultrafast gradient echo 3D sequence (MPRAGE) with PAT k-space-based algorithm GRAPPA. The parameters included: echo time = 3.31 ms; repetition time = 2530 ms; matrix size = 256 × 256; field of view (FOV) = 256 mm; slice thickness = 1 mm. The DWI sequence consisted of 64 transverse slices with no gaps and 2.0 mm nominal isotropic resolution (TR/TE = 8600/93 ms, FOV = 244 × 244, data matrix = 96 × 96, zero-filled and reconstructed to 256 × 256). Diffusion weighting was applied along 64 directions with a *b* factor = 700 s/mm^2. One minimally weighted volume (b$_0$) was acquired within each DWI dataset. The total scan time to acquire the DWI dataset was 4 min., 52 s. A high resolution T2 scan was also obtained to align with the DWI images.

Diffusion tensor imaging preprocessing

An in-house script was used to correct for eddy current distortions and head motion. This script registered each diffusion-weighted volume to the baseline volume using FSL (http://fsl.fmrib.ox.ac.uk) linear registration software "FLIRT". Motion correction was not performed.

Whole brain tractography

For the purposes of this study, we used two-tensor tractography to determine white matter tracts/bundles. As compared to single tensor tractography, two-tensor tractography offers a better fiber representation in both fiber branching and fiber crossing by computing two tensors for each voxel [66]. We generated fiber tracts from DWI images using the Unscented Kalman Filter (UKF) based on two-tensor tractography algorithm [67]. Tract seeding was completed in every voxel where the primary single tensor FA value was larger than .18, with each voxel seeded 10 times. Fibers between neighboring voxels were traced following the direction of the primary tensor component. Fibers were terminated when the primary tensor FA value was less than .15.

FreeSurfer parcellations and registration to DTI space

We used FreeSurfer software (http://surfer.nmr.mgh.harvard.edu) to obtain regions of interest via an automated approach, which parcellated the cortical and white matter regions. We applied FreeSurfer software to segment T1-weighted SPGR images into 34 bilateral, cortical and white matter regions for each participant [68]. The label map with FreeSurfer-generated regions of interest was registered to the DWI space by first diffeomorphically registering a T2 image in the same space as the SPGR image to the baseline DWI image of the same participant using the FLIRT algorithm of the FSL software [69], and then applying this diffeomorphism to register the FreeSurfer-generated label map to the DWI space for the same participant. We performed this transformation of the FreeSurfer label map to DWI space for each participant.

White matter query language

White matter query language (WMQL) was used to extract fiber tracts from the two-tensor whole brain tractography [70]. WMQL was designed to use neuroanatomical definitions of white matter to estimate fiber tracts [47]. Fiber tract definitions were based on cortical regions known to be connected via these fiber bundles, as well as on white matter regions where the fiber tract is expected to project. These definitions used the FreeSurfer-generated parcellations of cortical and white matter regions [70]. We implemented WMQL queries to extract the left and right hemisphere CB, ILF, SLF II, and thalamo-frontal tracts. Because the WMQL approach does not rely on a specific atlas, label maps other than those generated by FreeSurfer can also be used. We extracted the right and left hemisphere UF and IFOF from the 2-tensor whole brain tractography using a label map with manually drawn ROIs. The DTI metrics of FA, AD, and RD were extracted from the entire fiber tract and the mean values were computed. WMQL also allowed us to calculate the number of streamlines for each tract, and only tracts with more than 10 streamlines were reported. Two-tensor tractography was first used in a study on first-episode schizophrenia [71], and in later studies combining two-tensor tractography with WMQL queries [48, 70]. It has not, until this study, been used in 22q11.2DS.

Statistical analyses

The data were examined for normality in order to ensure they met criteria for the assumptions of statistical tests to be used. For variables that did not meet the assumption of normality (i.e., skewness and/or kurtosis <1.0), we applied a log transformation to normalize the data. For data that remained nonnormal after transformation, we created standardized residuals so that nonparametric tests could be used. Where appropriate, analysis of covariance (ANCOVA) and multivariate analyses of covariance (MANCOVAs), using either hemispheric white matter volume or FSIQ as covariates, were used to investigate possible differences between groups on DTI metrics and social brain measures, respectively. Follow up ANOVAs examined which dependent variables drove the significant differences in DTI metrics and scores on social brain measures. In the Results section, we report on DTI metrics that passed Bonferroni correction for multiple comparisons on each hemispheric tract, as well as subscales of social brain measures that passed Bonferroni correction for each measure. Individual Bonferroni correction thresholds varied according to the number of dependent variables within each measure. We also used Pearson correlations to examine relationships between significantly different DTI tract metrics and social brain measures. We used Spearman correlations for variables that remained nonnormal after log transformation. Finally, we used zero-inflated Poisson (ZIP) regressions to analyze the associations between social measures and positive prodromal symptoms, and DTI tracts and positive prodromal symptoms. All data were analyzed using SPSS v. 23 or Stata v. 12.0.

Results

DTI tract differences

To explore group differences in DTI metrics, we conducted a multivariate analysis of covariance (MANCOVA), using hemispheric white matter volume as a covariate, to compare participants with 22q11.2DS and controls. Table 2 presents the descriptive statistics for all DTI metrics, and Table 3 includes results of the MANCOVA. Compared to controls, participants with 22q11.2DS showed a significant increase in left FA, suggesting increased white matter integrity, and a significant decrease in left RD (suggesting decreased white matter integrity) within the IFOF; a significant increase in right hemisphere FA (increased white matter integrity) and a significant decrease in right RD (decreased white matter integrity) within the CB; a significant increase in right hemisphere FA (increased white matter integrity) and a significant decrease in right hemisphere RD (decreased white matter integrity) within the thalamo-frontal tract; and a significant decrease in right hemisphere RD for the ILF. Results for the SLF did not pass the Bonferroni correction.

Nonparametric Mann–Whitney U tests were conducted for the non-normally distributed right hemisphere IFOF RD ($p < .0001$) and FA ($p = .001$), as well as the right hemisphere UF number of streamlines ($p = .010$), indicating group differences in these metrics.

Table 2 Descriptive statistics for DTI metrics

	22q11.2DS		Control	
	M	*SD*	*M*	*SD*
Left hemisphere				
UF FA	.589	.036	.591	.027
UF RD	.000467	.0000424	.000471	.0000328
UF AD	.00136	.0000365	.00138	.0000342
UF number of stream-lines	129.179	119.85	152.774	100.28
IFOF FA	*.691*	*.025*	*.662*	*.029*
IFOF RD	*.000373*	*.0000282*	*.000414*	*.0000352*
IFOF AD	.00147	.0000373	.00148	.0000292
IFOF number of streamlines	336.927	242.56	421.000	187.77
CB FA	.608	.032	.599	.032
CB RD	.000429	.0000338	.000448	.0000349
CB AD	.00132	.0000355	.00135	.0000350
CB number of stream-lines	1228.754	398.591	1119.677	344.107
ILF FA	.645	.039	.640	.047
ILF RD	.000423	.0000535	.000430	.0000470
ILF AD	.00143	.0000514	.00146	.0000719
ILF number of stream-lines	20.158	18.817	11.000	9.501
SLF FA	.643	.034	.639	.041
SLF RD	.000418	.0000498	.000420	.0000482
SLF AD	.00141	.0000496	.00141	.0000519
SLF number of streamlines	66.774	55.734	108.355	79.342
Thalamo-frontal FA	.629	.022	.624	.016
Thalamo-frontal RD	.000407	.0000218	.000447	.0000182
Thalamo-frontal AD	.00132	.0000288	.00134	.0000223
Thalamo-frontal number of streamlines	760.772	335.754	726.871	218.347
Right hemisphere				
UF FA	.601	.045	.593	.027
UF RD	.000442	.0000449	.000456	.0000295
UF AD	.00133	.0000322	.00134	.0000254
UF number of stream-lines	*144.036*	*114.118*	*236.581*	*142.907*
IFOF FA	*.708*	*.027*	*.683*	*.027*
IFOF RD	*.000354*	*.0000310*	*.000386*	*.0000312*
IFOF AD	.00147	.0000359	.00148	.0000274
IFOF number of streamlines	350.255	2235.006	474.452	239.131
CB FA	*.609*	*.027*	*.588*	*.029*
CB RD	.000421	.0000304	.000451	.0000310
CB AD	.00130	.0000346	.00132	.0000298
CB number of stream-lines	*995.035*	*341.383*	*818.516*	*283.127*
ILF FA	.662	.024	.646	.033
ILF RD	*.000396*	*.0000307*	*.000419*	*.0000404*
ILF AD	.00140	.0000588	.00143	.0000393

Table 2 continued

	22q11.2DS		Control	
	M	*SD*	*M*	*SD*
ILF number of stream-lines	31.684	31.783	25.065	20.855
SLF FA	.649	.039	.656	.043
SLF RD	.000399	.0000370	.000401	.0000491
SLF AD	.00139	.0000582	.00142	.0000417
SLF number of streamlines	83.192	74.113	144.194	133.073
Thalamo-frontal FA	*.633*	*.019*	*.621*	*.023*
Thalamo-frontal RD	*.000401*	*.0000223*	*.000417*	*.0000241*
Thalamo-frontal AD	.00132	.0000226	.00132	.0000214
Thalamo-frontal num-ber of streamlines	821.088	318.348	769.516	239.898

DTI, diffusion tensor imaging; 22q11.2DS, 22q11.2 deletion syndrome; UF, uncinate fasciculus; IFOF, inferior fronto-occipital fasciculus; CB, cingulum bundle; ILF, inferior longitudinal fasciculus; SLF, superior longitudinal fasciculus; FA, fractional anisotropy; RD, radial diffusivity; AD, axial diffusivity

Bonferroni corrected statistically significant differences indicated in italics

Compared to controls, participants with 22q11.2DS showed a significant increase in the right hemisphere IFOF FA, and a significant decrease in right hemisphere IFOF RD and UF number of streamlines. Figure 1 depicts the reconstructed white matter tracts for which we found significant differences between groups.

Differences in social brain behavioral measures

To explore group differences in behavior-based social brain measures, we conducted an Analysis of Covariance (ANCOVA) to compare participants with 22q11.2DS and controls for scores on the SRS. We used FSIQ as a covariate to account for the fact that overall intelligence may affect social cognitive ability. Due to the nonnormality of the SRS variable, we applied a log transformation which normalized the SRS data. Descriptive statistics are presented in Table 4. Results indicated significantly higher (i.e., more impaired) scores in the group of individuals with 22q11.2DS (range = 17–140) compared to controls (range = 3–75) [$F(1, 83) = 16.352, p < .0001$].

We conducted a multivariate analysis of variance (MANOVA) to compare scores between groups on the JSS. Descriptive statistics are presented in Table 4. Results demonstrated no significant differences between groups on the social, cognitive, physical, and perceptual subscales of the JSS; therefore, we did not run an analysis to covary for FSIQ (Table 5). We conducted a nonparametric Mann–Whitney U test for the non-normally distributed JSS Impulsive scale; results also indicated no significant differences between groups ($p = .677$).

Finally, we conducted a MANCOVA using FSIQ as a covariate to compare scores between groups on the

Table 3 Results of MANCOVAs for DTI Tracts

Tract	Wilks' Lambda	*p* value	Dependent variable	*F* (df)	p value	Partial eta squared
Left UF	.899	.069	Fractional anisotropy	.004 (1, 84)	.948	.000
			Radial diffusivity	.095 (1, 84)	.758	.001
			Axial diffusivity	2.878 (1, 84)	.093	.033
			Number of streamlines	.001 (1, 84)	.976	.000
Right UF	.758	<.0001	Fractional anisotropy	1.308 (1, 84)	.256	.015
			Radial diffusivity	3.483 (1, 84)	.065	.040
			Axial diffusivity	4.344 (1, 84)	.040	.049
Left IFOF	.678	<.0001	Fractional anisotropy	26.542 (1, 83)	*<.0001*	.242
			Radial diffusivity	34.271 (1, 83)	*<.0001*	.292
			Axial diffusivity	.762 (1, 83)	.385	.009
			Number of streamlines	1.581 (1, 83)	.212	.019
Right IFOF	.681	<.0001	Axial diffusivity	1.457 (1, 83)	.231	.017
			Number of streamlines	3.111 (1, 83)	.081	.036
Left CB	.825	.003	Fractional anisotropy	4.387 (1, 85)	.039	.049
			Radial diffusivity	8.051 (1, 85)	.006	.087
			Axial diffusivity	4.091 (1, 85)	.046	.046
			Number of streamlines	8.681 (1, 85)	.004	.093
Right CB	.708	<.0001	Fractional anisotropy	14.008 (1, 85)	*<.0001*	.141
			Radial diffusivity	20.097 (1, 85)	*<.0001*	.191
			Axial diffusivity	4.739 (1, 85)	.032	.053
			Number of streamlines	19.858 (1, 85)	*<.0001*	.189
Left ILF	.810	.002	Fractional anisotropy	.181 (1, 85)	.671	.002
			Radial diffusivity	.107 (1, 85)	.744	.001
			Axial diffusivity	1.352 (1, 85)	.248	.016
			Number of streamlines	5.167 (1, 85)	.026	.057
Right ILF	.803	.001	Fractional anisotropy	7.705 (1, 85)	.007	.083
			Radial diffusivity	11.332 (1, 85)	*.001*	.118
			Axial diffusivity	5.246 (1, 85)	.024	.058
			Number of streamlines	.571 (1, 85)	.452	.007
Left SLF	.885	.046	Fractional anisotropy	.608 (1, 81)	.438	.007
			Radial diffusivity	.128 (1, 81)	.722	.002
			Axial diffusivity	.115 (1, 81)	.736	.001
			Number of streamlines	4.813 (1, 81)	.031	.056
Right SLF	.899	.072	Fractional anisotropy	.004 (1, 83)	.952	.000
			Radial diffusivity	.496 (1, 83)	.483	.006
			Axial diffusivity	2.787 (1, 83)	.099	.032
			Number of streamlines	4.252 (1, 83)	.042	.049
Left thalamo-frontal	.831	.004	Fractional anisotropy	4.347 (1, 85)	.040	.081
			Radial diffusivity	7.483 (1, 85)	.008	.059
			Axial diffusivity	.845 (1, 85)	.361	.010
			Number of streamlines	1.008 (1, 85)	.318	.012
Right thalamo-frontal	.870	.021	Fractional anisotropy	9.116 (1, 85)	*.003*	.097
			Radial diffusivity	9.911 (1, 85)	*.002*	.104
			Axial diffusivity	.731 (1, 85)	.395	.009
			Number of streamlines	2.485 (1, 85)	.119	.028

UF, uncinate fasciculus; IFOF, inferior fronto-occipital fasciculus; CB, cingulum bundle; ILF, inferior longitudinal fasciculus; SLF, superior longitudinal fasciculus

Bonferroni corrected statistically significant results indicated in italics (*p* < .004)

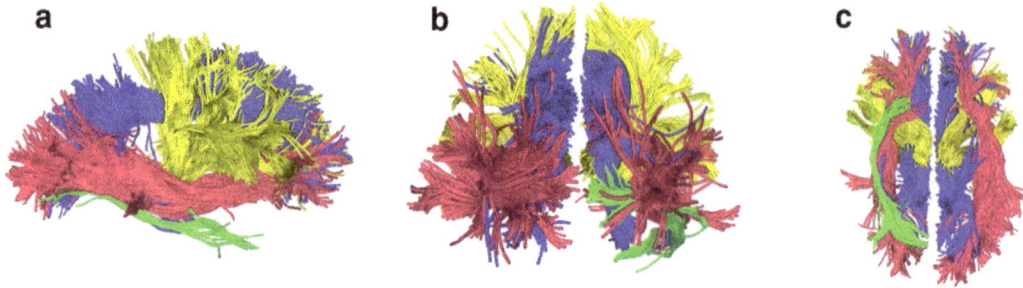

Fig. 1 Fiber tracts of interest. ILF = *green*, IFOF = *red*, thalamo-frontal connection = *yellow*, and CB = *blue*. **a** Right lateral view (**b**) posterior view (**c**) inferior view

Table 4 Descriptive statistics for social measures

Measure	22q11.2DS		Controls	
	M	SD	M	SD
SRS total	*73.321*	*3.896*	*18.433*	*5.323*
JSS social	2.930	2.412	1.700	1.841
JSS cognitive	3.982	2.066	2.900	2.057
JSS perceptual	1.298	1.773	.533	1.047
JSS impulsive	2.421	1.861	2.300	1.765
JSS physical	3.579	1.927	2.600	1.632
TEIQue emotion regulation	*3.949*	*1.196*	*5.247*	*.841*
TEIQue empathy	*3.452*	*1.043*	*5.196*	*.858*
TEIQue social awareness	*3.360*	*1.042*	*5.473*	*.965*
TEIQue emotion perception	*3.507*	*1.025*	*5.243*	*.841*

SRS, Social Responsiveness Scale, adult research version; JSS, Junior Schizotypy Scale; TEIQue, Trait Emotional Intelligence Questionnaire; 22q11.2DS, 22q11.2 deletion syndrome

Statistically significant differences indicated in italics

TEIQue. Descriptive statistics are presented in Table 4. Due to nonnormality of the social awareness variable, we ran an ANCOVA using FSIQ as a covariate for the log transformed version of this variable. Results indicated significant differences in scores between individuals with 22q11.2DS and controls (F [1, 83] = 13.395, p < .0001).

Therefore, parents/caregivers of individuals with 22q11.2DS rated them significantly lower than parents/caregivers of controls on three of the four facet scores of interest in this study; emotion regulation did not pass Bonferroni correction (Table 5).

Correlations between DTI tracts and social behavioral measures

We used Pearson correlations where appropriate and Spearman correlations for variables that remained nonnormal after log transformation to examine the associations between behavioral measures of social processing and the DTI tracts that had significantly differentiated the study groups. Results are displayed in Tables 6 and 7. Among participants with 22q11.2DS, marginally significant Bonferroni-corrected associations were found between the right UF number of streamlines and the JSS Social scale ($\rho = .260$, $p = .039$), the right UF number of streamlines and the TEIQue Social Awareness facet ($\rho = -.224$, $p = .050$), and the right IFOF RD and JSS Impulsive scale ($\rho = -.380$, $p = .006$). We noted significant Bonferroni-corrected positive correlations between the right thalamo-frontal tract RD and TEIQue Empathy facet ($r = .351$, $p = .001$), as well as between the right IFOF FA and the JSS Impulsive scale ($\rho = .412$, $p = .003$) and the right UF number of streamlines and

Table 5 Results of MANCOVA for social measures

Measure	Wilks' Lambda	p value	Dependent variable	F (df)	p value
Junior Schizotypy Scale	.934	.740	Social	1.128 (1, 31)	.296
			Cognitive	.003 (1, 31)	.958
			Perceptual	.417 (1, 31)	.523
			Physical	.016 (1, 31)	.901
TEIQue	.801	.001	Emotion regulation	5.667 (1, 83)	.020
			Empathy	14.618 (1,83)	*<.0001*
			Emotion perception	12.727 (1,83)	*.001*

TEIQue, Trait Emotional Intelligence Questionnaire

Bonferroni corrected significant results indicated in italics (*p* < .007)

Table 6 Pearson correlation coefficients for DTI tracts and social measures

Group	SRS	JSS social	JSS cognitive	JSS perceptual	JSS physical	JSS impulsive	TEIQue emotion perception	TEIQue social awareness	TEIQue empathy	TEIQue emotion regulation
22q11.2DS										
Right CB FA	.020	.263	.114	−.193	.229	.154	−.052	.039	−.205	.032
Right CB RD	−.068	−.290	−.152	.145	−.175	−.088	.043	−.017	.265	−.070
Left CB AD	.017	−.029	−.100	−.180	.163	.157	−.177	−.033	.025	−.194
Left IFOF FA	−.079	−.067	.019	−.305	−.032	−.091	.096	.060	−.081	−.056
Left IFOF RD	.087	−.006	.025	.216	−.007	.003	−.010	.003	.071	−.062
Right ILF RD	.162	−.049	.071	.122	−.192	.126	−.141	−.127	.244	−.208
Right thalamo-frontal RD	−.130	−.084	−.041	.233	−.034	.016	.082	.059	.351*	.017
Control										
Right CB FA	−.103	.028	−.056	−.186	−.148	−.225	−.088	−.062	−.060	−.207
Right CB RD	.094	.045	.037	.236	.087	.263	.058	.069	.057	.223
Left CB AD	−.028	.335	.099	.254	.196	.209	−.070	.050	.005	.037
Left IFOF FA	.054	−.080	.061	−.003	.359	−.211	−.112	.082	−.120	−.016
Left IFOF RD	−.038	.146	−.094	.041	−.304	.212	.110	−.069	.101	.001
Right ILF RD	−.055	.112	−.060	.299	−.090	.316	.064	.125	.028	.245
Right thalamo-frontal RD	−.078	.016	−.179	.093	.105	.242	.069	.080	−.139	.016

SRS, Social Responsiveness Scale; JSS, Junior Schizotypy Scale; TEIQue, Trait Emotional Intelligence Questionnaire; CB, cingulum bundle; IFOF, inferior fronto-occipital fasciculus; ILF, inferior longitudinal fasciculus; FA, fractional anisotropy; RD, radial diffusivity; AD, axial diffusivity

* $p < .01$

Table 7 Spearman correlation coefficients for DTI tracts and social measures

Group	SRS	JSS Social	JSS cognitive	JSS perceptual	JSS physical	JSS impulsive	TEIQue emotion perception	TEIQue social awareness	TEIQue empathy	TEIQue emotion regulation
22q11.2DS										
Right UF number streamlines	.396**	.260*	.100	.169	.061	.133	−.172	−.224*	−.362**	−.011
Right IFOF FA	.141	.179	.153	−.163	.200	.412**	−.075	−.043	−.189	.135
Right IFOF RD	−.097	−.142	−.148	.164	−.182	−.380*	.040	.005	.201	−.169
Control										
Right UF number streamlines	−.196	.217	−.411*	−.040	.265	.071	.138	.007	.019	.180
Right IFOF FA	−.066	−.032	.084	.408	.080	.049	−.004	.120	−.046	−.085
Right IFOF RD	.107	.029	−.052	−.408	−.039	−.109	−.032	−.071	.031	.068

SRS, Social Responsiveness Scale; JSS, Junior Schizotypy Scale; TEIQue, Trait Emotional Intelligence Questionnaire; UF, uncinate fasciculus; IFOF, inferior fronto-occipital fasciculus; FA, fractional anisotropy; RD, radial diffusivity

* p < .05

** p < .01

Table 8 Descriptive statistics for 22q11.2DS group by psychosis level

Demographic variable	22q11.2DS no psychosis ($n = 43$)	22q11.DS + prodromal psychosis ($n = 10$)	22q11.2DS + overt psychosis ($n = 4$)
Age [mean (SD)]	20.65 (2.15)	22.60 (2.50)	19.52 (1.76)
Gender [N (%)]			
Male	25 (58.1)	5 (50.0)	1 (25.0)
Female	18 (41.9)	5 (50.0)	3 (75.0)
FSIQ [mean (SD)]	*76.56 (12.33)*	71.00 (6.65)	*61.75 (5.32)*

22q11.2DS, 22q11.2 deletion syndrome; FSIQ, full scale IQ

Statistically significant differences indicated in italics ($p = .015$)

Table 9 Descriptive Statistics for DTI metrics by psychosis level

DTI metric	22q11.2DS no psychosis		22q11.DS + prodromal psychosis		22q11.2DS + overt psychosis	
	M	SD	M	SD	M	SD
RH UF number streamlines	145.488	123.879	165.000	91.459	103.750	38.638
RH IFOF FA	.702	.023	.715	.016	*.743*	*.053*
RH IFOF RD	.00036	.000026	.00034	.000023	*.00031*	*.000058*
RH CB FA	.609	.028	.062	.027	.587	.019
RH CB RD	.00042	.000031	.00041	.000030	.00043	.000032
RH ILF RD	.00039	.000028	.00038	.000039	.00039	.000035
LH IFOF FA	.692	.025	.688	.027	.679	.019
LH IFOF RD	.00037	.000028	.00037	.000032	.00038	.000026
LH CB AD	.00133	.000031	.00133	.000046	.00128	.000012

22q11.2DS, 22q11.2 deletion syndrome; RH, right hemisphere; IFOF, inferior fronto-occipital fasciculus; FA, fractional anisotropy; RD, radial diffusivity; CB, cingulum bundle; ILF, inferior longitudinal fasciculus; LH, left hemisphere; AD, axial diffusivity

Statistically significant differences identified in italics

Table 10 Results of MANOVA for psychosis level

Group	Wilks' Lambda	p value	DTI Tract	F (df)	p value
Psychosis level	.459	.005	RH UF number streamlines	.403 (2, 52)	.670
			RH IFOF FA	5.215 (2, 52)	.009
			RH IFOF RD	5.790 (2, 52)	.005
			RH CB FA	1.882 (2,52)	.162
			RH CB RD	.587 (2, 52)	.560
			RH ILF RD	.885 (2, 52)	.419
			LH IFOF FA	.542 (2, 52)	.585
			LH IFOF RD	.040 (2, 52)	.960
			LH CB AD	3.494 (2, 52)	.038
			RH thalamo-frontal RD	1.862 (2, 52)	.166

RH, right hemisphere; UF, uncinate fasciculus; IFOF, inferior fronto-occipital fasciculus; FA, fractional anisotropy; RD, radial diffusivity; CB, cingulum bundle; ILF, inferior longitudinal fasciculus; LH, left hemisphere

the SRS ($\rho = .396$, $p = .001$). We also found a significant Bonferroni-corrected negative correlation between the right UF number of streamlines and TEIQue Empathy facet ($\rho = -.362$, $p = .003$). There were no other significant relationships among the group of individuals with 22q11.2DS.

Among the control group, we found a marginally significant negative correlation after Bonferroni correction between the right UF number of streamlines and JSS Cognitive scale ($\rho = -.411$, $p = .017$). There were no other significant correlations between DTI tracts and social brain measures among the control group.

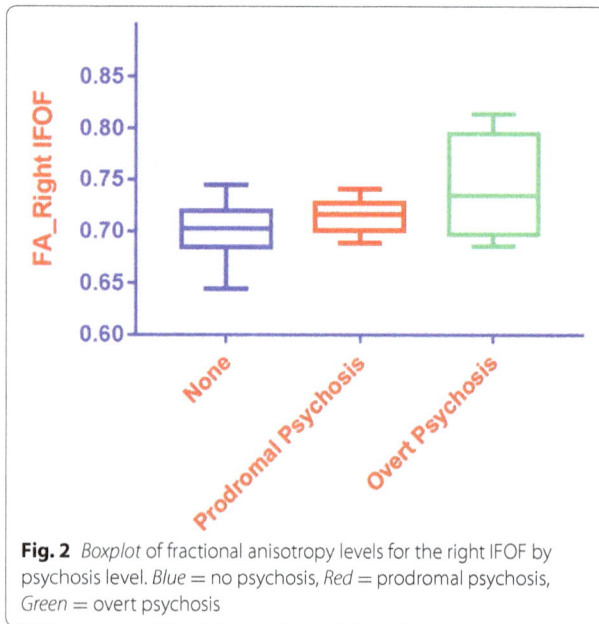

Fig. 2 *Boxplot* of fractional anisotropy levels for the right IFOF by psychosis level. *Blue* = no psychosis, *Red* = prodromal psychosis, *Green* = overt psychosis

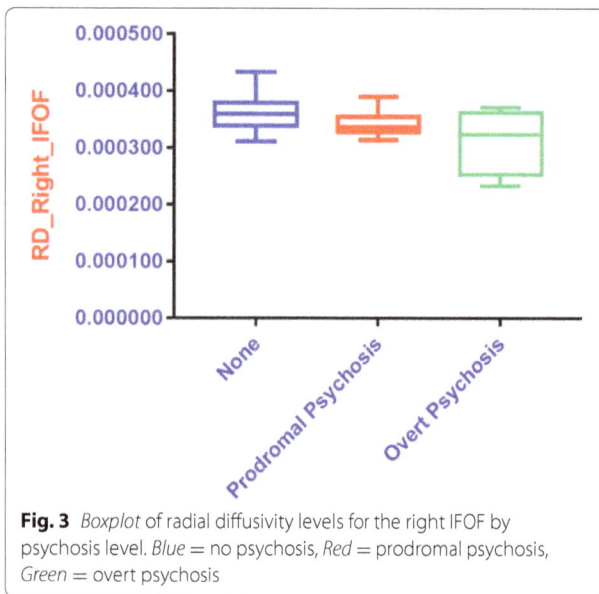

Fig. 3 *Boxplot* of radial diffusivity levels for the right IFOF by psychosis level. *Blue* = no psychosis, *Red* = prodromal psychosis, *Green* = overt psychosis

Associations between DTI metrics and symptoms of prodromal/overt psychosis

In order to examine whether the architecture of white matter tracts affects the development of prodromal symptoms, we ran ZIP regression analyses in order to determine whether there was a relationship between scores on a measure of prodromal symptoms (SIPS PS and SIPS NS) and DTI metrics. Results indicated that, after Bonferroni correction, several DTI metrics were significantly associated with positive symptoms of prodromal/overt psychosis, including left IFOF FA ($z = -3.41$,

$p = .001$) and right ILF RD ($z = -4.86$, $p < .0001$). DTI metrics that were significantly associated with negative symptoms of prodromal/overt psychosis (after Bonferroni correction) included the right IFOF RD ($z = -8.25$; $p < .0001$) and the right IFOF FA ($z = 7.50$, $p < .0001$).

Given these significant results, individuals with 22q11.2DS were further divided into three subgroups: those with no evidence of psychosis (22q11.2DS no psychosis); those with prodromal symptoms (22q11.2DS + prodromal psychosis) based on a score between 3 and 5 on any positive symptom item of the SIPS; and those with overt psychosis (22q11.2DS + overt psychosis) based on a diagnosis of psychotic disorder (Schizophrenia or Psychotic Disorder Not Otherwise Specified) from the SCID. Demographic information is presented in Table 8. We then conducted an exploratory MANOVA to compare individuals with 22q11.2DS with no psychosis to those with 22q11.2 and prodromal symptoms, and individuals with 22q11.2DS and overt psychosis on the DTI metrics that significantly differentiated individuals with 22q11.2DS from controls. Descriptive statistics for DTI metrics are presented in Table 9. Follow up ANOVAs indicated significant differences in the right hemisphere IFOF FA and RD (Table 10; Figs. 2, 3). Post-hoc Bonferroni-corrected analyses indicated that the group of individuals with 22q11.2DS and overt psychosis showed significant differences in DTI metrics as compared to the other two groups.

Conclusions

To our knowledge, this is the first study to use two-tensor tractography to examine the social brain among individuals with 22q11.2DS. Our results suggest significantly decreased left hemisphere RD in IFOF, and significantly increased FA in the IFOF among individuals with 22q11.2DS. We also found significantly decreased right hemisphere number of streamlines in UF, significantly increased number of streamlines in the CB, significantly decreased RD in IFOF, CB, ILF, and thalamo-frontal tract, while we found significantly increased FA in the IFOF, CB, and thalamo-frontal tract among individuals with 22q11.2DS. In addition, we found significant between group differences on social measures, particularly the SRS and TEIQue. Correlational analyses demonstrated very few associations between DTI tracts and social brain measures; the main significant findings were between the right thalamo-frontal tract RD and TEIQue Empathy facet, the right IFOF FA and the JSS Impulsive scale, the right UF number of streamlines and TEIQue Empathy facet, and the right UF number of streamlines and the SRS. Finally, ZIP regression analyses demonstrated significant associations between the presence of positive prodromal symptoms and left IFOF FA and right

ILF RD. Negative symptoms were associated with the right IFOF FA and RD metrics.

Alterations in IFOF, CB, and thalamo-frontal tract

In the present study, we found bilateral increases in FA of the IFOF, and right hemisphere increase in FA for the CB and thalamo-frontal tract among individuals with 22q11.2DS. This finding is somewhat unexpected, given previous findings of decreased FA in regions of the CB among individuals with schizophrenia [72] and individuals with 22q11.2DS [46, 73], as well as decreased FA in right hemisphere ATR/thalamo-frontal tract in individuals with ASD [53]. Interestingly, a few other studies of individuals with 22q11.2DS have demonstrated findings similar to ours. For example, Jalbrzikowski and colleagues' [74] whole brain analyses found overall increased FA in individuals with 22q11.2DS, regardless of age. The authors attributed this finding to a combination of decreased AD and RD, noting that increases in FA have been reported in individuals with other neurodevelopmental disorders [74]. While the cause of increased FA remains unknown, possible suggestions include decreases in axonal branching [75], flattened fibers that enable increased density of white matter [76], or decreased fiber crossing [77]. In a previous set of analyses by our group based on this cohort's assessments at the third time-point, we found increases in bilateral FA and decreases in bilateral RD in the ALIC, as well as decreases in left hemisphere RD in the UF [45]. We suggested an overall disruption of white matter connectivity as an explanation for these findings, noting that the observed increases in FA in ALIC were driven by the lower RD levels, which in turn suggested changes in myelin development of the ALIC [45]. It is possible that a similar change affected the IFOF and CB in our current set of analyses of Time 4 data.

As stated previously, the IFOF and CB are believed to underlie visual processing/facial emotion recognition and emotional information processing, respectively, whereas the thalamo-frontal/ATR region is believed to play a role in social cognition. These are domains of known difficulty in individuals with 22q11.2DS [39, 40], as well as individuals with ASD [38, 78–80]. Intriguingly, in a study of whole brain tractography in adults with ASD, Roine and colleagues [81] found higher mean FA values for individuals with ASD compared to typically developing controls. The authors suggest the possibility that abnormal synaptic pruning may play a role in the FA increase. They note that strong physical connectivity (e.g., between synapses and tracts) and low computational connectivity (e.g., information transfer) may reinforce each other, adding to the difficulty in differentiating signal from noise [81, 82]. Alternatively, the authors suggest a more strength-based

explanation. They note that that social skills and communication training prevalent in the population of individuals with ASD may lead to increased FA values in adults [81]. Research has demonstrated a link between learning a new skill and FA increases [83–85]. Many individuals with 22q11.2DS also participate in social skills or speech therapy/communication training. While these treatments were not examined in the present study, longitudinal studies that take into account the possible impact of social skills training or speech therapy interventions on white matter tracts is an area that warrants further investigation in the 22q11.2DS population.

Impairments in behavioral measures of social processing in 22q11.2DS

Our results also demonstrated more parent-rated impairments in social processing on the SRS and TEIQue among individuals with 22q11.2DS. These results are similar to those found by other studies. For example, Jalbrzikowski and colleagues [21] found significant impairment among individuals with 22q11.2DS as compared to typically developing controls on a measure of understanding another's intent and on an emotion recognition task [21]. Similarly, Campbell and colleagues [19] found that individuals with 22q11.2DS were less accurate than typically developing controls on measures of emotion identification and attribution [19]. Taken together, these social cognitive findings indicate that early identification of social impairments, particularly emotion identification and recognition, may provide an area for intervention in individuals with 22q11.2DS that could help to prevent or moderate future difficulty with social and adaptive functioning later in life.

Lack of correlations between DTI metrics and measures of social processing

In contrast to Jalbrzikowski and colleagues [74], we found only a few significant correlations between social brain measures and DTI metrics (right thalamo-frontal tract RD and TEIQue Empathy, right UF number of streamlines and TEIQue Empathy, right UF number of streamlines and SRS, right IFOF FA and JSS Impulsive), whereas a few others were marginally significant. This difference may be related to the different social measures utilized between studies. For example, Jalbrzikowski and colleagues (2014) found that increased AD in the left IFOF and left UF was associated with better scores on the awareness of social inference test (TASIT) in both individuals with 22q11.2DS and controls. In addition, increased AD in these same regions was also associated with better performance on the Penn Emotion Recognition Test (ER40) in individuals with 22q11.2DS [74]. Both the TASIT and ER40 are computerized measures of social processing concepts, as opposed to the parent and self-report measures of social processing utilized in our study. Therefore, our more indirect measures may be less sensitive to social processing abilities.

Differences in our findings may also be related to age differences between the samples. Our sample consisted more of young adult participants (mean age of 22q11.2DS group = 20.87, range = 17–25), whereas participants in the Jalbrzikowski et al. study were slightly younger and had a wider age range (mean age of 22q11.2DS group = 16.3 ± 4.3). Given that the developmental trajectory of brain white matter follows a U-shaped curve, with minimum MD and RD/maximum FA levels occurring around 30 years of age [86–88], it is possible that our older sample includes a greater number of individuals who have reached those levels, and may therefore help to explain our different results.

Associations between DTI metrics and symptoms of prodromal/overt psychosis

The presence of positive prodromal symptoms was related to DTI metrics of increased FA and in the left IFOF, and decreased RD in the right ILF, whereas presence of negative symptoms was associated with increases in FA, and decreases in RD of the IFOF. Taken together with Jalbrzikowski and colleagues [74] findings of a relationship between decreased AD in bilateral IFOF and increased positive symptom severity, these findings are intriguing, considering the IFOF's role in visual processing/facial emotion recognition and the difficulties with these types of tasks that are seen in individuals with schizophrenia [89]. Although we cannot infer a causal relationship, these findings lend support to the possibility that disrupted axonal coherence in the IFOF may underlie social cognitive impairment and psychotic symptoms in 22q11.2DS [74]. Longitudinal DTI studies could provide further insight as to whether this white matter disruption precedes the development of prodromal symptoms in individuals with 22q11.2DS.

Within the group of individuals with 22q11.2DS, our analysis of psychosis level, while exploratory, shows evidence of a possible biomarker for psychosis in that the right hemisphere IFOF FA was significantly increased, whereas right hemisphere IFOF RD was significantly decreased in individuals with overt psychosis, as compared to those with prodromal symptoms or no psychosis.

Limitations and suggestions

Our study does include several limitations. As previously noted, this study is a cross-sectional sample of an ongoing longitudinal study. As such, we are unable to draw any causal conclusions regarding the relationships we

did find between poor social processing and positive prodromal symptoms. Longitudinal studies that follow the progress of social processing difficulties and the development of prodromal symptoms in 22q11.2DS are needed to help further elucidate this relationship. Secondly, this study did include a relatively small sample size and our groups were unequal, with fewer participants in the control group. While we did find some between group differences, the study may have suffered from reduced statistical power. As a result, differences that may have appeared with a larger sample size may not have been detected. Similarly, our comparisons between individuals with 22q11.2DS and prodromal psychosis and those with overt psychosis also likely suffered from reduced statistical power, and therefore no final conclusions can be drawn from these particular results. Our sample also included some variability, in that approximately 47% of our participants with 22q11.2DS had either prodromal symptoms of psychosis or other psychiatric diagnoses (as noted in Table 1). While not entirely certain, it is possible that this variability diluted the association between the DTI findings and behavioral measures. While these diagnoses may have affected our findings, they are common in the 22q11.2DS population, and therefore were not used as covariates in statistical analyses. Moreover, the inclusion of siblings in the control sample may have posed a limitation in that siblings of individuals with schizophrenia have been reported to show alterations in social functioning and underlying white matter connectivity, potentially affecting their control status. However, as we note in Additional file 1, sibling controls and community controls did not differ in any social behavioral or DTI measure. In addition, our measures of social processing relied on parent and self-report questionnaires, which may not be particularly sensitive to the construct of interest.

Our study is the first that we know to report on two-tensor tractography of white matter tracts in the social brain. More studies using this methodology in individuals with 22q11.2DS are needed to ensure its reliability and validity in this population. Future studies would also benefit from equally sized, larger groups. In addition, studies that combine more direct theory of mind or social cognitive measures with a two-tensor tractography approach may be more sensitive to differences in the social brain network. While quite promising with a small sample size, replication of the results within right hemisphere FA and RD and their relationship to overt psychosis is also needed. Finally, while the current study provides some important findings, longitudinal studies that track white matter development of individuals with 22q11.2DS, particularly the social brain areas of IFOF and ILF, are needed to help identify further possible biomarkers for the development of psychotic symptoms in this population.

Abbreviations

22q11.2DS: chromosome 22q11.2 deletion syndrome; VCFS: velo-cardio-facial syndrome; ADHD: attention-deficit/hyperactivity disorder; ASD: autism spectrum disorder; FA: fractional anisotropy; RD: radial diffusivity; AD: axial diffusivity; CB: cingulum bundle; ALIC: anterior limb of the internal capsule; UF: uncinate fasciculus; SLF: superior longitudinal fasciculus; IFOF: inferior fronto-occipital fasciculus; ILF: inferior longitudinal fasciculus; ATR: anterior thalamic region; fMRI: functional magnetic resonance imaging; DTI: diffusion tensor imaging; FISH: fluorescence in situ hybridization; WAIS-III: Wechsler Adult Intelligence Scale, third edition; FSIQ: full scale IQ; VIQ: verbal IQ; PIQ: performance IQ; SRS: Social Responsiveness Scale; JSS: Junior Schizotypy Scale; TEIQue: Trait Emotional Intelligence Questionnaire; SIPS: structured interview for prodromal syndromes; MPRAGE: magnetization prepared rapid acquisition gradient echo; PAT: parallel acquisition techniques; GRAPPA: generalized autocalibrating partially parallel acquisitions; FOV: field of view; DWI: diffusion weighted image; UKF: unscented Kalman filter; SPGR: spoiled gradient recalled echo; FLIRT: FMRIB's linear image registration tool; WMQL: white matter query language; ROI: region of interest; ANOVA: analysis of variance; ANCOVA: analysis of covariance; MANOVA: multivariate analysis of variance; MANCOVA: multivariate analysis of covariance; ZIP: zero-inflated Poisson; TASIT: the awareness of social inference test; ER40: Penn Emotional Recognition Test.

Authors' contributions

AKO gathered background information, analyzed and interpreted data, and was a major contributor writing the manuscript. ZK, XG, AZ completed two-tensor tractography models and WMQL method. ZK and ILC wrote the imaging part of the methods section. CSG gathered background information. ILC, NM, XG, YR, and AZ were involved in the development of the two-tensor tractography protocol. KMA completed neuropsychological assessment with the participants. KMA and WF completed psychiatric interviews with the participants. MRK, SB, and MES served as consultants for the two-tensor tractography models. WRK designed the study, analyzed and interpreted data. All authors read and approved the final manuscript.

Author details

[1] Department of Psychiatry, SUNY Upstate Medical University, 750 E. Adams St., Syracuse, NY 13210, USA. [2] Department of Psychiatry, Brigham and Women's Hospital, Harvard Medical School, Boston, MA, USA. [3] Syracuse University, Syracuse, NY, USA. [4] Departments of Psychiatry and Neurology, Massachusetts General Hospital, Harvard Medical School, Boston, MA, USA. [5] Department of Radiology, Brigham and Women's Hospital, Harvard Medical School, Boston, MA, USA. [6] VA Boston Healthcare System, Harvard Medical School, Brockton, MA, USA.

Acknowledgements

Not applicable.

Competing interests

The authors declare that they have no competing interests.

Funding

This work was supported by funding from the National Institutes of Health Grant MH064824 to WRK and MH106793 to ZK.

References

1. Ryan AK, Goodship JA, Wilson DI, Philip N, Levy A, Seidel H, et al. Spectrum of clinical features associated with interstitial chromosome 22q11 deletions: a European collaborative study. J Med Genet. 1997; 34: 798–804. http://www.ncbi.nlm.nih.gov/pubmed/9350810.
2. Grati FR, Molina Gomes D, Ferreira JC, Dupont C, Alesi V, Gouas L, et al. Prevalence of recurrent pathogenic microdeletions and microduplications in over 9500 pregnancies. Prenat Diagn. 2015;35:801–9.
3. Shprintzen RJ. Velocardiofacial syndrome. Otolaryngol Clin North Am. 2000;33:1217–40. http://www.ncbi.nlm.nih.gov/pubmed/11449784.
4. Campbell LE, Azuma R, Ambery F, Stevens A, Smith A, Morris RG, et al. Executive functions and memory abilities in children with 22q11.2 deletion syndrome. Aust N Z J Psychiatry. 2010. doi:10.3109/00048670903489882.
5. Niklasson L, Gillberg C. The neuropsychology of 22q11 deletion syndrome. A neuropsychiatric study of 100 individuals. Res Dev Disabil. 2010. doi:10.1016/j.ridd.2009.09.001.
6. Woodin M, Wang PP, Aleman D, McDonald-McGinn D, Zackai E, Moss E. Neuropsychological profile of children and adolescents with the 22q11.2 microdeletion. Genet Med. 2001. doi:10.1097/00125817-200101000-00008.
7. Antshel KM, Shprintzen R, Fremont W, Higgins AM, Faraone SV, Kates WR. Cognitive and psychiatric predictors to psychosis in velocardiofacial syndrome: a 3-year follow-up study. J Am Acad Child Adolesc Psychiatry. 2010;49:333–44. http://www.ncbi.nlm.nih.gov/pubmed/20410726.
8. Arnold PD, Siegel-Bartelt J, Cytyrnbaum C, Teshima I, Schachar R. Velo-cardio-facial syndrome: implications of microdeletion 22q11 for schizophrenia and mood disorders. Am J Med Genet. 2001;105:354–62.
9. Baker KD, Skuse DH. Adolescents and young adults with 22q11 deletion syndrome: psychopathology in an at-risk group. Br J Psychiatry. 2005. doi:10.1192/bjp.186.2.115.
10. Jolin EM, Weller RA, Weller EB. Occurrence of affective disorders compared to other psychiatric disorders in children and adolescents with 22q11.2 deletion syndrome. J Affect Disord. 2012. doi:10.1016/j.jad.2010.11.025.
11. Antshel KM, Fremont W, Roizen NJ, Shprintzen R, Higgins AM, Dhamoon A, Kates WR. ADHD, major depressive disorder, and simple phobias are prevalent psychiatric conditions in youth with velocardiofacial syndrome. J Am Acad Child Adolesc Psychiatry. 2006. doi:10.1097/01.chi.0000205703.25453.5a.
12. Fabbro A, Rizzi E, Schneider M, Debbane M, Eliez S. Depression and anxiety disorders in children and adolescents with velo-cardio-facial syndrome (VCFS). Eur Child Adolesc Psychiatry. 2012. doi:10.1007/s00787-012-0273-x.
13. Tang SX, Yi JJ, Calkins ME, Whinna DA, Kohler CG, Souders MC, et al. Psychiatric disorders in 22q11.2 deletion syndrome are prevalent but undertreated. Psychol Med. 2014. doi:10.1017/S0033291713001669.
14. Antshel KM, Aneja A, Strunge L, Peebles J, Fremont WP, Stallone K, et al. Autistic spectrum disorders in velo-cardio facial syndrome (22q11.2 deletion). J Autism Dev Disord. 2007. doi:10.1007/s10803-006-0308-6.
15. Ousley OY, Smearman E, Fernandez-Carriba S, Rockers KA, Coleman K, Walker EF, Cubells JF. Axis I psychiatric diagnoses in adolescents and young adults with 22q11 deletion syndrome. Eur Psychiatry. 2013;28:417–22. doi:10.1016/j.eurpsy.2013.06.002.
16. Murphy KC, Jones LA, Owen MJ. High rates of schizophrenia in adults with velo-cardio-facial syndrome. Arch Gen Psychiatry. 1999;56:940–5. http://www.ncbi.nlm.nih.gov/pubmed/10530637.
17. Schneider M, Debbane M, Bassett AS, Chow EW, Fung WL, van den Bree M, et al. Psychiatric disorders from childhood to adulthood in 22q11.2 deletion syndrome: results from the International Consortium on Brain and Behavior in 22q11.2 Deletion Syndrome. Am J Psychiatry. 2014. doi:10.1176/appi.ajp.2013.13070864.
18. Campbell LE, Stevens AF, McCabe K, Cruickshank L, Morris RG, Murphy DG, Murphy KC. Is theory of mind related to social dysfunction and emotional problems in 22q11.2 deletion syndrome (velo-cardio-facial syndrome)? J Neurodev Disord. 2011;3:152. doi:10.1007/s11689-011-9082-7.
19. Campbell LE, McCabe KL, Melville JL, Strutt PA, Schall U. Social cognition dysfunction in adolescents with 22q11.2 deletion syndrome (velo-cardio-facial syndrome): relationship with executive functioning and social competence/functioning. J Intellect Disabil Res. 2015;59:845. doi:10.1111/jir.12183.
20. Ho JS, Radoeva PD, Jalbrzikowski M, Chow C, Hopkins J, Tran WC, et al. Deficits in mental state attributions in individuals with 22q11.2 deletion syndrome (velo-cardio-facial syndrome). Autism Res. 2012. doi:10.1002/aur.1252.
21. Jalbrzikowski M, Carter C, Senturk D, Chow C, Hopkins JM, Green MF, et al. Social cognition in 22q11.2 microdeletion syndrome: relevance to psychosis? Schizophr Res. 2012. doi:10.1016/j.schres.2012.10.007.
22. Green MF, Penn DL, Bentall R, Carpenter WT, Gaebel W, Gur RC, et al. Social cognition in schizophrenia: an NIMH workshop on definitions, assessment, and research opportunities. Schizophr Bull. 2008. doi:10.1093/schbul/sbm145.
23. Pinkham AE, Penn DL, Green MF, Buck B, Healey K, Harvey PD. The social cognition psychometric evaluation study: results of the expert survey and RAND panel. Schizophr Bull. 2014. doi:10.1093/schbul/sbt081.
24. Green MF, Horan WP, Lee J. Social cognition in schizophrenia. Nat Rev Neurosci. 2015. doi:10.1038/nrn4005

25. Senju A. Atypical development of spontaneous social cognition in autism spectrum disorders. Brain Dev. 2013. doi:10.1016/j.braindev.2012.08.002.

26. Lee KH, Farrow TF, Spence SA, Woodruff PW. Social cognition, brain networks and schizophrenia. Psychol Med 2004;34:391–400. http://www.ncbi.nlm.nih.gov/pubmed/15259824.

27. Schlaffke L, Lissek S, Lenz M, Juckel G, Schultz T, Tegenthoff M, et al. Shared and nonshared neural networks of cognitive and affective theory-of-mind: a neuroimaging study using cartoon picture stories. Hum Brain Mapp. 2015. doi:10.1002/hbm.22610.

28. Van Overwalle F, Baetens K, Marien P, Vandekerckhove M. Social cognition and the cerebellum: a meta-analysis of over 350 fMRI studies. Neuroimage. 2014. doi:10.1016/j.neuroimage.2013.09.033.

29. Ferrari PF. The neuroscience of social relations. A comparative-based approach to empathy and to the capacity of evaluating others' action value. Behaviour. 2014. doi:10.1163/1568539X-00003152.

30. Iacoboni M, Dapretto M. The mirror neuron system and the consequences of its dysfunction. Nat Rev Neurosci. 2006. doi:10.1038/nrn2024.

31. Bjorkquist OA, Herbener ES. Social perception in schizophrenia: evidence of temporo-occipital and prefrontal dysfunction. Psychiatry Res. 2013. doi:10.1016/j.pscychresns.2012.12.002.

32. Das P, Lagopoulos J, Coulston CM, Henderson AF, Malhi GS. Mentalizing impairment in schizophrenia: a functional MRI study. Schizophr Res. 2012. doi:10.1016/j.schres.2011.08.019.

33. Dodell-Feder D, Delisi LE, Hooker CI. The relationship between default mode network connectivity and social functioning in individuals at familial high-risk for schizophrenia. Schizophr Res. 2014. doi:10.1016/j.schres.2014.03.031.

34. Smith MJ, Schroeder MP, Abram SV, Goldman MB, Parrish TB, Wang X, et al. Alterations in brain activation during cognitive empathy are related to social functioning in schizophrenia. Schizophr Bull. 2015. doi:10.1093/schbul/sbu023.

35. Assaf M, Jagannathan K, Calhoun VD, Miller L, Stevens MC, Sahl R, et al. Abnormal functional connectivity of default mode sub-networks in autism spectrum disorder patients. Neuroimage. 2010. doi:10.1016/j.neuroimage.2010.05.067.

36. Bernhardt BC, Valk SL, Silani G, Bird G, Frith U, Singer T. Selective disruption of sociocognitive structural brain networks in autism and alexithymia. Cereb Cortex. 2014. doi:10.1093/cercor/bht182.

37. Hanson C, Hanson SJ, Ramsey J, Glymour C. Atypical effective connectivity of social brain networks in individuals with autism. Brain Connect. 2013. doi:10.1089/brain.2013.0161.

38. Kim SY, Choi US, Park SY, Oh SH, Yoon HW, Koh YJ, et al. Abnormal activation of the social brain network in children with autism spectrum disorder: an fMRI study. Psychiatry Investig. 2015. doi:10.4306/pi.2015.12.1.37.

39. Andersson F, Glaser B, Spiridon M, Debbane M, Vuilleumier P, Eliez S. Impaired activation of face processing networks revealed by functional magnetic resonance imaging in 22q11.2 deletion syndrome. Biol Psychiatry. 2008. doi:10.1016/j.biopsych.2007.02.022.

40. Schreiner MJ, Karlsgodt KH, Uddin LQ, Chow C, Congdon E, Jalbrzikowski M, Bearden CE. Default mode network connectivity and reciprocal social behavior in 22q11.2 deletion syndrome. Soc Cogn Affect Neurosci. 2014. doi:10.1093/scan/nst114.

41. Scariati E, Padula MC, Schaer M, Eliez S. Long-range dysconnectivity in fronal and midline structures is associated to psychosis in 22q11.2 deletion syndrome. J Neural Transm. 2016;123:823–39.

42. Barnea-Goraly N, Menon V, Krasnow B, Ko A, Reiss A, Eliez S. Investigation of white matter structure in velocardiofacial syndrome: a diffusion tensor imaging study. Am J Psychiatry. 2003;160:1863–9. http://www.ncbi.nlm.nih.gov/pubmed/14514502.

43. Kates WR, Olszewski AK, Gnirke MH, Kikinis Z, Nelson J, Antshel KM, et al. White matter microstructural abnormalities of the cingulum bundle in youths with 22q11.2 deletion syndrome: associations with medication, neuropsychological function, and prodromal symptoms of psychosis. Schizophr Res. 2015. doi:10.1016/j.schres.2014.07.010.

44. Kubicki M, McCarley R, Westin CF, Park HJ, Maier S, Kikinis R, et al. A review of diffusion tensor imaging studies in schizophrenia. J Psychiatr Res. 2007. doi:10.1016/j.jpsychires.2005.05.005.

45. Perlstein MD, Chohan MR, Coman IL, Antshel KM, Fremont WP, Gnirke MH, et al. White matter abnormalities in 22q11.2 deletion syndrome: preliminary associations with the Nogo-66 receptor gene and symptoms of psychosis. Schizophr Res. 2014. doi:10.1016/j.schres.2013.11.015.

46. Radoeva PD, Coman IL, Antshel KM, Fremont W, McCarthy CS, Kotkar A, et al. Atlas-based white matter analysis in individuals with velo-cardio-facial syndrome (22q11.2 deletion syndrome) and unaffected siblings. Behav Brain Funct. 2012. doi:10.1186/1744-9081-8-38.

47. Catani M, Thiebaut de Schotten M. A diffusion tensor imaging tractography atlas for virtual in vivo dissections. Cortex. 2008. doi:10.1016/j.cortex.2008.05.004.

48. Makris N, Preti MG, Wassermann D, Rathi Y, Papadimitriou GM, Yergatian C, et al. Human middle longitudinal fascicle: segregation and behavioral-clinical implications of two distinct fiber connections linking temporal pole and superior temporal gyrus with the angular gyrus or superior parietal lobule using multi-tensor tractography. Brain Imaging Behav. 2013. doi:10.1007/s11682-013-9235-2.

49. DeRosse P, Nitzburg GC, Ikuta T, Peters BD, Malhotra AK, Szeszko PR. Evidence from structural and diffusion tensor imaging for frontotemporal deficits in psychometric schizotypy. Schizophr Bull. 2015. doi:10.1093/schbul/sbu150.

50. Ashtari M. Anatomy and functional role of the inferior longitudinal fasciculus: a search that has just begun. Dev Med Child Neurol. 2012. doi:10.1111/j.1469-8749.2011.04122.x.

51. Ortibus E, Verhoeven J, Sunaert S, Casteels I, de Cock P, Lagae L. Integrity of the inferior longitudinal fasciculus and impaired object recognition in children: a diffusion tensor imaging study. Dev Med Child Neurol. 2012. doi:10.1111/j.1469-8749.2011.04147.x.

52. Cho Z, Law M, Chi J, Choi S, Park S, Kammen A, et al. An anatomic review of thalamolimbic fiber tractography: Ultra high resolution direct visualization of thalamolimbic fibers anterior thalamic radiation, superolateral and inferomedial forebrain bundle, and newly identified septum pellucidum tract. Word Neurosurg. 2015;83:54. doi:10.1016/j.wneu.2013.08.22.

53. Cheon K, Kim Y, Oh S, Park S, Yoon H, et al. Involvement of the anterior thalamic radiation in boys with high functioning autism spectrum disorders: a diffusion tensor imaging study. Brain Res. 2011. doi:10.1016/j.brainres.2011.08.20.

54. Skudlarski P, Jagannathan K, Calhoun VD, Hampson M, Skudlarska BA, Pearlson G. Measuring brain connectivity: diffusion tensor imaging validates resting state temporal correlations. Neuroimage. 2008. doi:10.1016/j.neuroimage.2008.07.063.

55. Teipel SJ, Bokde AL, Meindl T, Amaro E Jr, Soldner J, Reiser MF, et al. White matter microstructure underlying default mode network connectivity in the human brain. Neuroimage. 2010. doi:10.1016/j.neuroimage.2009.10.067.

56. Kates WR, Burnette CP, Bessette BA, Folley BS, Strunge L, Jabs EW, Pearlson GD. Frontal and caudate alterations in velocardiofacial syndrome (deletion at chromosome 22q11.2). J Child Neurol. 2004;19:337–42. http://www.ncbi.nlm.nih.gov/pubmed/15224707.

57. Kates WR, Burnette CP, Jabs EW, Rutberg J, Murphy AM, Grados M, et al. Regional cortical white matter reductions in velocardiofacial syndrome: a volumetric MRI analysis. Biol Psychiatry. 2001;49:677–84. http://www.ncbi.nlm.nih.gov/pubmed/11313035.

58. Aneja A, Fremont WP, Antshel KM, Faraone SV, AbdulSabur N, Higgins AM, et al. Manic symptoms and behavioral dysregulation in youth with velocardiofacial syndrome (22q11.2 deletion syndrome). J Child Adolesc Psychopharmacol. 2007. doi:10.1089/cap.2006.0023.

59. Wechsler D. Wechsler adult intelligence scale. 3rd ed. San Antonio: The Psychological Corporation; 1997.

60. Sattler JM. Assessment of children: cognitive applications. 4th ed. La Mesa: Jerome M. Sattler, Publisher, Inc.; 2001.

61. Constantino JN, Gruber CP. Social responsiveness scale (SRS) manual. Los Angeles: Western Psychological Services; 2005.

62. Constantino JN, Davis SA, Todd RD, Schindler MK, Gross MM, Brophy SL, et al. Validation of a brief quantitative measure of autistic traits: comparison of the social responsiveness scale with the autism diagnostic

interview-revised. J Autism Dev Disord. 2003;33:427–33. http://www.ncbi.nlm.nih.gov/pubmed/12959421.

63. DiDuca D, Joseph S. Assessing schizotypal traits in 13–18 year olds: revising the JSS. Personality Individ Differ. 1999. doi:10.1016/S0191-8869(98)00260-8.

64. Petrides KV. Technical manual for the Trait Emotional Intelligence Questionnaires (TEIQue). London: London Psychometric Laboratory; 2009.

65. Miller TJ, McGlashan TH, Rosen JL, Cadenhead K, Cannon T, Ventura J, et al. Prodromal assessment with the structured interview for prodromal syndromes and the scale of prodromal symptoms: predictive validity, interrater reliability, and training to reliability. Schizophr Bull. 2003;29:703–15. http://www.ncbi.nlm.nih.gov/pubmed/14989408.

66. Malcolm JG, Michailovich O, Bouix S, Westin CF, Shenton ME, Rathi Y. A filtered approach to neural tractography using the Watson directional function. Med Image Anal. 2010. doi:10.1016/j.media.2009.10.003.

67. Malcolm JG, Shenton ME, Rathi Y. Filtered multitensor tractography. IEEE Trans Med Imaging. 2010. doi:10.1109/TMI.2010.2048121.

68. Fischl B, van der Kouwe A, Destrieux C, Halgren E, Segonne F, Salat DH, et al. Automatically parcellating the human cerebral cortex. Cereb Cortex. 2004;14:11–22. http://www.ncbi.nlm.nih.gov/pubmed/14654453.

69. Smith SM, Jenkinson M, Woolrich MW, Beckmann CF, Behrens TE, Johansen-Berg H, et al. Advances in functional and structural MR image analysis and implementation as FSL. Neuroimage. 2004;23(Suppl 1):208–19. doi:10.1016/j.neuroimage.2004.07.051.

70. Wassermann D, Makris N, Rathi Y, Shenton M, Kikinis R, Kubicki M, Westin CF. On describing human white matter anatomy: the white matter query language. Med Image Comput Comput Assist Interv. 2013;16(Pt 1):647–54. http://www.ncbi.nlm.nih.gov/pubmed/24505722.

71. Rathi Y, Kubicki M, Bouix S, Westin CF, Goldstein J, Seidman L, et al. Statistical analysis of fiber bundles using multi-tensor tractography: application to first-episode schizophrenia. Magn Reson Imaging. 2011. doi:10.1016/j.mri.2010.10.005.

72. Whitford TJ, Lee SW, Oh JS, de Luis-Garcia R, Savadjiev P, Alvarado JL, et al. Localized abnormalities in the cingulum bundle in patients with schizophrenia: a diffusion tensor tractography study. Neuroimage Clin. 2014. doi:10.1016/j.nicl.2014.06.003.

73. Sundram F, Campbell LE, Azuma R, Daly E, Bloemen OJ, Barker GJ, et al. White matter microstructure in 22q11 deletion syndrome: a pilot diffusion tensor imaging and voxel-based morphometry study of children and adolescents. J Neurodev Disord. 2010. doi:10.1007/s11689-010-9043-6.

74. Jalbrzikowski M, Villalon-Reina JE, Karlsgodt KH, Senturk D, Chow C, Thompson PM, Bearden CE. Altered white matter microstructure is associated with social cognition and psychotic symptoms in 22q11.2 microdeletion syndrome. Front Behav Neurosci. 2014. doi:10.3389/fnbeh.2014.00393.

75. Hoeft F, Barnea-Goraly N, Haas BW, Golarai G, Ng D, Mills D, et al. More is not always better: increased fractional anisotropy of superior longitudinal fasciculus associated with poor visuospatial abilities in Williams syndrome. J Neurosci. 2007. doi:10.1523/JNEUROSCI.3591-07.2007.

76. Bode MK, Mattila ML, Kiviniemi V, Rahko J, Moilanen I, Ebeling H, et al. White matter in autism spectrum disorders—evidence of impaired fiber formation. Acta Radiol. 2011. doi:10.1258/ar.2011.110197.

77. Arlinghaus LR, Thornton-Wells TA, Dykens EM, Anderson AW. Alterations in diffusion properties of white matter in Williams syndrome. Magn Reson Imaging. 2011. doi:10.1016/j.mri.2011.07.012.

78. Ameis SH, Catani M. Altered white matter connectivity as a neural substrate for social impairment in Autism Spectrum Disorder. Cortex. 2015. doi:10.1016/j.cortex.2014.10.014.

79. Jou RJ, Jackowski AP, Papademetris X, Rajeevan N, Staib LH, Volkmar FR. Diffusion tensor imaging in autism spectrum disorders: preliminary evidence of abnormal neural connectivity. Aust N Z J Psychiatry. 2011. doi:10.3109/00048674.2010.534069.

80. Jou RJ, Mateljevic N, Kaiser MD, Sugrue DR, Volkmar FR, Pelphrey KA. Structural neural phenotype of autism: preliminary evidence from a diffusion tensor imaging study using tract-based spatial statistics. AJNR Am J Neuroradiol. 2011. doi:10.3174/ajnr.A2558.

81. Roine U, Roine T, Salmi J, Nieminen-Von Wendt T, Leppamaki S, Rintahaka P, et al. Increased coherence of white matter fiber tract organization in adults with Asperger syndrome: a diffusion tensor imaging study. Autism Res. 2013. doi:10.1002/aur.1332.

82. Belmonte MK, Allen G, Beckel-Mitchener A, Boulanger LM, Carper RA, Webb SJ. Autism and abnormal development of brain connectivity. J Neurosci. 2004. doi:10.1523/JNEUROSCI.3340-04.2004.

83. Schlegel AA, Rudelson JJ, Tse PU. White matter structure changes as adults learn a second language. J Cogn Neurosci. 2012. doi:10.1162/jocn_a_00240.

84. Scholz J, Klein MC, Behrens TE, Johansen-Berg H. Training induces changes in white-matter architecture. Nat Neurosci. 2009. doi:10.1038/nn.2412.

85. Takeuchi H, Sekiguchi A, Taki Y, Yokoyama S, Yomogida Y, Komuro N, et al. Training of working memory impacts structural connectivity. J Neurosci. 2010. doi:10.1523/JNEUROSCI.4611-09.2010.

86. Cohen AH, Wang R, Wilkinson M, MacDonald P, Lim AR, Takahashi E. Development of human white matter fiber pathways: from newborn to adult ages. Int J Dev Neurosci. 2016. doi:10.1016/j.ijdevneu.2016.02.002.

87. Imperati D, Colcombe S, Kelly C, Di Martino A, Zhou J, Castellanos FX, Milham MP. Differential development of human brain white matter tracts. PLoS ONE. 2011. doi:10.1371/journal.pone.0023437.

88. Westlye LT, Walhovd KB, Dale AM, Bjornerud A, Due-Tonnessen P, Engvig A, et al. Life-span changes of the human brain white matter: diffusion tensor imaging (DTI) and volumetry. Cereb Cortex. 2010. doi:10.1093/cercor/bhp280.

89. Kohler CG, Walker JB, Martin EA, Healey KM, Moberg PJ. Facial emotion perception in schizophrenia: a meta-analytic review. Schizophr Bull. 2010. doi:10.1093/schbul/sbn192.

Venlafaxine ameliorates the depression-like behaviors and hippocampal S100B expression in a rat depression model

Chang-Hong Wang[1†], Jing-Yang Gu[1†], Xiao-Li Zhang[1], Jiao Dong[1], Jun Yang[2,3], Ying-Li Zhang[1], Qiu-Fen Ning[1], Xiao-Wen Shan[1] and Yan Li[4*]

Abstract

Background: Accumulating evidence has indicated that S100B may be involved in the pathophysiology of depression. No published study has examined the effect of the antidepressant drug venlafaxine on S100B in animal models of depression. This study investigated S100B expression in the hippocampus and assessed the effect of venlafaxine on S100B mRNA level and protein expression in rats exposed to chronic unpredictable mild stress (CUMS).

Methods: Forty Sprague-Dawley rats were randomly divided into four groups as control, 0, 5 and 10 mg venlafaxine groups. The venlafaxine groups were exposed to CUMS from day 2 to day 43. Venlafaxine 0, 5 and 10 mg/kg were then administered from day 23 to day 43. We performed behavioral assessments with weight change, open-field and sucrose preference, and analyzed S100B protein expression and mRNA level in the hippocampus.

Results: The CUMS led to a decrease in body weight, locomotor activity and sucrose consumption, but venlafaxine treatment (10 mg) reversed these CUMS-induced decreases Also, CUMS increased S100B protein expression and mRNA level in the hippocampus, but venlafaxine treatment (10 mg) significantly decreased S100B protein expression and mRNA level, which were significantly lower than the other treatment groups, without significant difference between the 10 mg venlafaxine and the control groups.

Conclusions: Our findings showed that venlafaxine treatment (10 mg) may improve the depression-like behaviors and decrease over-expression of S100B protein and mRNA in the hippocampus in a rat model of depression.

Keywords: Venlafaxine, Stress, Depression, Hippocampus, S100B protein

Background

Major depressive disorder (MDD) is one of the most common, serious mood disorders with a high recurrence rate, representing a major socio-economical burden [1]. However, the pathogenic mechanisms are still unclear. Understanding the causes and neurobiological basis of depression remains a challenge. Recently, it has been suggested that mood disorders are characterized by disease-specific glial pathology [2, 3]. Post mortem studies showed reductions in glial cell density or glial cell numbers in prefrontal brain regions in patients with mood disorders [4], mainly displaying alterations of astrocytes and oligodendrocytes [5].

S100B is a glia-derived neurotrophic marker and an acidic and calcium-binding protein that is primarily produced by astrocytes and oligodendrocytes in the human brain [6]. Astrocytes are the main type of glial cells and are distributed throughout the nervous system. They have a role in the nutrition and protection of neurons and maintain brain and nervous system function. Under normal circumstances, high levels of S100B protein are mainly found in the cerebrospinal fluid (CSF), but low level of S100B in plasma and brain [7]. After brain injury, the activated microglia can secrete interleukin (IL) such as IL-1β, IL-6, tumor necrosis factor-α, and stimulate

*Correspondence: liyanzzu2009@126.com
†Chang-Hong Wang and Jing-Yang Gu contributed equally to this work
⁴ Department of Child and Adolescent, Public Health College, Zhengzhou University, 100 Kexue Road, Zhengzhou 450001, Henan, China
Full list of author information is available at the end of the article

the activation and proliferation of glial cells, resulting in a large amount of S100B [8]. In the serum and CSF of patients with major depression, S100B protein has been shown to be increased compared to levels in healthy controls [9, 10], although other studies did not demonstrate this difference in the CSF of MDD patients [11]. A postmortem study found that the density of S100B-immunopositive astrocytes is decreased in the CA1 pyramidal layer of the hippocampus in patients with MDD [12]. In some longitudinal studies, it was reported that higher S100B levels were decreased after treatment with antidepressants [13]. A recent meta-analysis by Schroeter et al. [3] revealed that S100B serum levels were consistently increased in acute major depressive or manic episodes, which was shown to be decreased after treatment with antidepressants, suggesting that S100B may be a biomarker for treatment outcomes in depression [14]. However, Ambrée et al. [15] reported low S100B levels in patients with depression, which predicted nonresponse to venlafaxine. Taken together, these studies suggest that the increased serum S100B levels may be involved in the pathophysiology of MDD and in pharmacological mechanisms of antidepressants.

The hippocampus is an important brain region that can regulate emotions and cognition [16]. Some studies have reported neurochemical changes mainly in the hippocampus in patients with depression [17]. The antidepressant venlafaxine, which is widely used to treat patients with depression, has unique chemical characteristics in inhibiting of 5-hydroxytryptamine (5-HT) and norepinephrine synaptosomal reuptake and increasing brain 5-HT levels more than fluoxetine [18]. To our knowledge, no published studies have directly examined the alteration of S100B mRNA level and protein expression in the hippocampus of depression patients or animal models and the influence of venlafaxine on them. We hypothesized that the anti-depressant activity of venlafaxine is associated with its effects on S100B mRNA level and protein expression in the hippocampus in a rat depression model induced by chronic unpredictable mild stress (CUMS).

Methods
Animals
Forty male Sprague-Dawley rats (provided by the Experimental Animal Center of Hebei Province, China), aged 8–10 weeks and weight 240–280 g (SCXK2003-1-003) were housed under standard laboratory conditions and maintained on a 12-h light–dark cycle with free access to food and water. The animals and experimental protocols were approved and supervised by the Institutional Animal Ethics Committee of the Xinxiang Medical University (with the ethical approval number 20090517) and followed the guidelines of the China National Science Academy for the use and care of experimental animals.

Chronic unpredictable mild stress (CUMS) model
The CUMS procedure was modified based on the methods in previous reports [19]. All rats in the treated groups received a variety of different stimuli from day 2 to day 43: (1) 45° cage tilt (for 24 h); (2) cold temperature swimming (water temperature 4 °C, 30 cm depth, every day for 5 min); (3) shaking (frequency: 1 per second, for 10 min); (4) tail clamp (nipped the rat's tail side of the body nearly 1/3 with large oval clamp for 1 min); (5) heat stress (rats placed in narrow-mouthed bottles at 45 °C for 5 min); (6) water deprivation (24 h); (7) food deprivation (24 h); (8) noise stimulation (1500 Hz at 95 dB for 1 h/day; (9) 120 min limit behavior (the heads of rats were fixed in the end of a cylinder without affecting their breathing); (10) wet bedding (250 ml of water added to the cage with sawdust, 24 h). The rats received one of these ten stimulation styles each day and each stimulus was applied two or three times with a completely random order. However, the same stimulus could not be used consecutively.

Drugs and drug treatment
Venlafaxine (Southwest Pharmaceutical Co., Ltd., Chengdu, China; Batch number: 080203) were dissolved in normal physiological saline. Rats were treated with venlafaxine at doses of 0, 5 or 10 mg/kg (1 ml/each rat) and were administered by oral gavage once a day for 21 days. The dosages of venlafaxine used in this study were chosen based on previous reports by Chen et al. [20] and Xing et al. [21].

The rats were randomly divided into four groups (n = 10/each group): (a) control group: rats were reared 3–4/cage, and were neither exposed to CUMS nor treated with venlafaxine. (b) active groups: rats were housed individually in the cage and were exposed to CUMS from day 2 to day 43. Then they were administered with different doses of venlafaxine (0, 5 or 10 mg/kg) from day 23 to day 43.

Behavioral assessment
Behavioral assessments were carried out on day 1, 22, 29, 36 and 43, which were shown in Fig. 1. The tests on day 1 and day 22 were used to examine whether the depression model was successful [19]. The tests on day 29, day 36 and day 43 were to estimate whether the depression-like behaviors was reversed by different doses of venlafaxine at different time points.

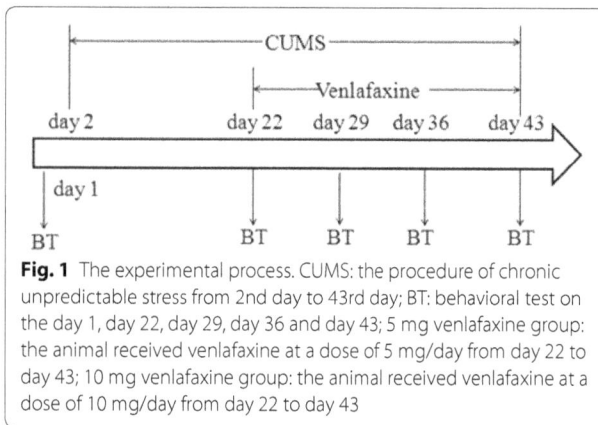

Fig. 1 The experimental process. CUMS: the procedure of chronic unpredictable stress from 2nd day to 43rd day; BT: behavioral test on the day 1, day 22, day 29, day 36 and day 43; 5 mg venlafaxine group: the animal received venlafaxine at a dose of 5 mg/day from day 22 to day 43; 10 mg venlafaxine group: the animal received venlafaxine at a dose of 10 mg/day from day 22 to day 43

The body weight and the open-field test

The body weight was measured before each the open-field test and at day 1, 22, 29, 36 and 43, respectively to calculate the mean body weight change during the entirety of the experiment. The open-field test included the distance of horizontal motion, the number of vertical motion, which was used to monitor the motor ability and explorative ability of the rats in an unfamiliar environment.

Following [19], rats were individually placed in a small 100 cm × 100 cm × 40 cm Plexiglas cage and allowed 30 s to accommodate to the observation cage. The behavioral parameters of the open-field test were continuously measured for 5 min by three observers at the same time. In all the experiments, the scorers were blinded to animal treatment. Each rat was placed in the center of the open field; the distance of the horizontal motion was recorded by a data acquisition system (software of Smart 2008, Germany). The number of vertical motion (rearing times) was recorded by the trained observers. The vertical motion reflected explorative ability (curiosity) and horizontal motion referred to locomotor activity in an unfamiliar environment. Thus, the decrease of horizontal and vertical motion simulated the hypoactivity and anhedonia symptoms of depression.

Sucrose preference test

The sucrose preference test was performed as described previously [19, 22, 23], with minor modification. Decreased sucrose consumption was used to mimic the core symptoms of anhedonia in patients with depression. After deprivation of water and food for 12 h (21:00–09:00 h), rats were free to access either of two bottles containing 1% sucrose solution or water. The positions of the two bottles were switched after 30 min. The rats were housed in individual cages. After 1 h, the volumes of consumed sucrose solution and water were recorded. The sucrose preference ratio (SPR) was calculated according

to the following equation: SPR = sucrose intake (ml)/ sucrose intake (ml) + water intake (ml).

Immunohistochemistry

Experimental and control animals were sacrificed within 12 h following the last behavior test [23]. All rats were deeply anesthetized with intraperitoneal injection of 0.3 ml/100 g chloral hydrate. The brain was quickly removed, postfixed in 4% paraformaldehyde for 3–4 h, and kept overnight for 12 h. After dehydration and paraffinization, serial 5-μm-thick coronal sections were cut. Sections were incubated for 10 min in 3% hydrogen peroxide to eliminate endogenous peroxidases, and then incubated with rabbit anti-S100B polyclonal antibody (1:100; Santa Cruz Biotechnology, Santa Cruz, CA, USA) overnight at 4 °C. For negative controls, the antibody was replaced with normal goat serum. After removal of the primary antibody, the sections were all washed three times with PBS. Biotinylated goat anti-rabbit antibody (Bo Shi De, Wuhan, China) and streptavidin–biotin complex (Bo Shi De, Wuhan, China) were then each applied for 20 min at 20–37 °C. Color for the peroxidase-linked antibody was developed with diaminobenzidine (DAB) for 5 min at room temperature. Finally, they were photographed under a light microscope [24].

In situ hybridization

The method of in situ hybridization referred to the research of Bjørnebekk's et al. [25]. Paraffin sections were fixed to glass slides and washed in water, and treated with 3% hydrogen peroxide at room temperature for 10 min to inactivate endogenous peroxidase. After washing in distilled water three times, tissue sections were placed in 3% newly diluted pepsin with citric acid at room temperature for 30 min. After washing in PBS three times, each time for 5 min and in distilled water three times, sections were fixed in 1% paraformaldehyde/0.1 M PBS (pH 7.4) containing 1/1000 diethylpyrocarbonate at room temperature for 10 min. After washing in distilled water three times, each time for 5 min, the sections were placed in 20 μl pre-hybridization to solution at 38 °C for 2 h, and excess liquid was absorbed without washing. The sections were then placed in 20 μl hybridization solution (S100B oligonucleotide probe to target mRNA sequence was 5'-TTCCA TCAGT ATTCA GGGAG AGAGG GTGAC AAGCA-3'), and the coverslip was placed on the glass slide and hybridized overnight at 38 °C. After removing the coverslip, the sections were washed twice for 1 min with 2× saline-sodium citrate (SSC) buffer, once for 15 min with 0.5× SSC, and once for 15 min with 0.2× SSC at 37 °C. Sections were incubated orderly with blocking buffer at 37 °C for 30 min, biotinylated anti-mouse digoxin (Bo Shi De) for 1 h at 37 °C, streptavidin–biotin complex (Bo Shi De) for 20 min at 37 °C, biotin–peroxidase for 20 min at 37 °C, one drop DAB reagent for 20 min at room temperature. After washing in running water, sections were dehydrated and made transparent. Finally, the coverslip was placed on the glass slide. Sections were visualized with a light microscope. In the negative control, S100B oligonucleotide probes were replaced by 0.1 M PBS (pH 7.4).

The analysis of the sections in immunohistochemistry and In situ hybridization

The sections were located in 3.3–3.8 mm distance from bregma and used Lecia Image collection and analysis system (DM2000) to take the photographs of immunohistochemistry and in situ hybridization. The photographs were counted by means of Image pro-plus (6.0), which outcomes were adopt by the formula of Mean optical density (MOD) = Integral optical density (IOD)/Area. Four sections were selected to count each rat, and 10 rats were in each group.

Statistical analysis

To investigate the effects of different dose of venlafaxine on behavior tests and the change in the hippocampal S100B protein expression and mRNA level, we used repeated-measures ANOVA test for interactions of treatment grouping with changes in behavior tests and S100B expression and mRNA level, with baseline and post-treatment values as the dependent measures (within-subject factors). Post hoc comparisons between groups were made using the Bonferronni or Tukey post hoc analysis. In addition, we compared the post-treatment values in the four groups using a univariate analysis of covariance (ANCOVA) with baseline value as covariate. S100B data was analyzed by one-way ANOVA followed by Bonferronni or Tukey post hoc analysis. Data were presented as mean ± SD. Differences at $p < 0.05$ level were considered to be significant. All statistical analyses were performed using SPSS, version 17.0 (Chicago, IL, USA).

Results

Body weight

Figure 2 presents the mean body weight on each testing occasion for the different groups. At baseline, there was no statistical difference between the four groups in body weight (F = 0.152, df = 3,36, $p > 0.05$). After 21 days of CUMS, all three treated groups showed significantly lower body weight than control group (0 mg venlafaxine: t = 13.2; 5 mg venlafaxine: t = 10.9; 10 mg venlafaxine: t = 12.794, all $p < 0.001$).

On day 29, there was a significant difference among the four groups (F = 93.2, df = 3,36, $p < 0.001$) and a significant low body weight was found in the three treatment

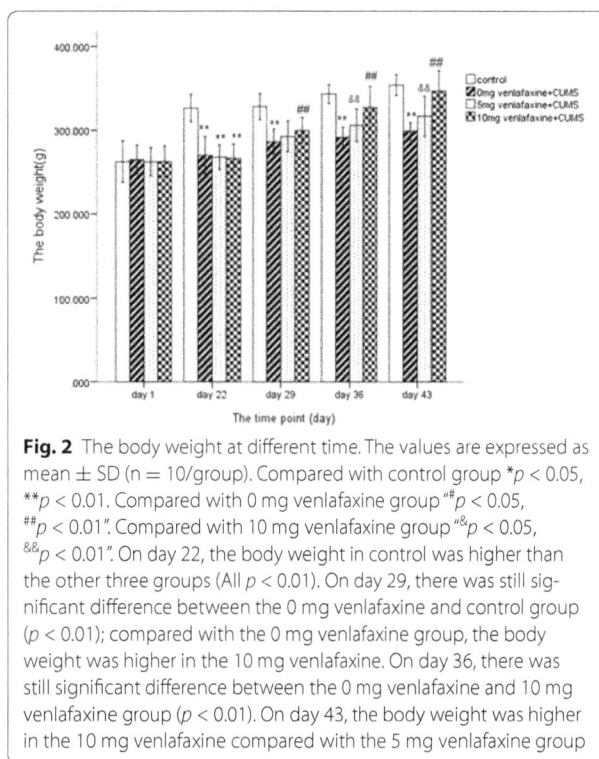

Fig. 2 The body weight at different time. The values are expressed as mean ± SD (n = 10/group). Compared with control group *$p < 0.05$, **$p < 0.01$. Compared with 0 mg venlafaxine group $^{#}p < 0.05$, $^{##}p < 0.01$". Compared with 10 mg venlafaxine group $^{&}p < 0.05$, $^{&&}p < 0.01$". On day 22, the body weight in control was higher than the other three groups (All $p < 0.01$). On day 29, there was still significant difference between the 0 mg venlafaxine and control group ($p < 0.01$); compared with the 0 mg venlafaxine group, the body weight was higher in the 10 mg venlafaxine. On day 36, there was still significant difference between the 0 mg venlafaxine and 10 mg venlafaxine group ($p < 0.01$). On day 43, the body weight was higher in the 10 mg venlafaxine compared with the 5 mg venlafaxine group

groups compared to control group ($p < 0.01$). On day 36, there was a significant difference among the four groups (F = 88.2, df = 3,36, $p < 0.001$) and high body weight was observed in the 10 mg venlafaxine group than that in the 5 mg venlafaxine group ($p < 0.001$). On day 43, there was a significant difference among the four groups (F = 97.0, df = 3,36, $p < 0.001$) and the body weight in 10 mg venlafaxine group was significantly greater than in the 5 mg venlafaxine group ($p < 0.001$); however, there was no significant difference between the 10 mg venlafaxine group and the control group ($p > 0.05$) (Additional file 1).

The open-field test

Figure 3 presents the open-field test results on each testing occasion for the different groups. At baseline, there was no statistical difference between the four groups in the distance of horizontal motion and rearing times among the four groups (F = 0.248, df = 3,36, $p > 0.05$; F = 1.282, df = 3,36, $p > 0.05$). After 21 days of CUMS, all three treated groups showed the decrease in distance of horizontal motion and rearing times compared to the control group (all $p < 0.001$).

On day 29, there was a significant difference in distance of horizontal motion, the rearing times among the four groups (F = 95.4, df = 3,36, $p < 0.001$; F = 25.0, df = 3,36, $p < 0.001$; respectively). Although the behaviors of open-field test have still significant difference between the

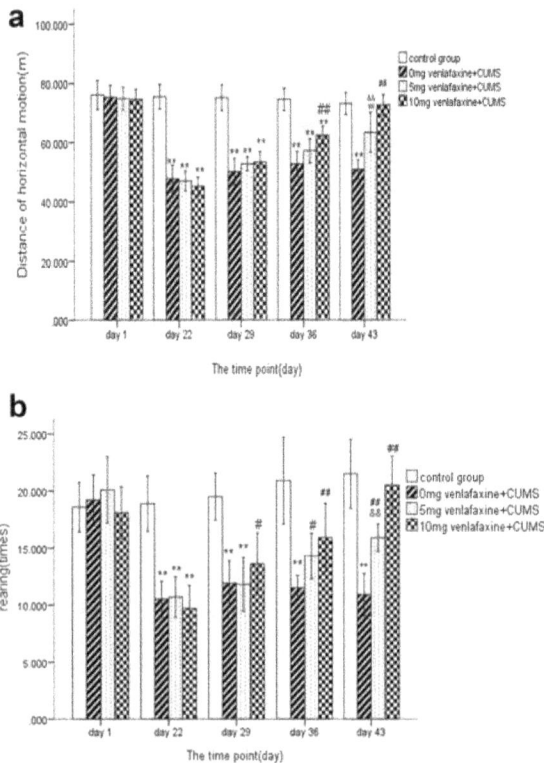

Fig. 3 Behaviors of the open-field test at different time. The values are expressed as mean ± SD (n = 10/group). Compared with control group "*p < 0.05, **p < 0.01". Compared with 0 mg venlafaxine group "#p < 0.05, ##p < 0.01". Compared with 10 mg venlafaxine group "&p < 0.05, &&p < 0.01". **a** Distance of horizontal motion; **b** rearing times. On day 22, there were significant differences among the control group and three treated groups in distance of horizontal motion, and rearing times (all p < 0.01). On day 29, there was still significant difference between the 0 mg venlafaxine and control group (p < 0.01). On day 36, there was still significant difference between the 0 mg venlafaxine and 10 mg venlafaxine group (p < 0.01). On day 43, the distance of horizontal motion and number of vertical motion was higher in the 10 mg venlafaxine compared with the 5 mg venlafaxine group (p < 0.01)

three treated groups and control group ($p < 0.01$), higher times was found in the number of rearing in venlafaxine group(10 mg) than that in venlafaxine group (0 mg) ($p < 0.05$).

On day 36, there was a significant difference in distance of horizontal motion and rearing times among the four groups (F = 61.8, df = 3,36, $p < 0.001$; F = 21.7, df = 3,36, $p < 0.001$; F = 100.8, df = 3,36, $p < 0.001$, respectively) and the activities of the venlafaxine group (0 mg) were significantly lower than that of venlafaxine groups (5 or 10 mg) (all $p < 0.05$). On day 43, there was a significant difference in distance of horizontal motion, the rearing times among the four groups (F = 51.9, df = 3,36, $p < 0.001$; F = 45.9, df = 3,36, $p < 0.001$) and significant

increase in the open-field tests was observed in venlafaxine group (10 mg) compared to venlafaxine group (5 mg) (all $p < 0.05$), but no significant differences in all open-field tests were observed between 10 mg venlafaxine group and control group (all $p > 0.05$) (Additional file 2).

Sucrose preference test

Figure 4 presents the sucrose preference test results on each testing occasion for the different groups. At baseline, there was no statistical difference in sucrose preference test among the four groups (F = 0.192, df = 3,36, $p > 0.05$). After 21 days of CUMS, all three treated groups showed significantly lower sucrose preference than control group (0 mg venlafaxine t = 13.104, $p < 0.001$; 5 mg venlafaxine t = 9.510, $p < 0.001$; 10 mg venlafaxine t = 9.955, $p < 0.001$).

On day 29, there was a significant difference among the four groups (F = 29.2, df = 3,36, $p < 0.001$) and the control group still showed greater sucrose preference than the treated groups (all $p < 0.01$). On day 36, there was a significant difference among the four groups (F = 32.9, df = 3,36, $p < 0.001$) and both the 0 and 5 mg venlafaxine groups had lower sucrose preference than the 10 mg venlafaxine group (both $p < 0.001$). On day 43, there was a significant difference among the four groups (F = 22.8, df = 3,36, $p < 0.001$) and significant difference was observed between 10 versus 5 mg venlafaxine groups

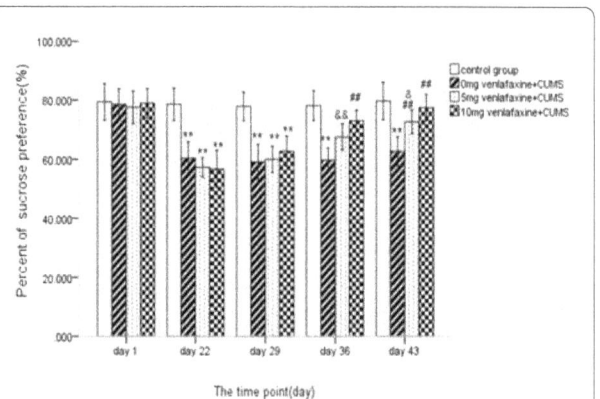

Fig. 4 The sucrose preference test at different time. The values are expressed as mean ± SD (n = 10/group). Compared with control group "*p < 0.05, **p < 0.01". Compared with 0 mg venlafaxine group "#p < 0.05, ##p < 0.01". Compared with 10 mg venlafaxine group "&p < 0.05, &&p < 0.01". On day 22, the sucrose preference in control was higher than the other three groups (all p < 0.01). On day 29, there was still significant difference between the 0 mg venlafaxine and control group (p < 0.01); compared with the 0 mg venlafaxine group, the sucrose preference was higher in the 10 mg venlafaxine (p < 0.01). On day 36, there was still significant difference between the 0 mg venlafaxine and 10 mg venlafaxine group (p < 0.01). On day 43, the sucrose preference was higher in the 10 mg venlafaxine compared with the 5 mg venlafaxine group (p < 0.01)

(all $p < 0.05$), but no significant difference was observed between 10 mg venlafaxine group and control group ($p > 0.05$) (Additional file 3).

Immunohistochemistry and in situ hybridization
Significant difference in S100B protein expression was observed in the four groups (F = 31.4, df = 3,36, $p < 0.001$). S100B protein expression in saline group was significantly higher than in the other three groups (all $p < 0.05$); however, no significant difference was noted between the control and 10 mg venlafaxine groups ($p > 0.05$). Further, S100B protein expression was significantly greater in the 5 mg venlafaxine group than in the control and 10 mg venlafaxine groups ($p < 0.001$; $p < 0.01$, respectively) (Figs. 5, 6). In addition, significant differences in S100B mRNA expression were observed among the four groups (F = 23.7, df = 3,36, $p < 0.001$), and the control group showed greater S100B mRNA expression than the other three groups (all $p < 0.05$). After 21 days of venlafaxine treatment, S100B mRNA expression was significantly greater in the 5 mg venlafaxine group than in the control and 10 mg venlafaxine groups ($p < 0.001$; $p < 0.01$, respectively); however, no significant difference was noted between the 10 mg venlafaxine and control groups ($p > 0.05$) (Figs. 7, 8) (Additional file 4).

Discussion
The CUMS-induced behavioral changes may simulate depression-like behaviors in individuals with depression, which is considered as one of the classical models [26].

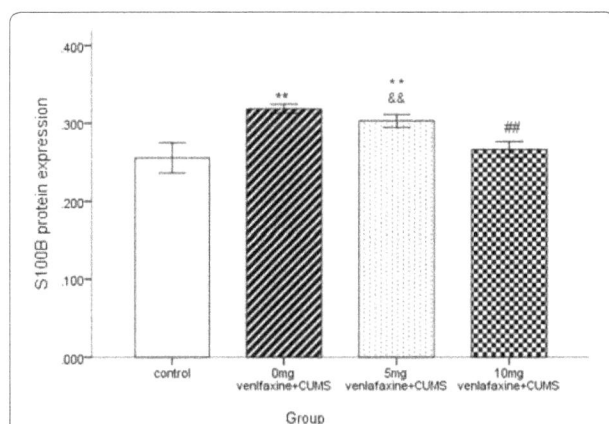

Fig. 5 Mean optical density for S100B protein in the hippocampus. The values are expressed as mean ± SD (n = 10/group). Compared with control group "*$p < 0.05$, **$p < 0.01$". Compared with 0 mg venlafaxine group "#$p < 0.05$, ##$p < 0.01$". Compared with 10 mg venlafaxine group "&$p < 0.05$, &&$p < 0.01$". The S100B protein in 0 mg venlafaxine was higher than the other three groups (all $p < 0.01$). There was significant difference between the 10 mg venlafaxine and control group ($p < 0.01$); compared with the 5 mg venlafaxine group, S100B protein was lower in the 10 mg venlafaxine ($p < 0.01$)

In our present study, following three weeks of chronic stress, decreases in distance of horizontal motion and the rearing times in an open-field suggested lowered motor ability and explorative ability. Body weight and sucrose consumption, similar to the symptoms of psychomotor inhibition, anhedonia, and appetite decreases in depression [1], were decreased in the treated groups compared to the control group. Taken together, CUMS-induced behavioral changes in our present study paralleled the symptoms of depression in humans.

The present results in this animal model of depression confirm that both 5 and 10 mg venlafaxine administration improved the depression-like behaviors at day 36 and day 43 after 2- and 3-week treatments. Moreover, venlafaxine treatment (10 mg) produced anti-depression effects better than 5 mg venlafaxine treatment at both time points. Interestingly, the depression-like behaviors in rats were reversed fully to normal levels by 21-day treatment of 10 mg venlafaxine, suggesting that high dose of venlafaxine may produce better therapeutic effects than low dose.

A further finding of our present study is that S100B expression and mRNA levels were markedly increased in the hippocampus of the CUMS model of depression suggesting that the depression-like behaviors induced by CUMS might be associated with the elevated S100B mRNA level and protein expression in the hippocampus. Our results were consistent with two previous studies by Gosselin et al. [27], who reported an increase in the intensity of S100b immunoreactivity in prefrontal cortex region, the basolateral amygdala as well as in the hippocampus, and by Ye et al. [28], who reported that CUMS produced increased S100b expression in rat hippocampus.

As mentioned previously, S100B is considered as a potential biomarker of structural brain damage and disease activity [29]. S100B displays neuroprotective or neurodegenerative effects depending on its concentration. At nanomolar concentrations, S100B has been shown to have neurotrophic effects [30], whilst at elevated concentrations (micromolar) is neurotoxic participating in a cascade of events leading to cell death or apoptosis [31]. Numerous studies have shown that S100B is altered in both serum and CSF of patients with mood disorders [3, 32]. Increased S100B levels have been reported in CSF in drug-free mild to moderate depressive patients compared with euthymic patients [33]. Moreover, S100B levels were decreased following successful treatment with antidepressant [34]. The most recent meta-analysis including a very high number of subjects has shown that fluctuations in serum levels of S100B seem to be state markers for major depression [35]. Furthermore, S100B serves as a biochemical predictor of behavioral responses to chronic

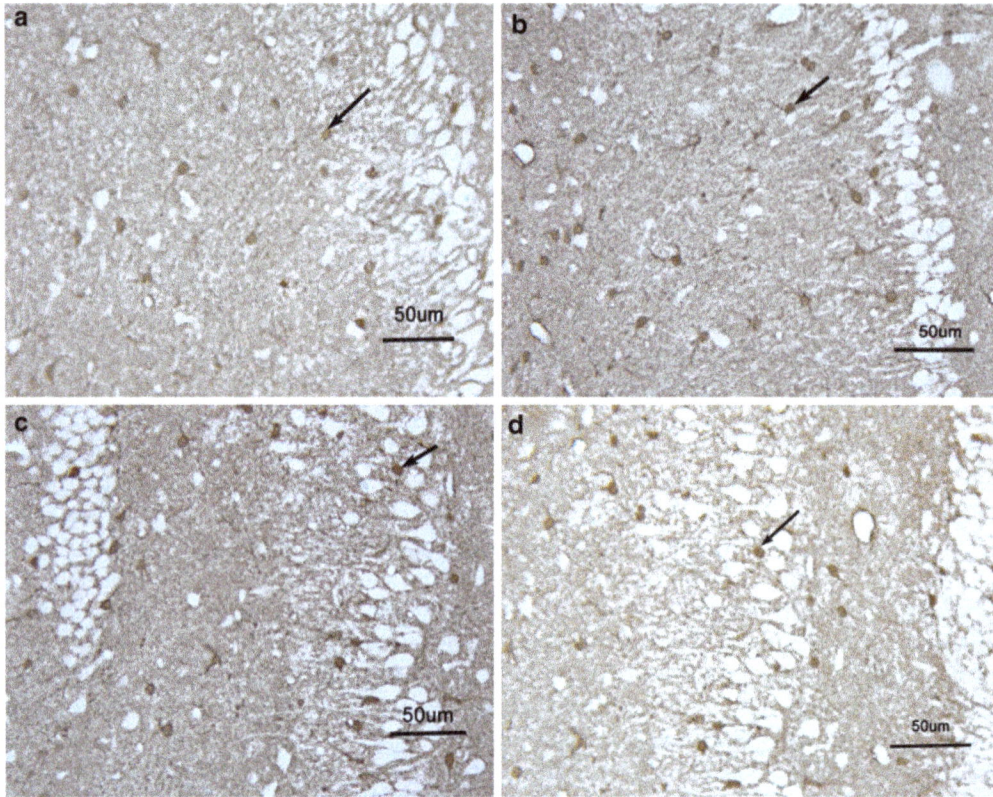

Fig. 6 S100B protein pictures in the immunohistochemistry. **a** Control group; **b** 0 mg venlafaxine group; **c** 5 mg venlafaxine group; **d** 10 mg venlafaxine group. The amplification factor of each picture was ×200; the *scale bars of every picture* were 50 μm; →: positive staining

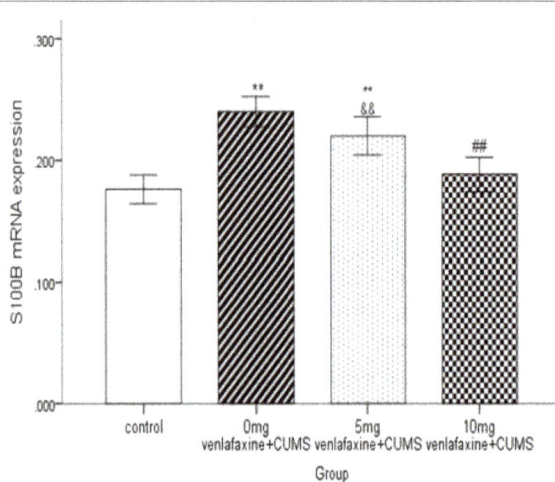

Fig. 7 Mean optical density for S100B mRNA in the hippocampus. The values are expressed as mean ± SD (n = 10/group). Compared with control group "*$p < 0.05$, **$p < 0.01$". Compared with 0 mg venlafaxine group "#$p < 0.05$, ##$p < 0.01$". Compared with 10 mg venlafaxine group "&$p < 0.05$, &&$p < 0.01$". The S100B mRNA level in 0 mg venlafaxine was higher than the other three groups (all $p < 0.01$). The significant difference had been found between the 10 mg venlafaxine and 5 m venlafaxine ($p < 0.01$); compared with the 0 mg venlafaxine group, there was no significance in the 10 mg venlafaxine ($p < 0.01$)

fluoxetine treatment [36]. Hence, it has been proposed that S100B serum and CSF levels may represent a suitable surrogate marker of glial damage or dysfunction in mood disorders [3, 8]. However, a recent postmortem analysis showed that the numerical density of S100B-immunopositive astrocytes was bilaterally decreased in the CA1 pyramidal layer of the hippocampus in MDD and bipolar disorder (BD) patients compared to controls [12]. The authors assume that reduced glial S100B-immunostaining in the hippocampus of MDD and BD patients is rather caused by an increased release of S100B from glial cells than by reduced cellular S100B expression, because of the observed increase in levels of S100B in the peripheral blood and CSF of MDD and BD patients [8, 10, 14]. Taken together, our finding of increased S100B expression and mRNA levels in the hippocampus of The CUMS model of depression suggests that that S100B overexpression may be a significant marker related to the pathophysiology of the depression.

Interestingly, we found that high dose of venlafaxine at 10 mg not only reversed the CUMS induced behavioral changes in rats, but also reduced increased levels of S100B mRNA level and protein expression. We speculate

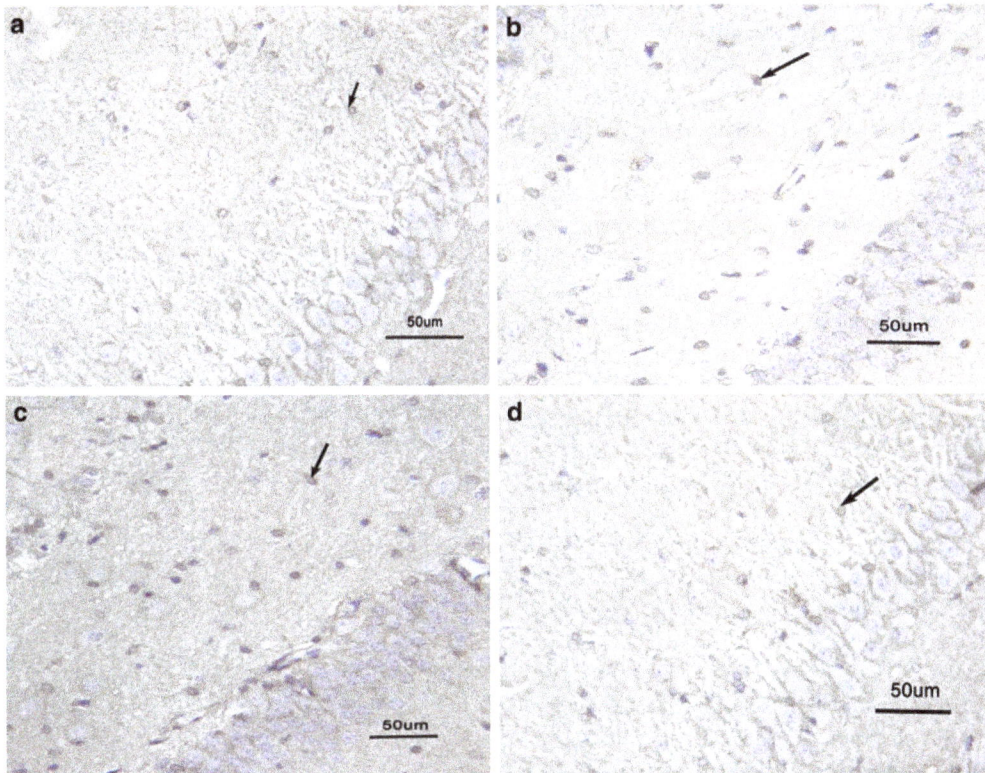

Fig. 8 S100B mRNA pictures in situ hybridization. **a** Control group; **b** 0 mg venlafaxine group; **c** 5 mg venlafaxine group; **d** 10 mg venlafaxine group. The amplification factor of each picture was ×200; the scale bars of every picture were 50 μm; →: positive staining

that venlafaxine may ameliorate the depression-like behaviors by influencing the expression of S100B in the hippocampus.

It was reported that S100B protein stimulated secretion of pro-inflammatory cytokines including IL-1β, IL-6, IL-8 and tumor necrosis factor (TNF)-α through activated glial cells [37, 38], acting as proinflammatory molecule [39]. Therefore, the increased S100B expression in our model of depression may originate from the activated glial cells of the hippocampus and elevate the release of pro-inflammatory cytokines. Recent studies reported that vatairea macrocarpa lectin (VML) caused an enhancement of S100B levels, trigger neuroinflammatory response in mouse hippocampus and exhibited a depressive-like activity [40], suggesting close relationships between the increased S100B and neuroinflammatory markers in the hippocampus and depressive-like behaviors. Some studies have indicated that higher blood levels of pro-inflammatory cytokines TNF-α and IL-6 in drug-free patients with depression [41, 42]. Moreover, the pro-inflammatory cytokines levels were normalized once antidepressant treatment was administered [43]. In addition, it has been demonstrated that the selective serotonin reuptake inhibitors (SSRIs) and serotonin–norepinephrine reuptake inhibitors (SNRIs) exerted anti-inflammatory effects in vivo [44, 45]. Furthermore, Ohgi et al. [46] examined the effects of SSRIs and SNRIs on lipopolysaccharide-induced depression in mice, and found that the two types of antidepressants have anti-inflammatory effects by decreasing TNF-α and increasing IL-10 levels in serum. Also, it has been reported that venlafaxine has an anti-inflammatory effect by the way of suppression on interferon-γ/IL-10 production ratio. The increased hippocampal levels of pro-inflammatory cytokines have been found in the CUMS model of depression, and the improvement of CUMS-induced depression-like behaviors are associated with a reduction of pro-inflammatory cytokines in the rat hippocampus [47, 48]. In addition, the astrocytes have been damaged and their immunoreactivity decrease in the hippocampus of rats exposed to the CUMS [28, 49]. Taken together, we speculate that chronic stress may lead to damage of astrocytes and the hippocampus, causing increases in S100B, which in turn may result in pro-inflammatory cytokines and depression-like symptoms in the CUMS model of depression. After treatment with venlafaxine, the increased expression of S100B mRNA and protein levels was decreased and the release of proinflammatory cytokine declined in the hippocampus, leading to improvements in the depression-like behaviors. However, the mechanisms underlying venlafaxine effects on depression-like behaviors deserve future investigation.

Several limitations of the study should be noted here. First, our study was focused on a single molecular investigation of S100B; however, numerous neurotrophic factors are involved in brain activities. It has been known that there is an interrelationship between different neurotrophins, such as interactions between BDNF and S100B [50]. Second, all the drugs were administered by oral gavage, a very invasive route of administration and source of stress for the animals. Consequently, the oral gavage could be a reason for weight loss observed in the treated rats. A group of naive animals should have been included in the experimental protocol to assess the effect of the stress of the gavage procedure on the evaluated parameters.

In summary, we found that chronic stress led to depression-like behaviors and increased S100B expression and mRNA levels in the hippocampus, suggesting that increased S100B may be relevant to the pathology of depression. Venlafaxine treatment (10 mg) improved these chronic stress induced depression-like behaviors and decreased the elevated S100B levels to the normal range. We speculate that venlafaxine may ameliorate the depression-like behaviors by influencing the expression of S100B in the hippocampus, which may work through its anti-inflammatory effect. However, this is only our speculation. The inter-relationships between increased S100B levels and pro-inflammatory cytokines in the hippocampus and depression deserves further investigation, and especially whether the anti-inflammatory effects of venlafaxine may contribute to its effects on the reduction of S100B level and reversal of the depression-like behaviors warrant further studies.

Additional files

Additional file 1. The data of S100B protein and mRNA.

Additional file 2. The data of body weight.

Additional file 3. The data of sucrose preference.

Additional file 4. The data of open-field test.

Abbreviations

CUMS: chronic unpredictable mild; MDD: major depression disorder; BD: bipolar disorder; CSF: cerebrospinal fluid; IL: interleukin; TNF: tumor necrosis factor; SSRIs: selective serotonin reuptake inhibitors; SNRIs: serotonin norepinephrine reuptake inhibitors; PBS: phosphate buffer saline; MOD: mean optical density; IOD: integral optical density; VML: vatairea macrocarpa lectins.

Authors' contributions

LY and WCH conceived of the study, and participated in its design and coordination and funds collection. WCH and GJY participated in data collection and helped to draft the manuscript. ZXL and DJ participated in the methods of Immunohistochemistry and based in situ hybridization. YJ and

ZYL participated in data collection and statistical analysis. NQF and SXW participated in the design of the study and performed the statistical analysis. All authors read and approved the final manuscript.

Author details

[1] Department of Psychiatry, The Second Affiliated Hospital of Xinxiang Medical University, Xinxiang 453002, Henan, China. [2] Standard Technological Co. Ltd. (Xinxiang Institute for New Medicine), Xinxiang 453003, Henan, China. [3] Xinjiang Hongda Food & Beverage Co. Ltd., Xinjiang 043102, Shanxi, China. [4] Department of Child and Adolescent, Public Health College, Zhengzhou University, 100 Kexue Road, Zhengzhou 450001, Henan, China.

Acknowledgements

This work was supported by Henan Key Laboratory of Biological Psychiatry. Xiang-Yang Zhang participated and made a lot of work in the revision of the manuscript. He is from Department of Psychiatry and Behavioral Sciences, The University of Texas Health Science Center at Houston, UT Houston Medical School. Professor Xiang-Yang Zhang is a Distinguished Professor in Second Affiliated Hospital of Xinxiang Medical College.

Competing interests

The authors declare that they have no competing interests.

Funding

The design of the study and collection, analysis, and interpretation of data and in writing the manuscript of this work were supported by grants from the Medical Technology Foundation of Henan Province (142300410025 and 112102310211), Science Technology Department of Technology research projects in Henan Science (102101310400), Scientific Research Fund of Xinxiang Medical University (2013ZD117), research innovation support plan project of Xinxiang Medical School graduate student (YJSCX201243Y) and National Science Fund Foundation of China (81671346).

References

1. Greenberg PE, Kessler RC, Birnbaum HG, Leong SA, Lowe SW, Berglund PA, et al. The economic burden of depression in the United States: how did it change between 1990 and 2000? J Clin Psychiatry. 2003;64(12):1465–75.
2. Rajkowska G. Postmortem studies in mood disorders indicate altered numbers of neurons and glial cells. Biol Psychiatry. 2000;48(8):766–77.
3. Schroeter ML, Abdul-Khaliq H, Sacher J, Steiner J, Blasig IE, Mueller K. Mood disorders are glial disorders: evidence from in vivo studies. Cardiovasc Psychiatry Neurol. 2010;2010:780645.
4. Cotter D, Mackay D, Landau S, Kerwin R, Everall I. Reduced glial cell density and neuronal size in the anterior cingulate cortex in major depressive disorder. Arch Gen Psychiatry. 2001;58(6):545–53.
5. Vostrikov VM, Uranova NA, Orlovskaya DD. Deficit of perineuronal oligodendrocytes in the prefrontal cortex in schizophrenia and mood disorders. Schizophr Res. 2007;94(1–3):273–80.
6. Steiner J, Bernstein HG, Bielau H, Berndt A, Brisch R, Mawrin C, et al. Evidence for a wide extra-astrocytic distribution of S100B in human brain. BMC Neurosci. 2007;8:2.
7. Haglid KG, Yang Q, Hamberger A, Bergman S, Widerberg A, Danielsen N. S-100beta stimulates neurite outgrowth in the rat sciatic nerve grafted with acellular muscle transplants. Brain Res. 1997;753:196–201.
8. Akuzawa S, Kazui T, Shi E, Yamashita K, Bashar AH, Terada H. Interleukin-1 receptor antagonist attenuates the severity of spinal cord ischemic injury in rabbits. J Vasc Surg. 2008;48(3):694–700.

9. Hetzel G, Moeller O, Evers S, Erfurth A, Ponath G, Arolt V, et al. The astroglial protein S100B and visually evoked event-related potentials before and after antidepressant treatment. Psychopharmacology. 2005;178(2–3):161–6.

10. Schroeter ML, Steiner J. Elevated serum levels of the glial marker protein S100B are not specific for schizophrenia or mood disorders. Mol Psychiatry. 2009;14(3):235–7.

11. Schmidt FM, Mergl R, Stach B, Jahn I, Schönknecht P. Elevated levels of cerebrospinal fluid neuron-specific enolase (NSE), but not S100B in major depressive disorder. World J Biol Psychiatry. 2015;16(2):106–13.

12. Gos T, Schroeter ML, Lessel W, Bernstein HG, Dobrowolny H, Schiltz K, et al. S100B-immunopositive astrocytes and oligodendrocytes in the hippocampus are differentially afflicted in unipolar and bipolar depression: a postmortem study. J Psychiatr Res. 2013;47(11):1694–9.

13. Arolt V, Peters M, Erfurth A, Wiesmann M, Missler U, Rudolf S, et al. S100B and response to treatment in major depression: a pilot study. Eur Neuropsychopharmacol. 2003;13(4):235–9.

14. Schroeter ML, Abdul-Khaliq H, Krebs M, Diefenbacher A, Blasig IE. Serum markers support disease specific glial pathology in major depression. J Affect Disord. 2008;111(2–3):271–80.

15. Ambrée O, Bergink V, Grosse L, Alferink J, Drexhage HA, Rothermundt M, et al. S100B Serum levels predict treatment response in patients with melancholic depression. Int J Neuropsychopharmacol.2015; 19(3):pyv103.

16. Femenía T, Gómez-Galán M, Lindskog M, Magara S. Dysfunctional hippocampal activity affects emotion and cognition in mood disorders. Brain Res. 2012;1476:58–70.

17. Eriksson TM, Delagrange P, Spedding M, Popoli M, Mathé AA, Ögren SO, et al. Emotional memory impairments in a genetic rat model of depression: involvement of 5-HT/MEK/Arc signaling in restoration. Mol Psychiatry. 2012;17(2):173–84.

18. Fenli S, Feng W, Ronghua Z, Huande L. Biochemical mechanism studies of venlafaxine by metabonomic method in rat model of depression. Eur Rev Med Pharmacol Sci. 2013;17(1):41–8.

19. Li ZY, Zheng XY, Gao XX, Zhou YZ, Sun HF, Zhang LZ, et al. Study of plasma metabolic profiling and biomarkers of chronic unpredictable mild stress rats based on gas chromatography/mass spectrometry. Rapid Commun Mass Spectrom. 2010;24(24):3539–46.

20. Chen Z, Xu H, Haimano S, Li X, Li XM. Quetiapine and venlafaxine synergically regulate heme oxygenase-2 protein expression in the hippocampus of stressed rats. Neurosci Lett. 2005;389(3):173–7.

21. Xing Y, He J, Hou J, Lin F, Tian J, Kurihara H. Gender differences in CMS and the effects of antidepressant venlafaxine in rats. Neurochem Int. 2013;63(6):570–5.

22. Banasr M, Valentine GW, Li XY, Gourley SL, Taylor JR, Duman RS. Chronic unpredictable stress decreases cell proliferation in the cerebral cortex of the adult rat. Biol Psychiatry. 2007;62(5):496–504.

23. Luo Y, Kuang S, Xue L, Yang J. The mechanism of 5-lipoxygenase in the impairment of learning and memory in rats subjected to chronic unpredictable mild stress. Physiol Behav. 2016;167:145–53.

24. Li H, Zhang L, Huang Q. Differential expression of mitogen-activated protein kinase signaling pathway in the hippocampus of rats exposed to chronic unpredictable stress. Behav Brain Res. 2009;205(1):32–7.

25. Bjørnebekk A, Mathé AA, Brené S. The antidepressant effects of running and escitalopram are associated with levels of hippocampal NPY and Y1 receptor but not cell proliferation in a rat model of depression. Hippocampus. 2010;20(7):820–8.

26. Surget A, Saxe M, Leman S, Ibarguen-Vargas Y, Chalon S, Griebel G, et al. Drug-dependent requirement of hippocampal neurogenesis in a model of depression and of antidepressant reversal. Biol Psychiatry. 2008;64(4):293–301.

27. Gosselin RD, Gibney S, O'Malley D, Dinan TG, Cryan JF. Region specific decrease in glial fibrillary acidic protein immunoreactivity in the brain of a rat model of depression. Neuroscience. 2009;159(2):915–25.

28. Ye Y, Wang G, Wang H, Wang X. Brain-derived neurotrophic factor (BDNF) infusion restored astrocytic plasticity in the hippocampus of a rat model of depression. Neurosci Lett. 2011;503(1):15–9.

29. Rothermundt M, Falkai P, Ponath G, Abel S, Bürkle H, Diedrich M, Siegmund A, Pedersen A, Maier W, Schramm J, Suslow T, Ohrmann P, Arolt V, et al. Glial cell dysfunction in schizophrenia indicated by increased S100B in the CSF. Mol Psychiatry. 2004;9(10):897–9.

30. Haglid KG, Yang Q, Hamberger A, Bergman S, Widerberg A, Danielsen N. S-100beta stimulates neurite outgrowth in the rat sciatic nerve grafted with acellular muscle transplants. Brain Res. 1997;753(2):196–201.

31. Donato R, Sorci G, Riuzzi F, Arcuri C, Bianchi R, Brozzi F, et al. S100B's double life: intracellular regulator and extracellular signal. Biochim Biophys Acta. 2009;1793(6):1008–22.

32. Schroeter ML, Steiner J, Mueller K. Glial pathology is modified by age in mood disorders—a systematic meta-analysis of serum S100B in vivo studies. J Affect Disord. 2011;134(1–3):32–8.

33. Grabe HJ, Ahrens N, Rose HJ, Kessler C, Freyberger HJ. Neurotrophic factor S100beta in major depression. Neuropsychobiology. 2001;44:88–90.

34. Schroeter ML, Sacher J, Steiner J, Schoenknecht P, Mueller K. Serum S100B represents a new biomarker for mood disorders. Curr Drug Targets. 2013;14(11):1237–48.

35. Polyakova M, Sander C, Arelin K, Lampe L, Luck T, Luppa M, et al. First evidence for glial pathology in late life minor depression: S100B is increased in males with minor depression. Front Cell Neurosci. 2015;9:406.

36. Benton CS, Miller BH, Skwerer S, Suzuki O, Schultz LE, Cameron MD, et al. Evaluating genetic markers and neurobiochemical analytes for fluoxetine response using a panel of mouse inbred strains. Psychopharmacology (Berl). 2012;221(2):297–315.

37. Li Y, Barger SW, Liu L, Mrak RE, Griffin WS. S100beta induction of the proinflammatory cytokine interleukin-6 in neurons. J Neurochem. 2000;74(1):143–50.

38. Dowlati Y, Herrmann N, Swardfager W, Liu H, Sham L, Reim EK, et al. A meta-analysis of cytokines in major depression. Biol Psychiatry. 2010;67(5):446–57.

39. Sorci G, Giovannini G, Riuzzi F, Bonifazi P, Zelante T, Zagarella S, et al. The danger signal S100B integrates pathogen- and danger-sensing pathways to restrain inflammation. PLoS Pathog. 2011;7(3):e1001315.

40. Gonçalves FM, Freitas AE, Peres TV, Rieger DK, Ben J, Maestri M, et al. Vatairea macrocarpa lectin (VML) induces depressive-like behavior and expression of neuroinflammatory markers in mice. Neurochem Res. 2013;38(11):2375–84.

41. De Souza DF, Wartchow K, Hansen F, Lunardi P, Guerra MC, Nardin P, et al. Interleukin-6-induced S100B secretion is inhibited by haloperidol and risperidone. Prog Neuropsychopharmacol Biol Psychiatry. 2013;43:14–22.

42. Liu Y, Ho RC, Mak A. Interleukin (IL)-6, tumour necrosis factor alpha (TNF-α) and soluble interleukin-2 receptors (sIL-2R) are elevated in patients with major depressive disorder: a meta-analysis and meta-regression. J Affect Disord. 2012;139(3):230–9.

43. Hiles SA, Baker AL, de Malmanche T, Attia J. Interleukin-6, C-reactive protein and interleukin-10 after antidepressant treatment in people with depression: a meta-analysis. Psychol Med. 2012;42(10):2015–26.

44. Horikawa H, Kato TA, Mizoguchi Y, Monji A, Seki Y, Ohkuri T, et al. Inhibitory effects of SSRIs on IFN-γ induced microglial activation through the regulation of intracellular calcium. Prog Neuropsychopharmacol Biol Psychiatry. 2010;34(7):1306–16.

45. Kubera M, Lin AH, Kenis G, Bosmans E, van Bockstaele D, Maes M. Anti-Inflammatory effects of antidepressants through suppression of the interferon-gamma/interleukin-10 production ratio. J Clin Psychopharmacol. 2001;21(2):199–206.

46. Ohgi Y, Futamura T, Kikuchi T, Hashimoto K. Effects of antidepressants on alternations in serum cytokines and depressive-like behavior in mice after lipopolysaccharide administration. Pharmacol Biochem Behav. 2013;103(4):853–9.

47. Lu J, Shao RH, Hu L, Tu Y, Guo JY. Potential antiinflammatory effects of acupuncture in a chronic stress model of depression in rats. Neurosci Lett. 2016;618:31–8.

48. Wang N, Yu HY, Shen XF, Gao ZQ, Yang C, Yang JJ, et al. The rapid antidepressant effect of ketamine in rats is associated with down-regulation of pro-inflammatory cytokines in the hippocampus. Ups J Med Sci. 2015;120(4):241–8.

49. Ayuob NN, Ali SS, Suliaman M, El Wahab MG, Ahmed SM. The antidepressant effect of musk in an animal model of depression: a histopathological study. Cell Tissue Res. 2016;366(2):271–84.

50. Cicek IE, Cicek E, Kayhan F, Uguz F, Erayman I, Kurban S, et al. The roles of BDNF, S100B, and oxidative stress in interferon-induced depression and the effect of antidepressant treatment in patients with chronic viral hepatitis: a prospective study. J Psychosom Res. 2014;76(3):227–32.

Cognitive-enhancing and antioxidant activities of the aqueous extract from *Markhamia tomentosa* (Benth.) K. Schum. stem bark in a rat model of scopolamine

Radu Ionita[1], Paula Alexandra Postu[1], Galba Jean Beppe[2,3*], Marius Mihasan[1], Brindusa Alina Petre[4*], Monica Hancianu[5], Oana Cioanca[5] and Lucian Hritcu[1*]

Abstract

Background: Plants of the genus *Markhamia* have been traditionally used by different tribes in various parts of West African countries, including Cameroun. *Markhamia tomentosa* (Benth.) K. Schum. (Bignoniaceae) is used as an antimalarial, anti-inflammatory, analgesic, antioxidant and anti-Alzheimer agent. The current study was undertaken in order to investigate its anti-amnesic and antioxidant potential on scopolamine-induced cognitive impairment and to determine its possible mechanism of action.

Methods: Rats were pretreated with the aqueous extract (50 and 200 mg/kg, p.o.), for 10 days, and received a single injection of scopolamine (0.7 mg/kg, i.p.) before training in Y-maze and radial arm-maze tests. The biochemical parameters in the rat hippocampus were also assessed to explore oxidative status. Statistical analyses were performed using two-way ANOVA followed by Tukey's post hoc test. F values for which $p < 0.05$ were regarded as statistically significant.

Results: In the scopolamine-treated rats, the aqueous extract improved memory in behavioral tests and decreased the oxidative stress in the rat hippocampus. Also, the aqueous extract exhibited anti-acetylcholinesterase activity.

Conclusions: These results suggest that the aqueous extract ameliorates scopolamine-induced spatial memory impairment by attenuation of the oxidative stress in the rat hippocampus.

Keywords: *Markhamia tomentosa* stem bark extract, Scopolamine, Spatial memory, Oxidative stress, Acetylcholinesterase, Alzheimer's disease

Background

Alzheimer's disease (AD) is considered to be the most common form of dementia relating to memory and cognitive decline. AD is a progressive neurodegenerative disorder in which dementia symptoms gradually worsen over a number of years [1].

The biochemical hallmarks of AD include the accumulation of the amyloid-beta (Aβ) peptide oligomers and soluble hyperphosphorylated tau proteins [2]. AD is also accompanied by the loss of the cholinergic markers in vulnerable neurons and the degeneration of basal forebrain cortical cholinergic neurons in end–stage AD patients [3]. The memory loss and cognitive impairments are strongly related to changes in the acetylcholinesterase (AChE) activity [4]. Moreover, AChE can increase the rate of fibrillation by binding amyloid-β-associated proteins as potent amyloid-promoting factors [5]. Thus, the cholinergic hypothesis led to the development of clinically effective therapeutics for AD [6].

*Correspondence: galbajeanbeppe@yahoo.com; brindusa.petre@uaic.ro; hritcu@uaic.ro
[1] Department of Biology, Alexandru Ioan Cuza University of Iasi, Bd. Carol I, No. 11, 700506 Iasi, Romania
[3] Department of Biological Sciences, Faculty of Science, University of Maroua, PO Box, 814, Maroua, Cameroon
[4] Department of Chemistry, Alexandru Ioan Cuza University of Iasi, Bd. Carol I, No. 11, 700506 Iasi, Romania
Full list of author information is available at the end of the article

Scopolamine, a muscarinic acetylcholine receptor (MAChR) antagonist, can block the cholinergic function of the central nervous system by targeting M1AChR and M2AChR. It has been reported that scopolamine can induce anterograde memory impairment, particularly short-term memory and learning acquisition [7]. Moreover, scopolamine can significantly increase the activity of AChE and malondialdehyde (MDA) levels in the cortex and hippocampus, and oxidative stress in the brain [8, 9].

Oxidative stress is an important factor in the pathophysiology of neurodegenerative disorders, including AD [10]. Oxidative damage triggers the pathogenesis and cognitive disturbances in AD [11]. AD is highly related to cholinergic deficits and intracellular oxidative stress. Scopolamine-induced AD model is a valuable animal model for screening anti-AD drugs [12].

Markhamia tomentosa (Benth.) K. Schum. commonly known in west Cameroon as "bobedu, abbe or mawelu" is a shrub or tree that belongs to the family Bignoniaceae [13]. Previously, we demonstrated that the methanolic extract of *M. tomentosa* leaves (50, 100 and 200 mg/kg) possess in vivo analgesic and anti-inflammatory effects in healthy rats and mice as claimed by the traditional practitioners [13]. In addition, we suggested that anti-inflammatory and analgesic effects of the methanolic extract are attributed to the inhibition of serotonin, histamine, prostaglandin and morphinomimetic action.

The root bark of *M. tomentosa* has been in vitro screened for AChE and butyrylcholinesterase inhibitory activity [14, 15]. The authors suggested that this plant could be considered for further studies in the management of early stages of AD. Moreover, ethanolic extract of *M. tomentosa* leaves (50, 100 and 150 mg/kg) was reported to prevent gastric mucosal ulceration in stomachs of the Wistar rats supported a scientific base for the traditional use of this plant [16]. Ibrahim et al. [17] demonstrated that the leaf extract of *M. tomentosa* has shown antiproliferative and apoptosis profile on the HeLa cells, but not in the MCF-7 breast cancer cell line and normal Vero cell line. Furthermore, the methanolic extract of *M. tomentosa* possesses in vitro high antioxidant activity as evidenced by DPPH TLC screening [18]. In this study, the results of DPPH assay at 33.33 µg/mL indicated maximum antioxidant activity at 80%. The aforementioned results indicated that the extract of *M. tomentosa* could be a source of natural antioxidants useful for preventing oxidative stress damage with relevance AD condition.

Recently, Ibrahim et al. [14] reported in a review that the main phytochemical identified constituents of *Markhamia* species were phenylpropanoid glycosides,

terpenoids, phytosterols, lignans, and flavonoids. Verbascoside, one of the main active phenylpropanoid glycoside from *M. tomentosa* leaves, was reported to reverse memory impairment induced by a combination of D-gal and $AlCl_3$ in a senescent mouse model [19]. Isoverbascoside, another phenylpropanoid glycoside from *M. tomentosa* leaves, ameliorated cognitive deficits in AD-like rat model induced by administration of Aβ1–42 through blocking of amyloid deposition, reversing cholinergic and hippocampal dopaminergic neuronal function [20]. Oleanolic acid, a triterpene identified in the stem bark of *M. tomentosa*, exhibited neuroprotective effects and improved Aβ-induced memory deficits in mice [21, 22]. Palmitone, a lignin isolated from the stem heartwood of *M. tomentosa*, exhibited neuroprotective effects and prevents pentylenetetrazole-induced neuronal damage in the CA3 hippocampal region of the prepuberal Wistar rats [23]. Lapachol and its furano derivatives, a quinone isolated from the stem bark of *M. tomentosa*, displayed significant anxiolytic and antidepressant effects in mice [24]. Finally, luteolin, a flavonoid identified from the *M. tomentosa* leaves, ameliorated memory impairment in streptozotocin-induced AD rat model [25]. Although the identified compounds from *M. tomentosa* had significant activity in AD, there is no study clarifying the possible cognitive-enhancing and antioxidant potentials of the aqueous extract from *M. tomentosa* stem bark in a rat model of scopolamine. Therefore, we investigated the possible memory-enhancing effects of the aqueous extract from *M. tomentosa* stem bark in memory-impaired rats and its possible mechanism on the levels of biochemical parameters in the rat hippocampus of the scopolamine model.

Methods
Plant collection and extraction

Markhamia tomentosa (Benth.) K. Schum. (Bignoniaceae) stem bark was collected from Yaoundé, Cameroon in June 2010. Identification and authentication of the plant material were done at the National Herbarium, Yaoundé, Cameroon where a voucher specimen (N°1974/SRFK) was registered and deposited for ready reference. Air-dried stem bark of *M. tomentosa* was reduced to fine powder (1000 g) and macerated in 10 L of distilled water for 48 h at room temperature and then the mixture was filtered through Whatman filter paper no. 3. The aqueous extract was then lyophilized to obtain powder used for our various tests. Percentage yield (w/w) of 3.70% was obtained. The dried extract was dissolved in distilled water and administered by gastric gavage to animals at the doses of 50 and 200 mg/kg body weight.

HPLC–DAD analysis

HPLC analysis of the aqueous extract from *M. tomentosa* stem bark was performed using a Thermo UltiMate3000 gradient chromatograph equipped with quaternary pumps controlled by Chromeleon interface, an autosampler and multidiode array detector (DAD). Solvents were filtered using a Millipore system and analysis was performed on an Accucore XL C18 column (150 × 4.6 mm, 4 μm). All the samples were filtered through 0.22 μm filter before being analyzed. The mobile phase was acetonitrile (A) and water containing 0.1% acetic acid (B) and the composition gradient was: 10–23% (A) in 5 min; 23% (A) isocratic for 10 min and then 23–35% (A) in 12 min; 35–70% (A) for 5 min. The injection volume was 20 μL scanning absorbance wavelengths from 240 to 520 nm, typical for phenols including flavonols, flavones, hydroxycinnamic acids, and anthocyanins. The flow rate increased from 0.2 to 1 mL/min. HPLC grade solvents and bidistilled water were used in the chromatographic studies. All chromatographic experiments were performed at 25 °C. Standard curves for authentic samples of the polyphenols were obtained from purchased reagents (Sigma Chemical Co., USA) of analytical or high-performance liquid chromatography (HPLC) grade. Each solution was injected in triplicate and the calibration curves were constructed with the averages. A stock solution of the investigated samples was obtained by dissolving 1.915 mg of dry extract in 1 mL of HPLC grade methanol. Different amounts (1–20 μL) were injected by the autosampler. The final results represent the mean of three to five measurements.

Animals

Twenty male Wistar rats weighing 350 ± 10 g (4–5-month-old) at the start of the experiment were used. The animals were housed in a temperature and light-controlled room (22 °C, a 12-h cycle starting at 08:00 h) and were fed and allowed to drink water ad libitum. The experiments were conducted in the quiet laboratory between hours of 10:00–16:00 h. The rats were divided into four groups (five animals per group): (1) the control group received the distilled water treatment; (2) the scopolamine (Sco)-alone-treated group received the distilled water treatment, as negative control; (3) the scopolamine-treated group received 50 mg/kg of the aqueous extract from *M. tomentosa* stem bark treatment [Sco+ME (50 mg/kg)]; (4) the scopolamine-treated group received 200 mg/kg of the aqueous extract from *M. tomentosa* stem bark treatment [Sco+ME (200 mg/kg)]. The aqueous extract from *M. tomentosa* stem bark was dissolved in distilled water. The administration of the distilled water and the aqueous extract was performed by 15-gauge oral gavage needle (Instech, Plymouth Meeting,

PA). The volume administered was 10 mL/kg of body weight, daily, for 10 consecutive days. Moreover, animals received extract treatment during training in the Y-maze and the radial arm-maze tasks. The aqueous extract doses (50 and 200 mg/kg) used in this experiment were chosen since they have been demonstrated by our group to provide significant analgesic and anti-inflammatory effects as claimed by traditional healers [13]. Scopolamine hydrobromide (Sigma-Aldrich, Germany) was dissolved in an isotonic solution (0.9% NaCl) and 0.7 mg/kg scopolamine was injected intraperitoneally (i.p.), 30 min before the behavioral testing in the Y-maze and radial arm-maze tasks. Rats were treated in accordance with the guidelines of animal bioethics from the act on animal experimentation and animal health and welfare from Romania and all procedures were in compliance with Directive 2010/63/ EU of the European Parliament and of the Council of 22 September 2010 on the protection of animals used for scientific purposes.

Y-maze task

Short-term memory was assessed by spontaneous alternation behavior in the Y-maze task. The Y-maze used in the present study consisted of three arms (35 cm long, 25 cm high and 10 cm wide) and an equilateral triangular central area. 30 min after the aqueous extract from *M. tomentosa* stem bark administration, rats were placed at the end of one arm and allowed to move freely through the maze for 8 min. An arm entry was counted when the hind paws of the rat were completely within the arm. Spontaneous alternation behavior was defined as entry into all three arms on consecutive choices. The number of maximum spontaneous alternation behaviors was then the total number of arms entered minus two and percent spontaneous alternation was calculated as (actual alternations/maximum alternations) × 100. The maze was cleaned with a 10% ethanol solution and dried with a cloth before the next animal was tested. Spontaneous alternation behavior is considered to reflect spatial working memory, which is a form of short-term memory [26, 27].

Radial arm-maze task

The radial arm-maze used in the present study consisted of eight arms, numbered from 1 to 8 (48 × 12 cm), extending radially from a central area (32 cm in diameter). The apparatus was placed 40 cm above the floor and surrounded by various extra-maze visual cues placed at the same position during the study. At the end of each arm, there was a food cup that had a single 50 mg food pellet. Prior to the performance of the maze task, the animals were kept on restricted diet and body weight was maintained at 85% of their free-feeding weight over a week period, with water being available ad libitum. Before the actual training began, three or four rats were simultaneously placed in the radial maze and allowed to explore for 5 min and take food freely. The food was initially available throughout the maze but was gradually restricted to the food cup. The animals were trained for 4 days to run to the end of the arms and consume the bait. To evaluate the basal activity of rats in radial eight arm-maze, the rats were given one training trial per day to run to the end of the arms and consume the bait. The training trial continued until all the five baits had been consumed or until 5 min has elapsed. After adaptation, all rats were trained with one trial per day. Briefly, 30 min after the aqueous extract from *M. tomentosa* stem bark administration, each animal was placed individually in the center of the maze and subjected to working and reference memory tasks, in which same 5 arms (no. 1, 2, 4, 5 and 7), were baited for each daily training trial. The other 3 arms (no. 3, 6 and 8) were never baited. An arm entry was counted when all four limbs of the rat were within an arm. Measures were made of the number of working memory errors (entering an arm containing food, but previously entered), reference memory errors (entering an arm that was not baited). The maze was cleaned with a 10% ethanol solution and dried with a cloth before the next animal was tested. Reference memory is regarded as a long-term memory for information that remains constant over repeated trials (memory for the positions of baited arms), whereas working memory is considered a short-time memory in which the information to be remembered changes in every trial (memory for the positions of arms that had already been visited in each trial) [26, 28].

Biochemical parameter assay

After the behavioral tests, all rats were deeply anesthetized (using sodium pentobarbital, 100 mg/kg b.w., i.p., Sigma-Aldrich, Germany), decapitated and whole brains were removed. The hippocampi were carefully excised. Each of the hippocampal samples was weighed and homogenized (1:10) with Potter Homogenizer coupled with Cole-Parmer Servodyne Mixer in ice-cold 0.1 M potassium phosphate buffer (pH 7.4), 1.15% KCl. The homogenate was centrifuged (15 min at $960 \times g$) and the supernatant was used for assays of AChE, SOD, and GPX specific activities, the total content of reduced GSH, protein carbonyl, and MDA levels.

Determination of hippocampal AChE activity

The activity of acetylcholinesterase (AChE) in the rat hippocampus was determined according to the method of Ellman et al. [29] using acetylthiocholine (ATC) as artificial substrate [30, 31]. The reaction mixture (600 μL final

volume) contained 0.26 M phosphate buffer with pH 7.4, 1 mM 5,5′-dithio-bis-2-nitrobenzoic acid (DTNB) and 5 mM ATC chloride. The assay was started by adding supernatant and following the developing of the yellow color at 412 nm for 10 min at room temperature. Suitable controls were performed for the non-enzymatic hydrolysis of ATC. The enzyme activity is expressed as nmol of ACT/min per/mg of protein.

Determination of hippocampal SOD activity

The activity of superoxide dismutase (SOD, EC 1.15.1.1) was assayed by monitoring its ability to inhibit the photochemical reduction of nitroblue tetrazolium (NBT). Each 1.5 mL reaction mixture contained 100 mM TRIS/HCl (pH 7.8), 75 mM NBT, 2 μM riboflavin, 6 mM EDTA and 200 μL of supernatant. Monitoring the increase in absorbance at 560 nm followed the production of blue formazan. One unit of SOD is defined as the quantity required to inhibit the rate of NBT reduction by 50% as previously described by Winterbourn et al. [32, 33]. The enzyme activity is expressed as units/mg protein.

Determination of hippocampal GPX activity

Glutathione peroxidase (GPX, E.C. 1.11.1.9) activity was analyzed by a spectrophotometric assay. A reaction mixture consisting of 1 mL of 0.4 M phosphate buffer (pH 7.0) containing 0.4 mM EDTA, 1 mL of 5 mM NaN_3, 1 mL of 4 mM glutathione (GSH), and 200 μL of supernatant was pre-incubated at 37 °C for 5 min. Then 1 mL of 4 mM H_2O_2 was added and incubated at 37 °C for further 5 min. The excess amount of GSH was quantified by the 5,5′-dithiobis-2-nitrobenzoic acid (DTNB) method as previously described by Sharma and Gupta [34, 35]. One unit of GPX is defined as the amount of enzyme required to oxidize 1 nmol GSH/min. The enzyme activity is expressed as units/mg protein.

Total hippocampal content of reduced GSH

Glutathione (GSH) was measured following the method of Fukuzawa and Tokumura [36, 37]. 200 μL of supernatant was added to 1.1 mL of 0.25 M sodium phosphate buffer (pH 7.4) followed by the addition of 130 μL DTNB 0.04%. Finally, the mixture was brought to a final volume of 1.5 mL with distilled water and absorbance was read in a spectrophotometer at 412 nm and results were expressed as μg GSH/μg protein.

Determination of hippocampal protein carbonyl level

The extent of protein oxidation in the hippocampus was assessed by measuring the content of protein carbonyl groups, using 2,4-dinitrophenylhydrazine (DNPH) derivatization as described by Oliver et al. [38] and following the indications of Luo and Wehr [39, 40]. Basically, the supernatant fraction was divided into two equal aliquots containing approximately 2 mg of protein each. Both aliquots were precipitated with 10% trichloroacetic acid (TCA, w/v, final concentration). One sample was treated with 2 N HCl, and the another sample was treated with an equal volume of 0.2% (w/v) DNPH in 2 N HCl. Both samples were incubated at 25 °C and stirred at 5 min intervals. The samples were then reprecipitated with 10% TCA (final concentration) and subsequently extracted with ethanol–ethyl acetate (1:1, v/v) and then reprecipitated at 10% TCA. The pellets were carefully drained and dissolved in 6 M guanidine hydrochloride with 20 mM sodium phosphate buffer, pH 6.5. Insoluble debris was removed by centrifugation at $13,000 \times g$ at 4 °C. The absorbance at 370 nm of the DNPH-treated sample vs. the HCl control was recorded, and the results are expressed as nmols of DNPH incorporated/mg of protein based on an average absorptivity of 21/mM cm for most aliphatic hydrazones.

Determination of MDA level

Malondialdehyde (MDA), which is an indicator of lipid peroxidation, was spectrophotometrically measured by using the thiobarbituric acid assay as previously described by Ohkawa et al. [41, 42]. 200 µL of supernatant was added and briefly mixed with 1 mL of 50% trichloroacetic acid in 0.1 M HCl and 1 mL of 26 mM thiobarbituric acid. After vortex mixing, samples were maintained at 95 °C for 20 min. Afterward, samples were centrifuged at $960 \times g$ for 10 min and supernatants were read at 532 nm. A calibration curve was constructed using MDA as standard and the results were expressed as nmol/mg protein.

Estimation of protein concentration

Estimation of protein was done using a bicinchoninic acid (BCA) protein assay kit (Sigma-Aldrich, Germany). The BCA protein assay is a detergent-compatible formulation based on BCA for the colorimetric detection and quantification of total protein, as previously described by Smith et al. [43, 44].

Statistical analysis

Behavioral scores within Y-maze and radial arm-maze tasks and biochemical data were analyzed by two-way analysis of variance (ANOVA) followed by Tukey post hoc test using GraphPad Prism 6 software for Windows, La Jolla California USA. In order to evaluate differences between groups in the radial arm-maze task, separate repeated-measures ANOVA were calculated on the number of working memory errors and the number of reference memory errors with group [Control, Sco, Sco+ME (50 mg/kg) and Sco+ME (200 mg/kg)] as

between-subject factor and days (1–7) as within-subjects factors. All results are expressed as a mean ± standard error of the mean (SEM). F values for which $p < 0.05$ were regarded as statistically significant. Pearson's correlation coefficient and regression analysis were used in order to evaluate the connection between behavioral measures, the antioxidant defense, and lipid peroxidation.

Results

Phytochemical screening

A stock solution of the investigated samples was obtained by dissolving 1.915 mg of dry extract in 1 mL of HPLC grade methanol. Different amounts (1–20 µL) were injected by the autosampler. The final results represent the mean of 3–5 measurements.

Regarding *M. tomentosa* stem bark there are no studies available in regards to the chemical composition of this vegetal product. Although some researchers have evaluated the biologic properties of *M. tomentosa* leaves extracts, there is no data confirming the presence of specific compounds, but rather major groups of substances. Thus, from the 14 standards used, we were able to identify and quantify catechin, epicatechin, rosmarinic acid and several catechin/epicatechin derivatives (without being able to specify which) as indicated in the chromatogram below (Fig. 1).

The amounts detected/mg of dry extract were: 541.5 µg/mg rozmarinic acid; 11.37 µg/mg (+)-catechin; 15.86 µg/mg procyanidin dimer; 42.47 µg/mg (−)-epicatechin and 14.65 µg/mg cyanidin trimmers. Such chemical composition is related to strong antioxidant and radical chelating activities, as many researchers state the importance of catechin derivatives in protective mechanisms [45].

Effect of the aqueous extract from *Markhamia tomentosa* stem bark on behavioral performance

In the Y-maze test, significant overall differences between groups ($F(3, 16) = 3.68$, $p < 0.01$) on the spontaneous alternation percentage were evidenced (Fig. 2a). The results suggest that scopolamine treatment decreased the spontaneous alternation percentage ($p < 0.01$) as compared to control group. The scopolamine treated rats with both doses of studied extract, but especially the dose of 200 mg/kg, displayed significant differences ($p < 0.001$) for spontaneous alternations percentage as compared to scopolamine-alone treated group.

In the radial arm-maze task, significant overall differences between groups ($F(3,16) = 43.64$, $p < 0.0001$) on the working memory were evidenced (Fig. 2b). Scopolamine significantly increased ($p < 0.0001$) the working memory errors as compared to control group. The scopolamine treated rats with both doses of the aqueous

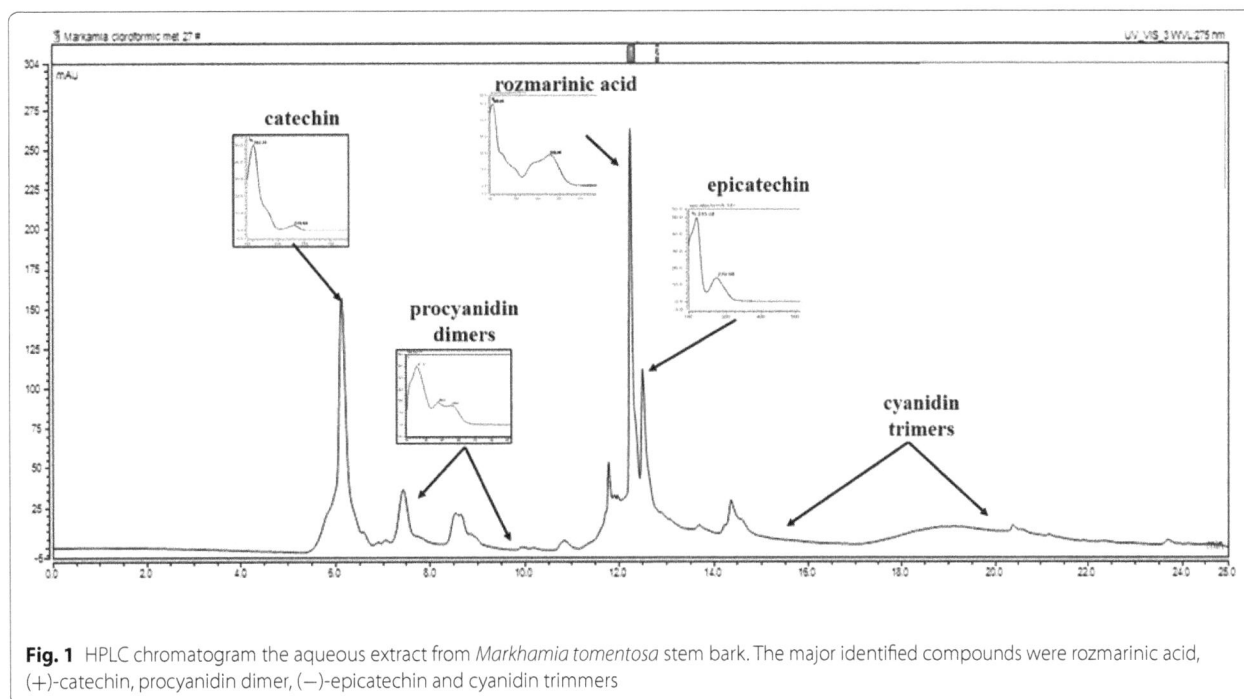

Fig. 1 HPLC chromatogram the aqueous extract from *Markhamia tomentosa* stem bark. The major identified compounds were rozmarinic acid, (+)-catechin, procyanidin dimer, (−)-epicatechin and cyanidin trimmers

extract showed a decreased (p < 0.0001) working memory errors as compared to scopolamine-alone treated group. Moreover, repeated-measures ANOVA revealed a significant group difference (F(3,252) = 34.62, p < 0.0001) for the working memory errors. Additionally, Tukey's post hoc analysis revealed a significant difference between group vs. working memory errors (p < 0.0001).

ANOVA revealed significant overall differences between groups (F(3,16) = 17.78, p < 0.0001) on the reference memory (Fig. 2c). Scopolamine significantly increased (p < 0.01) the reference memory errors as compared to control group. Rats in the scopolamine group pretreated with the extract showed a decreased (p < 0.0001) reference memory errors especially at the dose of 200 mg/kg as compared to scopolamine-alone treated group. Moreover, repeated-measures ANOVA revealed a significant group difference (F(3,252) = 3.31, p < 0.01) for the reference memory errors. Additionally, Tukey's post hoc analysis revealed a significant difference between group vs. reference memory errors (p < 0.0001).

Effect of the aqueous extract from *Markhamia tomentosa* stem bark on the AChE activity

For the AChE specific activity estimated in the rat hippocampal homogenates, significant overall differences between groups (F(3,16) = 9.00, p < 0.001) were evidenced (Fig. 3a). Scopolamine treatment increases the AChE specific activity (p < 0.01) as compared to control

group, while administration of the studied extract, in a dose of 50 mg/kg (p < 0.01), but especially at the dose of 200 mg/kg, decreased the AChE specific activity (p < 0.001) as compared to the scopolamine-alone treated group.

Effect of the aqueous extract from *Markhamia tomentosa* stem bark on the SOD and GPX activities

For the SOD specific activity estimated in the rat hippocampal homogenates, significant overall differences between groups (F(3,16) = 34.41, p < 0.0001) were noticed (Fig. 3b). While scopolamine treatment decreased SOD specific activity (p < 0.0001) as compared to control group, the administration of the aqueous extract in a dose of 50 mg/kg, significantly reverse the SOD activity (p < 0.001), but especially at the dose of 200 mg/kg (p < 0.0001), as compared to scopolamine-alone treated group.

In the rat hippocampal homogenates, significant overall differences between groups (F(3, 16) = 75.15, p < 0.0001) were evidenced for the GPX specific activity (Fig. 3c). Scopolamine group displayed markedly decline for the GPX specific activity (p < 0.0001) compared with control group. In addition, the results revealed that administration of the aqueous extract in a dose of 50 mg/kg (p < 0.01), but especially at the dose of 200 mg/kg (p < 0.001) could effectively reverse the GPX specific activity in scopolamine-induce decreasing of the GPX specific activity.

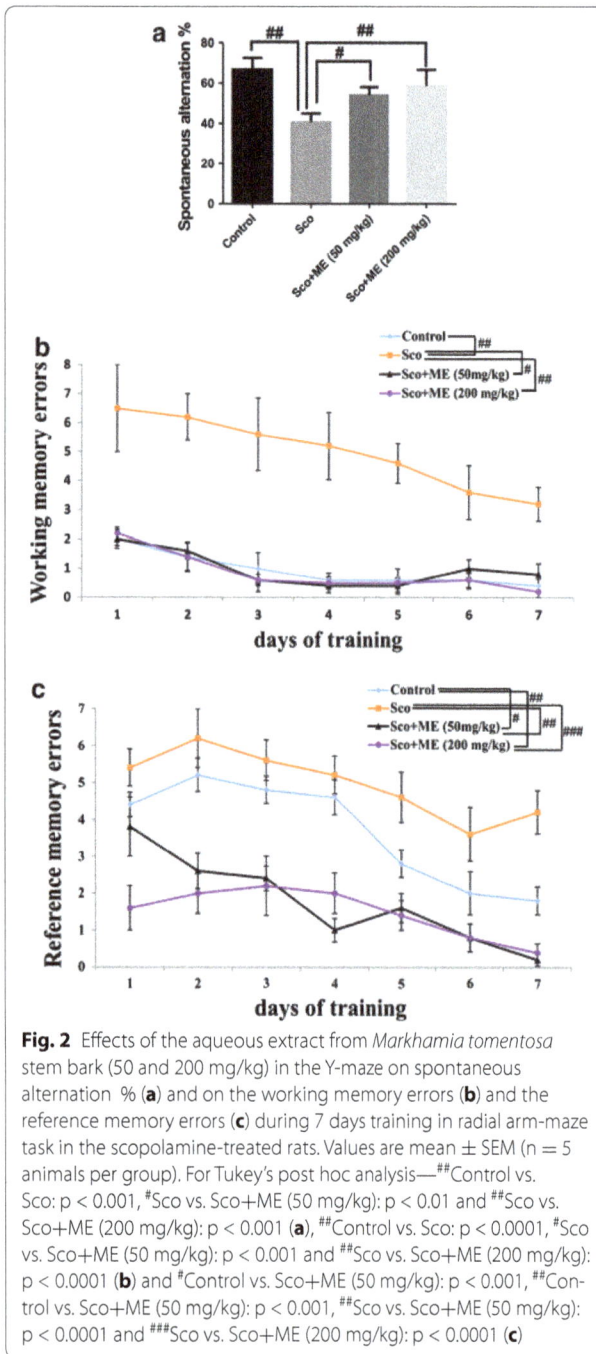

Fig. 2 Effects of the aqueous extract from *Markhamia tomentosa* stem bark (50 and 200 mg/kg) in the Y-maze on spontaneous alternation % (**a**) and on the working memory errors (**b**) and the reference memory errors (**c**) during 7 days training in radial arm-maze task in the scopolamine-treated rats. Values are mean ± SEM (n = 5 animals per group). For Tukey's post hoc analysis—##Control vs. Sco: p < 0.001, #Sco vs. Sco+ME (50 mg/kg): p < 0.01 and ##Sco vs. Sco+ME (200 mg/kg): p < 0.001 (**a**), ##Control vs. Sco: p < 0.0001, #Sco vs. Sco+ME (50 mg/kg): p < 0.001 and ##Sco vs. Sco+ME (200 mg/kg): p < 0.0001 (**b**) and #Control vs. Sco+ME (50 mg/kg): p < 0.001, ##Control vs. Sco: p < 0.001, ##Sco vs. Sco+ME (50 mg/kg): p < 0.0001 and ###Sco vs. Sco+ME (200 mg/kg): p < 0.0001 (**c**)

Effect of the aqueous extract from *Markhamia tomentosa* stem bark on the total content of reduced GSH, protein carbonyl, and MDA levels

In the rat hippocampal homogenates, significant overall differences between groups (F(3, 16) = 57.92, p < 0.01) were displayed for the total content of reduced GSH (Fig. 3d). The total content of reduced GSH decreased in scopolamine group (p < 0.01) as compared to control

group. Treatment with both doses of 50 mg/kg (p < 0.01) and 200 mg/kg (p < 0.001) of the aqueous extract to scopolamine administered rats significantly increased GSH content over normal levels.

For the protein carbonyl level measured in the rat hippocampal homogenates, significant overall differences between groups (F(3, 16) = 37.84, p < 0.0001) were revealed (Fig. 3e). Protein carbonyl level showed a significant increase (p < 0.0001) as compared to control group. Treatment of the aqueous extract, either with 50 mg/kg (p < 0.0001) and 200 mg/kg (p < 0.00001) to scopolamine administered rats significantly reduced protein carbonyl level close to normal levels.

For the lipid peroxidation (MDA) level measured in the rat hippocampal homogenates, significant overall differences between groups (F(3, 16) = 62.99, p < 0.0001) were evidenced (Fig. 3f). Administration of scopolamine resulted in increasing of the MDA level (p < 0.0001) as compared to control group. The results also revealed that in the scopolamine treated group, administration of the aqueous extract, at the doses of 50 mg/kg (p < 0.0001) and 200 mg/kg (p < 0.00001), markedly decreased MDA level under normal levels.

Importantly, when linear regression was determined, significant correlations between the spontaneous alternation percentage vs. AChE (n = 20, r = −0.657, p < 0.01) (Fig. 4a), spontaneous alternation percentage vs. MDA (n = 20, r = −0.664, p < 0.01) (Fig. 4b), working memory errors vs. AChE (n = 20, r = 0.856, p < 0.0001) (Fig. 4c), working memory errors vs. MDA (n = 20, r = 0.969, p < 0.001) (Fig. 4d), reference memory errors vs. AChE (n = 20, r = 0.826, p < 0.001) (Fig. 4e) and reference memory errors vs. MDA (n = 20, r = 0.966, p < 0.0001) (Fig. 4f) were evidenced.

Additionally, a significant correlation was evidenced by determination of the linear regression between SOD vs. MDA (n = 20, r = −0.953, p < 0.0001) (Fig. 5a), GSH vs. MDA (n = 20, r = −0.766, p < 0.001) (Fig. 5b), protein carbonyl vs. MDA (n = 20, r = 0.877, p < 0.001) (Fig. 5c) and AChE vs. MDA (n = 20, r = 0.877, p < 0.0001) (Fig. 5d). However, the significant correlation between MDA levels and behavioral measures, as well as MDA and biochemical measures, consistently displayed three rats all scopolamine-treated that were driving the significant relationship.

Discussion

In the present study, a series of experiments were designed in order to investigate the cognitive improvement of the aqueous extract from *M. tomentosa* stem bark in a scopolamine-induced a rat model of cognitive impairment in vivo.

Scopolamine is a muscarinic acetylcholine receptor (MAChR) antagonist known to block signals underlying

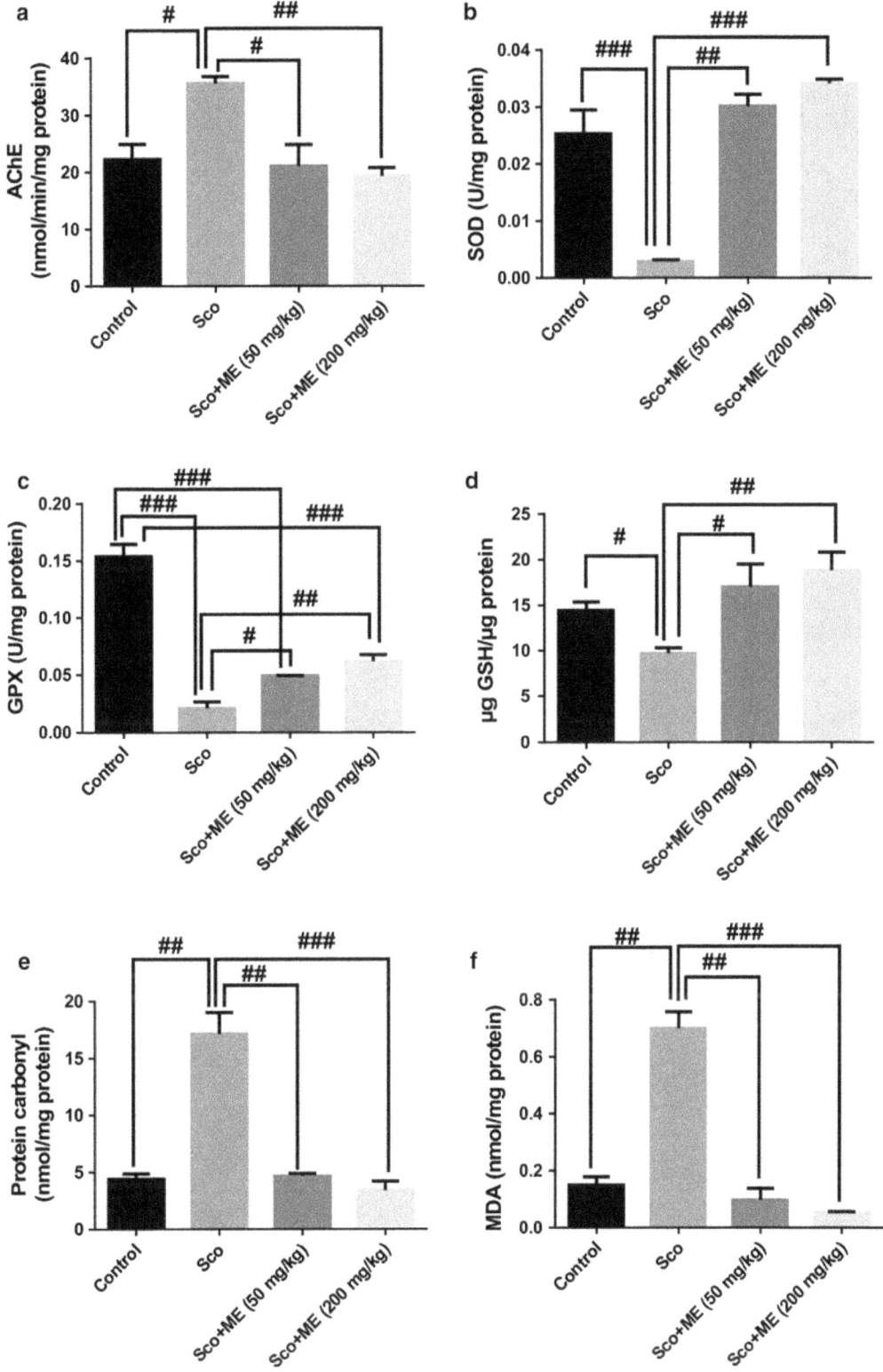

(See figure on previous page.)

Fig. 3 Effects of the aqueous extract from *Markhamia tomentosa* stem bark (50 and 200 mg/kg) on AChE (**a**), SOD (**b**) and GPX (**c**) specific activities, on reduced GSH (**d**), protein carbonyl (**e**) and MDA (**f**) levels in the scopolamine-treated rats. Values are mean ± SEM. (n = 5 animals per group). For Tukey's post hoc analysis—[#]Control vs. Sco: p < 0.01, [#]Sco vs. Sco+ME (50 mg/kg): p < 0.01 and [##]Sco vs. Sco+ME (200 mg/kg): p < 0.001 (**a**), [###]Control vs. Sco: p < 0.0001, [##]Sco vs. Sco+ME (50 mg/kg): p < 0.001 and [###]Sco vs. Sco+ME (200 mg/kg): p < 0.0001 (**b**), [###]Control vs. Sco: p < 0.0001, [###]Control vs. Sco+ME (50 mg/kg): p < 0.0001, [###]Control vs. Sco+ME (200 mg/kg): p < 0.0001, [#]Sco vs. Sco+ME (50 mg/kg): p < 0.01 and [##]Sco vs. Sco+ME (200 mg/kg): p < 0.001 (**c**), [#]Control vs. Sco: p < 0.01, [#]Sco vs. Sco+ME (50 mg/kg): p < 0.01 and [##]Sco vs. Sco+ME (200 mg/kg): p < 0.001 (**d**), [##]Control vs. Sco: p < 0.0001, [##]Sco vs. Sco+ME (50 mg/kg): p < 0.0001 and [###]Sco vs. Sco+ME (200 mg/kg): p < 0.00001 (**e**) and [##]Control vs. Sco: p < 0.0001, [##]Sco vs. Sco+ME (50 mg/kg): p < 0.0001 and [###]Sco vs. Sco+ME (200 mg/kg): p < 0.00001 (**f**)

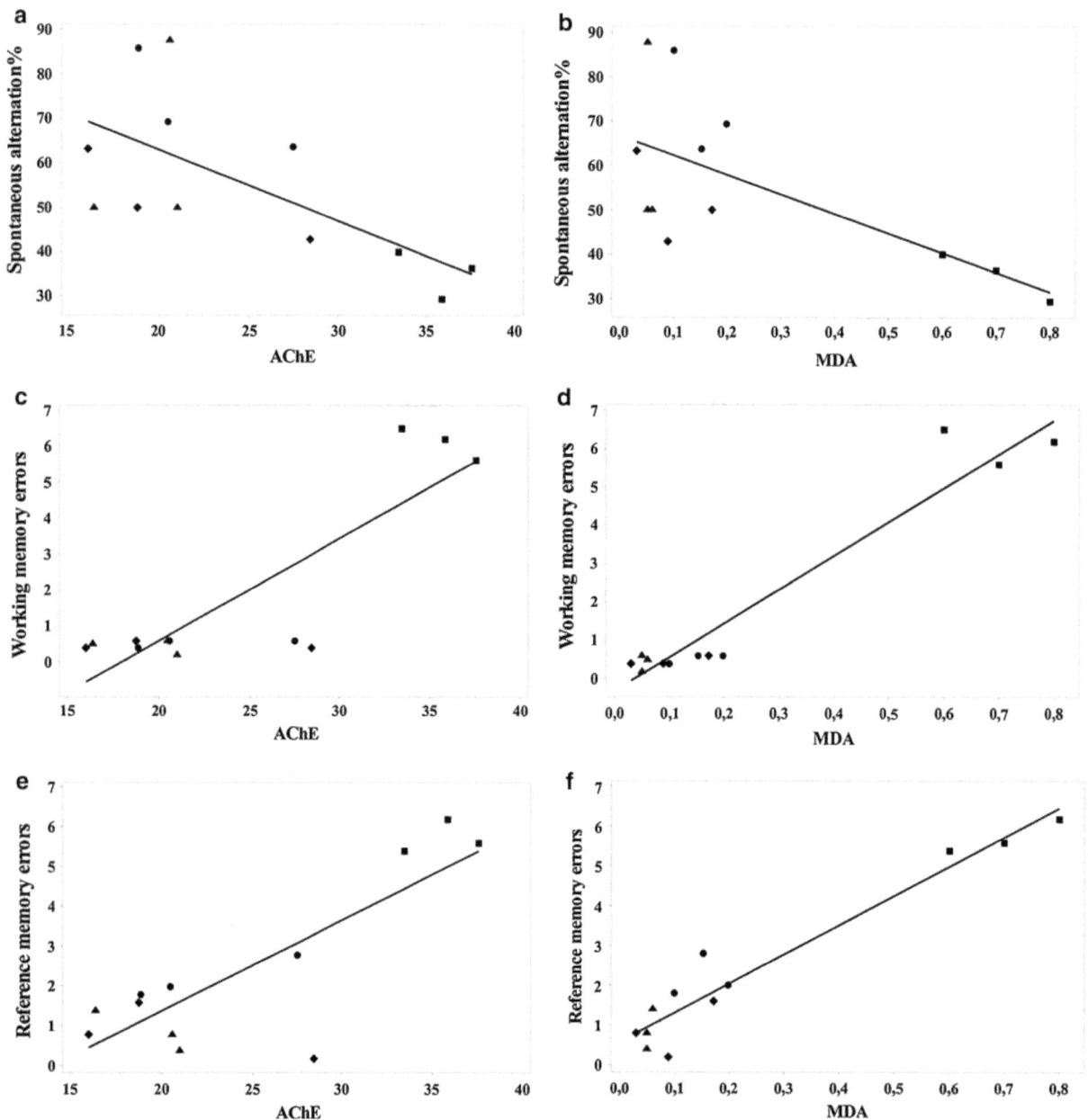

Fig. 4 Pearson's correlation between the spontaneous alternation percentage vs. AChE (**a**), spontaneous alternation percentage vs. MDA (**b**), working memory errors vs. AChE (**c**), working memory errors vs. MDA (**d**), reference memory errors vs. AChE (**e**) and reference memory errors vs. MDA (**f**) in control group (*filled circle*), scopolamine alone treated-group (*filled square*), Sco+ME (50 mg/kg) group (*filled diamond*) and Sco+ME (200 mg/kg) group (*filled triangle*)

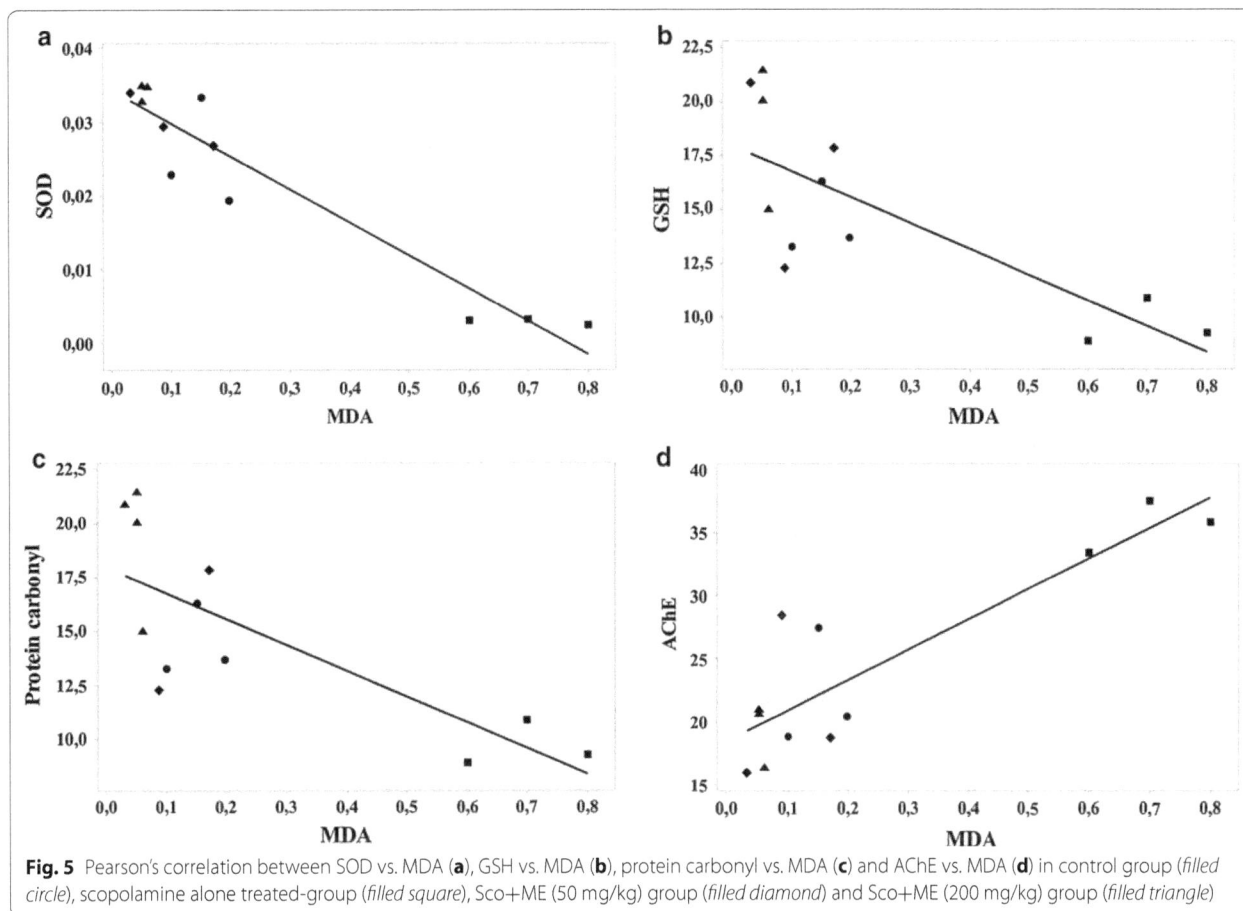

Fig. 5 Pearson's correlation between SOD vs. MDA (**a**), GSH vs. MDA (**b**), protein carbonyl vs. MDA (**c**) and AChE vs. MDA (**d**) in control group (*filled circle*), scopolamine alone treated-group (*filled square*), Sco+ME (50 mg/kg) group (*filled diamond*) and Sco+ME (200 mg/kg) group (*filled triangle*)

memory [46]. Our results are in line with previous data showing that the rats with a model of scopolamine-impaired memory significantly decreased their scores during training sessions within Y-maze and radial arm-maze tests [47–49]. Administration of the aqueous extract from *M. tomentosa* stem bark at both doses improved the impairment effect of scopolamine on memory formation, suggesting that the aqueous extract could act as an unspecific enhancer of the cholinergic activity.

The possible underlying mechanism of the aqueous extract action could be the increase of the brain cholinergic receptor sensitivity or the decrease of the AChE activity. Sugisaki et al. [50] reported that hippocampal-dependent memory is dependent by the increasing of extracellular acetylcholine (ACh) level. Also, the cholinergic synaptic transmission could by impaired by an overexpression of AChE activity-induced decreasing of ACh level [51]. AChE activity estimated in the rat hippocampal homogenates was significantly increased by scopolamine as compared to control group. The aqueous extract administration significantly decreased the AChE activity in the scopolamine-treated rats, suggesting that the aqueous extract may confer anti-amnesic effects.

Similarly, strong inhibition of the brain AChE activity was evidenced by administration of different herbal extracts in the scopolamine treated-rats [52, 53].

As an argument supporting this mechanism, the HPLC–DAD analysis of the aqueous extract from *M. tomentosa* stem bark showed that the most important group of components isolated were water-soluble polyphenolic derivatives (catechins, hydroxycinnamic acid compounds), mainly rozmarinic acid (541.5 µg/mg of dry extract), (+)-catechin (11.37 µg/mg of dry extract), procyanidin dimer (15.86 µg/mg of dry extract), (−)-epicatechin (42.47 µg/mg of dry extract) and cyaniding trimmers (14.65 µg/mg of dry extract). We can thus suggest that the effect of the aqueous extract on memory formation may be due to the presence of polyphenolic compounds such as rosmarinic acid and (−)-epicatechin.

It has been reported that rosmarinic acid exerted various beneficial biological effects such as antioxidant and neuroprotective effects and anti-AChE activity [54–56]. Also, rosmarinic acid has positive effects on learning and memory in the SAMP8 mouse model of accelerated aging [57] and decreased memory deficits in ischemic mice [58]. Furthermore, Zhang et al. [59] demonstrated that epicatechin plus treadmill exercise are neuroprotec¯ tive against moderate-stage amyloid precursor protein/ presenilin 1 mice. Also, epicatechin display a potent anti-AChE activity as previously reported [60]. Tseng et al. [61] reported that (−)-epigallocatechin-3-gallate prevents the reserpine-induced impairment of short-term social memory in rats most probably through its powerful antioxidant activities.

One of the important mechanism in the development and progression of AD is oxidative stress. In the present study, scopolamine decreased SOD, GPX, and GSH and increased the MDA and protein carbonyl levels in the rat hippocampal homogenates. It has been documented that scopolamine administration induced a neurochemical alteration in the brain along with changes in oxidative status of the brain [9]. Thus, scopolamine created an imbalance between antioxidant and oxidant defense systems which may be responsible for observed impairment of memory in rats. Furthermore, many studies have reported that the scopolamine-induced amnesic rats show similar patterns of memory impairments and oxidative damage with amnestic mild cognitive impairment (MCI) patients [62]. Evidence suggested that different plant extracts have potent anti-amnesic effects that may be mediated by improving the brain oxidative status [63–65]. Consequently, the aqueous extract treatment restored the antioxidants status as evidenced by an increase of SOD, GPX, and GSH while the levels of MDA (lipid peroxidation) and protein carbonyl significantly decrease which supports its antioxidant property.

Moreover, we found a significant correlation between the spontaneous alternation percentage vs. AChE, spontaneous alternation percentage vs. MDA, working memory errors vs. AChE, working memory errors vs. MDA, reference memory errors vs. AChE, reference memory errors vs. MDA, SOD vs. MDA, GSH vs. MDA, protein carbonyl vs. MDA and AChE vs. MDA when linear regression was determined. These results could suggest that the increase of behavioral scores in the Y-maze and the radial arm-maze tests along with the decrease of AChE activity, and also the MDA content and protein carbonyl level could be correlated with the involvement of the aqueous extract in neuroprotection against scopolamine-induced oxidative stress generation in the rat hippocampus.

Conclusions

In summary, the obtained results suggest that the aqueous extract from *M. tomentosa* stem bark (50 and 200 mg/kg) exerts its anti-amnesic effects through modulation of the antioxidant activity in the hippocampus of the rat model of scopolamine. Therefore, the aqueous extract may possibly be used as a promising natural product for the prevention of memory disorders and AD.

Abbreviations
AD: Alzheimer's disease; Aβ: amyloid-beta peptide; Aβ1–42: amyloid-beta peptide 1–42; ACh: acetylcholine; AChE: acetylcholinesterase; ANOVA: analysis of variance; BCA: bicinchoninic acid; DAD: multidiode array detector; DPPH TLC: 2,2-diphenyl-1-picrylhydrazyl thin-layer chromatography; DNPH: 2,4-dinitrophenylhydrazine; DTNB: 5,5′-dithiobis-2-nitrobenzoic acid; GPX: glutathione peroxidase; GSH: glutathione; HPLC: high-performance liquid chromatography; MAChR: muscarinic acetylcholine receptor; MDA: malondialdehyde; NBT: nitroblue tetrazolium; SOD: superoxide dismutase.

Authors' contributions
RI, GJB, PAP, MM, BAP, OC and LH performed the experimental studies and drafted the manuscript. LH, MM, MH and OC played roles in the writing and editing of the manuscript. LH on OC participated in the design and coordination of the study, supervised the study and revised the manuscript. All authors read and approved the final manuscript.

Author details
[1] Department of Biology, Alexandru Ioan Cuza University of Iasi, Bd. Carol I, No. 11, 700506 Iasi, Romania. [2] Laboratory of Animal Physiology, Faculty of Science, University of Yaoundé I, PO Box, 812, Yaoundé, Cameroon. [3] Department of Biological Sciences, Faculty of Science, University of Maroua, PO Box, 814, Maroua, Cameroon. [4] Department of Chemistry, Alexandru Ioan Cuza University of Iasi, Bd. Carol I, No. 11, 700506 Iasi, Romania. [5] Faculty of Pharmacy, University of Medicine and Pharmacy "Gr. T. Popa", 16 University Str., 700115 Iasi, Romania.

Acknowledgements
Not applicable.

Competing interests
The authors declare that they have no competing interests.

Funding
Galba Jean Beppe was supported by Doctoral scholarship Eugen Ionescu (2012/2013), Alexandru Ioan Cuza University, Iasi, Romania.

References
1. Palop JJ, Mucke L. Network abnormalities and interneuron dysfunction in Alzheimer disease. Nat Rev Neurosci. 2016;17(12):777–92.
2. Ittner LM, Götz J. Amyloid-β and tau-a toxic pas de deux in Alzheimer's disease. Nat Rev Neurosci. 2011;12(2):67–72.
3. Mufson EJ, Counts SE, Perez SE, Ginsberg SD. Cholinergic system during the progression of Alzheimer's disease: therapeutic implications. Expert Rev Neurother. 2008;8(11):1703–18.
4. Araujo JA, Studzinski CM, Milgram NW. Further evidence for the cholinergic hypothesis of aging and dementia from the canine model of aging. Prog Neuro Psychopharmacol Biol Psychiatr. 2005;29(3):411–22.
5. Inestrosa NC, Alvarez A, Pérez CA, Moreno RD, Vicente M, Linker C, Casanueva OI, Soto C, Garrido J. Acetylcholinesterase accelerates assembly of amyloid-β-peptides into Alzheimer's fibrils: possible role of the peripheral site of the enzyme. Neuron. 1996;16(4):881–91.
6. Craig LA, Hong NS, McDonald RJ. Revisiting the cholinergic hypothesis in the development of Alzheimer's disease. Neurosci Biobehav Rev. 2011;35(6):1397–409.
7. Navarro NM, Krawczyk MC, Boccia MM, Blake MG. Extinction and recovery of an avoidance memory impaired by scopolamine. Physiol Behav. 2017;171:192–8.
8. Tao L, Xie J, Wang Y, Wang S, Wu S, Wang Q, Ding H. Protective effects of aloe-emodin on scopolamine-induced memory impairment in mice and H_2O_2-induced cytotoxicity in PC12 cells. Bioorganic Med Chem Lett. 2014;24(23):5385–9.

9. Haider S, Tabassum S, Perveen T. Scopolamine-induced greater alterations in neurochemical profile and increased oxidative stress demonstrated a better model of dementia: a comparative study. Brain Res Bull. 2016;127:234–47.

10. Jomova K, Vondrakova D, Lawson M, Valko M. Metals, oxidative stress and neurodegenerative disorders. Mol Cell Biochem. 2010;345(1):91–104.

11. Qunxing D, Edgardo D, Jeffrey NK. Oxidative damage, protein synthesis, and protein degradation in Alzheimers disease. Curr Alzheimer Res. 2007;4(1):73–9.

12. Subedi L, Venkatesan R, Park YU, Kim SY. Lactucopicrin suppresses oxidative stress initiated by scopolamine-induced neurotoxicity through activation of NRF2 pathway. FASEB J. 2016;30(Suppl 1):lb511.

13. Temdie RJG, Fotio LA, Dimo T, Beppe JG, Tsague M. Analgesic and anti-inflammatory effects of extracts from the leaves of Markhamia tomentosa (Benth.) K. Schum (Bignoniaceae). Pharmacologia. 2012;3:565–73.

14. Ibrahim MB, Kaushik N, Sowemimo AA, Odukoya OA. Review of the phytochemical and pharmacological studies of the Genus Markhamia. Pharmacogn Rev. 2016;10(19):50–9.

15. Elufioye TO, Obuotor EM, Sennuga AT, Agbedahunsi JM, Adesanya SA. Acetylcholinesterase and butyrylcholinesterase inhibitory activity of some selected Nigerian medicinal plants. Rev Bras de Farmacogn. 2010;20:472–7.

16. Sofidiya MO, Agunbiade FO, Koorbanally NA, Sowemimo A, Soesan D, Familusi T. Antiulcer activity of the ethanolic extract and ethyl acetate fraction of the leaves of Markhamia tomentosa in rats. J Ethnopharmacol. 2014;157:1–6.

17. Ibrahim B, Sowemimo A, Spies L, Koekomoer T, van de Venter M, Odukoya OA. Antiproliferative and apoptosis inducing activity of Markhamia tomentosa leaf extract on HeLa cells. J Ethnopharmacol. 2013;149(3):745–9.

18. Aladesanmi AJ, Iwalewa EO, Adebajo AC, Akinkunmi EO, Taiwo BJ, Olorunmola FO, Lamikanra A. Antimicrobial and antioxidant activities of some Nigerian medicinal plants. Afr J Tradit Complement Altern Med. 2007;4(2):173–84.

19. Peng X-M, Gao L, Huo S-X, Liu X-M, Yan M. The mechanism of memory enhancement of acteoside (verbascoside) in the senescent mouse model induced by a combination of D-gal and AlCl₃. Phytother Res. 2015;29(8):1137–44.

20. Wu C-R, Lin H-C, Su M-H. Reversal by aqueous extracts of Cistanche tubulosa from behavioral deficits in Alzheimer's disease-like rat model: relevance for amyloid deposition and central neurotransmitter function. BMC Complement Altern Med. 2014;14:202.

21. Cho SO, Ban JY, Kim JY, Jeong HY, Lee IS, Song K-S, Bae K, Seong YH. Aralia cordata protects against amyloid β protein (25–35)-induced neurotoxicity in cultured neurons and has antidementia activities in mice. J Pharmacol Sci. 2009;111(1):22–32.

22. Yoo K-Y, Park S-Y. Terpenoids as potential anti-Alzheimer's disease therapeutics. Molecules. 2012;17(3):3524.

23. Cano-Europa E, González-Trujano ME, Reyes-Ramírez A, Hernández-García A, Blas-Valdivia V, Ortiz-Butrón R. Palmitone prevents pentylenetetrazole-caused neuronal damage in the CA3 hippocampal region of prepubertal rats. Neurosci Lett. 2010;470(2):111–4.

24. Eyong KO, Foyet HS, Eyong CA, Sidjui LS, Yimdjo MC, Nwembe SN, Lamshöft M, Folefoc GN, Spiteller M, Nastasa V. Neurological activities of lapachol and its furano derivatives from Kigelia africana. Med Chem Res. 2013;22(6):2902–11.

25. Wang H, Wang H, Cheng H, Che Z. Ameliorating effect of luteolin on memory impairment in an Alzheimer's disease model. Mol Med Rep. 2016;13(5):4215–20.

26. Aydin E, Hritcu L, Dogan G, Hayta S, Bagci E. The effects of inhaled Pimpinella peregrina essential oil on scopolamine-induced memory impairment, anxiety, and depression in laboratory rats. Mol Neurobiol. 2016;53:6557–67.

27. Jackson LL. VTE on an elevated maze. J Comp Psychol. 1943;36:99–107.

28. Olton DS, Samuelson RJ. Remembrance of places passed: spatial memory in rats. J Exp Psychol Anim Behav Process. 1976;2:97–116.

29. Ellman G, Courtney K, Andres VJ, Feather-Stone R. A new and rapid colorimetric determination of acetylcholinesterase activity. Biochem Pharmacol. 1961;7:88–95.

30. Srikumar B, Ramkumar K, Raju T, Shankaranarayana R. Assay of acetylcholinesterase activity in the brain. Brain Behav. 2009;1:142–4.

31. Mokhtari Z, Baluchnejadmojarad T, Nikbakht F, Mansouri M, Roghani M. Riluzole ameliorates learning and memory deficits in Aβ25–35-induced rat model of Alzheimer's disease and is independent of cholinoceptor activation. Biomed Pharmacother. 2017;87:135–44.

32. Winterbourn C, Hawkins R, Brian M, Carrell R. The estimation of red cell superoxide dismutase activity. J Lab Clin Med. 1975;85(2):337.

33. Arjmand Abbassi Y, Mohammadi MT, Sarami Foroshani M, Raouf Sarshoori J. Captopril and valsartan may improve cognitive function through potentiation of the brain antioxidant defense system and attenuation of oxidative/nitrosative damage in STZ-induced dementia in rat. Adv Pharm Bull. 2016;6(4):531–9.

34. Sharma M, Gupta YK. Chronic treatment with trans resveratrol prevents intracerebroventricular streptozotocin induced cognitive impairment and oxidative stress in rats. Life Sci. 2002;71(21):2489–98.

35. Bagci E, Aydin E, Mihasan M, Maniu C, Hritcu L. Anxiolytic and antidepressant-like effects of Ferulago angulata essential oil in the scopolamine rat model of Alzheimer's disease. Flavour Fragr J. 2016;31(1):70–80.

36. Fukuzawa K, Tokumura A. Glutathione peroxidase activity in tissues of vitamin E-deficient mice. J Nutr Sci Vitaminol. 1976;22(5):405–7.

37. Hritcu L, Ionita R, Motei DE, Babii C, Stefan M, Mihasan M. Nicotine versus 6-hydroxy-L-nicotine against chlorisondamine induced memory impairment and oxidative stress in the rat hippocampus. Biomed Pharmacother. 2017;86:102–8.

38. Oliver CN, Ahn BW, Moerman EJ, Goldstein S, Stadtman ER. Age-related changes in oxidized proteins. J Biol Chem. 1987;262(12):5488–91.

39. Luo S, Wehr NB. Protein carbonylation: avoiding pitfalls in the 2,4-dinitrophenylhydrazine assay. Redox Rep. 2009;14(4):159–66.

40. Navarro-Yepes J, Anandhan A, Bradley E, Bohovych I, Yarabe B, de Jong A, Ovaa H, Zhou Y, Khalimonchuk O, Quintanilla-Vega B, et al. Inhibition of protein ubiquitination by paraquat and 1-methyl-4-phenylpyridinium impairs ubiquitin-dependent protein degradation pathways. Mol Neurobiol. 2016;53(8):5229–51.

41. Ohkawa H, Ohishi N, Yagi K. Assay for lipid peroxides in animal tissues by thiobarbituric acid reaction. Anal Biochem. 1979;95(2):351–8.

42. Suchal K, Malik S, Khan SI, Malhotra RK, Goyal SN, Bhatia J, Kumari S, Ojha S, Arya DS. Protective effect of mangiferin on myocardial ischemia-reperfusion injury in streptozotocin-induced diabetic rats: role of AGE-RAGE/MAPK pathways. Sci Rep. 2017;7:42027.

43. Smith PK, Krohn RI, Hermanson GT, Mallia AK, Gartner FH, Provenzano MD, Fujimoto EK, Goeke NM, Olson BJ, Klenk DC. Measurement of protein using bicinchoninic acid. Anal Biochem. 1985;150(1):76–85.

44. Reichelt WN, Waldschitz D, Herwig C, Neutsch L. Bioprocess monitoring: minimizing sample matrix effects for total protein quantification with bicinchoninic acid assay. J Ind Microbiol Biotechnol. 2016;43:1271–80.

45. Kim H-S, Quon MJ, Kim J-a. New insights into the mechanisms of polyphenols beyond antioxidant properties; lessons from the green tea polyphenol, epigallocatechin 3-gallate. Redox Biol. 2014;2:187–95.

46. Blokland A. Scopolamine-induced deficits in cognitive performance: a review of animal studies. Scopolamine Rev. 2005;1:1–76.

47. Ishola IO, Adamson FM, Adeyemi OO. Ameliorative effect of kolaviron, a biflavonoid complex from Garcinia kola seeds against scopolamine-induced memory impairment in rats: role of antioxidant defense system. Metab Brain Dis. 2017;32(1):235–45.

48. Pahwa P, Goel RK. Asparagus adscendens root extract enhances cognition and protects against scopolamine induced amnesia: an in silico and in vivo studies. Chem Biol Interact. 2016;260:208–18.

49. Zhao X, Liu C, Qi Y, Fang L, Luo J, Bi K, Jia Y. Timosaponin B-II ameliorates scopolamine-induced cognition deficits by attenuating acetylcholinesterase activity and brain oxidative damage in mice. Metab Brain Dis. 2016;31(6):1455–61.

50. Sugisaki E, Fukushima Y, Fujii S, Yamazaki Y, Aihara T. The effect of coactivation of muscarinic and nicotinic acetylcholine receptors on LTD in the hippocampal CA1 network. Brain Res. 2016;1649:44–52.

51. Cohen JE, Zimmerman G, Melamed-Book N, Friedman A, Dori A, Soreq H. Transgenic inactivation of acetylcholinesterase impairs homeostasis in mouse hippocampal granule cells. Hippocampus. 2008;18(2):182–92.

52. Ozarowski M, Mikolajczak PL, Piasecka A, Kujawski R, Bartkowiak-Wieczorek J, Bogacz A, Szulc M, Kaminska E, Kujawska M, Gryszczynska A, et al. Effect of *Salvia miltiorrhiza* root extract on brain acetylcholinesterase and butyrylcholinesterase activities, their mRNA levels and memory evaluation in rats. Physiol Behav. 2017. doi:10.1016/j.physbeh.2017.02.019.

53. Qu Z, Zhang J, Yang H, Gao J, Chen H, Liu C, Gao W. *Prunella vulgaris* L., an edible and medicinal plant, attenuates scopolamine-induced memory impairment in rats. J Agric Food Chem. 2017;65(2):291–300.

54. Furtado RA, Oliveira BR, Silva LR, Cleto SS, Munari CC, Cunha WR, Tavares DC. Chemopreventive effects of rosmarinic acid on rat colon carcinogenesis. Eur J Cancer Prev. 2015;24(2):106–12.

55. Ono K, Li L, Takamura Y, Yoshiike Y, Zhu L, Han F, Mao X, Ikeda T, J-i Takasaki, Nishijo H, et al. Phenolic compounds prevent amyloid β-protein oligomerization and synaptic dysfunction by site-specific binding. J Biol Chem. 2012;287(18):14631–43.

56. Ertas A, Boga M, Yilmaz MA, Yesil Y, Tel G, Temel H, Hasimi N, Gazioglu I, Ozturk M, Ugurlu P. A detailed study on the chemical and biological profiles of essential oil and methanol extract of *Thymus nummularius* (Anzer tea): rosmarinic acid. Ind Crops Prod. 2015;67:336–45.

57. Farr SA, Niehoff ML, Ceddia MA, Herrlinger KA, Lewis BJ, Feng S, Welleford A, Butterfield DA, Morley JE. Effect of botanical extracts containing carnosic acid or rosmarinic acid on learning and memory in SAMP8 mice. Physiol Behav. 2016;165:328–38.

58. Fonteles AA, de Souza CM, de Sousa Neves JC, Menezes APF, do Carmo MRS, Fernandes FDP, de Araújo PR, de Andrade GM. Rosmarinic acid prevents against memory deficits in ischemic mice. Behav Brain Res. 2016;297:91–103.

59. Zhang Z, Wu H, Huang H. Epicatechin plus treadmill exercise are neuroprotective against moderate-stage amyloid precursor protein/presenilin 1 mice. Pharmacogn Mag. 2016;12(46):139–46.

60. Kim JH, Choi GN, Kwak JH, Jeong HR, Jeong C-H, Heo HJ. Neuronal cell protection and acetylcholinesterase inhibitory effect of the phenolics in chestnut inner skin. Food Sci Biotechnol. 2011;20(2):311–8.

61. Tseng H-C, Wang M-H, Soung H-S, Chang Y, Chang K-C. (−)-Epigallocatechin-3-gallate prevents the reserpine-induced impairment of short-term social memory in rats. Behav Pharmacol. 2015;26(8-Special Issue Pharmacological Approaches To The Study Of Social Behaviour-Part 3: Drug Effects):741–7.

62. Lee M-R, Yun B-S, Park S-Y, Ly S-Y, Kim S-N, Han B-H, Sung C-K. Anti-amnesic effect of Chong–Myung–Tang on scopolamine-induced memory impairments in mice. J Ethnopharmacol. 2010;132(1):70–4.

63. Foyet HS, Ngatanko Abaïssou HH, Wado E, Asongalem Acha E, Alin C. *Emilia coccinae* (SIMS) G extract improves memory impairment, cholinergic dysfunction, and oxidative stress damage in scopolamine-treated rats. BMC Complement Altern Med. 2015;15:333.

64. Mohammadpour T, Hosseini M, Naderi A, Karami R, Sadeghnia HR, Soukhtanloo M, Vafaee F. Protection against brain tissues oxidative damage as a possible mechanism for the beneficial effects of *Rosa damascena* hydroalcoholic extract on scopolamine induced memory impairment in rats. Nutr Neurosci. 2015;18(7):329–36.

65. Manal FE-K, Ebtesam MA-O, Ahmed EAM. Neuroprotective effects of *Citrus reticulata* in scopolamine-induced dementia oxidative stress in rats. CNS Neurol Disord: Drug Targ. 2015;13(4):684–90.

Transgenerational effects of paternal heroin addiction on anxiety and aggression behavior in male offspring

Mohd Zaki Farah Naquiah[1,2], Richard Johari James[1,2*], Suraya Suratman[2], Lian Shien Lee[1], Mohd Izhar Mohd Hafidz[3], Mohd Zaki Salleh[1,2] and Lay Kek Teh[1,2*]

Abstract

Background: Heroin addiction is a growing concern, affecting the socioeconomic development of many countries. Little is known about transgenerational effects on phenotype changes due to heroin addiction. This study aims to investigate changes in level of anxiety and aggression up to four different generations of adult male rats due to paternal exposure to heroin.

Methods: Male Sprague–Dawley rats were exposed with heroin intraperitoneally (i.p.) twice-daily for 14 days with increasing dosage regimen (F0-heroin). Male Sprague–Dawley rats (6-weeks-old) were divided into: (1) heroin exposed group (F0-heroin) and (2) control group treated with saline solution (F0-control). The dosage regime started with the lowest dose of 3 mg/kg per day of heroin followed by 1.5 mg/kg increments per day to a final dose of 13.5 mg/kg per day. Offspring were weaned on postnatal day 21. The adult male offspring from each generation were then mated with female-naïve rats after 2 weeks of heroin absence. Open field test and elevated plus maze test were used to study the anxiety level, whereas resident intruder test was used to evaluate aggression level in the addicted male rats and their offspring.

Results: Heroin exposure in male rats had resulted in smaller sizes of the litters compared to the control. We observed a higher anxiety level in the F1 and F2 progenies sired by the heroin exposed rats (F0) as compared to the control rats. Paternal heroin exposure also caused significantly more aggressive offspring in F1 compared to the control. The same pattern was also observed in the F2.

Conclusion: Our results demonstrated that the progenies of F1 and F2 sustained higher levels of anxiety and aggression which are due to paternal heroin exposure.

Keywords: Transgenerational effects, Paternal heroin addiction, Male offspring, Anxiety, Aggression

Background

Substance abuse and addiction is one of the serious public health concerns around the world. As reported by The World Drug Report [1], the global prevalence of opiates abusers is 16.5 million worldwide. In Malaysia, heroin is the most abused drugs with a percentage of 64.84 % and males constitute the biggest percentage of abusers each year [2].

The impact of various psychoactive substances on aggressive behavior had been studied previously, due to the documented rise in drug abusers involved in crime. Several drug related factors may contribute to this occurrence, e.g. pharmacological effects of the drug, substance-induced psychological or biological changes, and withdrawal effects [3]. Occasional use of opiates results in pleasure and euphoria [4, 5]. However, chronic exposure to heroin leads to complex changes in mood and behavior, and its abrupt withdrawal may cause adverse

*Correspondence: ritchjj@yahoo.fr; tehlaykek2016@gmail.com
[1] Integrative Pharmacogenomics Institute (iPROMISE), Level 7, FF3, Universiti Teknologi MARA Selangor, Puncak Alam Campus, 42300 Bandar Puncak Alam, Selangor, Malaysia
Full list of author information is available at the end of the article

after effects i.e. elevated aggression [6] and heightened pain sensitivity [7].

Over the last few decades, there have been several studies of how parental drug abuse may affect their progenies. While most of these studies focused on susceptibility to drug use, others have looked into behavioral, molecular and physiological changes in the offspring. Among them were studies looking at the impact of maternal opioid use on fetal development [8–10]. These studies documented long term consequences on fetal cognitive function including gender-specific modifications in specific emotional and social behaviors [11, 12]. Byrnes et al. [11] has also demonstrated an upregulation of dopamine and opioid-related genes in both mother and child, indicating transgenerational epigenetic effect. A delayed onset of puberty was observed in adolescent male rats exposed to morphine [13]. Mating between the male rats treated with heroin and naïve female rats resulted in smaller litter size. Upon maturation to the adult stage, the offspring displayed significant alteration in endocrine parameters, including gender specific changes in the adrenal weights, luteinizing hormone, and hypothalamic b-endorphin [14].

This study aims to examine the effects of paternal exposure to heroin on anxiety and aggression in the offsprings up to three generations (first generation—F1, second generation—F2 and third generation—F3).

Methods
Animals
A total of 64 male and 48 female Sprague–Dawley rats weighing 130–150 g were used. For F0, rats were divided into two experimental groups, with eight rats per group (heroin and control (saline) group). Rats were allowed to acclimatize for 2 weeks prior to experimental procedure and were placed in individual cages. Throughout the experiment, rats were maintained in a temperature and humidity controlled environment (24 °C $\pm$ 3.55 $\pm$ 1 %) in a 12:12 h light: dark cycle (lights on at 7:00 a.m.) and were given fresh water and standard rat chow ad libitum. All experiments were performed in accordance with the guidelines and approval from the Animal Ethics Committee of Universiti Teknologi MARA (UiTM) (46/2014).

Drug preparation
Heroin hydrochloride was obtained from LIPOMED (Switzerland). Heroin of 1 mg/ml concentration was prepared daily before injection by dissolving in 0.9 % normal saline heated to 40–50 °C.

Heroin exposure
Intraperitoneal injections with heroin were given to F0-heroin (F0-H) rats twice daily at 9:00 a.m. and 6:00

p.m., with a 27 gauge 1/2 inch (12 mm) needle for 14 consecutive days. A dose of 3 mg/kg on the first day and then increasing by 1.5 mg/kg per day to a final dose of 13.5 mg/kg per day were administered to the rats [15]. Escalating dose regimen was adopted in order to mimic the different phases of addiction in human. The control rats were injected with the same amount of saline.

Breeding
F0 rats were mated with heroin-naïve female rats at 2 weeks post heroin regime (Fig. 1). Withdrawal symptoms were observed during the 2-week period and female rats were introduced as withdrawal symptoms cease. Behavioral tests were then conducted on the rats before they were euthanized on week 11. Male pups were reared by their biological mothers and weaned on postnatal day 21. One male rat was randomly selected from each mother for behavioral testing, and was placed in individual cages each (n = 8). After the F1 rats reached sexual maturation, they were then mated with heroin-naïve female rats to produce F2 (Fig. 2). Behavioral testing commenced at 10 weeks of age. These procedures were then repeated in F2. F2 offspring (F3) were then tested with behavior tests at the age of 10 weeks (Fig. 3). All animals were raised in a similar and controlled environment across all generations.

Behavior testing
Elevated plus maze (EPM) apparatus
The elevated plus maze was constructed of wood and consisted of two open arms, OA (50 × 10 cm) and closed arms, CA (50 × 10 × 40 cm) set in a plus shape. The maze was elevated 50 cm from the floor with an open roof. The activities of the rats were recorded by an overhead camera attached on the ceiling and scoring was analyzed using ANY-maze Video Tracking System software (ANY-maze, Stoelting Co.). The test started with the rats being placed at the center region, facing the OA and were allowed to explore the maze for 5 min. The number of entries to the OA (the percentage of the total number of arm entries) and the total time spent in these arms of the maze were taken as an anxiety index (the higher the index, the lower the anxiety). To measure locomotion, the total number of entries for each arm was taken. An entry was counted when the four paws of the rats were placed in the arms. The maze was cleaned with 70 % ethanol between each trial.

Open field (OF) apparatus
To further analyze the anxiety behavior, the animals were tested in the OF for 5 min. The test was carried out in an arena (50 × 50 × 30 cm) divided into 25 squares (10 × 10 cm). Each of the rats was placed in the center

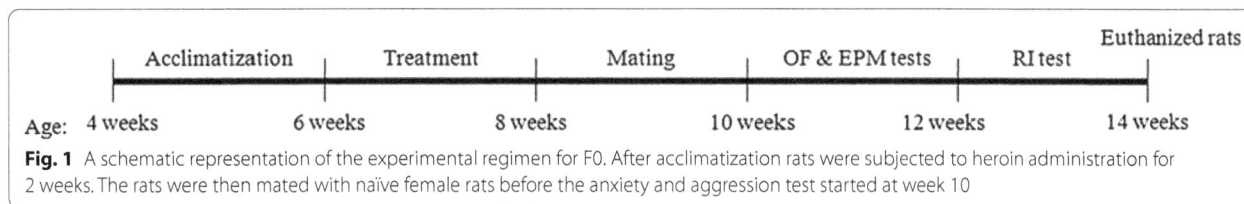

Fig. 1 A schematic representation of the experimental regimen for F0. After acclimatization rats were subjected to heroin administration for 2 weeks. The rats were then mated with naïve female rats before the anxiety and aggression test started at week 10

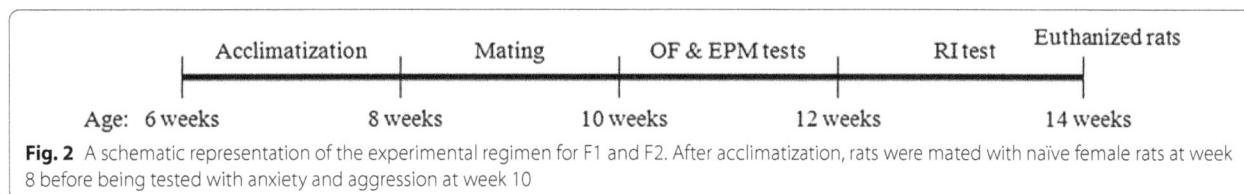

Fig. 2 A schematic representation of the experimental regimen for F1 and F2. After acclimatization, rats were mated with naïve female rats at week 8 before being tested with anxiety and aggression at week 10

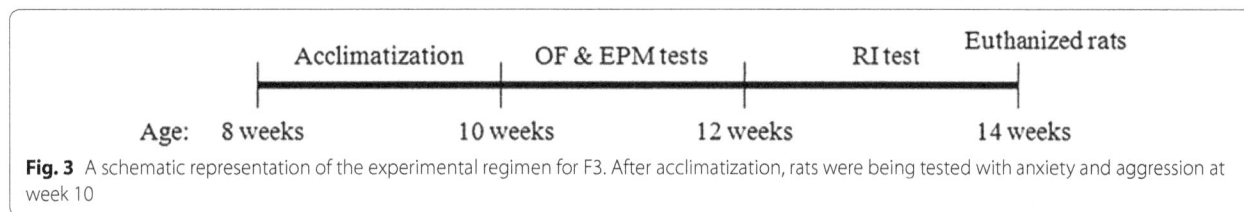

Fig. 3 A schematic representation of the experimental regimen for F3. After acclimatization, rats were being tested with anxiety and aggression at week 10

and was allowed to explore the arena for 5 min and the time spent in the center of the arena was recorded. After 5 min, the rat was then returned to its home cage and the open field was cleaned with 70 % ethyl alcohol and permitted to dry between tests.

Resident-intruder test
In this test, the resident male rats were housed in observation cages (80 × 55 × 50 cm) with a female rat as companion for a week before the test begins to facilitate territorial behavior. As territoriality is based on the presence of olfactory cues, the bedding of the cage was not changed during the week prior to testing. An hour before the test started, the companion female was removed. New male rat (intruder) was then introduced into the resident rat's cage and the test was started. The resident's reaction, i.e. non-social activities (attention, rear, sniff, walk, and body care), social activities (approach, follow, walk away, social sniff, genital sniff, and mount), and aggression (tail swish, lateral threat, bite, and clinch/fight), towards the intruder rat was recorded over 10 min. After the test was completed, the intruder rat was removed and the male resident was reunited with its female companion.

Statistical analysis
Data are presented as mean ± SEM normal distribution was tested using Kolmogorov–Smirnov test. The data were compared between groups in the same generation using student's t test. One-way ANOVA followed by Dunnett's or Tukey's post hoc tests were used for comparison within group for the variables studied in the behavioral test. Statistical significance were set at $p < 0.05$. Statistical parameters were determined using SPSS 20.0 (IBM Corporation, Armonk, NY, USA).

Results
Effects of paternal heroin exposure on litter size and body weight of first and second generation pups
The effects of paternal heroin exposure in F0 were apparent in the mean litter size of the first generation (Table 1). Number of offspring in heroin exposed male rat was significantly fewer than that of control group (p = 0.001, 95 % CI 3.07, 8.18). However, this pattern was not observed in second and third generations of the heroin exposed rats.

Effects of paternal heroin exposure on behavior of rats in the elevated plus-maze (EPM)
As depicted in Fig. 4a, heroin exposure in F0 resulted in a significantly lower percentage of the open arms entries (p = 0.001, 95 % CI 22.99, 66.1), which indicates anxiety effect of heroin withdrawal. In addition, heroin exposed rats spent shorter time in the open arm of the EPM (p = 0.001, 95 % CI 6.90, 15.5). A similar effect was found in the percentage of entries into the open arm of the maze in the first generation offspring of heroin exposed

Table 1 Average number of offspring for four generations of the experimental group

Generations	Average number of offspring	
	Control	Heroin
F0	11 ± 0.44	6 ± 1.04*
F1	11 ± 0.48	12 ± 0.32
F2	10 ± 0.29	10 ± 0.39
F3	11 ± 0.27	10 ± 0.33

This table represents the mean pups count per litter at postnatal day 21 (PND21) and postnatal day 90 (PND90)

* Statistically significant difference of p < 0.05 as compared to the control group

rats (F1-Heroin) compared to the offspring of vehicle-treated group (p = 0.001, 95 % CI 32.87, 60.52). Consistent with these results, rats of the F1-Heroin had a lower

percentage of time spent in the open arms of the maze in Fig. 4b when compared to offsprings of control group (F1-control) (p = 0.001, 95 % CI 49.05, 69.41). Interestingly, the second generation (F2) of the male addicted rats exhibit similar pattern with the first generation with a lower OA entries in F2-heroin (p = 0.001, 95 % CI 3.38, 10.41) as compared to control. However, the time spent in the OA was not significant in the F2 generation (p = 0.216, 95 % CI −0.92, 3.54). The difference between mean OA entries (%) and time spent in OA (%) in heroin and control group in F3 generation, on the other hand, was not statistically significant.

Effects of paternal heroin exposure which were investigated using elevated plus maze (EPM) test indicated no significant differences for the open arms (CA) entries between the heroin exposed rats with its offspring (One-way ANOVA, $p > 0.001$). However, a significant

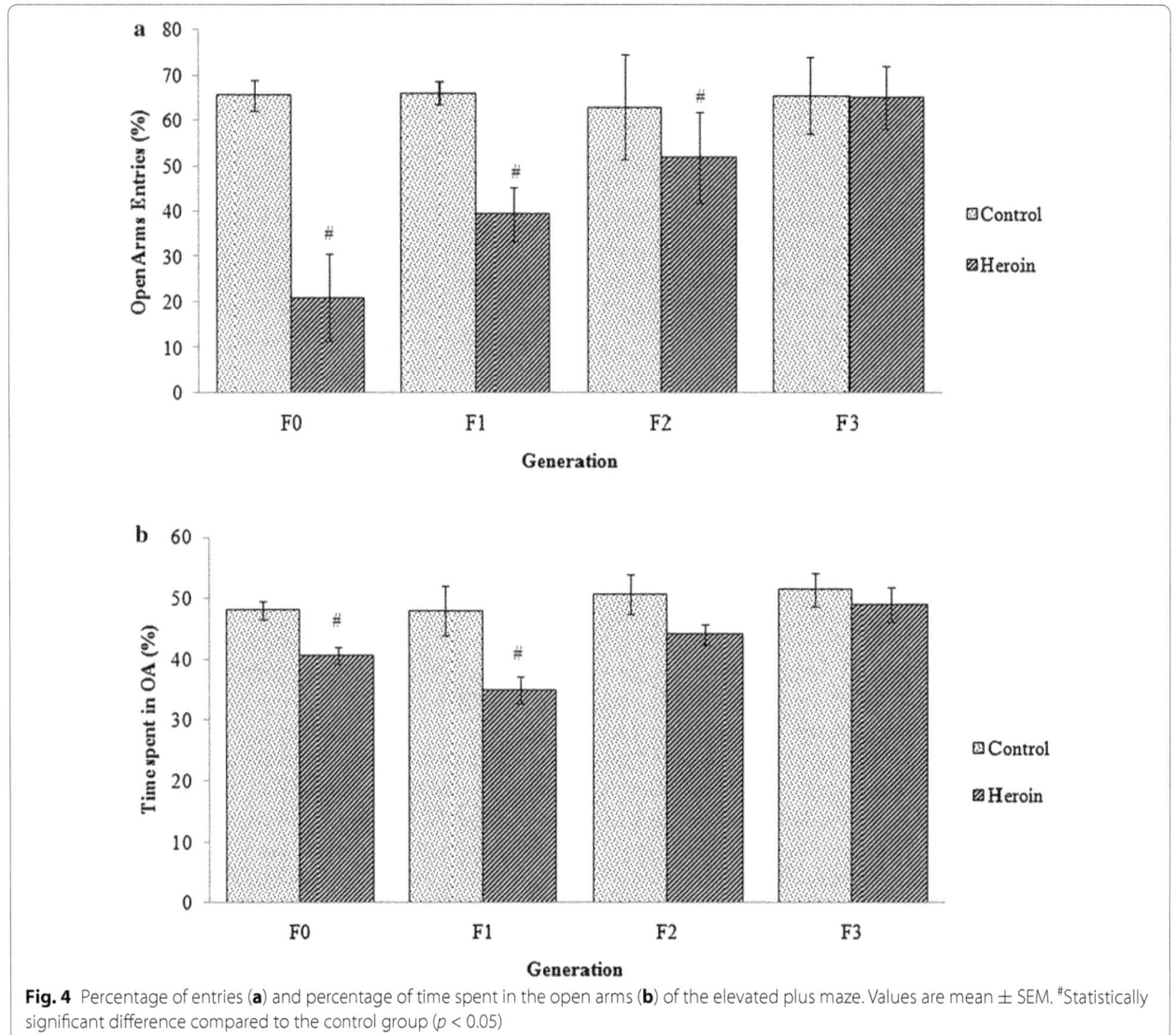

Fig. 4 Percentage of entries (**a**) and percentage of time spent in the open arms (**b**) of the elevated plus maze. Values are mean ± SEM. #Statistically significant difference compared to the control group ($p < 0.05$)

difference was seen between the heroin exposed rats and its third generation (F3). This shows that the behavior pattern was passed down only to F1 and F2 but not to its subsequent generation.

Effects of paternal exposure of heroin on the percentage of time spent and entries into the central zone of arena in the open field (OF) test

Number of entries into the central zone and percentage of time spent in the central zone are presented in Fig. 5. Heroin exposed rats showed statistically significant decrease (p = 0.001, 95 % CI 4.15, 7.85) in the number of entries into the central area compared to the control group (Fig. 5a). In addition, the offspring of F0-heroin rats exhibited significantly lower entries into the central area (p = 0.01, 95 % CI 1.27, 7.72), as compared to F1-control. Furthermore, a statistically significant difference was also observed between the second generations

of the heroin exposed rats and control rats (F2-heroin and F2-control) in the number of entries in the center of the OF (p = 0.017, 95 % CI 0.26, 2.23). This pattern however was not seen in F3 generation, which showed no statistically significant difference between F3-heroin and F3-control in both parameters measured.

Percentage of time spent in the center of OF is depicted in Fig. 5b. F0-heroin rats spent less time in the center zone as compared to F0-C during withdrawal phase (p = 0.001, 95 % CI 31.51, 35.31). Interestingly, F1-heroin also exhibited significantly shorter time spent in the center of OF than the F1-control (p = 0.001, 95 % CI 31.04, 34.29). In contrast, no statistical differences were found on the time spent by rats in the central square between F2-heroin and F2-control (p = 0.39, 95 % CI −2.29, 0.96). Both groups of the F3 generation exhibited no significant differences, indicating that the anxiety pattern has normalized towards control.

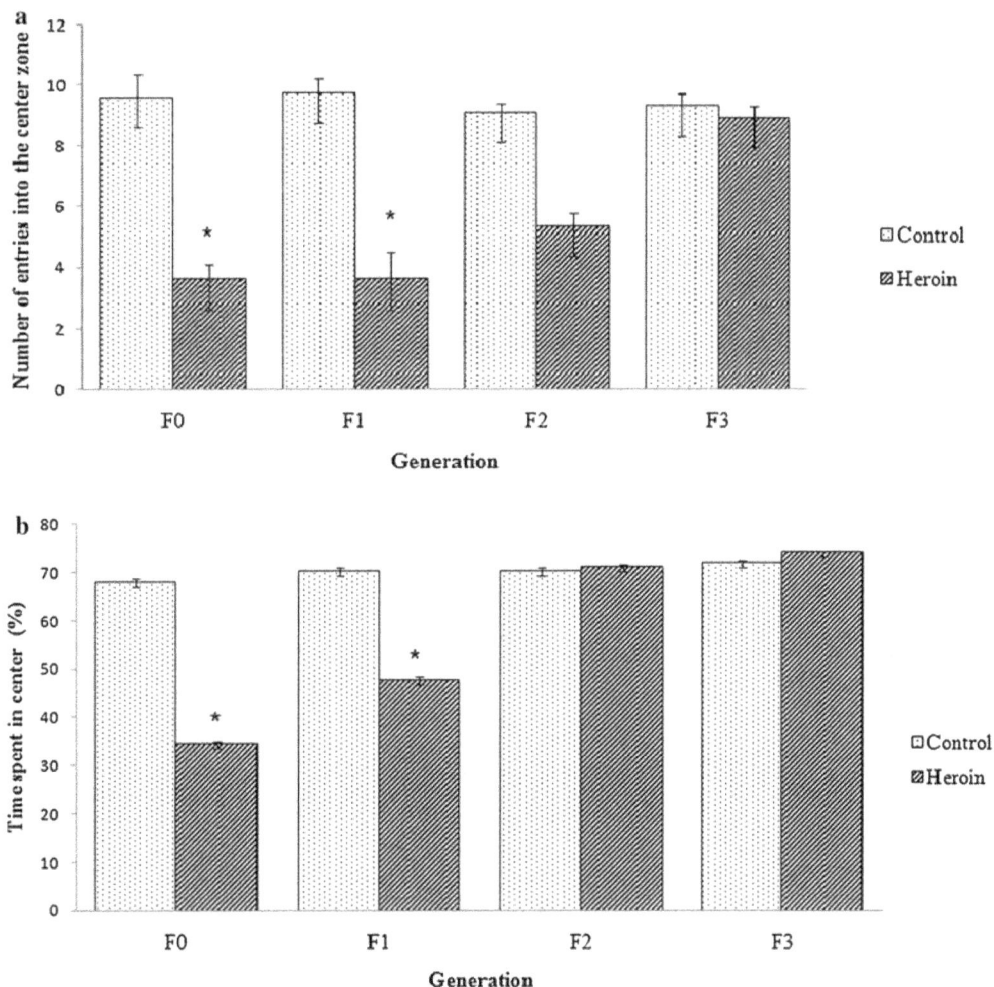

Fig. 5 Number of entries in the center (**a**) and percentage of time spent in the center (**b**) in the open field test. Values are mean ± SEM. *Statistically significant difference compared to the control group (p < 0.05)

It was found that anxiety behavior between the F0-heroin and F1-heroin groups were similar (post hoc, $p > 0.005$), implicating that transgenerational anxiety effects from the paternal to the descendants sustained over two generations.

Effects of paternal exposure of heroin in resident intruder (RI) test

Long-term behavioral effects of exposure to heroin in the first generation (F0) were then evaluated. Table 2 shows behavior phenotypes that were observed in this study: non-social activities, social activities, and aggressive behavior. Heroin exposed rats exhibited a pattern of pathological aggression as shown in tail swish, lateral threat, bite, and clinch/bite behavior during adulthood in RI test ($p < 0.005$). In non-social parameters, significant differences were exhibited in attention, rear, and body care behavior with heroin exposed male rats displaying higher frequency of these behaviors ($p < 0.05$). In social parameters, significant differences between the heroin exposed rats and control rats were displayed in approach, walk away, and social sniff ($p < 0.05$). In addition, in the aggression parameter, F0-heroin and F0-control exhibited a significantly difference in all of the parameters observed ($p < 0.05$), with F0-heroin displayed a higher frequency displaying the behaviors.

It was then further evaluated whether the next generation would also be affected by the previously heroin exposed father. Rats in the second generation (F1-heroin) showed higher frequency in non-social and social activity than the controls. In addition, the F1-Heroin also exhibited an increase in aggression parameters observed. This behavioral pattern was also observed in the third generation, F2-Heroin. However, in F3 generation, lower aggression behavior was observed.

As shown in Table 3, F0-heroin rats not only attack its intruder frequently, but also showing longer duration of attack towards the intruder and made a significantly longer time in clinch and fight. This pattern was exhibited by F1-heroin and F2-heroin. However, F3-heroin displayed a shorter time of attack towards the intruder, almost similar to F3-control.

Discussion

Drug abuse is an increasing societal burden. While it has been well documented that maternal opioids abuse during pregnancy results in detrimental effects in the offspring, less is understood about the contribution of paternal drug abuse on the next generation. The present study focused on paternal effects of heroin exposure during adolescence towards progenies i.e. F1, F2, and F3 generations.

Table 2 Behavioral observations from resident intruder test showing the mean for each group

Behavior	Frequency							
	F0-C	F0-H	F1-C	F1-H	F2-C	F2-H	F3-C	F3-H
Non-social activity								
Attention	30.62	24.83*	30.06	24.17*	30.50	24.17*	29.31	27.41
Rear	0.62	5.75*	0.87	5.5*	1.57	5.71*	0.88	1.31
Sniff	23.0	20.87	22.87	21	23.13	19.87	20.11	20.72
Walk	22.50	22.25	22.87	21.62	22.37	21.87	23.3	22.92
Body care	1.25	4.87*	1.37	5.1*	1.50	5.12*	2.31	6.22*
Social activities								
Approach	8.50	20.37*	7.5	21.62*	8.25	21.0*	9.22	15.51*
Follow	1.87	1.62	2.37	1.28*	4.0	2.25*	2.35	3.42
Walk away	2.50	10.12*	2.50	9.87*	2.62	0.62	3.16	4.26
Social sniff	23.25	39.62*	23.0	40.50*	23.0	28.12	23.16	27.17*
Genital sniff	8.62	9.87	8.75	10.50	7.37	10.62*	8.65	8.88
Mount	0.63	1.37	0.63	1.50	0.75	0.87	0.71	0.91
Aggression								
Tail swish	0.75	3.75*	1.25	4.12*	1.25	3.87*	0.65	1.31
Lateral threat	0.37	3.62*	0.63	3.63*	0.37	3.62*	0.39	0.61
Bite	2.37	9.25*	2.37	9.50*	2.87	9.12*	2.73	5.28*
Clinch/fight	1.25	7.5*	1.50	7.50*	1.62	2.50	1.45	3.32*

Data are given as mean frequencies. Student's t test: the asterisk means statistically significant difference compared to control rats ($p < 0.05$)

Table 3 Duration of the ethological measures

Behavior	Duration (s)							
	F0-C	F0-H	F1-C	F1-H	F2-C	F2-H	F3-C	F3-H
Non-social activity								
Attention	86.75	72.00	85.50	68.75*	86.75	68.75	71.83	70.05
Rear	1.63	7.13*	1.50	7.13*	1.31	7.00	5.79	6.22
Sniff	70.00	42.13*	69.00	41.88*	68.25	39.88	45.25	42.41
Walk	39.50	32.13	39.13	31.35	39.13	34.63	34.86	34.54
Body care	2.46	19.13*	1.51	19.20*	2.39	19.63*	16.05	17.57
Social activities								
App	9.00	20.13*	10.06	20.15*	9.50	20.00*	18.13	19.08
Follow	1.47	1.38	1.66	1.53	2.06	1.75	1.97	2.07
Walk away	1.94	12.56*	2.30	12.71*	2.51	2.47	10.70	11.64
Social sniff	88.63	161.38*	94.63	162.13*	86.88	78.88	144.94	150.52*
Genital sniff	29.13	48.50*	30.50	49.46*	29.75	52.00*	47.60	49.80
Mount	1.49	3.50	1.49	3.40	1.49	1.51	1.75	1.63
Aggression								
Tail swish	0.61	5.23*	0.94	5.43*	1.00	5.29*	4.60	5.03
Lateral threat	0.56	3.13*	0.93	3.08	0.31	3.17*	2.53	2.73
Bite	2.81	8.74*	2.45	8.25*	2.59	7.41	6.41	6.71
Clinch/fight	0.88	23.00*	1.21	23.00*	0.96	23.75*	19.14	21.14

Durations taken for the behavioral observations from resident intruder test showing the mean for each group. Student's t test: the asterisk means statistically significant different from control rats ($p < 0.05$)

The results of the present study demonstrated that heroin exposure produced adverse effect on the litter sizes (F1) as compared to saline administered group. The litter sizes of heroin treated rats were significantly lower than in control group (mean pup = 10). Our results were similar to other studies on fetal effects of opiate and other toxicants administration that caused abnormalities in their offspring such as decreased in the size of litters and lost in weight [14, 16–18]. Upon entering the human body, heroin is metabolized into 6-acetylmorphine (6-a. m.) and morphine, which will then be converted to morphine-3-glucuronide and morphine-6-glucuronide [19]. One of the possibilities that may leads to this paternal effects is that morphine may act directly as a mutagen on sperms, but the mechanisms of action has yet to be determined. In addition, the viability of sperms might also be affected after exposure to heroin [20]. Accumulation of the mu opioid receptors as well as endogenous expression of beta-endorphin in the male reproductive tract proposed that paternal gametes are receptive to endogenous and exogenous opioids [21]. μ-, κ-, and Δ opioid receptors are present in oocytes, most likely for mediating oocyte maturation [22]. Hence, the presence of opioid receptors on gametes not only maintains proper functions and development, but may lead to transgenerational inheritance [23]. Several previous studies have demonstrated that drug abusing behavior could lead to subtle

mutations in the sperms [16, 24–26]. Furthermore, it has been determined previously that drugs and other toxicants will accumulate in the semen and some may even bind to receptors on the sperms [27–30]. These studies suggested that abused substances may cause alterations in sperms thus influencing the development of the offspring, or transported to the ova via the seminal fluid, or by directly binding to the sperms and then affecting the development of the conceptus.

Research has shown that prenatal exposure to drugs of abuse can have long-term effects on the behavior of offspring [31]. Most of the previous studies focused on the impact of exposure of mothers to opioids such as heroin, morphine, and codeine during pregnancy, and its possible effects on prenatal opioid exposed offspring [32–34]. Other studies on congenital deficiencies, behavioral disorders, learning and memory impairment in offspring of addicted fathers have also been reported [11, 35]. This current study provides additional information that highlights the impact of heroin exposure of the father up to four generations of the offspring in terms of anxiety and aggressive behavior. OF and EPM are commonly used to measure anxiety-related behaviors in laboratory rodents. In EPM, anxiety-like behaviors are characterized by a lower frequency of entries and also shorter time spent in the open arms. To further validate the anxiety behavior, rats were then tested in the OF test. In OF, the anxiety behavior is characterized by a lower percentage of entries and shorter time spent in the center zone of the arena. Our results indicated that heroin addicted male rats were more anxious in both the OF box and EPM tasks which are in accordance with other studies using female addicted rats [11, 33]. Repeated heroin use leads to changes in the anatomy and physiology of the brain, consequently affecting the abilities in decision making, self-regulation behavior and response to stressful situations (Drug Policy Alliance, 2016). Additionally, it could lead to significant levels of tolerance and physical dependence. In this study, anxiety behavior in heroin induced male rats and its male progenies were increased as compared to the control rats. The offspring of the heroin exposed fathers displayed differences in several measures of behavioral tasks that look into anxiety level during the EPM and OF tests. Higher entries in the closed arms that were observed in the present study were also reported by Ahmadalipour et al. [36] using morphine induced female rats. We have further evaluated the anxiety level of the second generation of male heroin addicted rats. F2-heroin exhibited a statistically significant lower percentage of entries in the open arm of the EPM compared to F2-control. Interestingly, there was no significant difference in time spent in the OA between the two groups. The same pattern was also seen in the OF test. This indicates the rats of the F2-Heroin have an increase in exploratory behavior in the novel environment that has been introduced, despite the lower entries in the open arms and open arena. Notably, the anxiety levels in the third generation were reduced as compared to their father.

Anxiety is generally believed to be associated with aggressive behavior [37]. Thus, we evaluated whether there is an association between aggression and anxiety-like behavior in an animal model. The current findings demonstrate significant transgenerational effects of male rats addicted with heroin in the RI test. Heroin addicted rats are more aggressive than the controls in the RI test with a significant difference on several parameters that measures aggression i.e. tail swish, lateral threat, bite and clinch. These effects occurred in the absence of any direct exposure to heroin, and provide evidence that its administration may give psychological impacts on the addicts. From a pharmacological perspective, aggressive behavior can be escalated either by low acute heroin doses or during withdrawal from prolonged administration to repeated high heroin doses, presumably based on separate neural mechanisms. Interestingly, the male offspring of the heroin exposed rats displayed more aggressive responses towards the intruders when compared with the age-matched offspring of saline administered rats. This can be suggested as transgenerational effects of adolescent drug use, even in the absence of continued

use. This pattern can also be observed in the F2 generation but certain behaviors were not significantly different with the F2-control. However, the F3 generation of the heroin administered rats displayed a much lower aggressive response as compared to the previous generations.

Interestingly, rats that displayed heightened anxiety-like behavior exhibited higher aggression level, as indicated by the reduced time spent in the open arms of the EPM test as well as decreased ambulatory activities in the OF test. The mechanisms of heroin exposure towards the evolutionary phase of the gestational period and offspring's anxiety and aggression level remains unknown and needs further investigation. Many drugs including morphine may be mutagenic which often cause a minor but significant change in the physiological parameters, behaviors and neuroendocrine parameters [38].

In previous studies, possible effects of addicted father towards children were less considered. Thus, the results of this current study can be one of the supporting data highlighting the effects of heroin addicted fathers on children. It can be postulated that epigenetic mechanisms could be involved in transgenerational effects of heroin exposed paternal rats.

Epigenetic factors such as histone modifications (e.g. acetylation) have been implicated in the behavior of addiction [39]. In some instances, histone modifications alter the accessibility of DNA, hence affecting gene expression. DNA methylation (the addition of a methyl group to cytosine nucleotides, converting them to 5-methylcytosine) is another epigenetic process that has been shown to be involved in modulating behavior in response to substance abuse. For example, DNA methylation as well as histone acetylation represent key factors in regulating the *BDNF* gene, which encodes brain-derived neurotrophic factor (BDNF), a protein that is involved in numerous neurological conditions such as schizophrenia, depression, epilepsy, Alzheimer's disease, obesity and drug addiction at many stages of development [40].

As yet, no study has tracked the epigenetic effects on behavior of descendants of heroin abused fathers through the generations. Research is underway to examine the epigenetic influences on longstanding aggression behavior as a result of transgenerational substance abuse.

Conclusions

The idea that maternal heroin abuse can impact phenotype of subsequent generations is not new. Data from our studies however, highlighted the effects of paternal heroin exposure on progenies. Our findings have shown that heroin exposure can affect the levels of anxiety and aggression in the F0 generation. Of note, these effects were also observed in both the first (F1) and second (F2) generations, suggesting multigenerational and transgenerational effects triggered by adolescent exposure to heroin. Further investigations by our group are currently under way to understand the mechanisms involved in these observed effect.

Abbreviations

°C: degree celcius; a.m.: ante meridiem; ANOVA: analysis of variance; EPM: elevated plus maze; F0: first generation; F1: second generation (offspring of F0); F2: third generation (offspring of F1); F3: fourth generation (offspring of F2); g: gram; h: hour; kg: kilogram; ml: mililiter; mg: miligram; OF: open field; PND: postnatal day; RI: resident intruder; S.E.M: standard error mean.

Authors' contributions

MZFN carried out the animal behavioral studies and drafted the manuscript. LSL and MIMH participated in the animal behavioral experiments. SS helped in the data analysis of the animal behavioral studies and in drafting the manuscript. RJJ participated in the design and coordination of the study and helped to draft the manuscript. MZS helped to draft the manuscript. LKT conceived of the study, served as principal investigator throughout its execution and helped to draft the manuscript. All authors read and approved the final manuscript.

Author details

[1] Integrative Pharmacogenomics Institute (iPROMISE), Level 7, FF3, Universiti Teknologi MARA Selangor, Puncak Alam Campus, 42300 Bandar Puncak Alam, Selangor, Malaysia. [2] Faculty of Pharmacy, Universiti Teknologi MARA Selangor, Puncak Alam Campus, 42300 Bandar Puncak Alam, Selangor, Malaysia. [3] Comparative Medicine and Technology Unit, Institute Bioscience, Universiti Putra Malaysia, 43400 Serdang, Selangor, Malaysia.

Acknowledgements

This study was supported by a grant from the Ministry of Higher Education Malaysia (600-RMI/ERGS 5/3 (35/2013). The authors thank the staffs in the Laboratory Animal Facility and Management unit for excellent care of the animals and husbandry advice. Special thanks to members of iPROMISE for the technical support.

Competing interests

The authors declare that they have no competing interests.

Funding

This study was supported by a grant from the Ministry of Higher Education Malaysia (600-RMI/ERGS 5/3 (35/2013). The funder is not involved in the design of the study and collection, analysis, and interpretation of data and in writing the manuscript.

References

1. World Drug Report 2015. United Nations Office on drugs and crimes. 2015.
2. Malaysian National Anti-drug Agency. http://www.adk.gov.my/web/english/. Accessed 28 Jan 2016.
3. Hoaken PNS, Stewart SH, Sherry H. Drugs of abuse and the elicitation of human aggressive behavior. Addict Behav. 2003;28(9):1533–54.
4. Heroin facts. http://www.drugpolicy.org/drug-facts/heroin-facts Accessed 28 Jan 2016.
5. NIDA InfoFacts: heroin. http://www.drugabuse.gov/publications/drug-facts/heroin. Accessed 28 Jan 2016.
6. Tidey JW, Miczek KA. Heightened aggressive behavior during morphine withdrawal: effects of d-amphetamine. Psychopharmacology. 1992;107:297–302.
7. Miczek KA, Weerts EM, DeBold JF. Alcohol, benzodiazepine-GABAA receptor complex and aggression: ethological analysis of individual differences in rodents and primates. J Stud Alcohol. 1993;Suppl 11:170–9.
8. Hutchings DE. Methadone and heroin during pregnancy: a review of behavioral effects in human and animal offspring. Neurobehav Toxicol Teratol. 1982;4(4):429–34.
9. Malanga CJ 3rd, Kosofsky BE. Mechanisms of action of drugs of abuse on the developing fetal brain. Clin Perinatol. 1999;26(1):17–37.
10. Vathy I. Prenatal opiate exposure: long-term CNS consequences in the stress system of the offspring. Psychoneuroendocrinology. 2002;27(1):273–83.
11. Byrnes JJ, Babb JA, Scanlan VF, Byrnes EM. Adolescent opioid exposure in female rats: transgenerational effects on morphine analgesia and anxiety-like behavior in adult offspring. Behav Brain Res. 2011;218:200–5.
12. Johnson NL, Carini L, Schenk ME, Stewart M, Byrnes EM. Adolescent opiate exposure in the female rat induces subtle alterations in maternal care and transgenerational effects on play behavior. Front Psychiatry. 2011;2:29.
13. Cicero TJ, Adams ML, Giordano A, Miller BT, O'Connor L, Nock B. Influence of morphine exposure during adolescence on the sexual maturation of male rats and the development of their offspring. J Pharmacol Exp Ther. 1991;256:1086–93.
14. Cicero TJ. Basic endocrine pharmacology of opioid agonist and antagonist. In: Furr GJA, Wakeling AE, editors. Pharmacology and clinical uses of inhibitors of hormone secretion and action. London: Bailiere Tindall; 1987. p. 518–37.
15. Zheng T, Liu L, Aa J, Wang G, Cao B, Li M, Shi J, Wang X, Zhao C, RongrongGu JZ, Xiao W, Xiaoyi Yu, Sun R, Zhou Y, Zuo Y, Zhu X. Metabolic phenotype of rats exposed to heroin and potential markers of heroin abuse. Drug Alcohol Depend. 2013;127:177–86.
16. Abel EL. Paternal exposure to alcohol. In: Sonderegger TV, editor. Prenatal substance abuse: research findings and clinical implications. Baltimore: John Hopkins University Press; 1992. p. 1320–62.
17. Abel EL. Rat offspring sired by males treated with alcohol. Alcohol. 1993;10:237–42.
18. Day J, Savani S, Krempley BD, Nguyen M, Kitlinska JB. Influence of paternal preconception exposures on their offspring: through epigenetics to phenotype. Am J Stem Cells. 2016;5(1):11–8.
19. Aderjan RE, Skopp G. Formation and clearance of active and inactive metabolites of opiates in humans. Ther Drug Monit. 1998;20:561–9.
20. Carrel DT. Paternal influences on human reproductive success. Cambridge: Cambridge University Press; 2013.
21. Albrizio M, Guaricci AC, Calamita G, Zarrilli A, Minoia P. Expression and immunolocalization of the mu-opioid receptor in human sperm cells. Fertil Steril. 2006;86:1776–9.
22. Agirregoitia E, Peralta L, Mendoza R, Exposito A, Ereno ED, Matorras R, Agirregoitia N. Expression and localization of opioid receptors during the maturation of human oocytes. Reprod Biomed Online. 2012;24:550–7.
23. Yohn NL, Bartolomei MS, Blendy JA. Multigenerational and transgenerational inheritance of drug exposure: the effects of alcohol, opiates, cocaine, marijuana, and nicotine. Prog Biophys Mol Biol. 2015;118:21–33.
24. Badr FM, Badr RS. Induction of dominant lethal mutations in male mice nu ethyl alcohol. Nature. 1975;253:134–6.
25. Cohen FL. Paternal contributions to birth defects. Nurs Clin North Am. 1986;21:49–64.
26. Narod SA, Douglas GE, Nestmann ER, Blakey DH. Human mutagens: evidence from paternal exposure. Environ Mol Mutagen. 1988;11:401–15.
27. Borski AA, Pulaski EJ, Kimbrough JC, Fusillo MH. Prostatic fluid, semen, and prostatic tissue concentrations of major antibiotics following intravenous administration. Antibiot Chemother. 1954;4:905–10.
28. Gerber N, Lynn RK. Excretion of methadone in semen from methadone addicts: comparison with blood levels. Life Sci. 1976;19:787–92.
29. Leger RM, Swanson BN, Gerber N. The excretion of 5, 5-deiphenylhydantoin in the semen of man and the rabbit: comparison with plasma concentrations of the drug. Proc West Pharmacol Soc. 1977;20:69–72.
30. Yazigi RA, Odem RR, Polakoski KL. Demonstration of specific binding of cocaine to human spermatozoa. J Am Med Assoc. 1991;226:1956–9.
31. Che Y, Sun H, Tan H, Peng Y, Zeng T, Ma Y. The effect of prenatal morphine exposure on memory consolidation in the chick. Neurosci Lett. 2005;380(3):300–4.
32. Slamberova R, Schindler CJ, Pometlova M, Urkuti C, Purow-Sokol JA, Vathy I. Prenatal morphine exposure differentially alters learning and memory in male and female rats. Physiol Behav. 2001;73:93–103.

33. Tsang D, Ng SC. Effect of antenatal exposure to opiates on the development of opiate receptors in rat brain. Brain Res. 1980;188:199–206.

34. Byrnes EM. Transgenerational consequences of adolescent morphine exposure in female rats: effects on anxiety-like behaviors and morphine sensitization in adult offspring. Psychopharmacology. 2005;182:537–44.

35. Sarkaki A, Assaei R, Motamedi F, Badavi M, Pajouhi N. Effect of parental morphine addiction on hippocampal long-term potentiation in rats offspring. Behav Brain Res. 2008;186:72–7.

36. Ahmadalipour A, Sadeghzadeh J, Vafaei AA, Bandegi AR, Mohammadkhani R, Rashidy-Pour A. Effects of environmental enrichment on behavioral deficits and alterations in hippocampal BDNF induced by prenatal exposure to morphine in juvenile rats. Neuroscience. 2015;305:372–83.

37. Rylands AJ, Hinz R, Jones M, Holmes SE, Feldmann M, Brown G, McMahon AW, Talbot PS. Pre-and postsynaptic serotonergic differences in males with extreme levels of impulsive aggression without callous unemotional traits: a positron emission tomography study using 11 C-DASB and 11 C-MDL100907. Biol Psychiatry. 2012;72(12):1004–11.

38. Friedler G. Effects of limited paternal exposure to xenobiotic agents on the development of progeny. Neurobehav Toxicol Teratol. 1985;7:739–43.

39. Nestler EJ. Epigenetic mechanisms of drug addiction. Neuropharmacology. 2014;76:259–68.

40. Mitchelmore C, Gede L. Brain derived neurotrophic factor: epigenetic regulation in psychiatric disorders. Brain Res. 2014;1586:162–72.

Acute immobilization stress following contextual fear conditioning reduces fear memory: timing is essential

Akemi Uwaya[1], Hyunjin Lee[1], Jonghyuk Park[2], Hosung Lee[3], Junko Muto[4], Sanae Nakajima[5], Shigeo Ohta[1] and Toshio Mikami[6*]

Abstract

Background: Histone acetylation is regulated in response to stress and plays an important role in learning and memory. Chronic stress is known to deteriorate cognition, whereas acute stress facilitates memory formation. However, whether acute stress facilitates memory formation when it is applied after fear stimulation is not yet known. Therefore, this study aimed to investigate the effect of acute stress applied after fear training on memory formation, mRNA expression of brain-derived neurotrophic factor (BDNF), epigenetic regulation of BDNF expression, and corticosterone level in mice in vivo.

Methods: Mice were subjected to acute immobilization stress for 30 min at 60 or 90 min after contextual fear conditioning training, and acetylation of histone 3 at lysine 14 (H3K14) and level of corticosterone were measured using western blot analysis and enzyme-linked immunosorbent assay (ELISA), respectively. A freezing behavior test was performed 24 h after training, and mRNA expression of BDNF was measured using real-time polymerase chain reactions. Different groups of mice were used for each test.

Results: Freezing behavior significantly decreased with the down-regulation of BDNF mRNA expression caused by acute immobilization stress at 60 min after fear conditioning training owing to the reduction of H3K14 acetylation. However, BDNF mRNA expression and H3K14 acetylation were not reduced in animals subjected to immobilization stress at 90 min after the training. Further, the corticosterone level was significantly high in mice subjected to immobilization stress at 60 min after the training.

Conclusion: Acute immobilization stress for 30 min at 60 min after fear conditioning training impaired memory formation and reduced BDNF mRNA expression and H3K14 acetylation in the hippocampus of mice owing to the high level of corticosterone.

Keywords: Histone acetylation, Fear conditioning, Stress, Corticosterone

Background

Adrenal glands release corticosterone in response to stress, and this hormone plays an important role in memory formation [1, 2]. It triggers the transcription of brain-derived neurotrophic factor (BDNF) via the activation of the N-methyl-D-aspartic acid (NMDA) receptor.

The contextual fear conditioning test is a well-established paradigm to investigate the neural mechanisms of learning and memory [3, 4]. Animals subjected to fear training showed enhanced expression of BDNF and an increase in freezing time after 24 h [5]; however, animals with impaired BDNF function due to *BDNF* gene knockout [6, 7] or treatment with an anti-BDNF neutralizing antibody [8] showed deteriorated memory, indicating that BDNF is critical for memory formation.

During memory formation, BDNF expression is mostly regulated by epigenetic modification, especially histone

*Correspondence: mikami@nms.ac.jp
[6] Department of Health and Sport Science, Nippon Medical School, 1-7-1, Sakaiminami machi, Mushasino-shi, Tokyo 180-0023, Japan
Full list of author information is available at the end of the article

acetylation. Histone acetylation is associated with the regulation of the transcription of genes encoding proteins related to memory formation, thereby improving it [9–12]. For example, contextual fear training increases histone acetylation [3] and BDNF promoter binding to acetylated histone [12], followed by the consolidation of memory [12]; further, inhibition of histone deacetylation facilitates memory formation [9], indicating that the regulation of BDNF via histone acetylation plays an important role in memory formation [3, 13].

Chronic stress deteriorates cognition, and stress-induced deficits of cognition are attributed to epigenetic modifications such as increase in histone deacetylation and methylation [14]. On the other hand, when animals are subjected to acute stress, memory formation improves. That is, in the contextual fear conditioning test, acute stress applied before fear training facilitates memory [15]. Further, histone acetylation in the hippocampus regulates memory formation [16]. However, whether acute stress impairs or facilitates memory formation when stress is applied after fear training is not yet known. This study aimed to investigate the effect of acute stress applied after fear training on contextual fear memory formation in mice. To this end, we selected a contextual fear memory paradigm and histone acetylation marks because memory formation induced by contextual fear conditioning training requires histone acetylation, which occurs during a short period following such training [3].

Methods

Animals

All experimental procedures and animal treatments were performed in accordance with the laboratory animal manual guidelines of Nippon Medical School. This study was approved by the Animal Care and Use Committee of Nippon Medical School (Tokyo, Japan) and the approval number was 24-029. Male C57/BL6 mice (Sankyo Lab Service, Japan), aged 10 weeks and weighing 24.1 ± 0.75 g, were used. These animals were housed under a 12-h light/dark schedule and given access to rodent chow (Oriental Yeast Co., Japan) and water ad libitum.

Experimental Protocol

We performed six experiments. Each experiment was designed and performed based upon the results of previous experiments and used a separate group of mice.

Experiment 1: contextual fear conditioning training

Mice were randomly divided into six groups: no training, 0, 30, 60, 90, and 120 min. The mice were sacrificed to collect hippocampus samples at 0, 30, 60, 90, or 120 min after contextual fear conditioning training to examine

acetylated H3K14 and acetylated H4K5 (Fig. 1a). The no training mice were allowed to explore the training chamber, but did not receive any foot shock. The hippocampus samples of the no training mice were collected immediately after removal from the contextual fear conditioning chamber.

Contextual fear conditioning was applied according to published protocols with slight modifications [17]. The mice were transported to an animal experimental laboratory and allowed to acclimate for at least 30 min prior to contextual fear conditioning training. The mice were then placed in the foot shock system model MK-450MSQ (Muromachi Kikai CO. LTD, Japan) and allowed to explore for 2 min followed by three electric foot shocks (0.8 mA, 2-s duration and 2-min interval). Animals were left in the apparatus for a further minute before being removed.

Histone extraction was performed according to published protocols with slight modifications [17]. For histone extraction experiments, animals were sacrificed, and the brains were removed and hippocampi were dissected. Hippocampus samples were homogenized for 10 strokes in homogenizing buffer [250 mM sucrose (Wako, Japan), 50 mM Tris–HCl pH 7.5, 25 mM KCl (Kato Chemical Co., Inc., Japan), 0.5 mM phenylmethylsulfonyl fluoride (PMSF; Sigma, USA), 0.9 mM Na t-butyrate (Sigma), 1 % protein inhibitor cocktail (Sigma)] using a Dounce homogenizer. All steps were performed on ice, and all centrifugations were performed at 4 °C. Homogenized samples were centrifuged at $770 \times g$ for 1 min. The supernatant was removed and then re-suspended in 0.5 mL of 0.4 N H_2SO_4 for 30 min to extract histones. Samples were centrifuged at $14,000 \times g$ for 10 min. The supernatant was transferred to a fresh tube, and 250 μL of trichloroacetic acid (with 4 mg/mL deoxycholic acid) was added to the precipitated proteins. The precipitate was incubated on ice for 30 min and then centrifuged at $14,000 \times g$ for 30 min. The supernatant was discarded and the protein pellet was washed with 1 mL of acidified acetone (0.1 % HCl) and 1 mL of pure acetone for 5 min each, with centrifugation at $14,000 \times g$ for 5 min after each wash. The final protein pellet was resuspended in 10 mM Tris–HCl pH 8.0 and stored at −80 °C.

Experiment 2: measurement of freezing time and measuring mRNA levels by RT-PCR

Mice were randomly divided into six groups: no training, training, training + stress (60–90 min), training + stress (90–120 min), immobilization stress only, and naïve. Naïve mice were kept in their home cage until sample collection. The no training mice were exposed to the training chamber without footshock, and then returned to their home cage. Training mice were returned to their

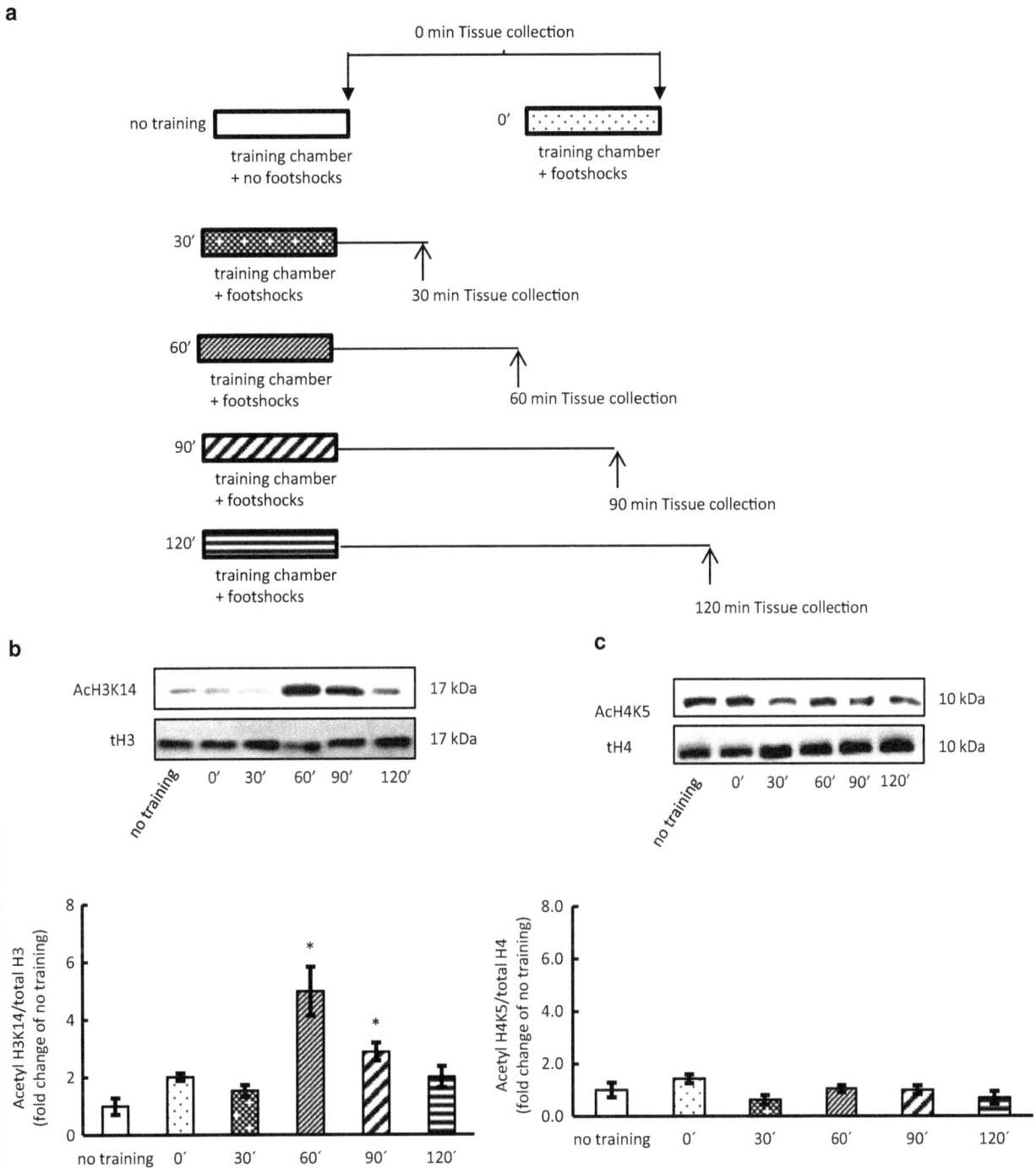

Fig. 1 Effect of contextual fear conditioning (Experiment 1). **a** Experimental protocol for contextual fear conditioning training. Hippocampus samples were collected at 0, 30, 60, 90, 120 min after contextual fear conditioning training. **b** Representative western blots for the acetylation of H3K14 in the hippocampus and quantification of immunoblot densities for mean (±SEM) acetylated H3K14 at each time point after the contextual fear conditioning training compared with that in mice without training (n = 3–4). **c** Representative western blots for acetylation of H4K5 in the hippocampus and quantification of immunoblot densities for mean (±SEM) acetylated H4K5 at each time point after the contextual fear conditioning training compared with that in mice without training (n = 3–4). Data are expressed as mean ± SEM. *$P < 0.05$ compared with no training

home cage immediately after contextual fear conditioning training. After contextual fear conditioning training, training + stress (60–90 min), and training + stress (90–120 min) mice were subjected to immobilization stress for 30 min, and then returned to their home cage. Immobilization stress only mice were subjected to immobilization stress for 30 min, and then returned to their home cage. Twenty-four hours after the training, all mice were subjected to the measurement of freezing time and sacrificed to collect hippocampus samples. The hippocampus samples were used for analyzing mRNA (Fig. 2a).

Immobilization stress was applied according to published protocols with slight modifications [18]. Mice were exposed to 30 min of immobilization in an immobilization cage (width: 3 cm, length: 3 cm, height: 7.5 cm) 60 or 90 min after contextual fear conditioning training.

Freezing behavior (defined as complete lack of movement, except for respiration) was measured by observing the animals for 3 min, 24 h after training. The absence of all non-respiratory movement was measured and hand-scored by trained observers. Memory was assessed as the percentage of time that the mice spent freezing when placed back in the training apparatus without receiving footshocks.

The mice were sacrificed by decapitation immediately after the fear conditioning behavioral test, and the hippocampi were isolated. Hippocampal BDNF mRNA (NCBI accession no. NM-007540.4) was measured. Total RNA was isolated using the RNeasy Mini Kit (QIAGEN, Germany) according to the manufacturer's instructions. RNA quantification was carried out by measuring absorption at 260 nm. Complementary DNA was generated from total RNA by reverse transcription (RT) using oligo(dT) [19] 12–18 primers (Invitrogen, USA) and superscript reverse transcriptase (Invitrogen, USA) in PCR thermal cycler DICE (Takara, Japan). The RT steps consisted of incubation at 37 °C for 10 min followed by incubation at 50 °C for 60 min. BDNF mRNA level in the hippocampus was measured by real-time quantitative PCR. Glyceraldehyde-3-phosphate dehydrogenase (GAPDH) served as an endogenous control. Quantification of the TaqMan® real-time PCR results was performed by plotting fluorescent signal intensity against the number of PCR cycles on a semi-logarithmic scale. The fluorescent probes and the forward and reverse primers were designed using Primer 3 software based on information from NCBI accession no. NM-007540.4 and synthesized by Hokkaido System Science (Hokkaido System Science Co., Japan). The primer and probe sequences were as follows: BDNF probe: 5'-ACACTTCCCGGGTGATGCTCAGCA-3', BDNF reverse primer: 5'-GAGGCTCCAAAGGCACTTGA-3', BDNF forward primer: 5'-ACCATAAGGACGCGGACT

TG-3', GAPDH probe: 5'-TGGATGGCCCCTCTGGA AAGCTG-3', GAPDH reverse primer: 5'-ATGTTCTGG GCAGCC-3', and GAPDH forward primer: 5'-CATC ACTGCCACCCAGAAGA-3'. The reaction protocol for real-time PCR consisted of 50 °C for 5 min followed by 95 °C for 5 min. This was followed by 40 cycles of a two-step PCR reaction consisting of 95 °C for 20 s and 60 °C for 1 min. The real-time PCR values for BDNF were corrected relative to the values for GAPDH.

Experiment 3: western blotting

Mice were randomly divided into seven groups: no training, training 90 min, training 120 min, training + stress (60–90 min), training + stress (90–120 min), immobilization stress only, and naïve. Naïve mice remained in their home cage until sample collection. The no training mice were sacrificed to collect hippocampus samples immediately after exposure to the training apparatus without footshock. Training 90 min and training 120 min mice were sacrificed to collect the hippocampus, 90 and 120 min after the training respectively. Training + stress (60–90 min) and training + stress (90–120 min) mice were sacrificed to collect the hippocampus immediately after the immobilization stress following training. The hippocampus samples were used for western blotting (Fig. 3a).

Extracted histone protein concentrations were measured using commercially available reagents (BCATM Protein Assay Reagents, Pierce, USA). Four volumes of sample buffer (final concentration 6.25 mM Tris–HCl, pH 6.8, 2 % sodium dodecyl sulfate (SDS, Wako), 10 % glycerol (Wako), 1.25 % 2-mercaptoethanol (Wako), 0.1 % bromophenol blue (Wako) was added to each sample. One microgram of protein for acetylation of H3K14 and H4K5, and 0.5 microgram of protein for total H3 and total H4 from each sample was loaded and run on a 4 % acrylamide stacking gel and 15 % acrylamide resolving gel. Proteins were transferred to polyvinylidene difluoride membranes, which were processed for immunoblotting. These membranes were first blocked in 3 % bovine serum albumin in Tris-buffered saline with Tween (TTBS) (150 mM NaCl, 20 mM Tris–HCl pH 7.5, 0.05 % Tween-20) for 60 min at room temperature and then incubated with primary antibody overnight at 4 °C. The primary antibodies and dilutions used were anti-histone H3 (1:500, Millipore), anti-acetyl-histone H3 (Lys14, 1:1000, Millipore), anti-histone H4 (1:500, Millipore), and anti-acetyl-histone H4 (Lys5, 1:1000, Millipore). Subsequently, membranes were washed with TTBS and incubated with secondary antibody for 2.5 h at room temperature. The secondary antibody used was anti-rabbit IgG, horseradish peroxidase-linked antibody (1:3000, Cell Signaling). Finally, membranes were washed with TTBS and

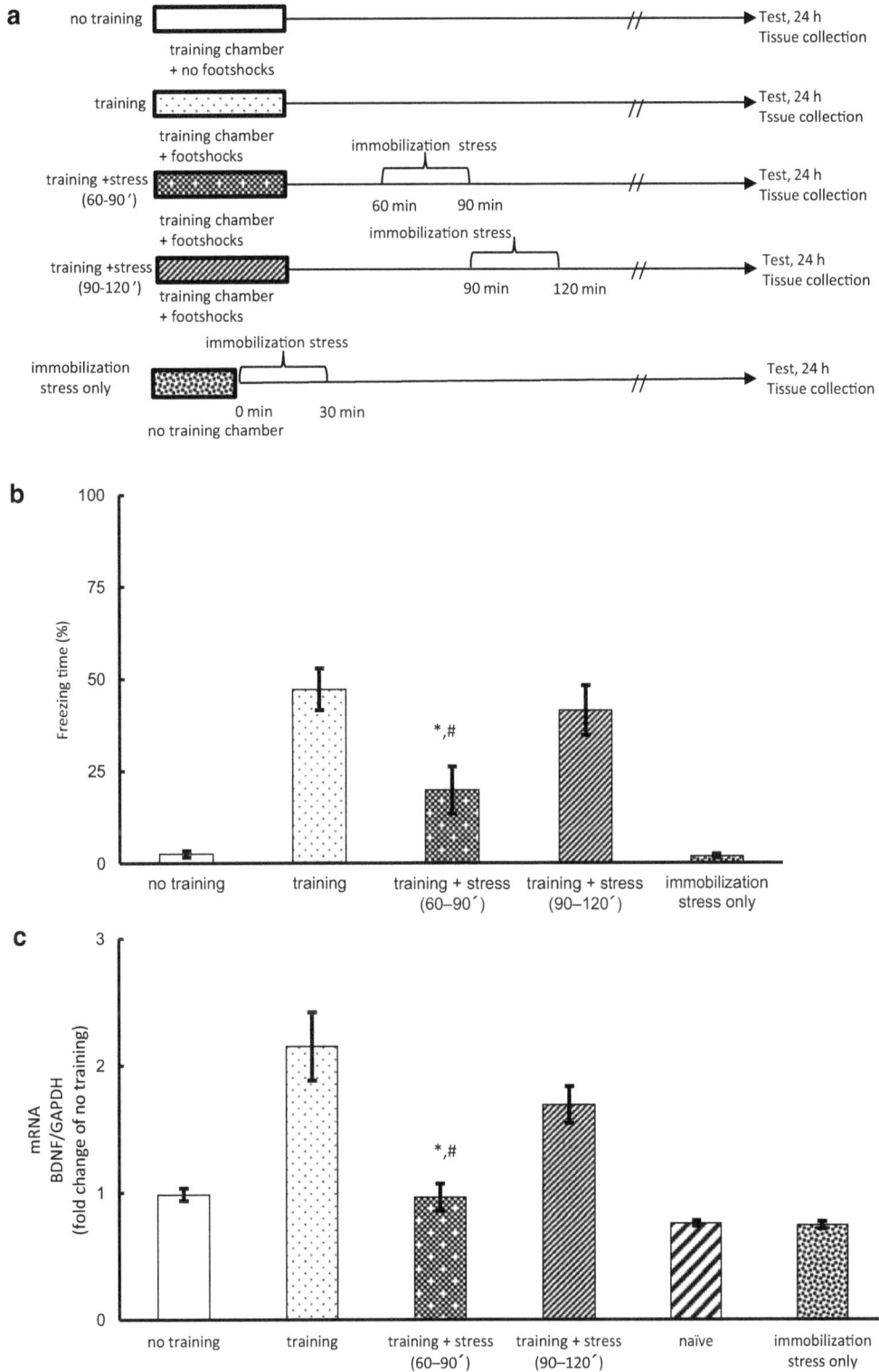

Fig. 2 Effect of acute immobilization stress after contextual fear conditioning (Experiment 2). **a** Experimental protocol for contextual fear conditioning training followed by stress and behavior tests. **b** Quantification of freezing behavior 24 h after the contextual fear conditioning training followed by immobilization stress (n = 10). **c** Quantification of BDNF/GAPDH mRNA ratio in the hippocampus (n = 5–8). The samples of naïve mice were collected the same day as the other groups. Naïve mice were not exposed to the training apparatus or immobilization stress. Data are expressed as mean ± SEM. *$P < 0.05$ compared with training group. #$P < 0.05$ compared with training + stress group (90–120 min)

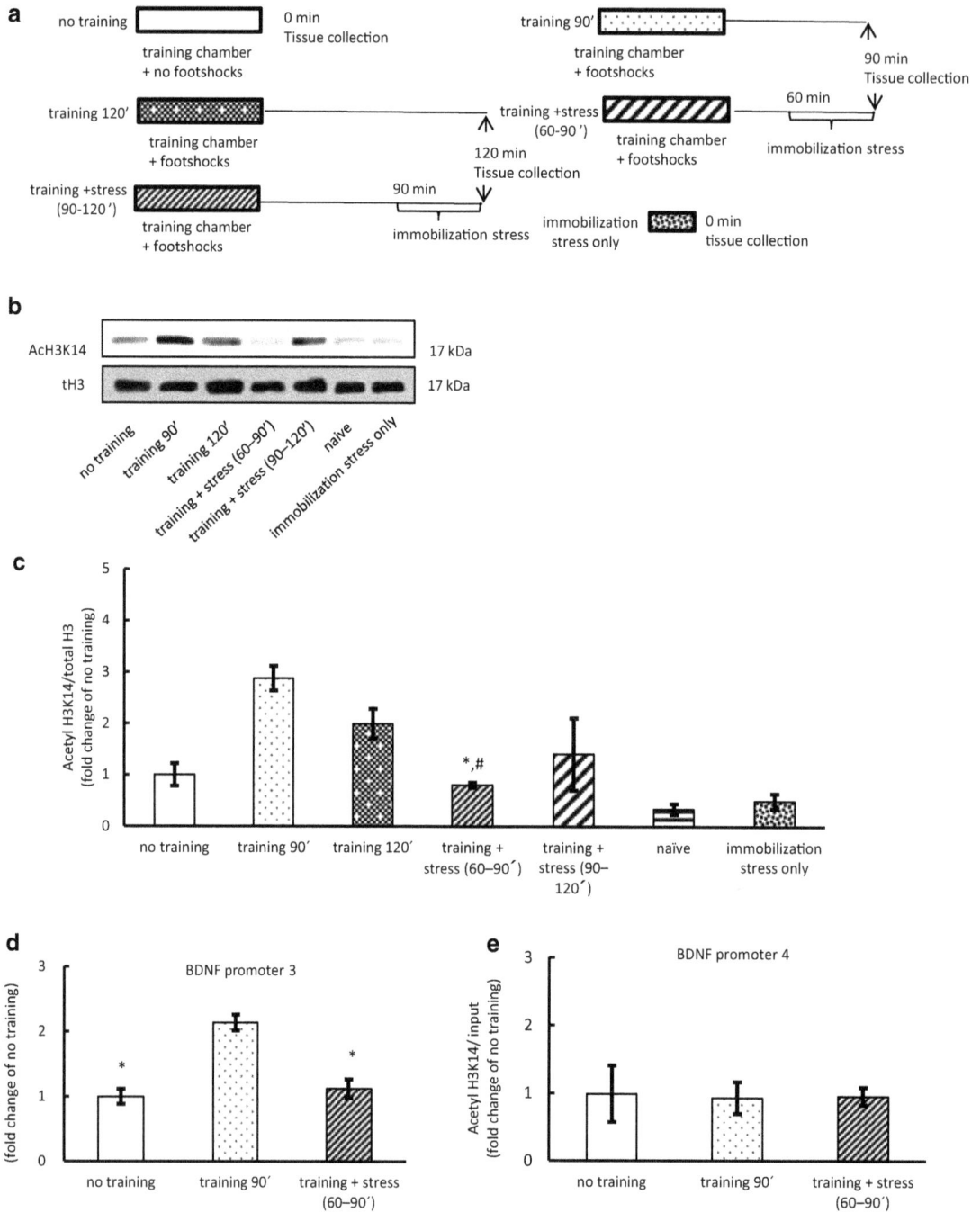

Fig. 3 Epigenetic modification of BDNF promoter via acute immobilization stress applied after fear training (Experiments 3 and 4). **a** Experimental protocol for contextual fear conditioning training followed by immobilization stress. **b** Representative western blots for the acetylation of H3K14 in the hippocampus at 90 and 120 min after the training and quantification of immunoblot densities for mean (± SEM) acetylated H3K14 at 90 and 120 min after the training compared with that in the without training group (n = 4–5). **c** Acetylated H3K14 levels in the hippocampus at *bdnf* promoter 3 at 90 min after the training compared with that in the no training group (n = 3–4). **d** Levels of H3K14 acetylation in the hippocampus at *bdnf* promoter 3 at 90 min after the training compared with that in the group without training (n = 3–4). **e** Levels of H3K14 acetylation in the hippocampus at *bdnf* promoter 4 at 90 min after the training compared with that in the group without training (n = 4). Data are expressed as mean ± SEM. *$P < 0.05$ compared with training 90 min. #$P < 0.05$ compared with training 120 min. Different sets of mice were used for western blotting and ChIP assay analyses

then immunolabeled using chemical luminescence with Immunostar LD (Wako, Tokyo). The luminescence was detected with an LAS 1000 mini-image analyzer (Fuji Film, Tokyo). Densitometric analysis was performed using Image Gauge ver. 4.0 (Fuji Film).

Experiment 4: chromatin immunoprecipitation (ChIP)

Mice were randomly divided into three groups: no training, training 90 min, and training + stress (60–90 min). Immediately after exposure to the training chamber without footshock, the no training mice were sacrificed to collect the hippocampus samples. Training 90 min mice were sacrificed to collect the hippocampus 90 min after the training. Training + stress (60–90 min) mice were sacrificed to collect the hippocampus immediately after the immobilization stress following training. The hippocampus samples were used for a chromatin immunoprecipitation (ChIP) assay.

ChIP was performed following a modified version of the Millipore ChIP kit protocol. Immediately after hippocampus tissue disruption, the sample was cross-linked in formalin for 15 min at room temperature. The crosslinking reaction was stopped by adding glycine at a final concentration of 0.125 M. The tissue was washed with cold PBS containing 1 mM PMSF and a protease inhibitor cocktail (Sigma). Then, the sample was homogenized in cell lysis buffer (10 mM Tris–HCl pH 8.0, 10 mM NaCl, 0.2 % NP-40, 1 mM PMSF and protease inhibitors cocktail) for 10 strokes using a Dounce homogenizer. The homogenized sample was centrifuged at $4000 \times g$ for 5 min at 4 °C, and the supernatant was removed. Nuclear lysis buffer (1 % SDS, 10 mM EDTA, 50 mM Tris–HCl pH 8.0, 1 mM PMSF and protease inhibitors cocktail) was added to the precipitate and incubated for 10 min on ice, followed by sonication using Bioruptor® (Cosmo Bio Co., Ltd.). Next, DNA fragments were centrifuged at $10,000 \times g$ for 15 min at 4 °C. Twenty microliters of lysate was saved as "input" for later normalization. The remaining lysate was diluted with ChIP dilution buffer (1.1 % Triton X-100, 0.01 % SDS, 1.2 mM EDTA, 167 mM NaCl, 16.7 mM Tris–HCl pH 8.0, 1 mM PMSF and protease inhibitor cocktail) at a 1:10 ratio. The chromatin solution was pre-cleared with 75 µL of protein A agarose/salmon sperm DNA (50 % slurry, Millipore) for 1 h at 4 °C and centrifuged at $3000 \times g$ for 5 min at 4 °C, with the supernatant recovered. This supernatant was immunoprecipitated overnight at 4 °C with 3 µL of antibody (H3K14, Millipore). After immunoprecipitation, the DNA-histone complex was collected with 60 µL of protein A agarose/salmon sperm DNA (50 % slurry) for 1 h at 4 °C, followed by one wash in low-salt buffer (0.1 % SDS, 1 % Triton

X-100, 2 mM EDTA, 20 mM Tris–HCl pH 8.0, 150 mM NaCl), one wash in high-salt buffer (0.1 % SDS, 1 % Triton X-100, 2 mM EDTA, 20 mM Tris–HCl pH 8.0, 500 mM NaCl), one wash in LiCl buffer (0.25 M LiCl, 1 % NP-40, 1 % deoxycholate Na, 1 mM EDTA, 10 mM Tris–HCl pH 8.0) and two washes in Tris–EDTA buffer pH 8.0 (Wako). The precipitated protein-DNA complexes were eluted from the antibody with elution buffer (1 % SDS, 50 mM NaHCO$_3$). The elution buffer was added to the input, and then incubated overnight at 65 °C in 200 mM NaCl to reverse the formaldehyde cross-links. Ten microliters of 0.5 M EDTA, 20 µL of 1 M Tris–HCl pH 6.5 and 2 µL of 10 mg/mL proteinase K (Sigma) were added to the elutes and incubated for 1 h at 45 °C. DNA was extracted using phenol/chloroform/isoamyl alcohol and then precipitated with ethanol. Next, quantitative PCR was performed with primers specific to the *bdnf* gene promoters. Specific primers were designed to amplify proximal promoter regions and used as described previously [14]. For *bdnf* P3, the forward primer was 5'-GTGAGA-ACCTGGGGCAAATC-3' and the reverse primer was 5'-ACGGAAAAGAGGGAGGGAAA-3'. For *bdnf* P4, the forward primer was 5'-CTTCTGTGTGCGTGAATTTG CT-3' and the reverse primer was 5'-AGTCCACGAGAG GGCTCCA-3'. Input and immunoprecipitated DNA amplification reactions were run in the presence of SYBR Green (real-time PCR master mix). The cumulative fluorescence for each amplification was normalized to the input amplification.

Experiment 5: measurement of plasma corticosterone

Mice were randomly divided into five groups: no training, training 90 min, training + stress (60–90 min), training + stress (90–120 min), and immobilization stress only. Ninety minutes after exposure the training chamber without footshock, the no training mice were sacrificed to collect the blood samples. Training 90 min mice were sacrificed to collect the blood 90 min after the training. Training + stress (60–90 min) and training + stress (90–120 min) mice were sacrificed to collect the blood immediately after the immobilization stress following training. Immobilization stress only mice were sacrificed to collect the blood sample immediately after the immobilization stress. The blood samples were used for corticosterone measurement (Fig. 4a).

Blood samples were collected after contextual fear training and immobilization stress. Plasma corticosterone levels were quantified by ELISA according to the instructions of the supplier (AssayMax Corticosterone ELISA Kit, AssayPro LLC, USA).

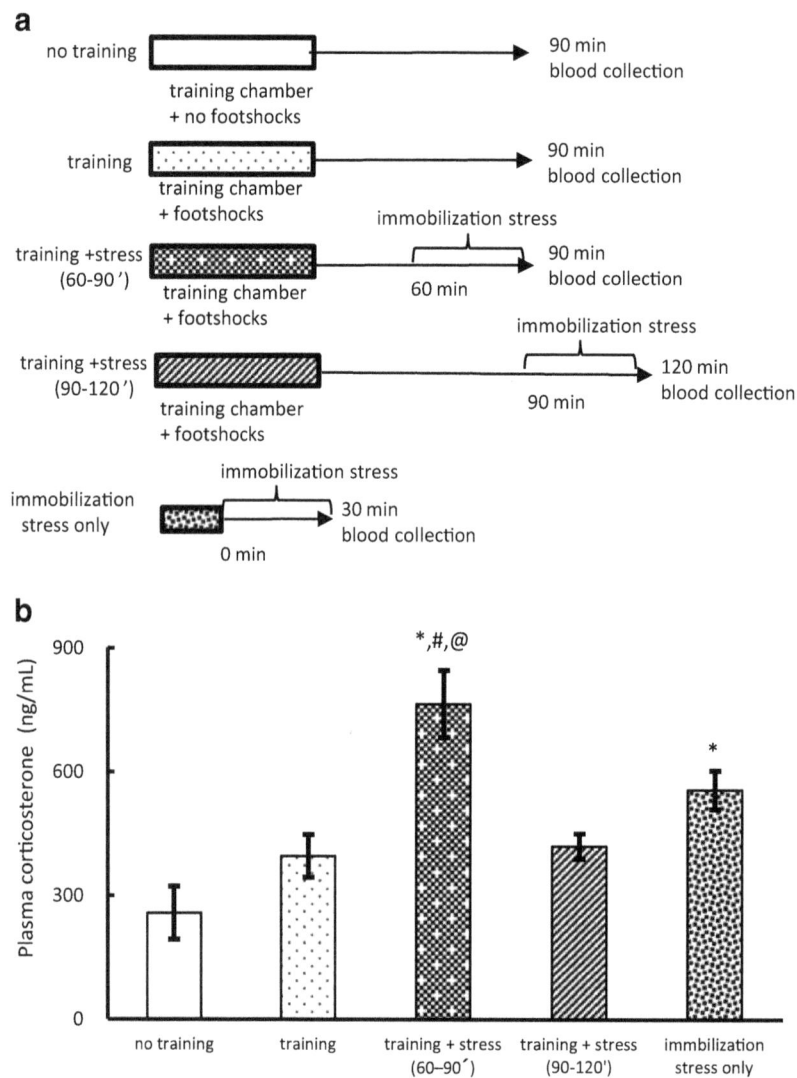

Fig. 4 Plasma corticosterone levels (Experiment 5). **a** Experimental protocol for blood sample collection. **b** Comparison of plasma corticosterone levels (n = 5). Data are expressed as mean ± SEM. *$P < 0.05$ compared with no training group. #$P < 0.05$ compared with training group. @$P < 0.05$ compared with training + stress group (90–120 min)

Experiment 6: effect of glucocorticoid receptor antagonist (mifeprostone) injection after contextual fear conditioning training

The glucocorticoid receptor antagonist mifepristone (mif, Sigma, 10 mg/kg) or vehicle (veh., propylene glycol, Wako) was injected subcutaneously 30 min after contextual fear conditioning training [20]. The mice were randomly divided into six groups: no training, training (veh), training (mif), training (veh) + stress, training (mif) + stress, and mif only. After exposure to the training chamber without footshock, the no training mice were returned to their home cage. Immediately after the injection of mifepristone (mif), mif only

mice were returned to their home cage. Thirty min after contextual fear conditioning training, the other groups of mice were injected with veh or mif as appropriate. Immediately after the injection, training (veh) and training (mif) mice were returned to their home cage. Training + stress (60–90 min) and training + stress (90–120 min) mice were subjected to immobilization stress for 30 min, then returned to their home cage. Twenty-four hours after training, all mice were subjected to the measurement of freezing time and sacrificed to collect hippocampus samples. The hippocampus samples were used for analyzing mRNA BDNF as in Experiment 2 (Fig. 5a).

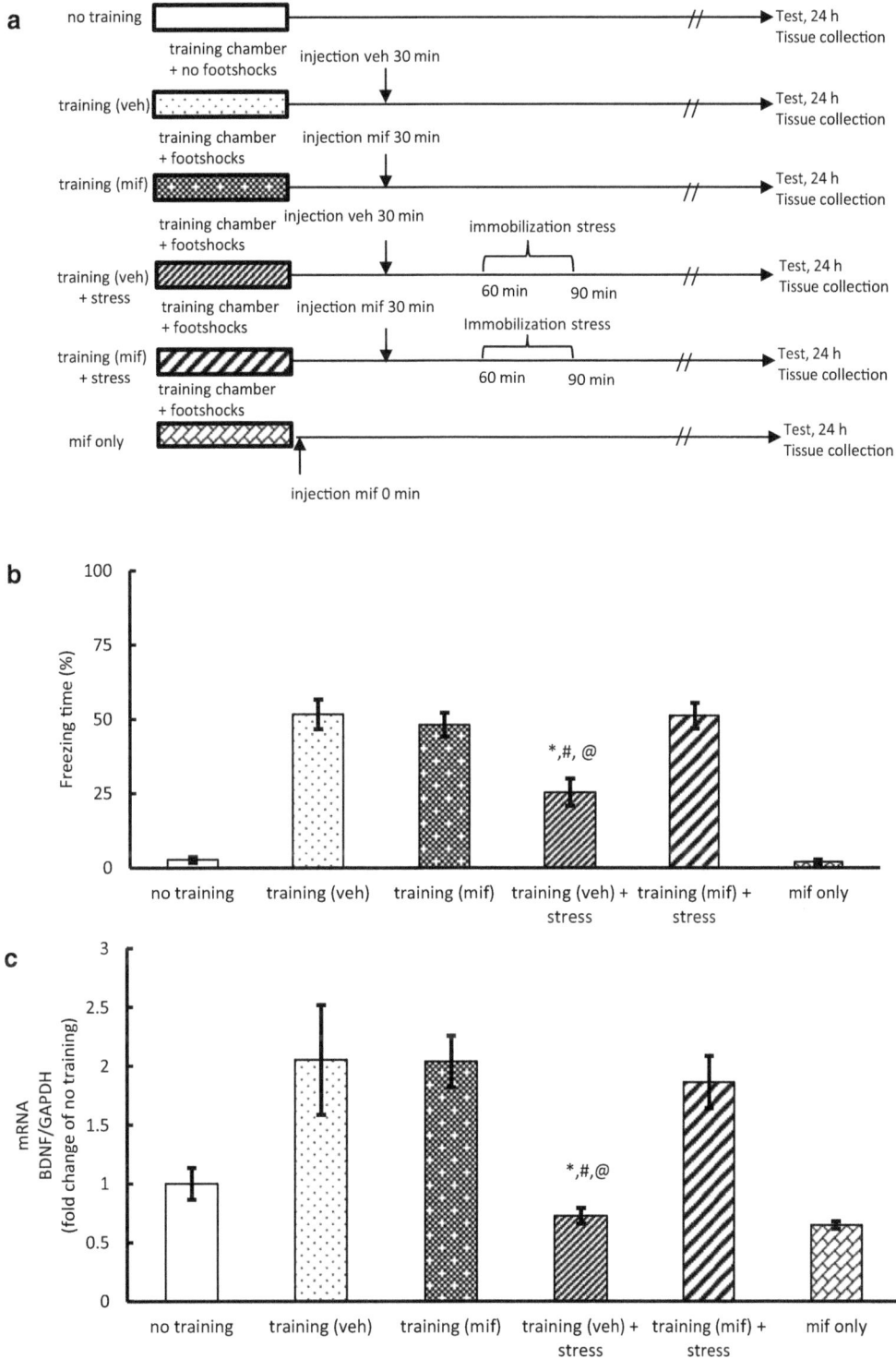

Fig. 5 Effect of glucocorticoid receptor antagonist (mifepristone) injection after contextual fear conditioning training (Experiment 6). **a** Experimental protocol for contextual fear conditioning training followed by stress and behavior tests **b** quantification of freezing behavior 24 h after the contextual fear conditioning training followed by immobilization stress (n = 9–11). **c** Quantification of BDNF/GAPDH mRNA ratio in the hippocampus (n = 6–8). *$P < 0.05$ compared with training (veh). #$P < 0.05$ compared with training (mif). @$P < 0.05$ compared with training (mif) + stress

Statistical analysis

All values are shown as the mean ± standard error of measurement (SEM). One-way analysis of variance (ANOVA), followed by the Tukey post hoc test was used for comparisons between groups. Statistical significance was accepted at $P < 0.05$. SPSS 21 software was used to perform the statistical analysis. Additional file 1: Table S1, Additional file 2: Table S2, Additional file 3: Table S3, Additional file 4: Table S4, Additional file 5: Table S5, Additional file 6: Table S6, Additional file 7: Table S7, Additional file 8: Table S8, Additional file 9: Table S9, Additional file 10: Table S10 show details of the Tukey post hoc tests.

Results

Time course of histone acetylation in the hippocampus (Experiment 1)

Memory formation induced by contextual fear conditioning training requires histone acetylation that occurs during a short period following such training [3]. To investigate the critical timing for histone acetylation following contextual fear training, we examined the time course change in histone acetylation after such training. Acetylation of H3 at lysine 14 (H3K14) in the hippocampus was significantly increased at 60 and 90 min after fear training ($F_{(5,17)} = 12.33$, $P < 0.05$; Fig. 1b, Additional file 1: Table S1). However, acetylation of H4 at lysine 5 (H4K5) did not change at any time point (Fig. 1c, Additional file 2: Table S2). These findings indicate that acetylation of H3K14, but not H4K5, is involved in memory formation, and that the critical timing for histone acetylation is from 60 to 90 min after the training.

Effect of acute immobilization stress after contextual fear conditioning (Experiment 2)

Based on our finding that H3K14 acetylation was enhanced from 60 to 90 min after the training, we examined whether freezing behavior was influenced when acute stress was applied while histone acetylation was elevated. For this purpose, the trained mice were subjected to 30 min of acute immobilization 60 or 90 min after fear training and then subjected to the measurement of freezing time 24 h later. Mice in the immobilization stress only group were subjected to immobilization stress for 30 min, without fear training beforehand. Immobilization at 60 min after fear training significantly reduced the freezing time as compared to that when the mice were subjected to training alone ($F_{(4,45)} = 78.73$, $P < 0.05$; Fig. 2b, Additional file 3: Table S3); however, immobilization applied at 90 min after fear training did not reduce the freezing time (Fig. 2b).

BDNF expression is critically involved in the consolidation phase of long-term memory [5]. Therefore, we analyzed the expression of BDNF mRNA. Hippocampus samples were collected immediately after the measurement of freezing time. Naïve mice did not explore the training apparatus, nor were they subjected to immobilization stress. Training and training + stress (90–120 min) mice showed significantly increased expression of BDNF mRNA compared with those without training (i.e., naïve, no training, and immobilization stress only mice), whereas mice in the training + stress (60–90 min) group did not show increased expression of BDNF mRNA ($F_{(5,34)} = 12.75$, $P < 0.05$; Fig. 2c, Additional file 4: Table S4). Taken together, the results indicate that immobilization stress affected expression of BDNF mRNA at 60–90 min, but not 90–120 min after fear training.

Epigenetic modification of BDNF promoter in response to acute stress applied after fear training (Experiment 3 and 4)

Based on the above findings, we examined whether immobilization following fear training influences epigenetic change via histone acetylation in BDNF transcription. At 90 and 120 min after fear training, a significant increase in the acetylation of H3K14 was noted compared with that in the groups without training. No significant difference was observed between training + stress (60–90 min) and training + stress (90–120 min) ($P = 0.228$); however, training + stress (60–90 min), but not training + stress (90–120 min), significantly reduced acetylation ($F_{(6,26)} = 19.47$, $P < 0.05$; Fig. 3c, Additional file 5: Table S5). These data suggested that around 60 min after fear training is a critical time for memory formation. Next, we analyzed H3K14 acetylated at BDNF promoters 3 and 4 in the hippocampus. Acetylation of H3K14 at promoter 3, but not at promoter 4, after training for 90 min was significantly elevated ($F_{(2,8)} = 22.86$, $P < 0.05$; Fig. 3d, Additional file 6: Table S6, Additional file 7: Table S7). In addition, training + stress (60–90′) reduced the acetylation of H3K14 at promoter 3 compared to that in the no training group ($F_{(2,8)} = 22.86$, $P < 0.05$; Fig. 3d). These results suggest that immobilization applied at 60 min after fear training might inhibit memory formation by suppressing the acetylation of H3K14 at BDNF promoter 3 in the hippocampus.

Effect of glucocorticoid on memory formation and BDNF expression (Experiment 5 and 6)

On the basis of the findings, we hypothesized that an increase in corticosterone due to immobilization would be the primary cause of a disturbance of memory formation, since corticosterone is one of the hormones regulating memory [21]. To evaluate our hypothesis, we measured plasma corticosterone levels 90 and 120 min after training. Mice in the training + stress (60–90 min) group showed a remarkable increase in the plasma corticosterone level as compared to that in the training, training + stress (90–120 min), and no training ($F_{(4,20)} = 11.05$, $P < 0.05$; Fig. 4b, Additional file 8: Table S8) mice. A significant difference was observed between the no training and immobilization stress only groups. However, no significant difference was noted among the training, training + stress (90–120 min), and immobilization stress only groups. The high level of corticosterone of training + stress (60–90 min) was probably due to the synergistic effect of training and immobilization stress from 60 to 90 min post training, which might block memory formation following contextual fear training.

This was confirmed by injecting the mice with mifepristone (mif), a glucocorticoid receptor antagonist, or vehicle (veh) at 30 min before immobilization stress (Experiment 6). Mice were subjected to 30 min of immobilization at 60 min after the training, and the freezing time was measured after 24 h (Fig. 5b). The freezing time significantly decreased in the mice in the training (veh) + stress group as compared to the trained mice without immobilization stress [i.e., training (veh) and training (mif)], whereas training (mif) + stress reverted the freezing time to that of the training (veh) mice ($F_{(5,55)} = 40.29$, $P < 0.05$; Fig. 5b, Additional file 9: Table S9). In addition, training (veh) + stress led to the downregulation of BDNF mRNA, and training (mif) + stress reverted the BDNF mRNA expression level to that of the training (veh) and the training (mif) levels ($F_{(5,34)} = 7.89$, $P < 0.05$; Fig. 5c, Additional file 10: Table S10). These findings indicate that the high level of corticosterone induced in response to acute stress impairs memory formation.

Discussion

Chronic stress is known to deteriorate cognition [14], whereas acute stress is known to have a positive effect on memory formation [15]. However, whether acute stress facilitates memory formation when stress is applied after fear training has not yet been determined. Our study showed that acute immobilization stress applied at 60 min but not 90 min post-training could affect freezing time (Fig. 2b, c), enabling us to speculate that the interference during the memory consolidation (60–90 min post-training) could impair memory formation, but that the interference following the memory consolidation (90–120 min post-training) could have no effect on the memory formation.

Several studies have shown that BDNF contributes to memory formation. For example, knockdown of hippocampal BDNF expression was shown to decrease the freezing behavior in the contextual fear conditioning test [7]. Inhibition of BDNF function by using neutralizing antibody against BDNF led to the formation of spatial

memory alone [8]. In this study, trained mice showed an increase in freezing behavior and hippocampal BDNF mRNA expression, whereas they were decreased in mice subjected to immobilization at 60 min after the training (Fig. 2b, c), indicating that around 60 min after fear training is critical for memory formation in mice.

BDNF transcription after fear training is epigenetically regulated, especially by histone acetylation [3]. There are many lysine residues on the N-terminal tails of histone H3 and H4; for this study we selected lysine 14 for histone H3 and lysine 5 for histone H4 because the sites are the closest N-terminal tails and acetylation specific [22], and acetylation of the sites increases in the hippocampus following contextual fear conditioning for the establishment of contextual fear memory [4]. Our data showed that fear training increases the acetylation of H3K14, but not of H4K5 (Fig. 1b, c) in the hippocampus; this result is consistent with those of previous studies [3, 9, 13]. In addition, 30 min of immobilization stress at 60 min after fear training, but not immobilization stress at 90 min, reduced the acetylation (Fig. 3b). Our chromatin chip assay showed that the binding of *bdnf* promoter 3 to H3K14 was increased following fear training and suppressed by the immobilization stress; however, no changes were noted in the function of promoter 4 (Fig. 3c, d). These findings suggest that fear memory formation might be mediated by the regulation of BDNF transcription via the acetylation of H3K14 at *bdnf* promoter 3. However, other epigenetic modifications are also required for memory formation. Gupta et al. indicated that histone methylation, especially trimethylation of histone H3 at lysine 4, is required for the accurate long-term consolidation of contextual fear memories [23]. Chwang et al. showed that histone H3 phosphorylation in hippocampal area CA1 is regulated after a behavioral fear-conditioning paradigm [17]. These findings indicate that, besides acetylation, other types of histone modifications (phosphorylation, methylation, etc.) need to be investigated following acute stress. Bredy et al. demonstrated that fear conditioning and extinction result in distinct patterns of histone acetylation of H3 and H4, and suggested that acetylated H3 increased after fear training, and that acetylated H4 increased after extinction training [24]. This study supported our finding that acetylated histone H4 was not involved BDNF gene expression in fear condition paradigm (Fig. 1c).

Chronic and acute actions of glucocorticoids on memory processes differ in many respects, including differences in behavior and the molecular mechanisms. In general, an increase in corticosterone due to chronic stress can be a cause of disturbance in memory formation [25]. In this study, acute immobilization at 60 min after fear conditioning training significantly increased plasma corticosterone levels as compared to those in trained mice (Fig. 4b). Furthermore, both freezing time and BDNF mRNA expression level of mice subjected to immobilization at 60 min were ameliorated by injecting a glucocorticoid receptor antagonist, mifepristone, 30 min before immobilization (Fig. 5b, c). However, the corticosterone level of mice subjected to immobilization at 90 min after the training reverted to the level in trained mice. These findings indicate that the impediment of memory formation by acute immobilization stress applied at 60 min after training can be attributed to a high level of corticosterone.

A possible mechanism of memory formation is that glucocorticoid released by fear training enhances the activation of NMDA receptors via glutamate and the transcription of BDNF by extracellular signal-regulated kinase [3]. Thus, glucocorticoid triggers the transcription of BDNF, resulting in enhanced memory. However, acute stress applied at 60 min after fear training might further increase the release of corticosterone from the adrenal cortex. When acute immobilization stress was applied at 60 min after fear training, the additional increase in corticosterone might have disrupted epigenetic modification associated with BDNF transcription, followed by the impairment of memory formation. Abrari et al. suggested that the administration of corticosterone after memory training enhanced memory formation in a dose-dependent manner, but excess administration of corticosterone reduced freezing behavior to the level noted in the vehicle control group [26]. These and our findings confirm that learning and synapse plasticity depend on the level of corticosterone: when its level is very low or high, memory formation is impaired, whereas an intermediate level of corticosterone facilitates memory formation [21].

To our knowledge, this is the first study to show that acute immobilization stress after contextual fear conditioning affects memory formation, including freezing behavior, BDNF mRNA expression, and acetylation of H3K14 and BDNF promoter 3 in the hippocampus. Owing to the high level of corticosterone, acute immobilization stress applied at 60 min after contextual fear training had an adverse effect, but not at 90 min after training. Facilitation or impairment of fearful memory formation depends on not only the timing of stress stimulation but also the level of corticosterone. This finding might be useful for memory study, including investigation of the mechanism underlying memory formation.

Conclusions

In this study, we investigated the effect of acute stress applied after fear training on memory formation, BDNF expression, epigenetic regulation of BDNF expression, and corticosterone level. Our results showed that 60 min after contextual fear training is the critical time for memory formation in mice. When acute immobilization stress was applied during this critical time, freezing behavior significantly decreased, along with reduction in BDNF mRNA expression and H3K14 acetylation in the hippocampus, owing to the high level of corticosterone.

Additional files

Additional file 1: Table S1. Tukey HSD for acetylation of H3K14 (Experiment 1).

Additional file 2: Table S2. Tukey HSD for acetylation of H4K5 (Experiment 1).

Additional file 3: Table S3. Tukey HSD for behavioral test 1 (Experiment 2).

Additional file 4: Table S4. Tukey HSD for BDNF analysis 1 (Experiment 2).

Additional file 5: Table S5. Tukey HSD for acetylation H3K14 (Experiment 3).

Additional file 6: Table S6. Tukey HSD for acetylation H3K14 at promoter 3 (Experiment 4).

Additional file 7: Table S7. Tukey HSD for acetylation H3K14 at promoter 4 (Experiment 4).

Additional file 8: Table S8. Tukey HSD for corticosterone analysis (Experiment 5).

Additional file 9: Table S9. Tukey HSD for behavioral test 2 (Experiment 6).

Additional file 10: Table S10. Tukey HSD for mRNA 2 (Experiment 6).

Abbreviations
H3K14: histone 3 at lysine 14; H4K5: histone 4 at lysine 5; ELISA: enzyme-linked immunosorbent assay; BDNF: brained-derived neurotrophic factor; RT-PCR: reverse transcription polymerase chain reaction; GAPDH: glyceraldehyde-3-phsphate dehydrogenase; NCBI: national center for biotechnology Information; MSF: phenylmethylsulfonyl fluoride; SDS: sodium dodecyl sulfate; TTBS: tris-buffered saline with Tween; ChIP: chromatin immunoprecipitation; PBS: phosphate buffered saline; mif: mifepristone; SEM: standard error of measurement; ANOVA: analysis of variance; NMDA: n-methyl-D-aspartic acid.

Authors' contributions
AU carried out all the study and drafted the manuscript. HL, JP, HL, JM, and SN participated in performance in vivo experiments. SO gave advice for the study and corrected the manuscript. TM made substantial contribution to conception and design of the study. All authors read and approved the final manuscript.

Authors' information
AU is a postgraduate of Nippon Medical School and studying in Department of Biochemistry and Cell Biology, Insstitute for Advanced Medical Sciences. HL is a postdoctoral research fellow of Department of Biochemistry and Cell Biology, Institute for Advanced Medical Sciences. JP is a graduate student of Jikei University School of Medicine and studying in Department of Laboratory Medicine. HL is a researcher assistant of Department of Cell Biology and Neuroscience, Juntendo Medical School. JM is a researcher of Graduate School of Health and Sports Science, Nippon Sport Science University. SN is a lecturer of health and sports sciences at Kyoritsu Women's Junior College. SO is the professor of Department of Biochemistry and Cell Biology, Institute for Advanced Medical Sciences, Nippon Medical School. TM is an associate professor of Department of Health and Sports Science, Nippon Medical School.

Author details

[1] Department of Biochemistry and Cell Biology, Institute for Advanced Medical Sciences, Nippon Medical School, 1-396 Kosugi-cho, Nakahara-ku, Kawasaki, Kanagawa 211-8533, Japan. [2] Department of Laboratory Medicine, The Jikei University School of Medicine, 3-25-8, Nishi-Shimbashi, Minato-ku, Tokyo 105-8641, Japan. [3] Department of Cell Biology and Neuroscience, Juntendo Medical School, 2-1, Hongo, Bunkyo-ku, Tokyo 113-8421, Japan. [4] Graduate School of Health and Sport Science, Nippon Sport Science University, 7-1-1 Fukasawa, Setagaya-ku, Tokyo 158-8508, Japan. [5] Kyoritsu Women's Junior College, 2-2-1 Hitotsubashi, Chiyoda-ku, Tokyo 101-8437, Japan. [6] Department of Health and Sport Science, Nippon Medical School, 1-7-1, Sakaiminami machi, Mushasino-shi, Tokyo 180-0023, Japan.

Acknowledgements

This study was supported by JSPS KAKENHI Grant Number 2350825.

Competing interests

The authors declare that they have no competing interests.

References

1. Wiegert O, Joels M, Krugers H. Timing is essential for rapid effects of corticosterone on synaptic potentiation in the mouse hippocampus. Learn Mem. 2006;13(2):110–3.
2. Reul JM, Chandramohan Y. Epigenetic mechanisms in stress-related memory formation. Psychoneuroendocrinology. 2007;32(Suppl 1):S21–5.
3. Levenson JM, et al. Regulation of histone acetylation during memory formation in the hippocampus. J Biol Chem. 2004;279(39):40545–59.
4. Park CS, Rehrauer H, Mansuy IM. Genome-wide analysis of H4K5 acetylation associated with fear memory in mice. BMC Genom. 2013;14:539–57.
5. Chen J, et al. Contextual learning induces an increase in the number of hippocampal CA1 neurons expressing high levels of BDNF. Neurobiol Learn Mem. 2007;88(4):409–15 **(Epub 2007 Aug 31)**.
6. Choi DC, et al. Prelimbic cortical BDNF is required for memory of learned fear but not extinction or innate fear. Proc Natl Acad Sci USA. 2010;107(6):2675–80. doi:10.1073/pnas.0909359107 **(Epub 2010 Jan 25)**.
7. Heldt SA, et al. Hippocampus-specific deletion of BDNF in adult mice impairs spatial memory and extinction of aversive memories. Mol Psychiatry. 2007;12(7):656–70 **(Epub 2007 Jan 30)**.
8. Xin J, et al. Involvement of BDNF signaling transmission from basolateral amygdala to infralimbic prefrontal cortex in conditioned taste aversion extinction. J Neurosci. 2014;34(21):7302–13. doi:10.1523/JNEUROSCI.5030-13.2014.
9. Maddox SA, Schafe GE. Epigenetic alterations in the lateral amygdala are required for reconsolidation of a pavlovian fear memory. Learn Mem. 2011;18(9):579–93.
10. Monsey MS, et al. Epigenetic alterations are critical for fear memory consolidation and synaptic plasticity in the lateral amygdala. PLoS One. 2011;6(5):e19958.
11. Roozendaal B, et al. Glucocorticoid effects on memory consolidation depend on functional interactions between the medial prefrontal cortex and basolateral amygdala. J Neurosci. 2009;29(45):14299–308.
12. Sui L, et al. Epigenetic regulation of reelin and brain-derived neurotrophic factor genes in long-term potentiation in rat medial prefrontal cortex. Neurobiol Learn Mem. 2012;97(4):425–40. doi:10.1016/j.nlm.2012.03.007 **(Epub 2012 Mar 24)**.
13. Levenson JM, Sweatt JD. Epigenetic mechanisms in memory formation (Review). Nat Rev Neurosci. 2005;6(2):108–18.
14. Tsankova NM, et al. Sustained hippocampal chromatin regulation in a mouse model of depression and antidepressant action. Nat Neurosci. 2006;9(4):519–25 **(Epub 2006 Feb 26)**.
15. Shors TJ, Weiss C, Thompson RF. Stress-induced facilitation of classical conditioning. Science. 1992;257(5069):537–9.
16. Lubin FD, Sweatt JD. The IkappaB kinase regulates chromatin structure during reconsolidation of conditioned fear memories. Neuron. 2007;55(6):942–57.
17. Chwang WB, et al. ERK/MAPK regulates hippocampal histone phosphorylation following contextual fear conditioning. Learn Mem. 2006;13(3):322–8.
18. Nakajima S, et al. Regular voluntary exercise cures stress-induced impairment of cognitive function and cell proliferation accompanied by increases in cerebral IGF-1 and GST activity in mice. Behav Brain Res. 2010;211(2):178–84.
19. Warner-Schmidt JL, Duman RS. VEGF is an essential mediator of the neurogenic and behavioral actions of antidepressants. Proc Natl Acad Sci USA. 2007;104(11):4647–52.
20. Zhou M, et al. Blocking mineralocorticoid receptors prior to retrieval reduces contextual fear memory in mice. PLoS One. 2011;6(10):e26220.
21. Sandi C. Glucocorticoids act on glutamatergic pathways to affect memory processes. Trends Neurosci. 2011;34(4):165–76.
22. Turner BM. Cellular memory and the histone code. Cell. 2002;111(3):285–91.
23. Gupta S, et al. Histone methylation regulates memory formation. J Neurosci. 2010;30(10):3589–99. doi:10.1523/JNEUROSCI.3732-09.2010.
24. Bredy TW, et al. Histone modifications around individual BDNF gene promoters in prefrontal cortex are associated with extinction of conditioned fear. Learn Mem. 2007;14(4):268–76 **(Print 2007 April)**.
25. McEwen BS, Sapolsky RM. Stress and cognitive function. Curr Opin Neurobiol. 1995;5(2):205–16.
26. Abrari K, Rashidy-Pour A, Semnanian S, Fahollahi Y. Post-training administration of corticosterone enhances consolidation of contextual fear memory and hippocampal long-term potentiation in rats. Neurobiol Learn Mem. 2009;91:260–5.

Sex differences in avoidance behavior after perceiving potential risk in mice

Sayaka Yokota[1], Yusuke Suzuki[2], Keigo Hamami[1], Akiko Harada[1] and Shoji Komai[1,3*] (iD)

Abstract

Background: Sex has been considered as a potential factor regulating individual behaviors in different contexts. Recently, findings on sex differences in the neuroendocrine circuit have expanded due to exact measurements and control of neuronal activity, while findings on sex differences in behavioral phenotypes are limited. One efficient way to determine the miscellaneous aspects of a sexually different behavior is to segment it into a set of simpler responses induced by discrete scenes.

Methods: In the present study, we conducted a battery of behavioral tests within a variety of unique risky scenes, to determine where and how sex differences arise in responses under those scenes.

Results: A significant sex difference was observed in the avoidance responses measured in the two-way active and the passive avoidance tests. The phenotype observed was higher mobility in male mice and reduced mobility in female mice, and required associative learning between an escapable risk and its predictive cue. This was limited in other scenes where escapable risk or predictive cue or both were missing.

Conclusions: Taken together, the present study found that the primary sex difference occurs in mobility in the avoidance response after perceiving escapable risks.

Keywords: Sex difference, Associative learning, Avoidance behavior, Mobility, Context, Behavioral test battery

Background

Sex has been considered as a potential variable regulating individual behavior in animals including humans under various contexts. Recently, sex differences in neuroendocrine circuits have been shown to exist even at a microscopic scale [1–5], owing to the development of techniques that allow for precise measurement and control of neuronal activity [1, 2, 6]. However, those phenotypes at a behavioral scale have been difficult to elucidate, since most behavior are composed of several responses closely associated with specific scenes [7–11]. To detect those unique responses, scene segmentation, i.e. to break down a general context into discrete behavioral tests would be a plausible approach. By identifying the responses and the conditions in which they occur,

phenotypes of a behavior could be determined. In the present study, we conducted a test battery probing the responses to a variety of risky contexts, to determine where and how sex differences arise in these responses under those test conditions in mice.

In particular, we determined whether sex differences arise in the avoidance response, since it constitutes major components of a behavior under escapable risks [10, 12–18]. Avoidance can be further segmented into two sub-components, active and passive avoidance, depending on the cue that prompts it [11, 12, 19]. Active avoidance occurs when animals attempt to move away from a risk, whereas in passive avoidance, animals try to maintain a safe distance from such a threat [12, 20, 21], in response to cues predicting an escapable risk after associative learning has occurred. For the former sub-component, a two-way active avoidance test was carried out. In this test, we measured the formation of the association between a conditioned stimulus and an escapable unconditioned stimulus in a context, with subsequent

*Correspondence: skomai@bs.naist.jp
[1] Graduate School of Biological Sciences, Nara Institute of Science and Technology, 8916-5 Keihanna Science City, Nara 630-0192, Japan
Full list of author information is available at the end of the article

active transfer during the tone allowing avoidance of the foot-shock simultaneously with the termination of the tone. For the latter, a passive avoidance test was used. In this test, we measured the formation of the association between a dark room and an inescapable foot-shock, and subsequent staying in the light compartment that constitutes the passive avoidance. Since associative learning is necessary to perceive a risk that are hidden in the environment [13], the formation of associative learning alone was also compared between sexes by using a fear-conditioning test including contextual fear conditioning and cued-fear conditioning. Three additional tests were prepared to confirm whether sex differences arise under the lack of escapable risks or risk prediction or both. In a light/light (L/L) test, risk-predicting cues were unavailable. For active and passive response to an aversive, inescapable scene, a forced-swim test and tail-suspension test were used. Further, sex differences in innate aversion were tested in a light/dark test (L/D), and the basal activity in a home cage was also compared between sexes.

Methods

Subjects

Subjects were sexually naïve, 7-week-old male and female C57BL/6N mice (Japan SLC, Shizuoka, Japan). Each animal was housed separately in a home cage in a standard laboratory environment, on a 12-h light/dark cycle, at a constant temperature (23–24 °C) and relative humidity (50–70%). Food (pellets; Japan SLC, Shizuoka, Japan) and water were available ad libitum. All behavioral tests were carried out in the light phase. We used different batches of mice for each behavioral test; the mice were randomly assigned to any one behavioral test when 8 weeks old, with 3–4 days of prior handling. Experiments were approved by the Animal Care Committee of Nara Institute of Science and Technology (the permit number: 1004) and conformed to all relevant regulatory standards.

Determination of the estrous cycle phases

We compared the behaviors between males and females and also between females in different phases of the estrous cycle, as it is well known that both human and rodent females alter their behavior depending on the estrous cycle phase [21–24].

For all female mice, estrous cycle phase was determined by vaginal smear cytology analyses during the 4 days prior to handling. Briefly, we rinsed the vagina with 150–200 μL sterile water. The smear was placed on a glass slide (FRC-01, Matsunami Glass industries, Osaka, Japan). After drying, 50 μL of Giemsa stain solution (Merck, Tokyo, Japan) was applied to the smear, which was left to stand for 10–20 min and then washed with distilled water. After drying, the smear was observed

under a light microscope (Nikon Diaphot 300, Nikon Corporation, Tokyo, Japan), and we then classified it as either proestrus, estrus, diestrus [25], or 'not determined' (nd) depending on the results of the analysis. To control for any behavioral effects of this procedure between sexes, males were also treated in the same way, with sterile water applied under the scrotum.

Behavioral tests

Two-way active avoidance test

Initially, we examined whether any sex differences occurred in active avoidance. In this test, 14 male and 16 female (3 proestrus, 6 estrus, and 7 diestrus) mice were used. The mice were required to learn the association between an auditory cue and a nociceptive foot-shock stimulus, and to then avoid the foot-shock by perceiving the auditory cue, across trials. The experimental procedure was based on a previous study [26]. Briefly, mice were placed in 1 of 2 adjacent compartments, separated by a partition, in a shuttle box (height = 185 mm, width = 300 mm, depth = 115 mm; Passive Avoidance System, Bio-Medica, Osaka, Japan). Constant luminance was maintained in both compartments. Immediately after the partition was removed, the mice could move freely between the two compartments. One minute after placement, the auditory cue was presented for 5 s in the shock compartment. The final 2 s of cue presentation were accompanied by the foot-shock. This procedure was repeated for 100 trials. The inter-trial interval was set at 20 ± 3 s. The active avoidance rate was defined as the number of entries into the safe compartment across 100 trials.

To ensure that the foot-shock did not disrupt their behavior, the current intensity of foot-shock for males and females was set at their pain threshold, which was determined in a pilot study (males = 0.11 ± 0.005 mA, females = 0.09 ± 0.003 mA). The threshold was determined as the average of individual thresholds within the group, and these were measured as the minimum current that induced a jumping response when the intensity was gradually increased from 0.089 mA by manually adjusting the current controller.

Passive avoidance test

In the active avoidance test, animals faced a threatening context in which their mobility (the active movement between compartments) constituted an adaptive behavior to avoiding a threat. Next, we performed the passive avoidance test to test whether any sex differences existed in a converse situation where the subject's immobility (staying in one compartment) would be more adaptive. Therefore, if a difference in the avoidance pattern between the sexes was observed in the active avoidance test, we predicted that the passive avoidance test would show the opposite result.

In the passive avoidance test, 11 male and 18 female (3 proestrus, 8 estrus, 6 diestrus, and 1 nd) mice were examined. While the experimental procedure was based on a previous study [27], the foot-shock current intensity was set at the pain threshold for both males and females similar to the active avoidance test (see above). The same shuttle box was used as in the active avoidance test, except that one compartment was darkened while normal illumination was maintained in the other.

This test comprised of training and test sessions. In the training session, mice learned the association between a dark compartment and foot-shock that would enable them to anticipate the upcoming foot-shock. The two compartments were initially separated by a partition. After a mouse was placed in the light compartment, the partition was removed. When the mouse entered the dark compartment, the partition was closed again. Ten seconds after entry, a foot-shock was applied for 2 s. Ten seconds later, the partition was opened and the mouse returned to the light compartment. Twenty-four hours after the training session, the test session was initiated. The partition was removed at the beginning of the session, and a mouse was then placed in the light compartment. The mouse could then move freely between the two compartments, and its behavior was recorded over 700 s. Since the latency to enter and the number of entries into the dark compartment should each reflect avoidance, both were measured from the recorded video. The latency ceiling was fixed at 700 s.

Fear-conditioning test

To test sex difference in associative learning, and how it may contribute to any observed differences in avoidance, we performed a fear-conditioning test based on a protocol [28].

Twelve male and 31 female (8 proestrus, 9 estrus, 10 diestrus, 4 nd) mice were used. All stimulus presentation was computer-controlled (Image FZC, O'Hara & Co., Tokyo, Japan). This test comprised of four sessions: training, contextual fear-conditioning (CXT), pre-auditory-cued fear-conditioning (pre-AUD), and auditory-cued fear-conditioning (AUD). The training session was carried out on day 1, and the remaining three sessions were conducted the next day.

In the training session, mice learned the association between a foot-shock and an accompanying cue. Mice were placed individually in an operant chamber (width = 120 mm, height and depth = 110 mm; O'Hara & Co.). After placement, contextual (a mixture of implicit cues, such as odor, field-view, and sound, in the chamber) cues were presented for 30 s. The last 2 s of auditory

(10 kHz, 75 dB) cue presentation were accompanied by a 0.75 mA foot-shock delivered from stainless steel bars on the floor. After the foot-shock, the mice were returned to their home cages. After the training session, it was expected that mice could anticipate the upcoming foot-shock whenever either cue was presented.

Twenty-four hours after the training session, mice were subjected to the CXT session. They were re-exposed to the same chamber and the same contextual cues, as in the training session. They spent 180 s in this chamber with neither an auditory cue nor a foot-shock.

Two hours later, the same mice were subjected to the pre-AUD and AUD sessions. They were placed in a novel chamber, which formed a triangular prism (side = 110 mm, height = 120 mm, O'Hara & Co.), for 360 s. To mask the olfactory cues, the chamber was cleaned with sodium hypochlorite before and after each use. The mice were re-exposed, 180 s after placement, to the same auditory cue as in the training session (AUD). To ensure that the mice were subjected to the AUD session without generalized contextual fear carried over from the preceding session, we also measured their response in the first 180 s (pre-AUD).

We measured freezing as a conditioned response in each mouse, as it is recognized as a behavioral index of associative learning. Behavior in the chamber was recorded at one frame per second, and a freezing response was defined as any instance when a difference of pixel intensities between two successive frames was less than 30% (Image FZC).

Light/dark and light/light test

In the active and passive avoidance tests, the perception of potential threats prompts the subsequent avoidance. We expected that if the perception of potential threats was influenced by a sex difference in both types of avoidance, the difference would be diminished in the absence of the perceived threat. Therefore, we carried out the light/dark (L/D) and light/light (L/L) tests as additional contexts. In the L/D and L/L tests, mice did not encounter the threat or the threat-predicting cue, respectively. The sessions and the measured behavior were the same as in the passive avoidance test (see above).

In the L/D test, 12 mice (6 male and 6 female) were used. The chamber was the same as in the passive avoidance test, except that the foot-shock was never applied. In the L/L test, 36 mice (6 male and 30 female) were used. The chamber was the same as in the active avoidance test, except that the auditory stimulus was never presented.

Tail suspension test

We tested whether a sex difference arises in the escape component using the tail suspension test (TST) and the forced swim test (FST). In both tests, mice faced an imminent threat, rather than a potential one.

The TST was used to examine 12 male and 17 female (5 proestrus, 6 estrus, 4 diestrus, 2 nd) mice. The experimental procedure was based on previous studies 29–31]. Briefly, mice were suspended by their tails from a fixture 35 cm above the floor for 360 s. Their behavior was recorded and analyzed by motion analysis software (Image FZC).

Since immobility indicates how individuals attempt to escape behavior from an imminent threat [13, 14, 32–34], we measured the immobility of the trunk, excluding slight movements of the limbs and tail, and calculated the total time spent immobile (immobility time) for data analysis. This procedure was conducted daily on 2 consecutive days.

Forced swim test

The FST was used to examine 12 male and 18 female (4 proestrus, 4 estrus, 7 diestrus, and 3 nd) mice. The experimental procedure was based on previous studies [29–31]. For 360 s, mice were placed in a glass beaker (diameter = 135 mm, height = 200 mm; Hario Glass Co., Tokyo, Japan), which was filled to a height of 130 mm with water at 25 ± 1 °C. Behavior in the pool was recorded and analyzed using Image FZC software. Immobility was measured as passive floating with slight movements of the limbs and tail, and the immobility time was calculated. This procedure was conducted daily on 2 consecutive days.

Measurement of basal activity in familiar home cage

We checked whether a sex difference arises in the basal activity in the familiar home cage in the absence of any threat. This test was used to examine 8 male and 8 female mice. Each mouse was housed in a separate standard laboratory home cage (width = 203 mm, height = 118 mm, depth = 133 mm) for 3 days. On the 4th day, their activity was measured for 1 min with a camera (1.3 million pixels, viewing angle of 78°, 30 frames/s). The mean velocity, total travel distance, and distance from the center were calculated from the track point on the body by Motion Analyzer (version 1.4.21.0, Keyence Co. Ltd., Osaka, Japan).

Data analysis

In all tests, we recorded 1–3 behavioral measures per test for each mouse, and then calculated the group mean with a 95% confidence interval (CI) for each of the following groups: males, females, and females in each estrous phase. We excluded subjects that exceeded 2 standard deviations of the group mean. For statistical analysis, females in specific estrous phases and all

females group were treated as independent groups whenever either was compared with males. We performed Shaffer's modified sequentially rejective Bonferroni procedure as a multiple comparison whenever we found statistical significance in 1- or 2-factorial analysis of variance (ANOVA). Alpha was set at 0.05. We calculated the effect size [Pearson's R on t test and the multiple comparisons, generalized eta-squared (η_G^2) on ANOVA] where η_G^2 is a recommended effect size statistic for various experimental designs [35], including the mixed design used in the present study. These effect size statistics are available indices that are standardized to quantify the practical magnitude of the relationship between independent and dependent variables, independent of the sample size, and thereby, enable results to be compared with other studies [35]. The magnitude of the effect size was interpreted as either small, medium, or large in accordance with the standard guidelines [36, 37]. The sex ratio (SR) = male/female * 100 was calculated from the group mean of males and that of females in each test. Statistical analysis was done by customized codes in MATLAB (MathWorks Inc., MA, US).

In the active avoidance test, we calculated the avoidance rate in 5 bins of 20 trials for each mouse, and the group mean for males, females, and females in each estrous phase. We performed a 2-way [sex (males, females) × bin (1st, 2nd, 3rd, 4th, 5th)] ANOVA for the avoidance rate. To compare males with females in each estrous phase, another 2-way [sex (males, proestrus, estrus, diestrus) × bin (1st, 2nd, 3rd, 4th, 5th)] ANOVA was performed.

In the passive avoidance test, we calculated the latency to enter and the number of entries into the dark compartment for each mouse in the test session, and then, the group mean for males, females, and females in each estrous phase. We performed a 2-sample t test (males vs. females) and a 1-way [sex (males, proestrus, estrus, diestrus)] ANOVA for latency. A 2-sample t test (males vs. females) for the number of transitions was also performed.

In the fear-conditioning test, we calculated the percentage of time spent freezing (freezing rate) for each mouse in each session, and then, the group mean for males, females, and females in each estrous phase. We performed a 2-way [sex (males or females) × session (training, CXT, pre-AUD, AUD)] ANOVA for the freezing rate. To compare males with females in each estrous phase, another 2-way [sex (males, proestrus, estrus, diestrus) × session (training, CXT, pre-AUD, AUD)] ANOVA was performed.

As in the passive avoidance test, we performed a 2-sample t test (males vs. females) for latency in the L/D and L/L tests.

In both the TST and FST, we calculated the immobility time for each mouse on both days. The group mean was then calculated for males, females, and females in each estrous phase. We performed 2-way [sex (males or females) × day (1st or 2nd)] ANOVA for immobility time. To compare males with females in each estrous phase, another 2-way [sex (males, proestrus, estrus, diestrus) × day (1st or 2nd)] ANOVA was performed.

For measurement of the basal activity in the familiar home cage, mean velocity, total travel distance, and distance from the center of the cage were measured. After the individual mean and the group mean were calculated, a 2-sample t test (males vs. females) was performed for each motion parameter.

Results

Two-way active avoidance test

The 2-way ANOVA comparing males to females for the active avoidance rate showed a significant interaction between sex and bin (each 20 trials) ($F_{4,104} = 4.20$, $p < 0.05$, $\eta_G^2 = 0.07$). The avoidance rate between the sexes within each bin was compared. Although the avoidance rate in the initial bin was similar between the sexes, in most of the subsequent bins, males exhibited a significantly higher avoidance rate than females ($p < 0.05$) (Fig. 1).

When we compared the avoidance rate between the bins within each sex, males exhibited a steeper learning curve than females (Fig. 1). In males, the avoidance rate for bin 5 was significantly higher than all of the previous bins ($p < 0.05$). Similarly, bins 3 and 4 showed significantly higher avoidance rates than observed during bins 1 and 2 ($p < 0.05$). By contrast, in females, the avoidance rate during bin 5 was only significantly higher than bins 1 and 2 ($p < 0.05$). Although bin 4 showed a significantly higher avoidance rate than the previous 3 bins ($p < 0.05$), the avoidance rate during bin 3 was only higher than bin 2 ($p < 0.05$).

The 2-way ANOVA comparing males to females in different estrous cycle for the active avoidance rate showed a significant interaction between sex/phase of estrous cycle and bin ($F_{12,96} = 2.28$, $p < 0.05$, $\eta_G^2 = 0.12$). Significant simple main effects of sex/phase of estrous cycle were observed at bins 2 and 5 (Additional file 1: Figure S1). Specifically, females in estrus exhibited a significantly lower avoidance rate than males in both bins ($p < 0.05$). Similarly, females in diestrus and proestrus showed a significantly lower avoidance rate than males in bins 2 and 5, respectively ($p < 0.05$).

The learning curve of the avoidance also significantly differed between males and females in each estrous phase (Additional file 1: Figure S1). Although males showed a steep learning curve as described above, females in proestrus exhibited an invariant avoidance rate across the bins.

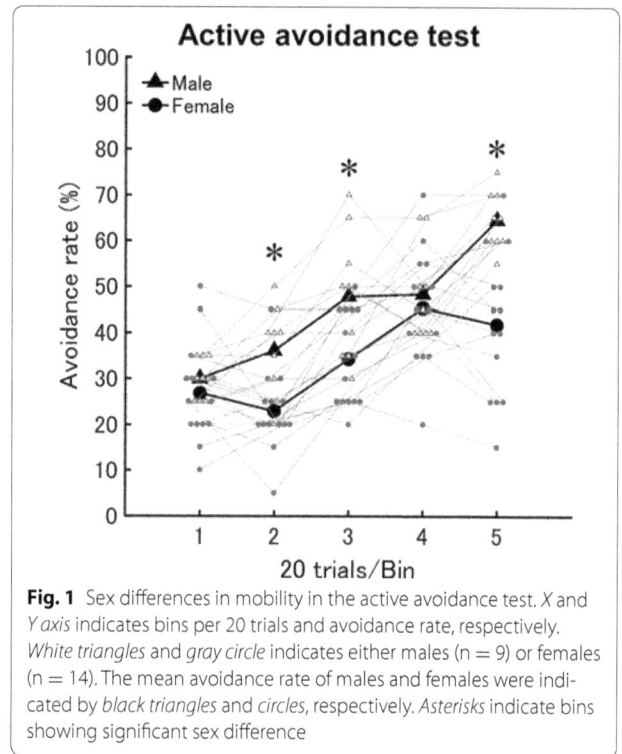

Fig. 1 Sex differences in mobility in the active avoidance test. *X* and *Y axis* indicates bins per 20 trials and avoidance rate, respectively. *White triangles* and *gray circle* indicates either males (n = 9) or females (n = 14). The mean avoidance rate of males and females were indicated by *black triangles* and *circles*, respectively. *Asterisks* indicate bins showing significant sex difference

For females in estrus, only bin 4 showed a significantly higher avoidance rate than bins 2 and 3. Similarly, for females in diestrus the avoidance rate during bins 4 and 5 was significantly higher than the rate during bins 1 and 2.

Passive avoidance test

Males exhibited a significantly higher number of entries into the dark compartment than females (2-sample t test; $t_{25} = 3.13$, $p < 0.05$, Pearson's $R = 0.53$, SR = 307.69%). When we compared the latency to enter the dark chamber between the sexes, we found that males also had significantly shorter latencies than females (2-sample t test; $t_{25} = 3.74$, $p < 0.05$, Pearson's $R = 0.60$, SR = 33.34%) (Fig. 2).

We also found a significant difference in latency between males and females in different phases of the estrous cycle (1-way ANOVA; $F_{3,22} = 6.08$, $p < 0.05$, $\eta_G^2 = 0.45$) (Additional file 2: Figure S2). The latency for females in each estrous group decreased in the following order: proestrus, estrus, and diestrus. Females in proestrus and estrus showed significantly longer latencies than males ($p < 0.05$, Pearson's $R = 0.60$ and 0.48, respectively) (Additional file 2: Figure S2).

Fear-conditioning test

The 2-way ANOVA for the freezing rate showed a significant interaction between sex and session, although

Passive avoidance test

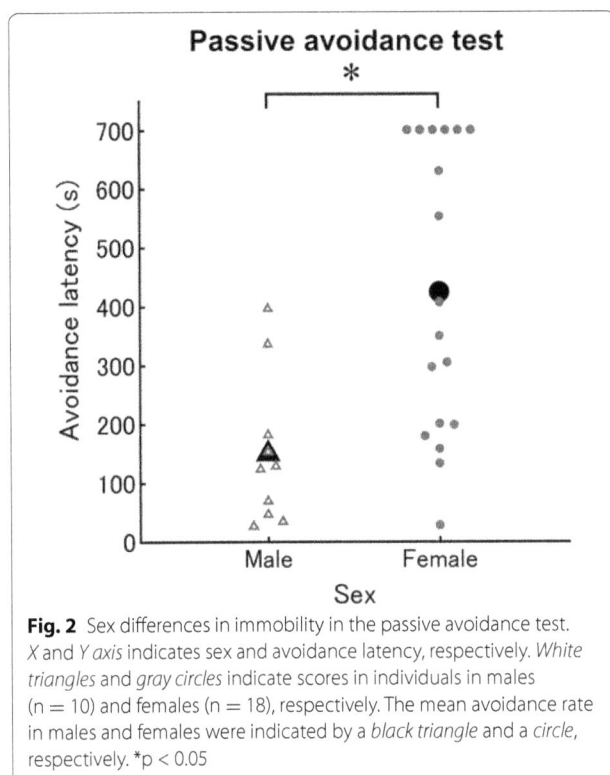

Fig. 2 Sex differences in immobility in the passive avoidance test. *X* and *Y* axis indicates sex and avoidance latency, respectively. *White triangles* and *gray circles* indicate scores in individuals in males (n = 10) and females (n = 18), respectively. The mean avoidance rate in males and females were indicated by a *black triangle* and a *circle*, respectively. *p < 0.05

the size of the effect was small ($F_{3,108} = 3.34$, $p < 0.05$, $\eta_G^2 = 0.05$) (Fig. 3, left panel).

When we compared the freezing rate between sexes within each session, we found a significant sex difference only in the AUD session ($p < 0.05$, Pearson's $R = 0.40$) (Fig. 3, left panel). The SRs during training, CXT, pre-AUD, and AUD were 63.47, 86.95, 21.05, and 39.73%, respectively. We also compared the freezing rate within females between sessions. The freezing rate in the AUD session was significantly higher than in the training and pre-AUD sessions ($p < 0.05$, Pearson's $R = 0.75$ and 0.57, respectively). Similar results were observed in the CXT session ($p < 0.05$, Pearson's $R = 0.73$ and 0.70, respectively), with no significant difference between the AUD and CXT sessions ($p > 0.05$, Pearson's $R = 0.01$). In contrast, the male freezing rate in the CXT session was significantly higher than in any other session ($p < 0.05$, Pearson's $R = 0.70$, 0.67, and 0.42 for training, pre-AUD and AUD, respectively), whereas the AUD session showed no significant difference when compared with the training and pre-AUD sessions ($p > 0.05$, Pearson's $R = 0.62$ and 0.55, respectively). When we compared the freezing rate between males and females in each estrous phase, neither a significant main effect of sex/ phase of estrous cycle ($F_{3,30} = 1.30$, $p > 0.05$, $\eta_G^2 = 0.04$)

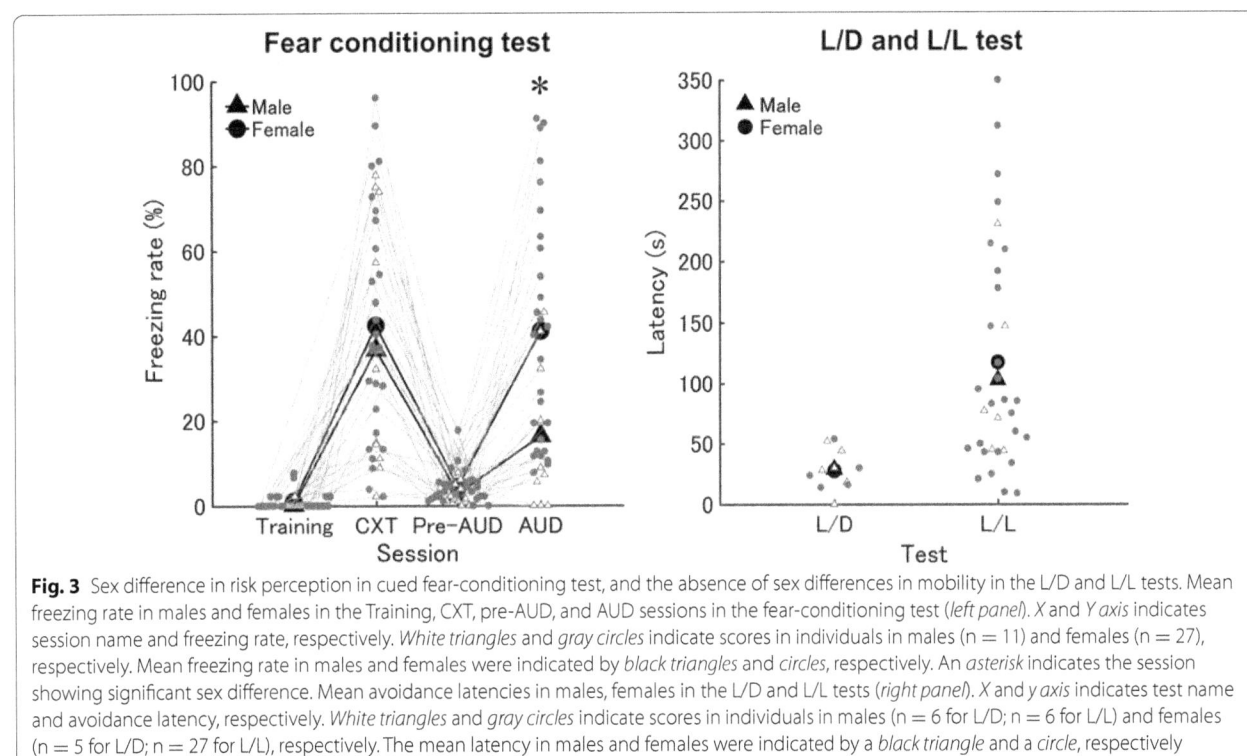

Fig. 3 Sex difference in risk perception in cued fear-conditioning test, and the absence of sex differences in mobility in the L/D and L/L tests. Mean freezing rate in males and females in the Training, CXT, pre-AUD, and AUD sessions in the fear-conditioning test (*left panel*). *X* and *Y* axis indicates session name and freezing rate, respectively. *White triangles* and *gray circles* indicate scores in individuals in males (n = 11) and females (n = 27), respectively. Mean freezing rate in males and females were indicated by *black triangles* and *circles*, respectively. An *asterisk* indicates the session showing significant sex difference. Mean avoidance latencies in males, females in the L/D and L/L tests (*right panel*). *X* and *y* axis indicates test name and avoidance latency, respectively. *White triangles* and *gray circles* indicate scores in individuals in males (n = 6 for L/D; n = 6 for L/L) and females (n = 5 for L/D; n = 27 for L/L), respectively. The mean latency in males and females were indicated by a *black triangle* and a *circle*, respectively

nor a significant interaction between group and session ($F_{9,90} = 1.16$, $p > 0.05$, $\eta_G^2 = 0.09$) was observed (Additional file 3: Figure S3).

We confirmed that mice could participate in the AUD session without a generalization of contextual fear memory from the preceding CXT session, because the freezing rate in neither males nor females differed between the training and pre-AUD sessions (see above). In addition, each contextual and auditory cue should independently induce the freezing response, because a contextual cue was sufficient for the mice to perceive the foot-shock in the CXT session. Likewise, an auditory cue was sufficient for foot-shock perception in the AUD session.

Although we found a significant interaction between sex and session, the magnitude of the effect of sex in this test was small according to the guideline (see "Methods"), even when it was compared to those in both avoidance tests. Thus, we concluded that the sex difference in associative learning was small.

L/D and L/L test

No significant sex difference was observed in either the L/D (2-sample t test; $t_{31} = 0.35$, $p > 0.05$, Pearson's $R = 0.05$, SR = 103.88%) or the L/L tests (2-sample t test; $t_9 = 0.10$, $p > 0.05$, Pearson's $R = 0.02$, SR = 87.41%) (Fig. 3, right panel).

Tail suspension test

For immobility during the TST, neither a significant interaction between sex and day ($F_{1,26} = 0.01$, $p = 0.92$, $\eta_G^2 = 0.00$) nor a significant main effect of sex ($F_{1,26} = 0.37$, $p = 0.55$, $\eta_G^2 = 0.01$) was observed (Fig. 4, left panel). The SR values were 98.35 and 98.25% on days 1 and 2, respectively. However, the immobility was significantly higher for both sexes on day 2 than on day 1 (main effect of day: $F_{1,27} = 96.15$, $p < 0.05$, $\eta_G^2 = 0.58$) (Fig. 4, left panel). This effect was also observed when we compared males with females in each estrous phase (main effect of day: $F_{1,23} = 65.83$, $p < 0.01$, $\eta_G^2 = 0.49$). Neither a significant main effect of sex/phase of estrous cycle ($F_{3,23} = 0.08$, $p = 0.97$, $\eta_G^2 = 0.01$) nor a significant interaction between sex/phase of estrous cycle and day ($F_{3,23} = 0.52$, $p = 0.67$, $\eta_G^2 = 0.02$) was observed (Additional file 4: Figure S4A, B).

Forced swim test

Results analyzing the immobility in the FST were similar to those in the TST. There was neither a significant interaction between sex and day ($F_{1,25} = 1.01$, $p = 0.32$, $\eta_G^2 = 0.01$) nor a significant main effect of sex ($F_{1,25} = 0.51$, $p = 0.48$, $\eta_G^2 = 0.01$) (Fig. 4, right panel). The SR values were 99.78 and 103.80% on days 1 and 2, respectively, and immobility increased significantly on day 2 in both sexes (main effect of day: $F_{1,25} = 149.20$, $p < 0.05$, $\eta_G^2 = 0.69$) (Fig. 4, right panel). This effect was also observed when

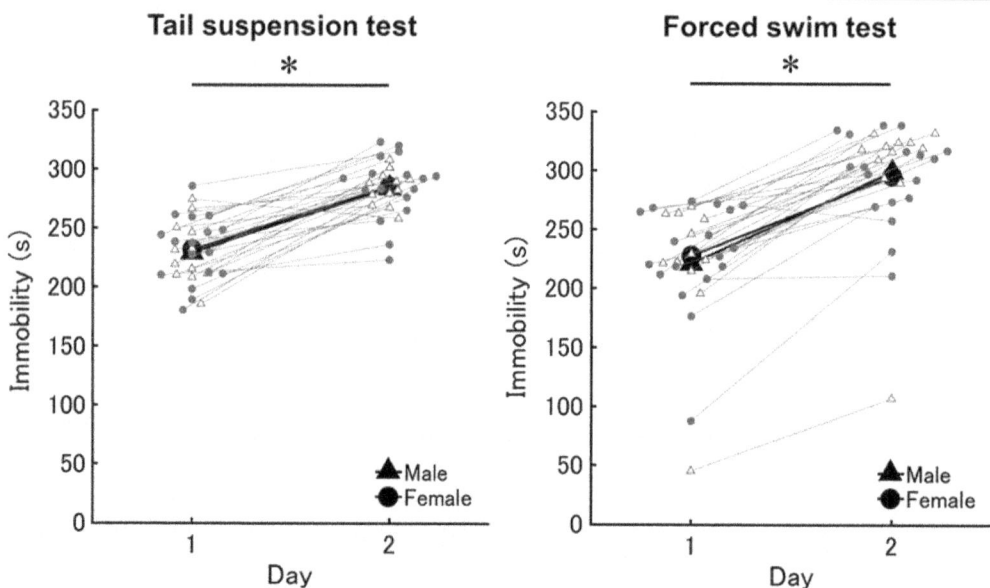

Fig. 4 Absence of sex differences in responses in the TST and FST. Mean immobility time in males and females across day 1 and 2 in the TST (*left panel*). Mean immobility time in males and females across day 1 and 2 in the FST (*right panel*). *X* and *Y* axis indicates day and immobility time, respectively. *White triangles* and *gray circles* indicate scores in individuals in males (n = 12 for TST; n = 12 for FST) and females (n = 17 for TST; n = 18 for FST), respectively. The mean immobility in males and females were indicated by *black triangles* and *circles*, respectively. Each *asterisk* indicates significant increasing the immobility from day 1 to 2

we compared males with females in each estrous phase (main effect of day: $F_{1,21} = 122.86$, $p < 0.05$, $\eta_G^2 = 0.51$) (Fig. 4, right panel). Although there was no significant main effect of sex/phase of estrous cycle ($F_{3,21} = 0.61$, $p = 0.62$, $\eta_G^2 = 0.06$), there was an apparent trend toward significance for the interaction between sex/phase of estrous cycle and day ($F_{3,21} = 2.56$, $p = 0.08$, $\eta_G^2 = 0.07$) (Additional file 4: Figure S4C, D).

Measurement of basal activity in familiar home cage

Each motion parameter (mean $\pm$ CI) in a familiar home cage was comparable between sexes. As such, no significant difference was observed in the mean velocity (male $= 43.76 \pm 7.91$ mm/s vs. female $= 38.60 \pm 7.48$ mm/s, $p > 0.05$, Pearson's $R = 0.23$, SR $= 113.54\%$), total distance travelled (male $= 2371.42 \pm 457.74$ mm vs. female $= 1795.86 \pm 615.33$ mm, $p > 0.05$, Pearson's $R = 0.36$, SR $= 132.05\%$), or distance from the center of the cage (male $= 69.57 \pm 7.37$ mm vs. female $= 75.54 \pm 4.71$ mm, $p > 0.05$, Pearson's $R = 0.32$, SR $= 92.07\%$).

Discussion

In this study, we investigated sex-mediated responses in behaviors under a variety of risks. Since a behavior is composed of a set of simpler responses toward a specific scene, scene segmentation, which involves breaking down a general context to each scene, would be an efficient way to extract subtle phenotypes in a behavior and their occurrence conditions. In line with this, we ran a battery of behavior tests modeling discrete types of risks. We hypothesized that avoidance response to an escapable risk would diverge between sexes. In the present battery of tests, avoidance was further segmented into active and passive sub-components, which were tested in the two-way active avoidance test and the passive avoidance test, respectively. Then, the fear-conditioning test was used to determine whether sex differences arise in the formation of associative learning alone, since it is necessary for responding to a predicted risk, and thereby required for learned avoidance behaviors [13]. The L/D and L/L tests were run as additional scenes in which the escapable risk and the risk-predicting cue were uncoupled. To check if sex differences arise in active and passive responding to an aversive, inescapable scene, the forced-swim test and tail-suspension test were done. Basal activity in a home cage was also compared between sexes.

Sex differences were shown to occur in the active as well as the passive avoidance tests. In general, the evidence suggested that males responded to a risk with higher mobility while females were less mobile after predicting an impending foot-shock from an associated cue. More specifically, in the active avoidance test,

males exhibited more transitions from the shock compartment to the safe compartment, as the avoidance rate in the last bin (trials 81–100) for males was nearly 150% of that shown by females. Similarly, in the passive avoidance test, transition to the dark compartment in males was almost 300% of that in females. Likewise, the latency of entry into the dark compartment for males was 30% of that of females. These differences could not be attributed to a difference in basic locomotor activity, because all motion parameters measured in the familiar home cage were comparable between sexes. Thus, we conclude that males express a higher exploratory avoidance than females in response to an escapable risk. These differences in mobility present an opportunity to learn to avoid the threat under the active avoidance test, but increase males' exposure to threat in the passive avoidance test.

When we consider the sexually different cognitive processing underlying the avoidance responses, we can assume that it requires a process from the perception of a potential risk to the subsequent execution of avoidance. Indeed, the perception of a potential risk relied on associative learning between a risk and a prediction cue in both types of avoidance tests. The sex difference in the active avoidance test was primarily observed in the later bins where the association between the cue and the threat was fully formed. In the fear-conditioning test, associative learning occurred despite an inability to carry out subsequent avoidance behavior. In this test, the higher freezing rates in females shown in auditory-cued fear conditioning might partially contribute to their immobility during avoidance. This is also supported by the results of the L/D and L/L tests, and is consistent with previous studies, which found no sex difference in tests with a lack of associative learning to perceive a potential risk, such as the elevated plus maze test [38, 39]. In the scenes with inescapable risks, sex differences disappeared as shown in the TST and the FST.

With regard to the neural mechanisms that induce these differences between sexes, the projection from the lateral habenula to the rostromedial tegmental nucleus in the midbrain is a possible candidate. The lateral habenula encodes both active and passive avoidance behavior associated with negative reward [40], and a sex difference has been observed in this region [41–43]. In addition, the lateral habenula shows a high expression of the estrogen receptor [43]. Estrogen facilitates anxiety-like behavior in a variety of tests including not only auditory-cued fear conditioning and passive avoidance tests, but also the elevated plus maze and open field test [44–46]. In addition to these anxiogenic effects, estrogen also decreases locomotor activity, such as the number of rotations in a running wheel or the travel distance in a new environment

[45, 46]. Thus, estrogen in the lateral habenula may account for the lower mobility in both types of avoidance in females in the estrus and proestrus phases.

In summary, the present study indicated that subtle divergences between sexes in sequentially varying behavior under risky contexts were successfully extracted by scene segmentation. We now know that sex-dependent divergences occur in the degree of locomotion in avoidance behaviors. Nevertheless, significant components would be still latent in a considerable number of behaviors. Hence, further study would be required for extracting them in order to comprehensively understand a behavior. For a general point of view to our behavior, we concluded the computational analysis of behavior needed to be established to understand our social behaviors like sex differences.

Additional files

Additional file 1: Figure S1. Sexually different mobility in the active avoidance test between male and females in each estrous phase. X and Y axis indicates bins per 20 trials and avoidance rate, respectively. (A) White triangles and dark gray circles, medium gray squares, and light gray diamonds indicates males (n = 9) or females in proestrus (n = 3), estrus (n = 5), and diestrus (n = 6). (B) The mean avoidance rate of males and females in each estrous phase were indicated by white triangles and dark gray circles, medium squares, and light diamonds, respectively. An asterisk and a dagger indicates the bin showing significant sex difference between male and females except in the proestrus phase, and that between male and females except in the diestrus phase, respectively.

Additional file 2: Figure S2. Sexually different immobility in the active avoidance test between male and females in each estrous phase. X and Y axis indicates sex and avoidance latency, respectively. White triangles, dark gray circles, medium gray squares, and light gray diamonds indicate scores in individuals in males (n = 10) and females in proestrus (n = 3), estrus (n = 8), and diestrus (n = 6) phase respectively. The mean avoidance rate in males and females in each estrus phase were indicated by a black triangle, circle, square, and diamond, respectively. Two asterisks indicate bins showing significant sex difference between male and females in proestrus, and male and females in estrus phase, respectively.

Additional file 3: Figure S3. Sexually different risk perception in cued fear-conditioning test between males and females in each estrous phase. X and Y axis indicates session name and freezing rate, respectively. (A) White triangles, dark gray circles, medium gray squares, and light gray diamonds indicate scores in individuals in males (n = 11) and females in proestrus (n = 8), estrus (n = 8), and diestrus (n = 7), respectively. (B) Mean freezing rate in males and females in each estrus phase were indicated by white triangles, dark gray circles, medium gray squares, and light gray diamonds respectively.

Additional file 4: Figure S4. Absence of sex differences between males and females in each estrous phase in responses in the TST (A, B) and FST (C, D). X and Y axis indicates day and immobility time, respectively. (A) White triangles, dark gray circles, medium gray squares, and light gray diamonds indicate scores in individuals in males (n = 12) and females in proestrus (n = 5), estrus (n = 6), and diestrus (n = 4) phase, respectively. (B) The mean immobility in males and females in each estrus phase were indicated by black triangles, dark gray circles, medium gray squares, and light gray diamonds, respectively. (C) Scores in individuals in males (n = 12) and females in proestrus (n = 4), estrus (n = 4) and diestrus (n = 7) were indicated by the same maker types with (A). (D) The mean immobility in males and females in each estrus phase were indicated by the same marker types with (B), respectively. Each asterisk indicates significant increasing the immobility from day 1 to 2.

Authors' contributions
We would like to thank Shanen Ganapathee for useful comments on this manuscript. SY, YS, AH, SK contributed to the conception or design of the work. SY, YS, HK contributed to the acquisition and analysis of the experimental data. SY, YS, SK wrote the manuscript. All authors read and approved the final manuscript.

Author details
[1] Graduate School of Biological Sciences, Nara Institute of Science and Technology, 8916-5 Keihanna Science City, Nara 630-0192, Japan. [2] Graduate School of Medicine, Kyoto University, Kyoto, Japan. [3] JST, PRESTO, Saitama, Japan.

Acknowledgements
We would like to thank Shanen Ganapathee for useful comments on this manuscript. And also we would like to thank JSPS for funding support on this work.

Competing interests
The authors declare that they have no competing interests.

Ethical statement
All experiments involving animals were approved by the Animal Care Committee of the Nara Institute of Science and Technology (permit number: 1004).

Funding
This study was supported by JSPS KAKENHI Grant (No. 25118009).

References
1. Cahill L. Why sex matters for neuroscience. Nat Rev Neurosci. 2006;7:477–84. doi:10.1038/nrn1909.
2. Kimchi T, Xu J, Dulac C. A functional circuit underlying male sexual behaviour in the female mouse brain. Nature. 2007;448:1009–14. doi:10.1038/nature06089.
3. Pasterski V, Hindmarsh P, Geffner M, Brook C, Brain C, Hines M. Increased aggression and activity level in 3- to 11-year-old girls with congenital adrenal hyperplasia (CAH). Horm Behav. 2007;52:368–74. doi:10.1016/j.yhbeh.2007.05.015.
4. Ronkainen H, Ylönen H. Behaviour of cyclic bank voles under risk of mustelid predation: do females avoid copulations? Oecologia. 1994;97:377–81. doi:10.1007/bf00317328.
5. Tan J, Ma Z, Gao X, Wu Y, Fang F. Gender difference of unconscious attentional bias in high trait anxiety individuals. PLoS ONE. 2011;6:e20305. doi:10.1371/journal.pone.0020305.
6. Forger NG, de Vries GJ. Cell death and sexual differentiation of behavior: worms, flies, and mammals. Curr Opin Neurobiol. 2010;20:776–83. doi:10.1016/j.conb.2010.09.006.
7. Benjamini Y, Lipkind D, Horev G, Fonio E, Kafkafi N, Golani I. Ten ways to improve the quality of descriptions of whole-animal movement. Neurosci Biobehav Rev. 2010;34:1351–65. doi:10.1016/j.neubiorev.2010.04.004.
8. Benjamini Y, Fonio E, Galili T, Havkin GZ, Golani I. Quantifying the buildup in extent and complexity of free exploration in mice. Proc Natl Acad Sci USA. 2011;108(Suppl 3):15580–7. doi:10.1073/pnas.1014837108.
9. Burgos-Artizzu XP, Dollár P, Lin D, Anderson DJ, Perona P. Social behavior recognition in continuous video. In: 2012 IEEE conference on computer vision and pattern recognition (CVPR). Piscataway: IEEE; 2012. p. 1322–9.
10. Neuberg SL, Kenrick DT, Schaller M. Human threat management systems: self-protection and disease avoidance. Neurosci Biobehav Rev. 2011;35:1042–51. doi:10.1016/j.neubiorev.2010.08.011.
11. Topál J, Csányi V. The effect of eye-like schema on shuttling activity of wild house mice (*Mus musculus domesticus*): context-dependent threatening aspects of the eyespot patterns. Anim Learn Behav. 1994;22:96–102. doi:10.3758/bf03199961.
12. Colwill RM, Creton R. Imaging escape and avoidance behavior in zebrafish larvae. Rev Neurosci. 2011;22:63–73. doi:10.1515/rns.2011.008.
13. Cryan JF, Holmes A. The ascent of mouse: advances in modelling human depression and anxiety. Nat Rev Drug Discov. 2005;4:775–90. doi:10.1038/nrd1825

14. Jesuthasan S. Fear, anxiety, and control in the zebrafish. Dev Neurobiol. 2012;72:395–403. doi:10.1002/dneu.20873.

15. Richter J, Hamm AO, Pane-Farre CA, Gerlach AL, Gloster AT, Wittchen HU, et al. Dynamics of defensive reactivity in patients with panic disorder and agoraphobia: implications for the etiology of panic disorder. Biol Psychiatry. 2012;72:512–20. doi:10.1016/j.biopsych.2012.03.035.

16. Rodgers RJ, Cao BJ, Dalvi A, Holmes A. Animal models of anxiety: an ethological perspective. Braz J Med Biol Res. 1997;30:289–304. doi:10.1590/s0100-879x1997000300002.

17. Rosen JB, Schulkin J. From normal fear to pathological anxiety. Psychol Rev. 1998;105:325–50. doi:10.1037/0033-295x.105.2.325.

18. Schlund MW, Cataldo MF. Amygdala involvement in human avoidance, escape and approach behavior. Neuroimage. 2010;53:769–76. doi:10.1016/j.neuroimage.2010.06.058.

19. Korte SM, De Boer SF, Bohus B. Fear-potentiation in the elevated plus-maze test depends on stressor controllability and fear conditioning. Stress. 1999;3:27–40. doi:10.1038/nature06089.

20. Barkus C, McHugh SB, Sprengel R, Seeburg PH, Rawlins JNP, Bannerman DM. Hippocampal NMDA receptors and anxiety: at the interface between cognition and emotion. Eur J Pharmacol. 2010;626:49–56. doi:10.1016/j.ejphar.2009.10.014.

21. Dohanich G. Ovarian steroids and cognitive function. Curr Dir Psychol Sci. 2003;12:57–61. doi:10.1111/1467-8721.01226.

22. Frohlich J, Morgan M, Ogawa S, Burton L, Pfaff D. Statistical analysis of hormonal influences on arousal measures in ovariectomized female mice. Horm Behav. 2002;42:414–23. doi:10.1006/hbeh.2002.1832.

23. Kuriyama H, Shibasaki T. Sexual differentiation of the effects of emotional stress on food intake in rats. Neuroscience. 2004;124:459–65. doi:10.1016/j.neuroscience.2003.12.012.

24. Miller G, Tybur JM, Jordan BD. Ovulatory cycle effects on tip earnings by lap dancers: economic evidence for human estrus? Evol Hum Behav. 2007;28:375–81. doi:10.1016/j.evolhumbehav.2007.06.002.

25. Caligioni CS. Assessing reproductive status/stages in mice. Curr Protoc Neurosci. 2009;. doi:10.1002/0471142301.nsa04is48 **(Appendix 4, Appendix 4I)**.

26. Chang T, Meyer U, Feldon J, Yee BK. Disruption of the US pre-exposure effect and latent inhibition in two-way active avoidance by systemic amphetamine in C57BL/6 mice. Psychopharmacology. 2007;191:211–21. doi:10.1007/s00213-006-0649-z.

27. Iso H, Simoda S, Matsuyama T. Environmental change during postnatal development alters behaviour, cognitions and neurogenesis of mice. Behav Brain Res. 2007;179:90–8. doi:10.1016/j.bbr.2007.01.025.

28. Nakazawa T, Komai S, Watabe AM, Kiyama Y, Fukaya M, Arima-Yoshida F, et al. NR2B tyrosine phosphorylation modulates fear learning as well as amygdaloid synaptic plasticity. EMBO J. 2006;25:2867–77. doi:10.1038/sj.emboj.7601156.

29. Kromer SA, Kessler MS, Milfay D, Birg IN, Bunck M, Czibere L, et al. Identification of glyoxalase-I as a protein marker in a mouse model of extremes in trait anxiety. J Neurosci. 2005;25:4375–84. doi:10.1055/s-2003-825414.

30. Jacobsen JP, Weikop P, Hansen HH, Mikkelsen JD, Redrobe JP, Holst D, et al. SK3K+ channel-deficient mice have enhanced dopamine and serotonin release and altered emotional behaviors. Genes Brain Beha. 2008;7:836–48. doi:10.1111/j.1601-183x.2008.00416.x.

31. McEuen JG, Semsar KA, Lim MA, Bale TL. Influence of sex and corticotropin-releasing factor pathways as determinants in serotonin sensitivity. Endocrinology. 2009;150:3709–16. doi:10.1210/en.2008-1721.

32. Imai S, Mamiya T, Tsukada A, Sakai Y, Mouri A, Nabeshima T, et al. Ubiquitin-specific peptidase 46 (Usp46) regulates mouse immobile behavior in the tail suspension test through the GABAergic system. PLoS ONE. 2012;7:e39084. doi:10.1371/journal.pone.0039084.

33. Adamec R, Head D, Blundell J, Burton P, Berton O. Lasting anxiogenic effects of feline predator stress in mice: sex differences in vulnerability to stress and predicting severity of anxiogenic response from the stress experience. Physiol Behav. 2006;88:12–29. doi:10.1016/j.physbeh.2006.03.005.

34. Adamec R, Head D, Soreq H, Blundell J. The role of the read through variant of acetylcholinesterase in anxiogenic effects of predator stress in mice. Behav Brain Res. 2008;189:180–90. doi:10.1016/j.bbr.2007.12.023.

35. Olejnik S, Algina J. Generalized eta and omega squared statistics: measures of effect size for some common research designs. Psychol Methods. 2003;8:434–47. doi:10.1037/1082-989x.8.4.434.

36. Cohen J. Statistical power analysis for the behavioral sciences. 2nd ed. Hillsdale: Lawrence Erlbaum Associates; 1988. doi:10.4324/9780203771587.

37. Field A. Discovering statistics using SPSS. 2nd ed. Thousand Oaks: Sage Publications; 2009. doi:10.1348/000709906X100611.

38. Chikahisa S, Sano A, Kitaoka K, Miyamoto K, Sei H. Anxiolytic effect of music depends on ovarian steroid in female mice. Behav Brain Res. 2007;179:50–9. doi:10.1016/j.bbr.2007.01.010.

39. O'Leary TP, Gunn RK, Brown RE. What are we measuring when we test strain differences in anxiety in mice? Behav Genet. 2013;43:34–50. doi:10.1007/s10519-012-9572-8.

40. Stamatakis AM, Stuber GD. Activation of lateral habenula inputs to the ventral midbrain promotes behavioral avoidance. Nat Neurosci. 2012;15:1105–7. doi:10.1038/nn.3145.

41. Brown LL, Siegel H, Etgen AM. Global sex differences in stress-induced activation of cerebral metabolism revealed by 2-deoxyglucose autoradiography. Horm Behav. 1996;30:611–7. doi:10.1006/hbeh.1996.0064.

42. Lonstein JS, De Vries GJ. Sex differences in the parental behaviour of adult virgin prairie voles: independence from gonadal hormones and vasopressin. J Neuroendocrinol. 1999;11:441–9. doi:10.1046/j.1365-2826.1999.00361.x.

43. Yokosuka M, Okamura H, Hayashi S. Postnatal development and sex difference in neurons containing estrogen receptor-alpha immunoreactivity in the preoptic brain, the diencephalon, and the amygdala in the rat. J Comp Neurol. 1997;389:81–93. doi:10.1002/(sici)1096-9861(19971208)389:1<81:aid-cne6>3.0.co;2-a.

44. Marcondes FK, Miguel KJ, Melo LL, Spadari-Bratfisch RC. Estrous cycle influences the response of female rats in the elevated plus-maze test. Physiol Behav. 2001;74:435–40. doi:10.1016/s0031-9384(01)00593-5.

45. Morgan MA, Pfaff DW. Effects of estrogen on activity and fear-related behaviors in mice. Horm Behav. 2001;40:472–82. doi:10.1006/hbeh.2001.1716.

46. Morgan MA, Pfaff DW. Estrogen's effects on activity, anxiety, and fear in two mouse strains. Behav Brain Res. 2002;132:85–93. doi:10.1016/s0166-4328(01)00398-9.

Visual food stimulus changes resting oscillatory brain activities related to appetitive motive

Takahiro Yoshikawa[1*], Masaaki Tanaka[2], Akira Ishii[2], Yoko Yamano[1] and Yasuyoshi Watanabe[2,3]

Abstract

Background: Changes of resting brain activities after visual food stimulation might affect the feeling of pleasure in eating food in daily life and spontaneous appetitive motives. We used magnetoencephalography (MEG) to identify brain areas related to the activity changes.

Methods: Fifteen healthy, right-handed males [age, 25.4 ± 5.5 years; body mass index, 22.5 ± 2.7 kg/m^2 (mean ± SD)] were enrolled. They were asked to watch food or mosaic pictures for 5 min and to close their eyes for 3 min before and after the picture presentation without thinking of anything. Resting brain activities were recorded during two eye-closed sessions. The feeling of pleasure in eating food in daily life and appetitive motives in the study setting were assessed by visual analogue scale (VAS) scores.

Results: The γ-band power of resting oscillatory brain activities was decreased after the food picture presentation in the right insula [Brodmann's area (BA) 13], the left orbitofrontal cortex (OFC) (BA11), and the left frontal pole (BA10). Significant reductions of the α-band power were observed in the dorsolateral prefrontal cortex (DLPFC) (BA46). Particularly, the feeling of pleasure in eating food was positively correlated with the power decrease in the insula and negatively with that in the DLPFC. The changes in appetitive motives were associated with the power decrease in the frontal pole.

Conclusions: These findings suggest automatic brain mechanics whereby changes of the resting brain activity might be associated with positive feeling in dietary life and have an impact on the irresistible appetitive motives through emotional and cognitive brain functions.

Keywords: Resting brain activity, Magnetoencephalography (MEG), Insula, Dorsolateral prefrontal cortex (DLPFC), Orbitofrontal cortex (OFC), Frontal pole

Background

Today's lifestyle provides ample opportunities for pleasurable but excessive food intake [1], which often leads to obesity and becomes a considerable health threat in susceptible individuals by raising the risk of chronic diseases such as diabetes mellitus, hypertension, heart disease, fatty liver, sleep apnea, and certain forms of cancer [2, 3]. Another health issue associated with modern dietary lifestyles is related to the physiological and psychological reductions in food intake that can be important contributors to sarcopenia in older individuals [4] as well as malnutrition in adolescents and young adult women [5]. Accordingly, from a public health perspective, it is imperative to clarify the control mechanisms involved in eating behaviors and to develop new strategies to encourage the consumption of proper nutrition. In particular, it is crucial to understand the neurobiological mechanisms by which the decision to start or stop eating comes about [6].

Eating behavior is affected by various physiological determinants including homeostatic requirements such as nutritional deficits, and is regulated by metabolic and neuroendocrine networks integrating central nervous

*Correspondence: tkhr6719@med.osaka-cu.ac.jp
[1] Department of Sports Medicine, Osaka City University Graduate School of Medicine, 1-4-3 Asahi-machi, Abeno-ku, Osaka, Osaka 545-8585, Japan
Full list of author information is available at the end of the article

pathways with signals from the periphery [7]. However, it is also known that human eating behaviors largely depend on cognitive (attention, learning, memory, and decision-making), sensory (visual, olfactory, taste, and somatosensory), and behavioral (motivational) processes [8, 9]. Additionally, fluctuations in mood and emotion can affect food choices and quantities [10]. Human eating behavior is thus extraordinarily complex, and disturbances in eating behaviors are difficult to treat.

Neuroimaging techniques have classically been employed to elucidate the neurological bases of eating behaviors. Positron emission tomography (PET) and functional magnetic resonance imaging (fMRI) have been utilized most frequently in research concerning eating behaviors. Hemodynamic changes are assessed as indicators of the changes of neural activation relating to cognition, emotion, and behaviors in various experimental conditions, including the fed state and stimuli (visual, olfactory, gustatory, and food intakes) [11]. In contrast, magnetoencephalography (MEG) monitors electrophysiological activities inside the brain by measuring electromagnetic fields using electric or magnetic sensors over the scalp surface [12–14]; it allows a quantitative assessment of oscillatory components in measured data, and synchronization of oscillatory neuronal firing represents a physiological coding mechanism to bind together spatially separated populations of neurons [15, 16]. Thus, brain activities are characterized by the presence of more and less regular oscillations in various frequency bands [16]. For example, a decrease of the α-band power suggests deactivated interaction between local negative feedback circuits in the thalamus and the cortex, while a decrease of the γ-band power indicates deactivated information processing reflecting reduced rapid synchronization among local brain areas [17, 18].

Recently, we applied the MEG analyses to research pertaining to the time course of neural processes for appetitive motives and self-control immediately after visual exposure to food pictures [19–21]. While most previous studies investigated ongoing neural networks during a sensory presentation relating to food, it is also valuable to focus on differences in resting brain activities before and after a series of visual stimuli using food images, by assessing changes in synchronization of oscillatory neuronal firing between these two conditions. Such differences, which could not be assessed by using fMRI or PET, might characterize involuntary residual effects in the resting brain activities that may persist after a cessation of visual food stimulation, and the lasting effects might transiently modify dietary emotion and cognition such as the appetitive motives or decisions to eat, and further impact the feelings of pleasure in a real dietary life in individuals who cannot help consuming too much or in those who cannot consume a sufficient amount of food.

In the present study, we measured resting brain activities by using MEG in fasting individuals who closed their eyes for 3 min before and after watching various food pictures presented every 2 s for 5 min. Throughout the experiment, the contents of the pictures were not disclosed to the study participants in advance, and they were instructed not to think of anything, including the pictures on the screen. We tried to identify the brain areas related to the residual effect on the resting brain activities by examining the differences in the oscillatory power between 2 eye-closed conditions, before and after the presentation of food pictures, using the time–frequency analyses of MEG. Next, we tried to determine whether the oscillatory power changes are associated with a transient change in appetitive motives spontaneously elicited by the visual presentation of food items. Additionally, in order to confirm the validity of our results in a real-life situation, we assessed the impact of the oscillatory power differences on practical factors related to appetitive motives and eating habits such as the feeling of pleasure in eating food in daily life. We hypothesized that, based on the previous literature when viewing food [11, 19–21], a short duration of visual food stimuli has a considerable impact on resting oscillatory brain activities which manifest as changes of powers across various time–frequency bands in emotional and cognitive brain areas.

Methods

Participants

In total, fifteen healthy male volunteers with normal body habitus [age, 25.4 ± 5.5 years; height, 171.3 ± 6.9 cm; body weight, 66.3 ± 11.7 kg; body mass index (BMI), 22.5 ± 2.7 kg/m^2 (mean $\pm$ SD)] were enrolled. Participants with a history of mental or neurological disorders, and those taking chronic medications that affect the central nervous system were excluded. All of the participants had normal or corrected-to-normal visual acuity and were right-handed. The study protocol was approved by the Ethics Committee of Osaka City University (license number 2811), and all participants provided written informed consent to participate in the study and were monetarily compensated. All procedures were done according to the research ethics of the Helsinki Declaration of 1975, and the applicable revisions at the time of the investigation [22].

Experimental design

The participants were enrolled in a randomized study consisting of two crossover experiments (food-picture and control experiments) (Fig. 1a). For 1 day before the visit, they were instructed to finish dinner by 9:00 p.m. and to fast overnight (they were only allowed to drink water), to avoid intensive physical and mental activities,

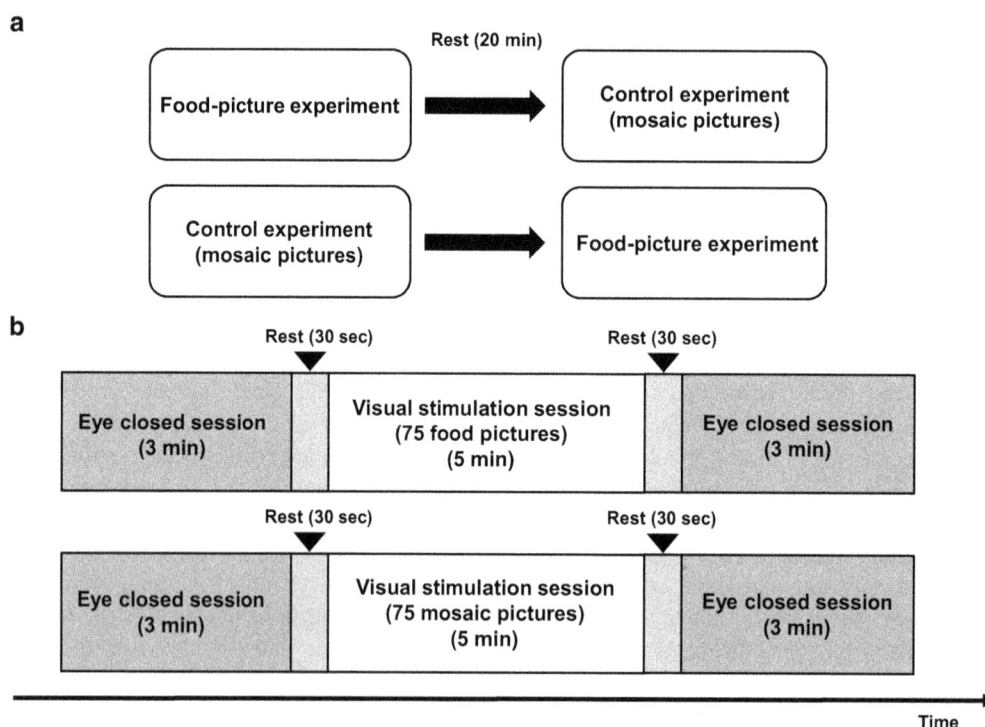

Fig. 1 Experimental design (**a**) and the procedure of experimental sessions (**b**). Participants were enrolled in a randomized study consisting of 2 crossover experiments (food-picture and control experiments), and asked to watch a series of pictures for 5 min (visual stimulation session) and to close their eyes for 3 min before and after the picture presentation (eye-closed sessions). Pictures of food items were presented as visual stimuli during the food-picture experiment, and mosaic pictures of food items were presented as visual stimuli during the control experiment. The contents of pictures were not disclosed to the study participants in advance

and to maintain normal sleeping hours. After they arrived at the laboratory in the morning, they were asked to report their physical condition including hunger. They rated their subjective level of hunger on a 5-point Likert-type scale ranging from 1 (*Yes, I am very hungry*) to 5 (*No, I am not hungry at all*). In addition, they were asked to rate their feeling of pleasure in eating food in daily life, using a unidimensional visual analogue scale (VAS), ranging from none (0 mm) to maximum (100 mm). Then, they were instructed to watch a series of pictures for 5 min (visual stimulation session) and to close their eyes for 3 min before and after the picture presentation (eye-closed sessions) (Fig. 1b). The contents of the pictures were not disclosed to the study participants in advance. The intersession intervals were set at approximately 30 s. Brain activities were recorded using MEG during these two eye-closed sessions. The pictures of food items were presented as visual stimuli during the food-picture experiment. In addition, the mosaic pictures created from the same pictures of food items were used as visual stimuli during the control experiment. During the visual stimulation sessions, while in the supine position on a bed, the participants were requested to keep both eyes open and

to fixate on a central point and to view the screen. During eye-closed sessions, they were instructed to close their eyes while in the same position as the visual stimulation session. Throughout the experiment, they were instructed not to think of anything, including the pictures on the screen. They were asked to rate their appetitive motives, using a VAS, ranging from none (0 mm) to maximum (100 mm) for each of the eye-closed and visual stimulation sessions in both experiments. This study was conducted in a quiet, temperature-controlled magnetically shielded room at Osaka City University Hospital.

Stimulus presentation

Visual stimulus presentation was performed similarly as described in our previous study [20]. Briefly, each visual stimulation session consisted of 75-picture sets of a 2-sec stimulation period followed by a 2-sec inter-stimulus interval (Fig. 2a, b). Fifteen pictures of typical modern Japanese food items were used, including steak, hamburger, fritter, chicken nugget, French fry, pizza, spaghetti, ice cream, and noodles [23]. After the experiment, each participant was asked to rate each picture for food preference in order to confirm that disliked

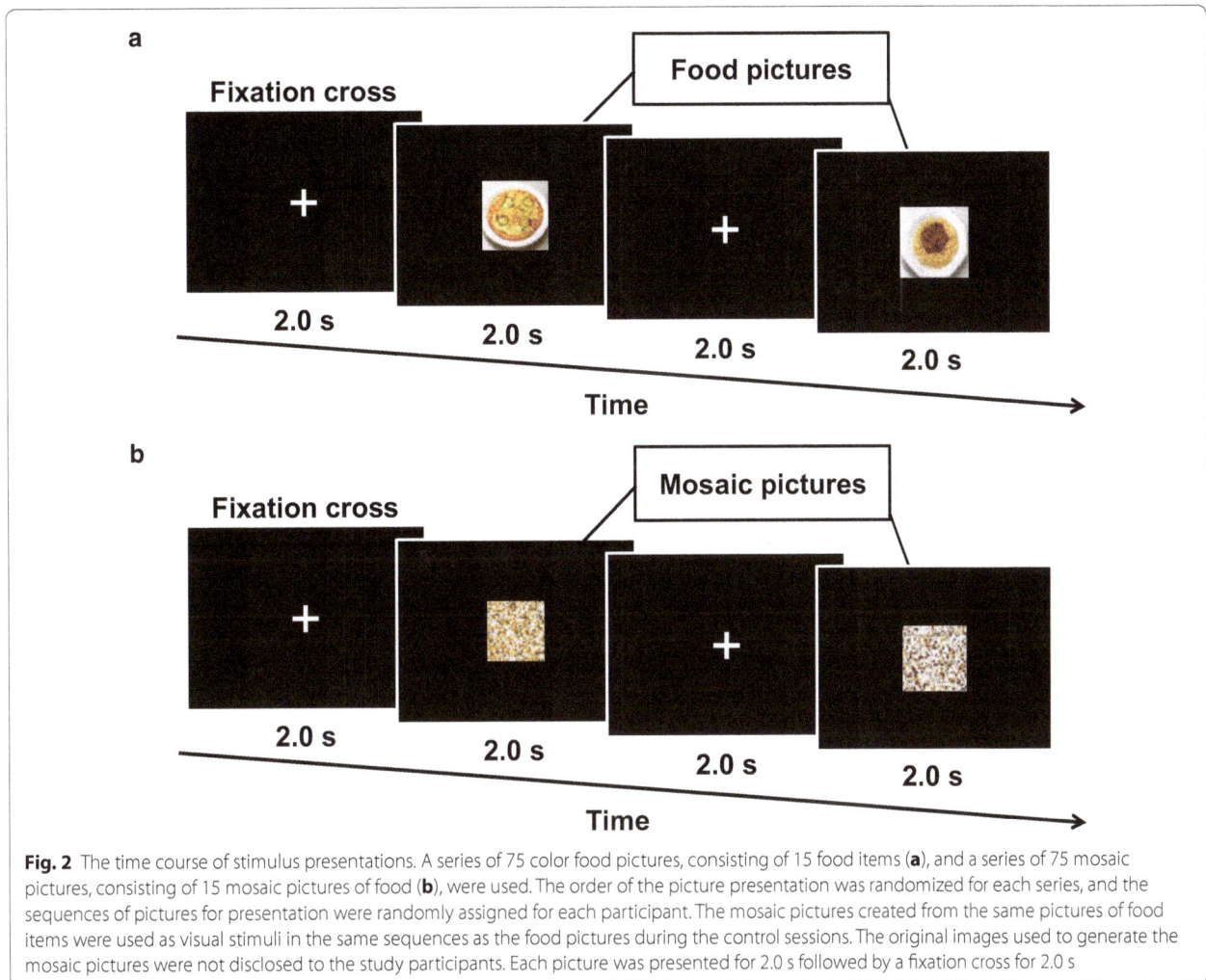

Fig. 2 The time course of stimulus presentations. A series of 75 color food pictures, consisting of 15 food items (**a**), and a series of 75 mosaic pictures, consisting of 15 mosaic pictures of food (**b**), were used. The order of the picture presentation was randomized for each series, and the sequences of pictures for presentation were randomly assigned for each participant. The mosaic pictures created from the same pictures of food items were used as visual stimuli in the same sequences as the food pictures during the control sessions. The original images used to generate the mosaic pictures were not disclosed to the study participants. Each picture was presented for 2.0 s followed by a fixation cross for 2.0 s

food items were not included. Each picture was used five times to construct the 75-picture set. The mosaic images of the original photographs (15 food items) were also used to control for luminance, color, and local features [24, 25]. Mosaic pictures were made using commercial software (Adobe® Photoshop Elements 6.0, Adobe Systems Inc., San Jose, CA). All of the food pictures were divided into a 30 × 30 grid and randomly reordered by a constant algorithm. This rearrangement made each picture unrecognizable as food. The original images used to generate the mosaic pictures were not disclosed to the study participants. The sequences of pictures for presentation were randomly assigned for each participant, but the same sequences were used for both food-picture and control experiments. These pictures were projected on a screen placed in front of the participants' eyes using a video projector (PG-B10S; SHARP, Osaka, Japan). The viewing angle of each picture was 18.4 × 14.0°.

MEG data acquisition

MEG data acquisition was performed using a whole-head type MEG system (MEG vision; Yokogawa Electric Corporation, Tokyo, Japan) with 160 channels. The signals were continuously recorded at a sampling rate of 1000 Hz in gradiometers 15.5 mm in diameter and 50 mm in baseline with a 0.3 Hz high-pass filter.

Structural MR images were obtained using a Philips Achieva 3.0TX (Royal Philips Electronics, Eindhoven, The Netherlands). Before MRI scanning, 5 adhesive markers (Medtronic Surgical Navigation Technologies Inc., Broomfield, CO) were attached to the skin of each participant's head (the first and second ones were located 10 mm in front of the left tragus and right tragus, the third at 35 mm above the nasion, and the fourth and fifth at 40 mm right and left of the third one), which were the former positions of MEG localization coils. MEG data were coregistered on MRI scans using information obtained from these markers and MEG localization coils.

MEG data analyses

MEG data analyses were performed similarly as described in our previous study [20]. Briefly, MEG signal data were analyzed offline after analogue-to-digital conversion. Magnetic noise originating outside the shield room was eliminated by subtracting the data obtained from reference coils using MEG 160 (Yokogawa Electric Corporation, Tokyo, Japan). Artifact rejection of MEG data was performed through careful visual artifact detection before band pass filtering and averaging. The MEG data were band-pass filtered by a fast Fourier transform using frequency trend (Yokogawa Electric Corporation) to obtain time–frequency band signals using a software, brain rhythmic analysis for MEG (BRAM; Yokogawa Electric Corporation) [26]. After the band pass filtering, the MEG data were split into segments of 1000 ms in length, and the segments were averaged.

Localization and intensity of the time–frequency power changes were assessed by BRAM software, which used narrow-band adaptive spatial filtering methods as an algorithm [26]. We used statistical parametric mapping (SPM8, Welcome Department of Cognitive Neurology, London, UK) in Matlab (Mathworks, Sherbon, MA) to analyze the MEG data. We initially performed normalization to the Montreal Neurological Institute (MNI) template of T1-weighed images [27] and smoothing (the normalized MEG data were filtered with a Gaussian kernel of 20 mm [full-width at half-maximum] in the x, y, and z axes [voxel dimension was $5.0 \times 5.0 \times 5.0$ mm]). The whole brain oscillatory powers for δ-band (1–4 Hz), θ-band (4–8 Hz), α-band (8–13 Hz), β-band (13–25 Hz), and γ-band (25–50 Hz) during the eye-closed session were measured on a region-of-interest basis. To investigate the alterations of the brain activities during the resting eye-closed condition after the visual stimulation session, we analyzed two contrast images: image after the visual stimulation of food pictures > image before the visual stimulation of food pictures; and image after the visual stimulation of mosaic pictures > image before the visual stimulation of mosaic pictures. The two contrast images were submitted to one sample t test on a voxel-by-voxel basis [28]. The threshold of individual analyses was set at $P < 0.05$ (corrected for multiple comparisons). Individual data were incorporated into a random-effect model so that inferences could be made at a population level [28]. The threshold of group analyses was set at $P < 0.05$ (corrected for multiple comparisons). Anatomical localizations of significant voxels within clusters were expressed in the form of MNI stereotactic spatial coordinates (x, y, z). In addition, these coordinates were converted to corresponding Brodmann's area (BA) by using the Talairach Daemon software [29].

Statistical analyses

Data are expressed as mean ± SD. Two-way analyses of variance followed by paired t test with Bonferroni correction were performed to examine the differences in VAS scores for appetitive motives among different sessions and experiments. Pearson's correlation analyses were used to examine whether the changes in the power of resting oscillatory brain activities by visual food presentation might be associated with subjective variables. All P values were two-tailed, and values less than 0.05 were considered statistically significant. Statistical analyses were performed using the SPSS 18.0 software package (SPSS, Inc., Chicago, IL).

Results

Decrease of resting oscillatory brain activities after visual food stimulation

Table 1 summarizes the results of spatial filtering analyses that show brain regions with a greater decrease of resting oscillatory band power during the eye-closed session after a cessation of visual food stimulation relative to that before the stimulation. These include the following 4 regions: (1) the right insula (BA13); (2) the right middle frontal gyrus (BA9 and 46) corresponding to the dorsolateral prefrontal cortex (DLPFC); (3) the left subcallosal gyrus (BA11) corresponding to the orbitofrontal cortex (OFC); and (4) the left superior frontal gyrus (BA10) corresponding to the frontal pole.

Rating scores of hunger before recordings of MEG, those of feeling of pleasure in eating food in daily life, and those of appetitive motives elicited spontaneously by presentation of food pictures—association with the decrease of resting oscillatory brain activities

Before the MEG recordings, all of the participants rated their subjective level of hunger as almost excessive [1.7 ± 0.6 (mean ± SD) on a 5-point Likert-type scale]. The mean VAS score of pleasure in eating food in daily life assessed was 78 ± 12 mm. They had considerable motives to eat during the visual stimulation in the food-picture experiment (Table 2). The subjective VAS scores for appetitive motives in the food-picture experiment were significantly higher than those in the control experiment ($P < 0.001$, main effect of experiment assessed by two-way analysis of variance), and the scores were significantly increased by the visual stimulation of food items ($P < 0.001$, main effect of session assessed by two-way analysis of variance; $P < 0.001$, assessed by post hoc paired t-test with Bonferroni correction). Correlation analyses revealed that the VAS scores for pleasure in eating food in daily life were positively associated with the decrease of the γ-band power of resting oscillatory brain activities in the right insula (BA13) ($r = 0.536$, $P = 0.040$)

Table 1 Brain regions that show a greater decrease of resting oscillatory band power during the eye-closed session (after a cessation of visual food stimulation) relative to that before the stimulation

Location	Frequency band (Hz)	Side	BA	MNI coordinate (mm)			Z value
				x	y	z	
DLPFC	4–8	R	9	52	28	40	3.78
OFC	8–13	L	11	−38	38	−15	3.94
DLPFC	8–13	R	46	42	48	20	3.57
Insula	25–50	R	13	42	−7	5	3.36
Insula	25–50	R	13	42	8	0	3.35
Frontal pole	25–50	L	10	−23	53	−5	2.93
OFC	25–50	L	11	−13	28	−10	2.76
DLPFC	25–50	R	9	27	53	40	2.71

x, y, z: stereotaxic coordinates of peak of activated clusters

BA Brodmann's area, MNI Montreal Neurological Institute, DLPFC dorsolateral prefrontal cortex, OFC orbitofrontal cortex, L left, R right

Random-effect analyses of 15 participants ($P < 0.05$, corrected for multiple comparisons at the voxel level)

Table 2 Subjective levels of appetitive motive

	Eye-closed session (before stimulation)	Visual stimulation session	Eye-closed session (after stimulation)
Food-picture experiment	34 ± 25	79 ± 17*	62 ± 26[†,‡]
Control experiment	37 ± 25	33 ± 28	32 ± 23

Data are expressed as mean ± SD (n = 15)

Participants were asked to rate their appetitive motive by using a visual analogue scale, ranging from none (0 mm) to maximum (100 mm)

Two-way analyses of variance followed by paired t test with Bonferroni correction were performed. Main effect of experiment, $P < 0.001$; main effect of session, $P < 0.001$; experiment × session interaction effect, $P < 0.001$

* $P < 0.001$ [visual stimulation session vs. eye-closed session (before stimulation)]

[†] $P = 0.007$ [visual stimulation session vs. eye-closed session (after stimulation)]

[‡] $P = 0.001$ [eye-closed session (before stimulation) vs. eye-closed session (after stimulation)]

(Fig. 3), and were inversely associated with that of α-band of resting oscillatory brain activities in the right DLPFC (BA46) ($r = -0.627$, $P = 0.012$) (Fig. 4), respectively. Significant correlations were found between the difference in the scores for appetitive motives during and after the food picture stimulation and the decrease of the γ-band power of resting oscillatory brain activities in the left frontal pole (BA10) ($r = 0.570$, $P = 0.027$) (Fig. 5). In addition, the decrease of the γ-band power of resting oscillatory brain activities in the left OFC (BA11) was negatively correlated with BMI ($r = -0.562$, $P = 0.029$) (Fig. 6).

Discussion

The present study demonstrates that a short duration of visual food stimuli has a considerable impact on resting oscillatory brain activities during eye closure in various emotional and cognitive brain areas such as the right insula (BA13), the right DLPFC (BA46), the left frontal pole (BA10) and the left OFC (BA11). Interestingly, the feelings of pleasure in eating food in daily life were positively associated with oscillatory power decreases in the insula, and negatively with those in DLPFC. Furthermore, in spite of the instruction not to think of anything including the pictures on the screen, the participants had appetitive motives spontaneously elicited by food picture stimulation, and the changes in appetitive motives were significantly related to the power decrease of the resting oscillatory brain activities in the left frontal pole.

One of the major findings is a significant decrease of the γ-band power of resting oscillatory brain activities in the right insula (BA13). Previous studies have suggested that this brain region performs a diversity of functions, some of which are linked to dietary lifestyle. For example, in our previous studies, equivalent current dipoles (ECDs) assessed by MEG were detected in the insula immediately (approximately 300 ms) after the onset of food picture presentation in response to viewing these pictures under the instruction to have appetitive motives in the fasting [19] or postprandial conditions [21]. These findings suggest the possible involvement of insula in the neural processes of the motivations to eat. Although the present study did not focus on the time course of the immediate neural responses after visual food stimuli nor on the neural

a
25-50 Hz
Peak (x, y, z) = (42, -7, 5), Insula, BA 13

b

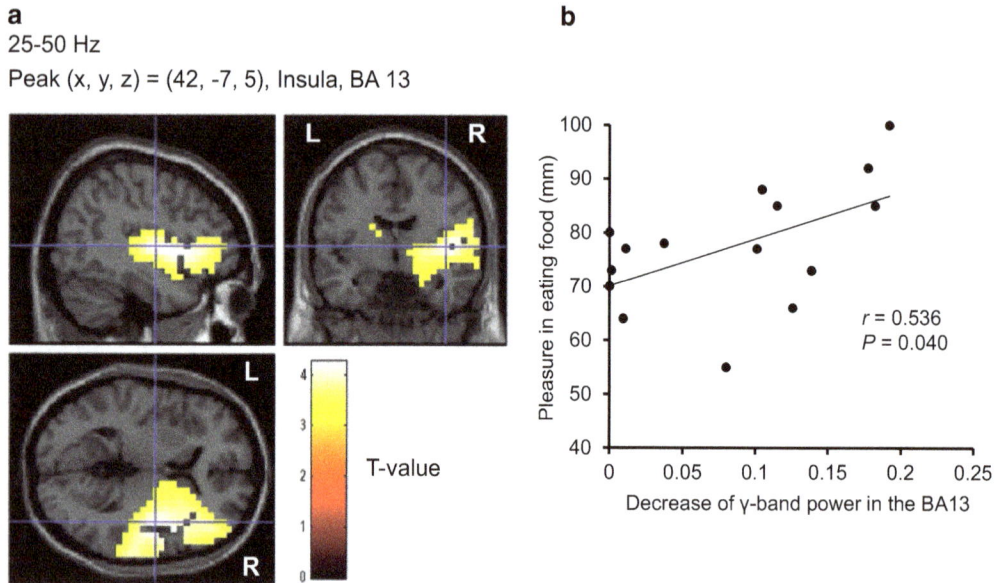

Fig. 3 Localization and intensity of the decrease of γ-band power during the eye-closed session after the cessation of the visual stimulation session, relative to the band power before the start of the visual stimulation session in the insula (BA13) (**a**) (random effect analyses of 15 participants, P < 0.05, corrected for multiple comparisons at voxel level) and association of the power decrease with the feeling of pleasure in eating food in daily life (**b**). **a** The results are superimposed on high-resolution MRIs averaged across all the participants. Sagittal (*upper left*), coronal (*upper right*), and axial (*lower left*) sections are shown. The *color bar* indicates T values. **b** Linear regression line, Pearson's correlation coefficient (*r*), and P value are shown. *BA* Brodmann's area, *R* right, *L* left

a
8-13 Hz
Peak (x, y, z) = (42, 48, 20), Frontal lobe, BA 46

b

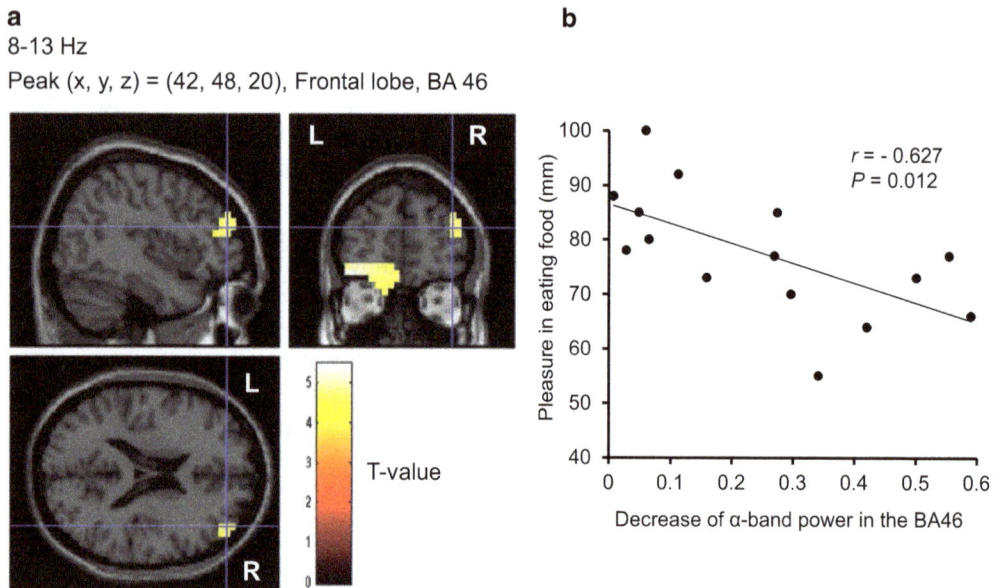

Fig. 4 Localization and intensity of the decrease of α-band power during the eye-closed session after the cessation of the visual stimulation session, relative to the band power before the start of the visual stimulation session in the DLPFC (BA46) (**a**) (random effect analyses of 15 participants, P < 0.05, corrected for multiple comparisons at voxel level) and association of the power decrease with the feeling of pleasure in eating food in daily life (**b**). **a** The results are superimposed on high-resolution MRIs averaged across all the participants. Sagittal (*upper left*), coronal (*upper right*), and axial (*lower left*) sections are shown. The *color bar* indicates T values. **b** Linear regression line, Pearson's correlation coefficient (*r*), and P value are shown. *BA* Brodmann's area, *DLPFC* dorsolateral prefrontal cortex, *R* right, *L* left

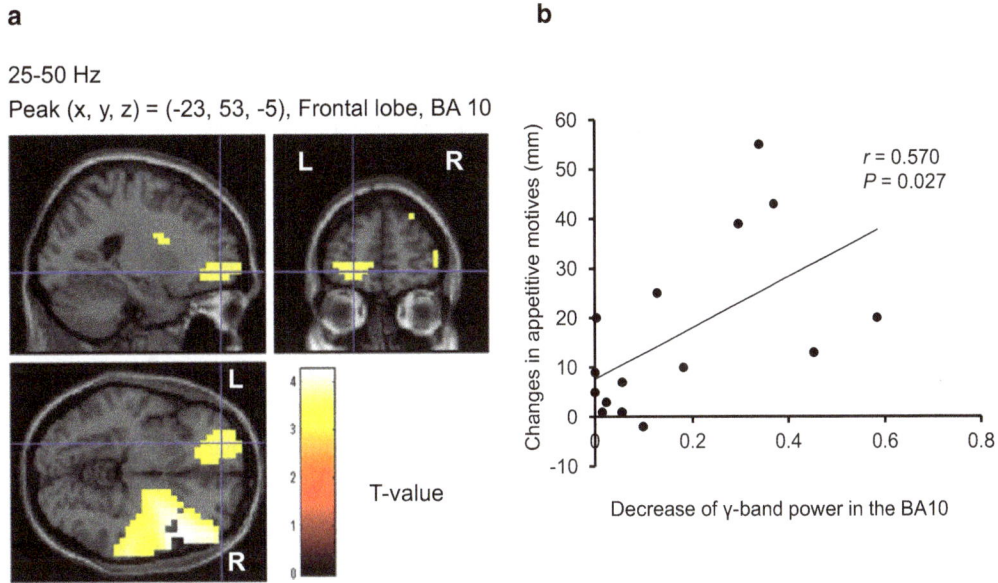

Fig. 5 Localization and intensity of the decrease of γ-band power during the eye-closed session after the cessation of the visual stimulation session, relative to the band power before the start of the visual stimulation session in the frontal pole (BA10) (**a**) (random effect analyses of 15 participants, $P < 0.05$, corrected for multiple comparisons at voxel level) and association of the power decrease with the changes in appetitive motives during and after visual food stimulation assessed by 100 mm VAS scores (**b**). **a** The results are superimposed on high-resolution MRIs averaged across all the participants. Sagittal (*upper left*), coronal (*upper right*), and axial (*lower left*) sections are shown. The *color bar* indicates T values. **b** Linear regression line, Pearson's correlation coefficient (*r*), and *P* value are shown. *BA* Brodmann's area, *R* right, *L* left, *VAS* visual analogue scale

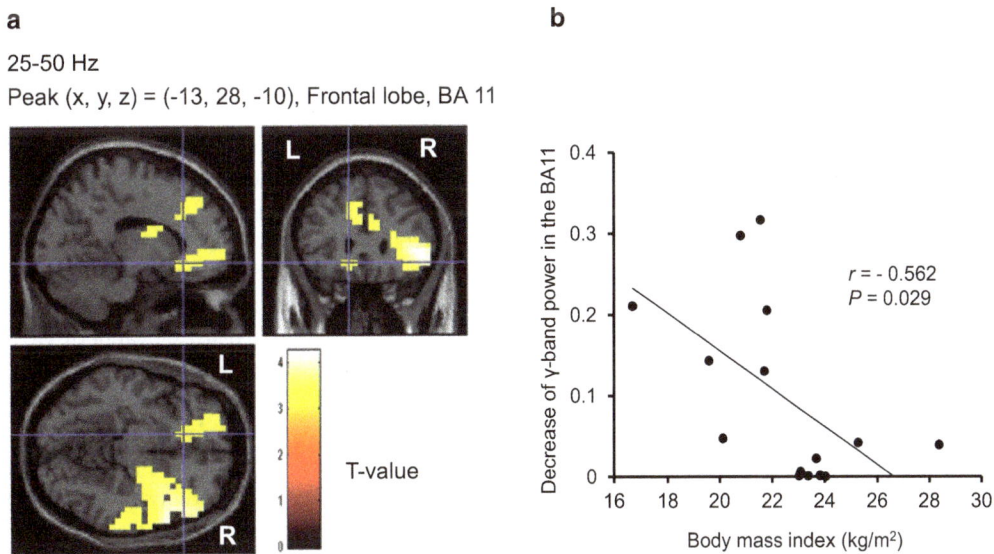

Fig. 6 Localization and intensity of the decrease of γ-band power during the eye-closed session after the cessation of the visual stimulation session, relative to the band power before the start of the visual stimulation session in the OFC (BA11) (**a**) (random effect analyses of 15 participants, $P < 0.05$, corrected for multiple comparisons at voxel level) and association of the power decrease with body mass index (**b**). **a** The results are superimposed on high-resolution MRIs averaged across all the participants. Sagittal (*upper left*), coronal (*upper right*), and axial (*lower left*) sections are shown. The *color bar* indicates T values. **b** Linear regression line, Pearson's correlation coefficient (*r*), and *P* value are shown. *BA* Brodmann's area, *OFC* orbitofrontal cortex, *R* right, *L* left

responses with having motivation to eat volitionally, a new evidence has surfaced that would support the involvement of insular activity even during the absence of visual food stimuli. Furthermore, the present study demonstrates the positive association of the resting brain activity in the insula with the feelings of pleasure in eating food in daily life. In line with this, functions of insula include the representation of pleasantness of flavor [30] and the control of habituation in food-related stimulation [31]. Considering these previous evidences, it is possible that the present residual insular activity as observed even after a cessation of stimulation might play a role in the formation of the positive emotional aspect (feeling of pleasure) in eating food and subsequently modify the habituation process of eating behaviors in daily dietary life.

Another finding in the present study was a significant decrease of the α-band power of resting oscillatory brain activities in the right DLPFC (BA46). In addition, the present study showed the inverse association of the resting brain activities in this brain region with the feelings of pleasure in eating food in daily life. In other words, the changes in the resting brain activity in the DLPFC tends to be more pronounced in individuals with less pleasure associated with eating food. Most of the previous studies demonstrated that the DLPFC plays a major role in the self-control in eating food as indicated by an association of the brain activities with the measure of ordinary eating behaviors such as cognitive restraints assessed using questionnaires [32, 33]. The present finding might imply that cognitive self-control of the desire for food might affect the expression of positive emotion to eat such as pleasure in eating food via this brain mechanism. Combined with the results in insular activity, the transient visual food stimuli could disturb the emotional and cognitive domains of the resting brain activities even in the absence of concurrent visual stimuli.

In the present study, it is important to note that the participants were asked not to think of anything about pictures in the stimulus presentation. Nevertheless, their appetitive motives were spontaneously elicited as assessed using the VAS, and interestingly, the changes in appetitive motives were positively associated with the power decrease of the resting oscillatory brain activities in the left frontal pole. The frontal poles have been reported to play roles in memory retrieval [34–36] as well as in memory encoding and recognition [36–38]. In addition to the functions of retrospective memory, the frontal poles are more involved with thinking about the future than about the past [39]. Based on the observed association with temporal fluctuations in appetitive scores of VAS, the frontal pole plays a role in subsequent planning, such as thinking about what to eat after a cessation of visual exposure of food items.

Previous neuroimaging studies have been inconsistent regarding structural and functional alterations in obesity. In particular, the OFC is one of major components of reward circuitry related to overeating palatable food and development of obesity [11, 40, 41]. In contrast, the OFC is reported to be an important structure in the termination of food intake, and disturbance in this function could contribute to overconsumption of food in obesity [42]. The present study demonstrated that the resting brain activity observed in the OFC is negatively correlated with the BMI. The range of the BMI in the present participants was less than 30 kg/m². Its physiological and clinical implications warrant further studies, particularly in more obese individuals.

Accumulating evidence suggests that visual afferent signals provide information to the central nervous system for appetite regulation even before food is ingested, and the limbic, paralimbic, and frontal brain circuits play important roles in neural processing during the visual stimuli in obese, healthy weight, and weight-loss populations [11, 43]. These brain regions are known to participate in emotional, salience, memory, reward, cognitive, and visual processing. In contrast, only a limited number of neuroimaging studies have addressed the residual effect of neural responses after the cessation of visual food stimulation like aftertaste [44]. Such a residual effect might be one of the important determinants of pleasure after a meal, possibly leading to a dietary learning process, irrespective of the type of sensation, and affect the decision to start or to stop eating subsequently [45]. Compared with traditional research, the present observation is unique because the essence of the study design was to examine the residual effect of neural responses to visual food stimuli by assessing the differences of the resting oscillatory brain activities before and after a series of visual presentations of food items. Collectively, the observed characteristics of the changes of resting brain activity before and after visual food stimulation might contribute to the formation of the feeling of pleasure in eating food and irresistible appetitive motives, and it might affect subsequent eating behaviors, possibly through emotional and cognitive functions including memory retrieval and future planning.

The present study has some potential limitations. First, we examined the brain activity in normal-weight young adults without apparent eating disorders during a fasted state. In order to clarify the impact of the changes of resting brain activities in general, further studies using similar MEG analytic methods in individuals with distorted eating habits and eating disorders in either the fasting state and/ or during satiety will be needed. Second, the design of the present study is to assess brain activity caused by visual food cues. Since eating behavior can be evoked through multiple sensory systems, in order to generalize the results of our data, future studies using other sensory modalities are essential. Third, a small number of subjects were recruited in the present study. A large population study will be necessary to confirm the present results. Fourth, the present instruction not to think of anything, including the pictures on the screen, might force the study participants to attempt to suppress their thoughts and feelings more than required. The observed brain areas related to self-control systems like DLPFC might not be in accordance with the original study purpose to identify brain areas of the resting brain activities simply when one closes his eyes without thinking anything. Fifth, it is more likely that, after the visual stimulation session, the hungry participants were 'replaying' in their heads the pictures of food that they saw a couple of minutes earlier. It is well known that experiencing an actual sensory stimulus or imagining the sensory stimulus activates the same brain areas. Sixth, in the present study, we did not measure brain activity during the 5-min visual food stimulation. Since the brain areas activated and the power changes obtained during stimulation might correlate with the power changes and activation locations after stimulation, it will be needed to compare the brain activities among before, during and after the visual food stimulation. Seventh, the analyses included a one-sample test on two contrasts involving time following food and mosaic pictures. A 2 (time) $\times$ 2 (stimuli) interaction effect should be tested to determine the specificity of the effect. Lastly, we cannot draw conclusions about cause-and-effect relationships because of the cross-sectional nature of our data.

Conclusions

The present findings raised the intriguing possibility that a series of visual food stimuli have a significant impact on resting oscillatory brain activities in the insula, DLPFC, OFC, and frontal pole. Since the changes of the resting brain activity are positively associated with positive emotion such as pleasure in eating food in daily life and appetitive motives, these changes are likely to determine subsequent eating behaviors. Although firm intention and conscious efforts are necessary for improvements in abnormal eating behavior and habits in a person's dietary lifestyle, it is also important to devote considerable attention to the characteristics of the automatic or unconscious brain mechanics after food-related stimulation in order to develop efficient strategies for optimizing dietary lifestyle in people who fall into overeating and anorexia against their will.

Abbreviations

BA: Brodmann's area; BMI: body mass index; BRAM: brain rhythmic analysis for MEG; DLPFC: dorsolateral prefrontal cortex; fMRI: functional magnetic resonance imaging; MEG: magnetoencephalography; MNI: Montreal Neurological Institute; MRI: magnetic resonance imaging; OFC: orbitofrontal cortex; PET: positron emission tomography; VAS: visual analogue scale.

Authors' contributions

TY and MT took part in planning and designing the experiment, collected the data, performed the data analyses and drafted the manuscript. AI took part in planning and designing the experiment, collected the data, and performed the data analyses. YY took part in performing data analyses and literature survey. YW took part in planning and designing the experiment and helped drafting the manuscript. All authors read and approved the final manuscript.

Author details

[1] Department of Sports Medicine, Osaka City University Graduate School of Medicine, 1-4-3 Asahi-machi, Abeno-ku, Osaka, Osaka 545-8585, Japan. [2] Department of Physiology, Osaka City University Graduate School of Medicine, 1-4-3 Asahi-machi, Abeno-ku, Osaka, Osaka 545-8585, Japan. [3] RIKEN Center for Life Science Technologies, 6-7-3 Minatojima-minamimachi, Chuo-ku, Hyogo 650-0047, Japan.

Acknowledgements

The authors would like to thank Manryoukai Imaging Clinic for MRI scans and Forte Science Communications for native English editorial help with the manuscript.

Competing interests

The authors declare that they have no competing interests.

Funding

This work was supported in part by the Grant-in-Aid for Scientific Research C (KAKENHI: 26350899) from Ministry of Education, Culture, Sports, Science and Technology (MEXT) of Japan. The funders had no roles in study design, data collection and analysis, decision to publish, or preparation of the manuscript.

References

1. Hill JO, Wyatt HR, Reed GW, Peters JC. Obesity and the environment: where do we go from here? Science. 2003;299(5608):853–5.
2. Must A, Spadano J, Coakley EH, Field AE, Colditz G, Dietz WH. The disease burden associated with overweight and obesity. JAMA. 1999;282(16):1523–9.
3. van der Klaauw AA, Farooqi IS. The hunger genes: pathways to obesity. Cell. 2015;161(1):119–32.
4. Roberts SB. Effects of aging on energy requirements and the control of food intake in men. J Gerontol A Biol Sci Med Sci. 1995;50:101–6.
5. Hoek HW. Incidence, prevalence and mortality of anorexia nervosa and other eating disorders. Curr Opin Psychiatry. 2006;19(4):389–94.
6. Smeets PA, Charbonnier L, van Meer F, van der Laan LN, Spetter MS. Food-induced brain responses and eating behaviour. Proc Nutr Soc. 2012;71(4):511–20.
7. Morton GJ, Cummings DE, Baskin DG, Barsh GS, Schwartz MW. Central nervous system control of food intake and body weight. Nature. 2006;443(7109):289–95.
8. Rolls ET. Understanding the mechanisms of food intake and obesity. Obes Rev. 2007;8(Suppl 1):67–72.
9. Berthoud HR. Metabolic and hedonic drives in the neural control of appetite: who is the boss? Curr Opin Neurobiol. 2011;21(6):888–96.
10. Singh M. Mood, food, and obesity. Front Psychol. 2014;5:925.
11. Carnell S, Gibson C, Benson L, Ochner CN, Geliebter A. Neuroimaging and obesity: current knowledge and future directions. Obes Rev. 2012;13(1):43–56.
12. Nunez PL, Srinivasan R. Electric fields of the brain. 2nd ed. Oxford: Oxford University Press; 2005.
13. Sekihara K, Nagarajan SS. Neuromagnetic source reconstruction and inverse modeling. In: He B, editor. Modeling and imaging of bioelectrical activity. New York: Kluwer Academic/Plenum Publishers; 2005. p. 213–50.
14. Hämäläinen M, Hari R, Ilmoniemi RJ, Knuutila J, Lounasmaa OV. Magnetoencephalography—theory, instrumentation, and applications to noninvasive studies of the working human brain. Rev Mod Phys. 1993;65(2):413–97.

15. Schnitzler A, Gross J, Timmermann L. Synchronised oscillations of the human sensorimotor cortex. Acta Neurobiol Exp (Wars). 2000;60(2):271–87.

16. Stam CJ. Use of magnetoencephalography (MEG) to study functional brain networks in neurodegenerative disorders. J Neurol Sci. 2010;289(1–2):128–34.

17. Pfurtscheller G, Lopes da Silva FH. Event-related EEG/MEG synchronization and desynchronization: basic principles. Clin Neurophysiol. 1999;110(11):1842–57.

18. Singer W. Synchronization of cortical activity and its putative role in information processing and learning. Annu Rev Physiol. 1993;55:349–74.

19. Yoshikawa T, Tanaka M, Ishii A, Watanabe Y. Immediate neural responses of appetitive motives and its relationship with hedonic appetite and body weight as revealed by magnetoencephalography. Med Sci Monit. 2013;19:631–40.

20. Yoshikawa T, Tanaka M, Ishii A, Fujimoto S, Watanabe Y. Neural regulatory mechanism of desire for food: revealed by magnetoencephalography. Brain Res. 2014;1543:120–7.

21. Yoshikawa T, Tanaka M, Ishii A, Watanabe Y. Suppressive responses by visual food cues in postprandial activities of insular cortex as revealed by magnetoencephalography. Brain Res. 2014;1568:31–41.

22. World Medical Association. World Medical Association Declaration of Helsinki: ethical principles for medical research involving human subjects. J Am Coll Dent. 2014;81(3):14–8.

23. Science and Technology Agency in Japan. Standard tables of food composition in Japan. 5th ed. Tokyo: Printing Bureau of the Ministry of Finance; 2005.

24. Allison T, McCarthy G, Nobre A, Puce A, Belger A. Human extrastriate visual cortex and the perception of faces, words, numbers, and colors. Cereb Cortex. 1994;4(5):544–54.

25. Nakamura K, Kawashima R, Sato N, Nakamura A, Sugiura M, Kato T, Hatano K, Ito K, Fukuda H, Schormann T, et al. Functional delineation of the human occipito-temporal areas related to face and scene processing. A PET study. Brain. 2000;123(Pt 9):1903–12.

26. Dalal SS, Guggisberg AG, Edwards E, Sekihara K, Findlay AM, Canolty RT, Berger MS, Knight RT, Barbaro NM, Kirsch HE, et al. Five-dimensional neuroimaging: localization of the time-frequency dynamics of cortical activity. Neuroimage. 2008;40(4):1686–700.

27. Evans AC, Kamber M, Collins DL, MacDonald D. An MRI-based probabilistic atlas of neuroanatomy. In: Shorvon SD, editor. Magnetic resonance scanning and epilepsy. New York: Plenum Press; 1994.

28. Friston KJ, Holmes AP, Worsley KJ. How many subjects constitute a study? Neuroimage. 1999;10(1):1–5.

29. Lancaster JL, Woldorff MG, Parsons LM, Liotti M, Freitas CS, Rainey L, Kochunov PV, Nickerson D, Mikiten SA, Fox PT. Automated Talairach atlas labels for functional brain mapping. Hum Brain Mapp. 2000;10(3):120–31.

30. de Araujo IE, Rolls ET, Kringelbach ML, McGlone F, Phillips N. Taste-olfactory convergence, and the representation of the pleasantness of flavour, in the human brain. Eur J Neurosci. 2003;18(7):2059–68.

31. Poellinger A, Thomas R, Lio P, Lee A, Makris N, Rosen BR, Kwong KK. Activation and habituation in olfaction—an fMRI study. Neuroimage. 2001;13(4):547–60.

32. Burger KS, Stice E. Relation of dietary restraint scores to activation of reward-related brain regions in response to food intake, anticipated intake, and food pictures. Neuroimage. 2011;55(1):233–9.

33. Hollmann M, Hellrung L, Pleger B, Schlögl H, Kabisch S, Stumvoll M, Villringer A, Horstmann A. Neural correlates of the volitional regulation of the desire for food. Int J Obes (Lond). 2012;36(5):648–55.

34. Tulving E, Kapur S, Markowitsch HJ, Craik FI, Habib R, Houle S. Neuroanatomical correlates of retrieval in episodic memory: auditory sentence recognition. Proc Natl Acad Sci USA. 1994;91(6):2012–5.

35. Düzel E, Picton TW, Cabeza R, Yonelinas AP, Scheich H, Heinze HJ, Tulving E. Comparative electrophysiological and hemodynamic measures of neural activation during memory-retrieval. Hum Brain Mapp. 2001;13(2):104–23.

36. Rugg MD, Fletcher PC, Frith CD, Frackowiak RS, Dolan RJ. Differential activation of the prefrontal cortex in successful and unsuccessful memory retrieval. Brain. 1996;119(Pt 6):2073–83.

37. Ranganath C, Johnson MK, D'Esposito M. Prefrontal activity associated with working memory and episodic long-term memory. Neuropsychologia. 2003;41(3):378–89.

38. Tulving E, Habib R, Nyberg L, Lepage M, McIntosh AR. Positron emission tomography correlations in and beyond medial temporal lobes. Hippocampus. 1999;9(1):71–82.

39. Okuda J, Fujii T, Ohtake H, Tsukiura T, Tanji K, Suzuki K, Kawashima R, Fukuda H, Itoh M, Yamadori A. Thinking of the future and past: the roles of the frontal pole and the medial temporal lobes. Neuroimage. 2003;19(4):1369–80.

40. Berridge KC, Ho CY, Richard JM, DiFeliceantonio AG. The tempted brain eats: pleasure and desire circuits in obesity and eating disorders. Brain Res. 2010;1350:43–64.

41. Small DM, Zatorre RJ, Dagher A, Evans AC, Jones-Gotman M. Changes in brain activity related to eating chocolate: from pleasure to aversion. Brain. 2001;124(Pt 9):1720–33.

42. Shott ME, Cornier MA, Mittal VA, Pryor TL, Orr JM, Brown MS, Frank GK. Orbitofrontal cortex volume and brain reward response in obesity. Int J Obes (Lond). 2015;39(2):214–21.

43. Pursey KM, Stanwell P, Callister RJ, Brain K, Collins CE, Burrows TL. Neural responses to visual food cues according to weight status: a systematic review of functional magnetic resonance imaging studies. Front Nutr. 2014;1:7.

44. James GA, Li X, DuBois GE, Zhou L, Hu XP. Prolonged insula activation during perception of aftertaste. Neuroreport. 2009;20(3):245–50.

45. Brunstrom JM. Dietary learning in humans: directions for future research. Physiol Behav. 2005;85(1):57–65.

Involvement of hippocampal acetylcholinergic receptors in electroacupuncture analgesia in neuropathic pain rats

Shu Ping Chen[1], Yu Kan[1], Jian Liang Zhang[1], Jun Ying Wang[1], Yong Hui Gao[1], Li Na Qiao[2], Xiu Mei Feng[1], Ya Xia Yan[1] and Jun Ling Liu[1]* 🄳

Abstract

Background: Cumulating evidence has shown a close correlation between electroacupuncture stimulation (EAS) frequency-specific analgesic effect and central opioid peptides. However, the actions of hippocampal acetylcholinergic receptors have not been determined. This study aims to observe the effect of different frequencies of EAS on the expression of hippocampal muscarinic and nicotinic acetylcholinergic receptors (mAChRs, nAChRs) in neuropathic pain rats for revealing their relationship.

Methods: Forty male Wistar rats were randomly and equally divided into sham, CCI model, 2, 2/15 and 100 HzEA groups. The neuropathic pain model was established by ligature of the left sciatic nerve to induce chronic constriction injury (CCI). EAS was applied to bilateral Zusanli (ST36) and Yanglingquan (GB34) for 30 min, once daily for 14 days except weekends. The mechanical pain thresholds (withdrawal latencies, PWLs) of bilateral hindpaws were measured. The expression levels of hippocampal M1 and M2 mAChR, and α4 and β2 nAChR genes and proteins were detected by quantitative RT-PCR and Western blot, separately. The involvement of mAChR and nAChR in the analgesic effect of EAS was confirmed by intra-hippocampal microinjection of M_1mAChR antagonist (Pirenzepine) and α4β2 nAChR antagonist (dihydro-beta-erythroidine) respectively.

Results: Following EAS, the CCI-induced increase of difference values of bilateral PWLs on day 6 and 14 was significantly reduced (P < 0.05), with 2/15 Hz being greater than 100 Hz EAS on day 14 (P < 0.05). After 2 weeks' EAS, the decreased expression levels of M1 mAChR mRNA of both 2 and 2/15 Hz groups and M1 mAChR protein of the three EAS groups, α4 AChR mRNA of the 2/15 Hz group and β2 nAChR protein of the three EAS groups were considerably increased (P < 0.05), suggesting an involvement of M1 mAChR and β2 nAChR proteins in EAS-induced pain relief. No significant changes were found in the expression of M2 mAChR mRNA and protein, α4 nAChR protein and β2 nAChR mRNA after CCI and EAS (P > 0.05). The analgesic effect of EAS was abolished by intra-hippocampal microinjection of M_1mAChR and α4β2 nAChR antagonists respectively.

Conclusions: EAS of ST36-GB34 produces a cumulative analgesic effect in neuropathic pain rats, which is frequency-dependent and probably mediated by hippocampal M1 mAChR and β2 nAChR proteins.

Keywords: Neuropathic pain, Electroacupuncture analgesia, Stimulating frequencies, Hippocampus, M1 muscarinic acetylcholinergic receptor (M1 mAChR), M2 mAChR, Alpha-4 nicotinic AChR (nAChR), Beta-2 nAChR

*Correspondence: 13521898023@163.com
[1] Department of Physiology, Institute of Acupuncture and Moxibustion, China Academy of Chinese Medical Sciences, 16 Nanxiaojie Street, Dongzhimennei, Beijing 100700, China
Full list of author information is available at the end of the article

Background

It has been well documented that chronic pain including neuropathic pain involves complex brain circuits for sensory, emotional, cognitive and interoceptive processing [1, 2]. The hippocampus, one of the limbic structures for antinociception [3], has been shown to undergo significant changes including reduction of hippocampal volume, learning and emotional deficits, sustained endocrine stress response, etc., in chronic pain syndrome patients [4–8], and abnormal expression of cytokine, extracellular signal-regulated kinase, neurokinin-1 (NK-1) receptor, etc., in experimental chronic neuropathic pain animals [9–11].

Among the neurotransmitters or mediators involving the chronic pain induced abnormal behavioral deficits, acetylcholine (ACh) is an important candidate in the hippocampus. Studies repeatedly demonstrated that cholinergic compounds produced antinociceptive effects in the rhesus monkey [12], cat [13] and rat [14–17]. Systemic administration of cholinesterase inhibitors which cross the blood brain barrier was found to produce analgesia and enhance analgesia from opiates [18, 19].

Early studies on acupuncture analgesia have already shown that hippocampal cholinergic activities are involved in acupuncture analgesia [20–22]. But, related researches are relatively fewer. In recent years, we demonstrated that both hippocampal and hypothalamic cholinergic activities were involved in the cumulative analgesia induced by repeated electroacupuncture stimulation (EAS) of "Zusanli" (ST36) and "Yanglingquan" (GB34) in rats with chronic constrictive injury (CCI) of the sciatic nerve [23, 24]. However, the detailed mechanisms underlying involvement of ACh in analgesia are still not clear.

Moreover, stimulating parameters, particularly the frequency, are important factors affecting the analgesic effect of EAS [25]. Chen and Wang [26] reported that in 252 cases of soft tissue injury-induced pain patients, 100 Hz EAS was significantly better than 2 Hz EAS in the cure rate and effective rate for pain. On the contrary, Zou et al. [27] observed that in 90 cases of acute arthritis patients, 2 Hz EAS was apparently better than 100 Hz EAS in pain-relief. Experimental studies also showed contradictory results about the analgesic effect of different frequencies of EAS in different acute pain models [28, 29].

In regard to the analgesic mechanisms of different EAS frequencies, majority of researches focused on the release of endogenous opioid peptides, one of which is Han's and his colleagues' well-known conclusion that 2 Hz EAS induced analgesia mediated by the release of met-enkephalin (M-ENK) and β-endorphin (β-EP), while 100 Hz EAS via dynorphin-A (DYN-A) in the central nervous system [30–34]. Latter, 5-HT in the brainstem

[35, 36], catecholamine [37, 38], hypothalamic substance P [39], cholecystokinin (CCK) and CCK-A and -B receptors [40] were found to be involved in the frequency-specific analgesic effect. However, to our knowledge, there have been no any reports on the cholinergic involvement of frequency-specific analgesic effect of EAS. For this reason, the present study was designed to observe the effect of EAS at different frequencies on pain behaviors and expressions of hippocampal muscarinic acetylcholine receptor (mAChR) and nicotinic acetylcholine receptor (nAChR) in CCI-induced neuropathic pain rats, thereby, to better our understanding on the mechanism of acupuncture in the management of neuropathic pain.

Methods

Animals and grouping

Male Wistar rats (230–270 g) were obtained from the Experimental Animal Center of Peking Union Medical College (Beijing, China), and housed within the animal care facilities in the Institute of Acupuncture and Moxibustion, China Academy of Chinese Medical Sciences. Rats were housed in a climate-controlled room on a 12 h light/dark cycle with food and water provided ad libitum. Animals were randomly divided into control (sham ligature), CCI model, CCI + 2 HzEA, CCI + 2/15 HzEA and CCI + 100 HzEA groups (n = 8 in each group). For verifying the effect of hippocampal mAChRs and nAChRs on EA analgesia, additional 30 male Wistar rats were randomized into control, model, saline-injection (saline), M1R-antagonist and nAChR-antagonist groups (n = 4 in each group). All experimental procedures were approved by the Institute of Acupuncture and Moxibustion of China Academy of Chinese Medical Sciences, and performed according to the "Guidelines for Laboratory Animal Care and Use" of the Chinese Ministry of Science and Technology (2006).

Neuropathic pain model and pain threshold detection

Following a 7-day environmental adaptation, rats were anesthetized (25 % urethane plus 1.5 % chloralose, 0.4 mL/100 g body weight) and received CCI of the sciatic nerve as previously described [41]. Briefly, the left posterolateral thigh was routinely sterilized, and a 2 cm incision was made through the skin. The left common sciatic nerve was exposed at mid-thigh by blunt dissection through the biceps femoris. Four constrictive ligatures (4–0 silk sutures) were tied around the nerve at the distal end close to the bifurcation site (about 1 mm space between every two ligatures). The ligature was alright until a moderate muscular contraction of the leg was seen. The same procedure was performed for rats in the control group but without nerve ligature. The incision was then closed using 5–0 silk sutures.

The paw withdrawal latency (PWL) (i.e., the mechanical pain threshold) of the bilateral hind paws was detected using a Dynamic Plantar Aesthesiometer (Ugo Basile, 37450, Italy) before CCI, 3 days after CCI, and 1, 6 and 14 days after EA treatment. Rats were placed on a metal mesh table and in an individual plexiglass housing at the same time. The steel rod (0.5 mm diameter) of 37450 was pushed up to the plantar surface of the hind paw with increasing force (2.5 g/s). The cutoff pressure was set to be 30 g and the threshold was recorded when the rat retracted its foot abruptly responding to the increased pressure. Thermal pain threshold was detected using PLANTAR TEST (Ugo Basile, 37370, Italy). The radiant heat source was focused on the plantar surface of the hindpaw, and light intensity was preset to obtain a baseline latency of approximately 15 s. Each rat underwent three trials with a 5-min inter-trial interval, and the mean value of these trials was used as the PWL. To minimize differences in individual animals, the difference value of PWL (PWLD) between the healthy and the affected hindpaws was calculated. Their hypersensitivities were defined as the presence of at least a 20 % decrease in pain threshold compared with pre-CCI baselines. Rats not exhibiting pain hypersensitivity after CCI were discarded.

Electroacupuncture intervention

Bilateral Zusanli (ST 36, 5 mm beneath the capitulum fibulae and lateral posterior to the knee-joint) and Yanglingquan (GB 34, about 5 mm superior-lateral to ST 36) were punctured with filiform needles (Gauge 28), respectively, and electrically stimulated using a HANS EA Apparatus (LH202, Beijing Huawei Industrial Developing Company, Beijing, China). EA (2 Hz, alternative 2/15, 100 Hz, 1 mA) was administered for 30 min, once per day for 1 or 2 weeks beginning from day 4 after surgery. For rats of hippocampal injection of M1mAChR and α4β2 nAChR antagonists, EA (2/15 Hz, 1 mA) was administered for 30 min, once daily for 5 days before the injection.

Intra-hippocampal injection

Under anesthesia with chloral hydrate (400 mg/kg i.p),the rat who experienced 3–5 days recovery from CCI operation was fixed in a stereotaxic instrument (Stoelting Co, USA) and stainless steel 26-gauge cannulae were implanted into the bilateral dorsal hippocampus (anteroposterior, −3.6 mm; medial-lateral, ± 3.1 mm; dorsoventral, −2.4 mm) according to Paxinos' and Watson's Atlas [The Rat Brain in Stereotaxic Coordinates, 6th edition from George Paxinos, Charles Watson], and fixed with dental cement. The stainless steel obdurator was remained in the cannulae before injection for preventing obstruction. After implantation of the cannula, each rat was

allowed to have a recovery period of at least 7 days before the experiments. For hippocampal injection, a mini-size pump (KDS310 Plus, kdScientific, USA) connected to the catheter was used for continuous infusion of antagonists [pirenzepine hydrochloride, M1mAChR selective antagonist, Sigma; dihydro-beta-erythroidine, an α4 β2 nAChR antagonist; Tocris, UK; dissolved in sterile saline to a concentration of 10 nmol/μL] or normal saline at a rate of 1 μL/h/hemisphere. The injector was remained connected for an additional 1 min to allow the drug diffusion away from the tip of the cannula. Before and 3−5 days after CCI surgery, 1, 3, and 5 days after hippocampal injections and EAS (2/15 Hz, 1 mA duration of 30 min), the thermal and mechanical pain thresholds were detected respectively. Rats with cannula-desquamation or death were excluded in the present study. The location of the intra-hippocampal catheter was confirmed by pantamine sky blue (0.2 %, 1 μL) microinjection after completion of the experiments.

Quantitative RT-PCR analysis

At the end of EA treatments, 6 randomly-selected rats of each group were deeply anesthetized with the anesthetics mentioned above, and the right hippocampus tissue was separated. Total RNA was extracted from the tissue using Trizol reagent (Invitrogen, USA). First-strand cDNA was synthesized by a reverse transcriptase kit (Invitrogen, USA) according to the manufacturer's instructions, and used as the template for quantitative RT-PCR analysis on a ABI 7500 fast real time system (Applied Biosystems, CA, USA), with β-actin as an internal control. Each reaction included 2 μl (25 ng/μl) of cDNA and was performed in triplicate.The primer sequences were as follows.

β-actin (NM_031144.3): 5′-GGAGATTACTGCCCTGG CTCCTA-3′ (Forward), 5′-GACTCATCGTACTCCTGC TTGCTG-3′ (Reverse) (bp:150); M1 mAChR (NM_ 080773.1): 5′-GCTGGAAGGAAGAAGAAGAGGAG GA-3′ (Forward), 5′-GCTGGAAGGAAGAAGAAGAGG AGGA (Reverse) (bp:160); M2 mAChR (NM_031061): 5′-CCATTCTCTTCTGGCAGTTCATCGT-3′ (Forward), TCTTTATTCTACTCTTGCTTGCCCG (Reverse) (bp: 183); β2 nAChR (NM_019297.1): 5′-CGGGAAGCA GTGGATGGCGTA -3′ (Forward), 5′-GTCCTCCCTCA CACTCTGGTCATCA-3′ (Reverse) (bp: 78); α4 nAChR (NM_024354.1): 5′-ATGGATGAAACCTACCTGATGA GCA-3′ (Forward), 5′-GCTGGGGGTTGTAGCAGGC AC-3′ (Reverse) (bp: 130). Cycling conditions were as follows: denaturation (95 °C for 10 min), amplification and quantitation (95 °C for 15 s, 60 °C for 60 s) repeated 40 times, and 72 °C for 32 s, with a single fluorescence measurement at the end of 72 °C for 32 s segment) repeated 35 times, a melting curve program (60–95 °C with a heating rate of 0.1 °C/s and continuous fluorescence measurement) and a cooling step to 40 °C. Quantitative RT-PCR data were normalized with β-actin mRNA levels. Relative mRNA levels were expressed as 2-ΔΔCt values.

Western blot analysis

Fresh contralateral hippocampal tissues were initially homogenized in lysis buffer containing a cocktail of phosphatase and proteinase inhibitors (Roche). Tissue protein concentrations were determined using the BCA protein assay kit (Pierce, Rockford). Protein samples(total 40 µg, 20 µl) were electrophoretically separated on a SDS-PAGE gel and transferred to polyvinylidene difluoride membranes (0.45 um pores; Millipore, Bedford, MA). The membranes were blocked with 2 % bovine serum albumin (BSA, Amresco, USA) solution for 2 h at room temperature (RT) and then incubated overnight at 4 °C with rabbit anti-M1 mAChR (1:2000, SC-9106, Santa) and mouse anti-M2 mAChR (1:2000, ab2805, Abcam), rabbit-anti- α-4nAChR (1:5000, Abcam, ab124832), rat anti-β2 nAChR (1:4000, ab24698, Abcam) primary antibodies. All antibodies were diluted in Tris-buffered saline solution containing 0.5 % Tween 20 (TBST) and 3.0 % BSA-TBSA. After washing in TBST, the blots were incubated with horseradish peroxidase (HRP)-conjugated secondary antibody for 2 h at RT (1:20,000; goat anti-rabbit immunoglobulin G; and 1:10,000: goat anti-mice IgG, 1:5000: goat anti-rat IgG). Following the rinse in TBST, the blots were developed using enhanced chemilluminescence for 1 min and exposed onto chemiluminescent films. For densitomentric analyses, the blots were scanned and quantified using TotalLab Quant analysis software (Totallab Limited, England), and the result was expressed as the ratio of target gene immunoreactivity to GAPDH immunoreactivity.

Statistical analysis

Data were expressed as mean ± standard deviation (mean ± SD). Data were analyzed via one-way ANOVA (for mRNA and protein expression) or two-way ANOVA (for pain thresholds) when appropriate, followed by least significant difference (LSD) tests for comparing data between groups. A value of $P < 0.05$ was considered statistically significant.

Results
Effect of EAS on pain threshold

As showed in Fig. 1 that after ligature of the sciatic nerve to induce CCI, the PWLDs were significantly increased in rats of the model group ($P < 0.05$, Fig. 1), suggesting a mechanical hypersensitivity 3 days after surgery. In comparison with the CCI model group, the PWLDs were pronouncedly decreased in rats of the CCI + EA2 Hz group and CCI + EA2/15 Hz group on day 6 and day 14 after CCI-operation ($P < 0.05$), and 2 Hz and 2/15 Hz EAS were notably superior to that of 100 Hz EAS in reducing PWLDS ($P < 0.05$, Fig. 1). In addition, the analgesic effect was gradually increased along with the extension of EA intervention, suggesting an accumulative effect of EA treatments.

Effect of EAS on hippocampal M1 and M2 mAChR gene and protein expression
M1 mAChR

In comparison with the control group, the expression levels of both M1 mAChR mRNA and protein in the hippocampus were significantly down-regulated ($P < 0.05$, Fig. 2a), suggesting an involvement of M1 mAChR in the nociceptive reactions following CCI. When compared with the CCI group, the expression

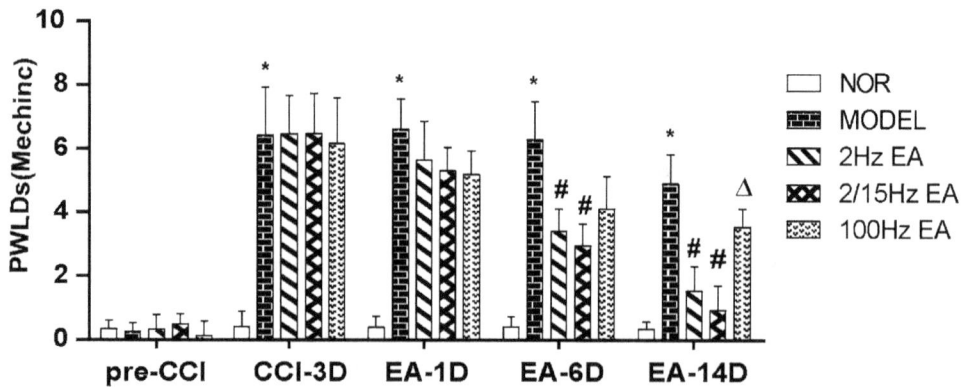

Fig. 1 Effect of different frequencies of electroacupuncture stimulation (EAS) of Zusanli (ST36) and Yanglingquan (GB34) on difference values of the bilateral hindpaw withdrawal latencies (PWLDs, mechanical pain threshold) in neuropathic pain rats (mean ± SD, g, n = 8 in each group); NOR normal group, Model group: CCI (chronic compressive injury), CCI + 2 Hz EAS group: 2 Hz EA, CCI + 2/15 Hz EAS group: 2/15 Hz EA, CCI + 100 Hz EAS group: 100 Hz EA (the same in Figs. 2, 3); *P < 0.05, vs the normal group; #P < 0.05, vs the model group; ΔP < 0.05, vs the 100 Hz EAS group

levels of M1 mAChR mRNA in both CCI + EA2 Hz and CCI + EA2/15 Hz groups and protein expression in CCI + EA2 Hz, CCI + EA2/15 Hz and CCI + EA100 Hz groups were considerably upregulated following 2 weeks' treatment (P < 0.05, Fig. 2b). The expression levels of M1 mAChR mRNA in both CCI + EA2 Hz group and CCI + EA2/15 Hz group were remarkably higher than that in the CCI + EA100 Hz group (P < 0.05, Fig. 2a). No significant differences were found among the three EAS groups in M1 mAChR protein expression levels, and between the CCI + EA2 Hz and CCI + EA2/15 Hz groups and between the CCI group and CCI + EA100 Hz groups in M1 mAChR mRNA expression levels (P > 0.05).

M2 mAChR

Compared to the control group, there were no apparent changes in the expression levels of both M2 mAChR mRNA and protein in the hippocampus after CCI surgery (P > 0.05, Fig. 2c, d). In comparison to the CCI group, no obvious changes were found in the expression levels of both M2 mAChR mRNA and protein after EAS (P > 0.05, Fig. 2c, d).

Effect of EAS on hippocampal α4 and β2 nAChR gene and protein expression

α4 nAChR

Quantitative real-time PCR detection of both α4 nAChR and β2 nAChR mRNA showed that only α4 nAChR mRNA expression in the hippocampus was significantly down-regulated after CCI in the CCI group (P < 0.05, Fig. 3a), while β2 nAChR mRNA expression had no marked changes in the CCI and the three EAS groups (P > 0.05, Fig. 3c). Following EAS, α4 nAChR mRNA expression level was obviously up-regulated in the CCI + EA2/15 Hz group (P < 0.05, Fig. 3a), not in the CCI + 2 Hz and CCI + 100 Hz groups (P > 0.05).

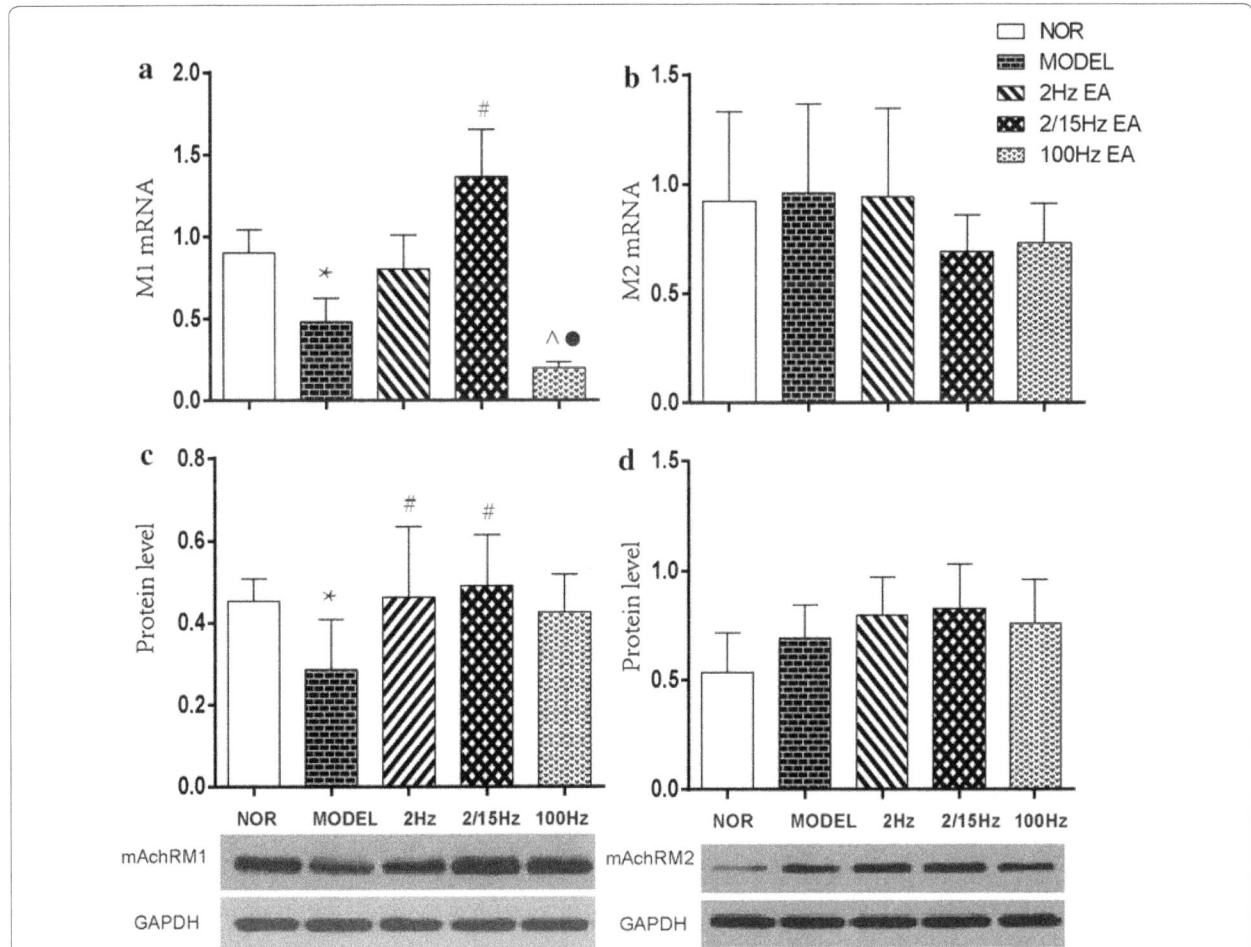

Fig. 2 Effect of different frequencies of EAS of ST36-GB34 on expression of M1 and M2 AChR mRNA and proteins in the hippocampus in neuropathic pain rats (mean ± SD, n = 6 in each group); **a** M1 AChR mRNA, **b** M1 AChR protein; **c** M2 AChR mRNA, **d** M2 AChR protein; *P < 0.05, vs the normal group; #P < 0.05, vs the model group; ^P < 0.05, vs the 2 Hz EAS group; •P < 0.05, vs the 2/15 Hz EAS group

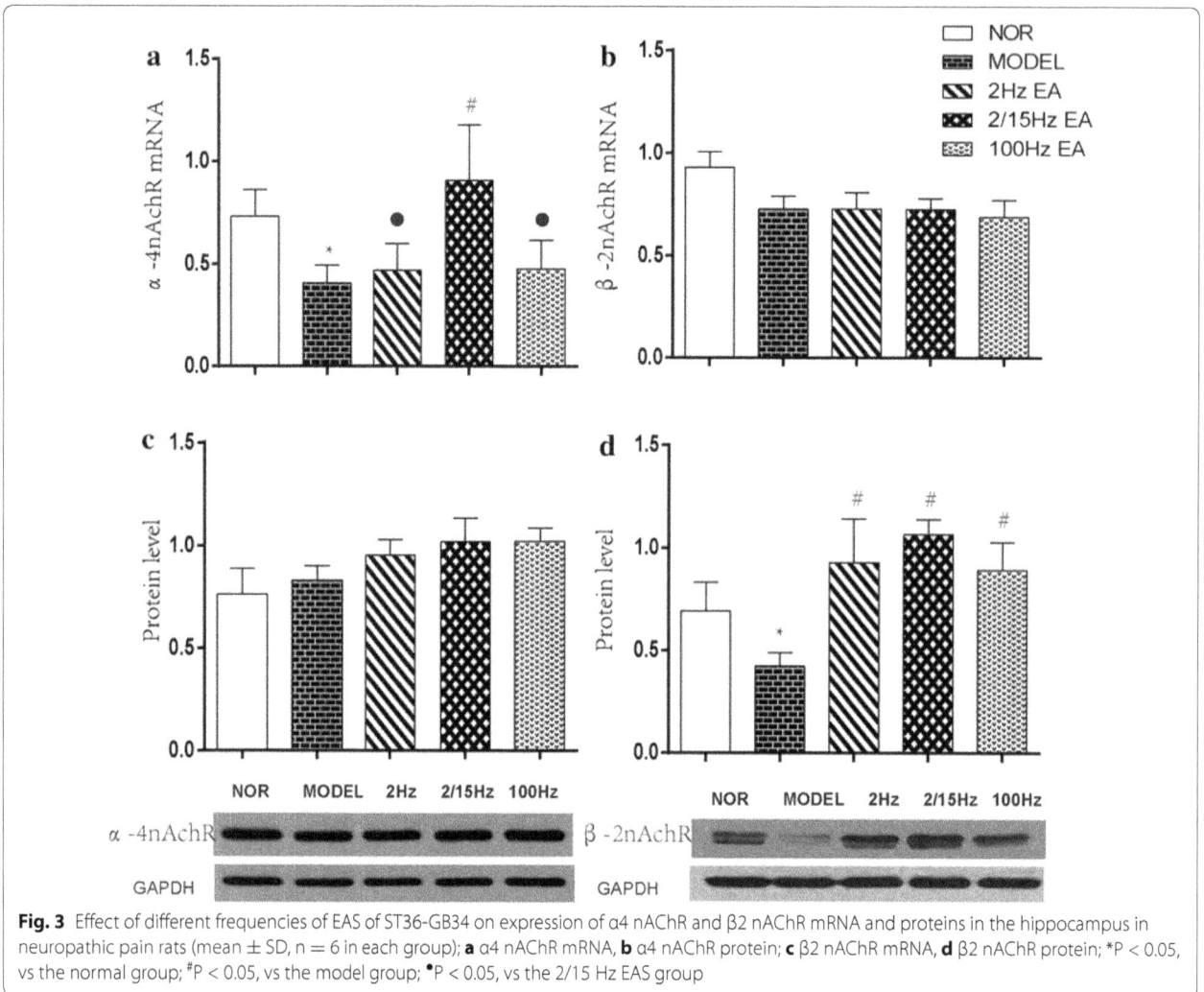

Fig. 3 Effect of different frequencies of EAS of ST36-GB34 on expression of α4 nAChR and β2 nAChR mRNA and proteins in the hippocampus in neuropathic pain rats (mean ± SD, n = 6 in each group); **a** α4 nAChR mRNA, **b** α4 nAChR protein; **c** β2 nAChR mRNA, **d** β2 nAChR protein; *P < 0.05, vs the normal group; #P < 0.05, vs the model group; •P < 0.05, vs the 2/15 Hz EAS group

β2 nAChR

Western blot detection displayed that hippocampal α4 nAChRprotein expression had no apparent changes after CCI in the CCI and the three EAS groups (P > 0.05, Fig. 3b), while β2 nAChR protein expression was significantly down-regulated in the CCI group (P < 0.05, Fig. 3d). After EAS, β2 nAChR protein expression levels of the CCI + EA2 Hz, CCI + EA2/15 Hz and CCI + EA100 Hz groups were considerably upregulated (P < 0.05, Fig. 3d). No significant differences were found among the three EAS groups in the expression of β2 nAChR protein (P > 0.05).

Effect of hippocampal injection of M1mAChR and α4β2 nAChR antagonist on EA analgesia

Results of Fig. 4 showed that the PWLDs of the model group at time-points of 6 h, 1, 3 and 5 days after CCI were significantly increased in the model group (P < 0.001). Compared to the model group, the

PWLD was significantly decreased in the EA + saline group (P < 0.05) but not in the EA + Pirenzepine and EA + DHβE groups on day 5 after EAS (P > 0.05), suggesting a reduction of EA analgesia after intra-hippocampal injection of M1mAChR and α4β2 nAChR antagonists.

Discussion

Findings of the present study revealed that after one and two weeks' EAS at 2 Hz and alternative frequencies of 2/15 Hz but not 100 Hz, the mechanical pain thresholds were significantly increased, and the effects of 2 and 2/15 Hz were superior to that of 100 Hz EAS beginning on day 6 and significantly on day 14 after EAS, meaning a better analgesic effect of lower frequency EAS in neuropathic pain rats. These results are basically identical to Zou's and colleagues' outcomes acquired in acute arthritis patients [27], Romita's and colleagues' study [42] and Li's [16], Mayor's [43], and Wang's [29] reviews about experimental studies, but different to Chen's and Wang's

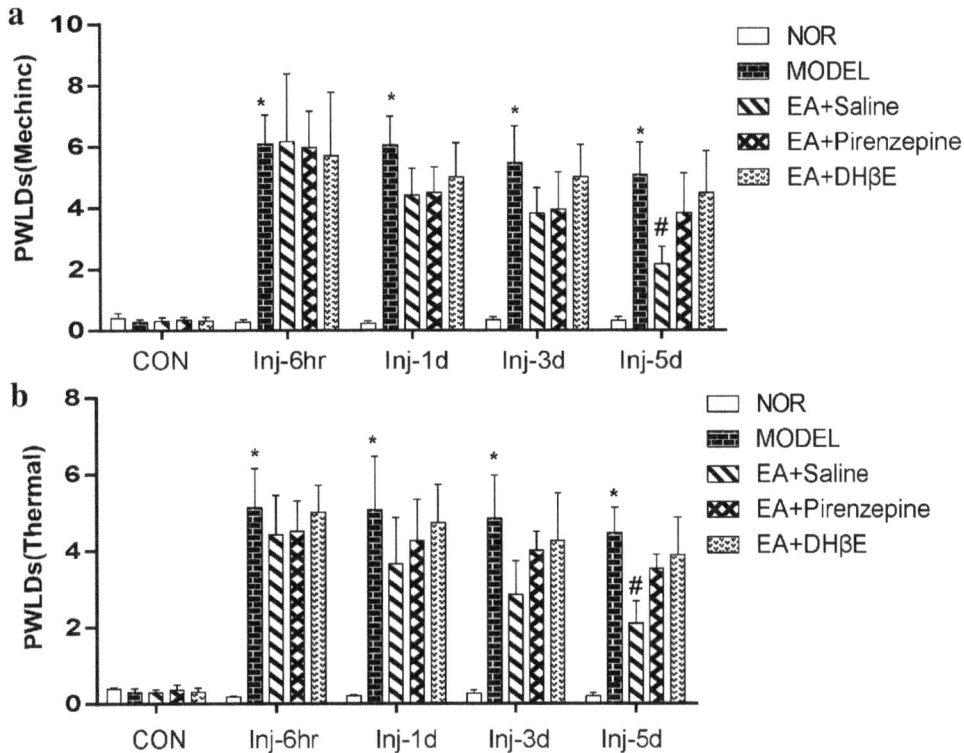

Fig. 4 Effect of intra-hippocampal injection of M1mAChR selective antagonist (pirenzepine hydrochloride) and α4β2 nAChR antagonist (Dihydro-beta-erythroidine, DHβE) on pain threshold (**a** mechanic, g; **b** thermal, sec) in neuropathic pain rats (mean ± SD, n = 4 in each group); *P < 0.05, vs the normal group; #P < 0.05, vs the model group

outcomes obtained in soft tissue injury patients which 100 Hz EAS was better than 2 Hz in pain relief [26] and also different to Hahm's [28] and Chang's and colleagues' [44] results in which a comparable pain relief of 2 Hz and 100 Hz EAS was observed in ankle sprain rats and inflammatory pain mice.

Results of real-time RT-PCR and WB of the present study showed that following 2 weeks' EAS, both 2 and 2/15 Hz could obviously reverse CCI-induced decrease of M1mAChR mRNA and protein expression, and so did 100 Hz EAS in upregulating M1mAChR protein expression. The effects of 2/15 Hz EAS were notably better than those of 100 Hz EAS in upregulating M1 mAChR mRNA and α4 nAChR mRNA expression, displaying a closer correlation between the EA analgesia at 2/15 Hz and M1 mAChR and β2 nAChR protein expression levels in CCI rats, rather than M2 mAChR protein expression. Following intra-hippocampal microinjection of M1 mAChR antagonist Pirenzepine and α-4β-2nAChR antagonist DHβE, both the increased thermal pain and mechanical pain thresholds were suppressed, denoting an involvement of hippocampal M1 mAChR and α-4β2 nAChR in mediating the cumulative analgesic effect of EAS.

It is well known that the gene expression contains both transcription and transduction, and changes of the target genes detected by PCR only reflects up- or down-regulation of a molecule at the transcription level with no relevance to physiological functions, while the relative expression of proteins detected by WB is simply referred to protein transduction, and directly involves functional activities. Thus, it is understandable that the expression levels of genes and proteins of α4 nAChR and β2 nAChR did not show a positive correlation. No selective antagonists for simple α4 nAChR and simple β2 nAChR were found, we were forced to observe the effect of α4β2 nAChR antagonist on EA analgesia.

Studies using retrograde tracing and excitotoxin lesions [45], ChAT and/or AChE pharmacohistochemical regimen [46] and co-cultured slices of septum and hippocampus (not single cultures of hippocampus) in combination with immunocytochemistry for choline acetyltransferase (AChT) [47] demonstrated that the hippocampal formation is innervated primarily by cholinergic neurons located in the vertical limb of the diagonal band and in the medial septum. It also has been shown that the cholinergic, opioidergic and GABAergic systems of the hippocampus were involved in the modulation of antinociception, and the cholinergic transmission may activate the release of endorphins/enkephalin from interneurons of the dorsal hippocampus to inhibit GABAergic neurons, resulting in antinociception [48].

The hippocampus expresses a broad range of mAChRs, with the M1 and M3 receptors being mainly expressed on principal neurons and M2 and M4 receptors on interneurons [49, 50]. However, only fewer studies have shown roles of different subunits of hippocampal mAChRs and nAChR in pain modulation. For instance, intra-CA3 microinjection of ACh or ACh agonist pilocarpine and mAChRs antagonist atropine showed that hippocampal mAChRs were complicated in the modulation of the nociceptive response by modulating the electrical activities of pain-excited or -inhibited neurons in the hippocampal CA1 and CA3 regions of normal rats experiencing electrical stimulation of the ischial nerve [16, 51]. The hippocampal M1 mAChR was shown to be involved in moderate pain reactions in repeated intraperitoneal injection-induced moderate pain in C57BL/6J mice [52].

The septo-hippocampal pathway was also thought to activate nAChRs, because intraperitoneal injection of nAChR antagonist chlorisondamine induced an antinociceptive effect in acute thermal (hot box) and persistent chemical (formalin test) pain rats [53]. At least three distinct functional nAChRsubtypes ($\alpha 7$, $\alpha 4$ $\beta 2$, $\alpha 3$ $\beta 4$) could be detected in the hippocampal region [54], and most of the rat hippocampal heteromeric nAChRs contain $\alpha 4$ and $\beta 2$ subunits, with the 3H] epibatidine –labeled $\alpha 4\beta 2$ and $\alpha 4\beta 2\alpha 5$ subtypes accounting for about 40 and 35 %, respectively [55]. In accordance with Mitsui's report [56], in spite of no obvious physical or neurological deficit in AChR knockout mice, pharmacological, biochemical, electrophysiological, neuroanatomical and behavioral analyses revealed that these AChR subunits may form a component of the nicotinic pain pathways modulating the antinociceptive effect of nicotine. Experimental results of tail-flick and hot-plate tests indicated that $\alpha 4$ $\beta 2$ nAChRs were important in mediating neuronal nicotinic analgesia in both spinal and supraspinal responses in knockin mice expressing hypersensitive $\alpha 4$ $\beta 2$ nicotinic receptors [57]. However, there still have been no any reports on gene and protein expression of hippocampal nicotinic receptors involving pain modulation up to now.

EAS frequency is considered to be an important parameter affecting its analgesic effect. Up to now, many studies focus on the low frequency 2–5 Hz, medium frequency 15–40 Hz, and high frequency 100–200 Hz for various pain models, which were chosen in consideration of nervous tissue responses. If the frequency is over

100 Hz, the reactions of the nerve tissue may not truthfully follow the electrical stimulation [25].

Using rat tail-flick tests, Silva et al. [58] observed that the analgesic effect of 2 Hz EAS of ST36 and Sanyinjiao (SP6) lasted longer than that of 100 Hz EAS. Intrathecal administration of antagonists of $\alpha 1$- (WB4101) and $\alpha 2$- (idazoxan) adrenoceptors and serotonergic (methysergide), opioid (naloxone), muscarinic (atropine), GABA (A) (bicuculline) and GABA (B) (phaclofen) receptors showed that the analgesic effect of 2 HZ EAS was inhibited by naloxone or atropine, being less intense and shorter after $\alpha 1$ or $\alpha 2$ inhibition, and lasting shorter after 5-HT, GABAA, or GABAB receptor suppression; while that of the 100 Hz EAS was less intense and shorter after opioid and muscarinic suppression, being less intense and longer after GABAB inhibition, shorter after 5-HT or GABAA inhibition, and remained unchanged after $\alpha 1$ or $\alpha 2$ inhibition. It suggests that the analgesic efficacy (intensity) of 2 Hz EAS depends on noradrenergic descending inhibition and involves spinal opioid and muscarinic mechanisms, whereas the duration of the analgesic effect relies on both noradrenergic and serotonergic descending control, and involves spinal GABAergic regulation. On the contrary, the analgesic efficacy of 100 Hz EAS involves spinal muscarinic, opioid, and GABAB activation, while the duration of the effects is affected by spinal serotonergic, muscarinic, opioid, and GABAA activation. Their further study [59] demonstrated that the cholinergic muscarinic, μ-opioid, GABAA and 5-HT1 mechanisms in the dorsal -anterior pretectal nucleus (APtN) and μ-opioid and 5-HT1 mechanisms in the ventral APtN were involved in 2 Hz EAS analgesia, while the μ-opioid and 5-HT1 mechanisms in the vAPtN but not in the dAPtN were complicated in 100 Hz EAS analgesia.

Recently, using cDNA microarray, Wang et al. [60] demonstrated in the rat that more genes were differentially regulated by 2 Hz EA than 100 Hz EA of ST36 and SP6 (154 vs. 66 regulated genes/ESTs) in the arcuate nucleus (Arc) region, especially those related to neurogenesis. Results of fMRI in combination with behavior tests showed that following 2 and 100 Hz EAS in the human body, the regional cerebral blood flow (CBF) signals revealed a trend of early activation with later inhibition; and a positive correlation between analgesia and the regional CBF change was observed in the anterior insula in the early stage, whereas a negative relationship was found in the parahippocampal gyrus in the later stage. TEAS analgesia was specifically associated with the default mode network and other cortical regions in the 2 Hz TEAS group, ventral striatum and dorsal anterior cingulate cortex in the 100 Hz TEAS group, respectively

[61]. Later, it was found in rhesus monkeys that 2 Hz but not 100 Hz TEAS evoked a significant increase in mu-opioid receptor (MOR) binding potential in the anterior cingulate cortex, caudate nucleus, putamen, temporal lobe, somatosensory cortex, and the amygdala which are related to pain and sensory processing [62]. These findings suggest that the mechanisms of low- and high-frequency EAS analgesia are different and partially overlapped.

Conclusions

Results of our present study showed that in neuropathic pain rats, repeated EA treatment at frequencies of 2 and 2/15 Hz, particularly the later (but not 100 Hz) has a cumulative analgesic effect, which is closely related to their effects in upregulating the expression of hippocampal M1 and β2 nAChR proteins, highlighting the involvement of muscarinic and nicotinic receptor subtypes in EA analgesia for the first time.

Abbreviations
CCI: chronic constrictive injury; EAS: electroacupuncture stimulation; PWL: paw withdrawal latency; PWLD: difference value of PWL; M1 mAChR: M1 muscarinic acetylcholinergic receptor; M2 mAChR: M2 muscarinic acetylcholinergic receptor,; α-4nAChR: alpha-4 nicotinic acetylcholinergic receptor; Beta-2 nAChR: beta-2 nicotinic acetylcholinergic receptor.

Authors' contributions
SPC and JLL wrote the manuscript. YK and SPC carried out the animal experiments, JLZ, JYW and YHG participated in partial experiments and executed statistical analysis, and LNQ and XMF helped the experiments. JLL contributed to the design of the study. All authors read and approved the final manuscript.

Author details
[1] Department of Physiology, Institute of Acupuncture and Moxibustion, China Academy of Chinese Medical Sciences, 16 Nanxiaojie Street, Dongzhimennei, Beijing 100700, China. [2] Department of Biochemistry and Molecular Biology, Institute of Acu-Moxibustion, China Academy of Chinese Medical Sciences, Beijing, China.

Acknowledgements
This study was jointly supported by National Natural Science Foundation of China (No.81273828, No.81202762, and No.30973796) and the Special Project of Chinese Medicine (973) of the National Basic Research Program of China (2007CB512505, 2013CB531904).

Competing interests
All authors declare that they have no any competing interests.

References
1. Simons LE, Elman I, Borsook D. Psychological processing in chronic pain: a neural systems approach. Neurosci Biobehav Rev. 2014;39:61–78.
2. Farmer MA, Baliki MN, Apkarian AV. A dynamic network perspective of chronic pain. Neurosci Lett. 2012;520(2):197–203.
3. Liu M-G, Chen J. Roles of the hippocampal formation in pain information processing. Neurosci Bull. 2009;25(5):237–66.
4. Pruessner M, Pruessner JC, Hellhammer DH, Bruce Pike G, Lupien SJ. The associations among hippocampal volume, cortisol reactivity, and memory performance in healthy young men. Psychiatry Res. 2007;155(1):1–10.
5. Zimmerman ME, Pan JW, Hetherington HP, Lipton ML, Baigi K, Lipton RB. Hippocampal correlates of pain in healthy elderly adults: a pilot study. Neurology. 2009;73:1567–70.
6. Mutso AA, Petre B, Huang L, Baliki MN, Torbey S, Herrmann K, et al. Reorganization of hippocampal functional connectivity with transition to chronic back pain. J Neurophysiol. 2014;111(5):1065–76.
7. Mutso AA, Radzicki D, Baliki MN, Huang L, Banisadr G, Centeno MV, et al. Abnormalities in hippocampal functioning with persistent pain. J Neurosci. 2012;32(17):5747–56.
8. Vachon-Presseau E, Roy M, Martel MO, Caron E, Marin MF, Chen J, et al. The stress model of chronic pain: evidence from basal cortisol and hippocampal structure and function in humans. Brain. 2013;136(Pt 3):815–27.
9. Al-Amin H, Sarkis R, Atweh S, Jabbur S, Saade N. Chronic dizocilpine or apomorphine and development of neuropathy in two animal models II: effects on brain cytokines and neurotrophins. Exp Neurol. 2011;228:30–40.
10. del Rey A, Yau HJ, Randolf A, Centeno MV, Wildmann J, Martina M, et al. Chronic neuropathic pain-like behavior correlates with IL-1 expression and disrupts cytokine interactions in the hippocampus. Pain. 2011;152:2827–35.
11. Duric V, McCarson KE. Persistent pain produces stress-like alterations in hippocampal neurogenesis and gene expression. J Pain. 2006;7(8):544–55.
12. Pert A. The cholinergic system and nociception in the primate: interactions with morphine. Psychopharmacologia. 1975;44(2):131–7.
13. Katayama Y, Watkins LR, Becker DP, Hayes RL. Non-opiate analgesia induced by carbachol microinjection into the pontine parabrachial region of the cat. Brain Res. 1984;296(2):263–83.
14. Hamm RJ, Knisely JS. Developmental differences in the analgesia produced by the central cholinergic system. Dev Psychobiol. 1987;20(3):345–54.
15. Jiao R, Yang C, Zhang Y, Xu M, Yang X. Cholinergic mechanism involved in the nociceptive modulation of dentate gyrus. Biochem Biophys Res Commun. 2009;379(4):975–9.
16. Li GZ, Liang QC, Jin YH, Yang CX, Zhang GW, Gao HR, et al. The effect of acetylcholine on pain-related electric activities in the hippocampal CA3 of rats. J Neural Transm. 2011;118(4):555–61.
17. Romano JA, Shih TM. Cholinergic mechanisms of analgesia produced by physostigmine, morphine and cold water swimming. Neuropharmacology. 1983;22(7):827–33.
18. Eisenach JC. Muscarinic-mediated analgesia. Life Sci. 1999;64(6–7):549–54.
19. Lewis JW, Cannon JT, Liebeskind JC. Involvement of central muscarinic cholinergic mechanisms in opioid stress analgesia. Brain Res. 1983;270(2):289–93.
20. Tang CM, Wei JH, Chen SS. Preliminary study on the involvement of hippocampus in electroacupuncture analgesia. Zhen Ci Ma Zui. 1979;2(1):58–61.
21. Xu G, Duanmu Z, Yin Q. The role of Ach in the central nerve system on pain modulation and analgesia. Zhen Ci Yan Jiu. 1993;18(1):1–5, 7.
22. Guan XM, Wang CY, Yu F. Correlation between central acytcholine and acupuncture analgesia. Zhen Ci Yan Jiu. 1991;16(2):129–37.
23. Wang JY, Liu JL, Chen SP, Gao YH, Meng FY, Qiao LN. Acupuncture effects on the hippocampal cholinergic system in a rat model of neuropathic pain. Neu Reg Res. 2012;7(3):212–8.
24. Wang JY, Meng FY, Chen SP, Gao YH, Liu JL. Analysis on Interrelation between electroacupuncture-induced cumulative analgesic effect and hypothalamic cholinergic activities in chronic neuropathic pain rats. Chin J Integr Med. 2012;18(9):699–707.
25. Han JS. Some factors affecting acupuncture-induced analgesia. Zhen Ci Yan Jiu. 1994;19(3, 4):1–4.
26. Chen HL, Wang QQ. Effect of different frequency electrical stimulation of acupoints on pain of acute soft tissue injury. J Chengdu Univer Trad Chin Med. 2006;29(4):29–31.
27. Zou R, Zhang HX, Zhang TF. Comparative study on treatment of acute gouty arthritis by electroacupuncture with different frequency. Chin J Clin Rehabil. 2006;10(43):188–9.
28. Hahm TS. The effect of 2 Hz and 100 Hz electrical stimulation of acupoint on ankle sprain in rats. J Korean Med Sci. 2007;22(2):347–51.
29. Wang YJ. An outline of experimental studies on the factors affecting electroacupuncture analgesia. Zhen Ci Yan Jiu. 1993;18(4):247–52.

30. Han JS, Wang Q. Mobilization of specific neuropeptides by peripheral stimulation of identified frequencies. News Physiol Sci. 1992;7(4):176–80.

31. Fei H, Sun SL, Han JS. New evidence supporting differential release of enkephalin and dynorphin by low and high frequency electro-acupuncture. Chin Sci Bull. 1988;33(9):703–5.

32. Fei H, Xie GX, Han JS. Low and high frequency electro-acupuncture stimulations release [met5] enkephalin and dynorphin A in rat spinal cord. Chin Sci Bull. 1987;32(21):1496–501.

33. Wang Y, Zhang Y, Wang W, Cao Y, Han JS. Effects of synchronous or asynchronous electroacupuncturestimulation with low versus high frequency on spinal opioid release and tail flick nociception. Exp Neurol. 2005;192(1):156–62.

34. Wang Q, Mao L, Han J. The arcuate nucleus of hypothalamus mediates low but not highfrequencyelectroacupunctureanalgesia in rats. Brain Res. 1990;513(1):60–6.

35. Zhang M, Han JS. 5-hydroxytryptamine is an important mediator for both high and low frequency electroacupuncture analgesia. Zhen Ci Yan Jiu. 1985;10(3):212–5.

36. Kwon YB, Kang MS, Son SS, Kim JT, Lee YH, Han HJ, Lee JH. Different frequencies of electroacupuncture modified the cellular activity of serotonergic neurons in brainstem. Am J Chin Med. 2000;28(3–4):435–41.

37. Kwon Y, Kang M, Ahn C, Han H, Ahn B, Lee J. Effect of high or low frequency electroacupuncture on the cellular activity of catecholaminergic neurons in the brain stem. Acupunct Electrother Res. 2000;25(1):27–36.

38. Shen EY, Lai YJ. The efficacy of frequency-specific acupuncture stimulation on extracellular dopamine concentration in striatum–a rat model study. Neurosci Lett. 2007;415(2):179–84.

39. Lin YP, Peng Y, Yi SX, Tang S. Effect of different frequency electroacupuncture on the expression of substance P and beta-endorphin in the hypothalamus in rats with gastric distension-induced pain. Zhen Ci Yan Jiu. 2009;34(4):252–7.

40. Ko ES, Kim SK, Kim JT, Lee G, Han JB, Rho SW, et al. The difference in mRNA expressions of hypothalamic CCK and CCK-A and -B receptors between responder and non-responder rats to high frequency electroacupuncture analgesia. Peptides. 2006;27(7):1841–5.

41. Bennett GJ, Xie YK. A peripheral mononeuropathy in rat that produces disorders of pain sensation like those seen in man. Pain. 1988;33:87–107.

42. Romita VV, Suk A, Henry JL. Parametric studies on electroacupuncture-like stimulation in a rat model: effects of intensity, frequency, and duration of stimulation on evoked antinociception. Brain Res Bull. 1997;42(4):289–96.

43. Mayor D. An exploratory review of the electroacupuncture literature: clinical applications and endorphin mechanisms. Acupunct Med. 2013;31(4):409–15.

44. Chang FC, Tsai HY, Yu MC, Yi PL, Lin JG. The central serotonergic system mediates the analgesic effect of electroacupuncture on ZUSANLI (ST36) acupoints. J Biomed Sci. 2004;11(2):179–85.

45. McKinney M, Coyle JT, Hedreen JC. Topographic analysis of the innervation of the rat neocortex and hippocampus by the basal forebrain cholinergic system. J Comp Neurol. 1983;217(1):103–21.

46. Woolf NJ, Eckenstein F, Butcher LL. Cholinergic systems in the rat brain: I. projections to the limbic telencephalon. Brain Res Bull. 1984;13(6):751–84.

47. Heimrich B, Frotscher M. Formation of the septohippocampal projection in vitro: an electron microscopic immunocytochemical study of cholinergic synapses. Neuroscience. 1993;52(4):815–27.

48. Favaroni Mendes LA. Menescal-de-Oliveira L. Role of cholinergic, opioidergic and GABA-ergic neuro-transmission of the dorsal hippocampus in the modulation of nociception in guinea pigs. Life Sci. 2008;83(19–20):644–50.

49. Levey AI, Edmunds SM, Koliatsos V, Wiley RG, Heilman CJ. Expression of m1-m4 muscarinic acetylcholine receptor proteins in rat hippocampus and regulation by cholinergic innervation. J Neurosci. 1995;15:4077–92.

50. Hajos N, Papp EC, Acsady L, Levey AI, Freund TF. Distinct interneuron types express m2 muscarinic receptor immunoreactivity on their dendrites or axon terminals in the hippocampus. Neuroscience. 1998;82:355–76.

51. Yang XF, Xiao Y, Xu MY. Both endogenous and exogenous ACh plays antinociceptive role in the hippocampus CA1 of rats. J Neural Transm. 2008;115(1):1–6.

52. Sase A, Khan D, Höger H, Lubec G. Intraperitoneal injection of saline modulates hippocampal brain receptor complex levels but does not impair performance in the Morris Water Maze. Amino Acids. 2012;43(2):783–92.

53. Bannon AW, Decker MW, Curzon P, Buckley MJ, Kim DJ, Radek RJ, et al. ABT-594 [(R)-5-(2-azetidinylmethoxy)-2-chloropyridine]: a novel, orally effective antinociceptive agent acting via neuronal nicotinic acetylcholine receptors: II. In vivo characterization. J Pharmacol Exp Ther. 1998;285(2):787–94.

54. Alkondon M, Alkondon M, Albuquerque EX. The nicotinic acetylcholine receptor subtypes and their function in the hippocampus and cerebral cortex. Prog Brain Res. 2004;145:109–20.

55. Lomazzo E, MacArthur L, Yasuda RP, Wolfe BB, Kellar KJ. Quantitative analysis of the heteromeric neuronal nicotinic receptors in the rat hippocampus. J Neurochem. 2010;115:625–34.

56. Mitsui T. Acetylcholine receptor knockout mice. Nihon Shinkei Seishin Yakurigaku Zasshi. 1999;19(5):233–8.

57. Damaj MI, Fonck C, Marks MJ, Deshpande P, Labarca C, Lester HA, et al. Genetic approaches identify differential roles for α4β2 nicotinic receptors in acute models of antinociception in mice. J Pharmacol Exp Ther. 2007;321(3):1161–9.

58. Silva JR, Silva ML, Prado WA. Analgesia induced by 2- or 100-Hz electroacupuncture in the rat tail-flick test depends on the activation of different descending pain inhibitory mechanisms. J Pain. 2011;12(1):51–60.

59. Silva ML, Silva JR, Prado WA. Analgesia induced by 2- or 100-Hz electroacupuncture in the rat tail-flick test depends on the anterior pretectal nucleus. Life Sci. 2013;93(20):742–54.

60. Wang K, Zhang R, He F, Lin LB, Xiang XH, Ping XJ, et al. Electroacupuncture frequency-related transcriptional response in rat arcuate nucleus revealed region-distinctive changes in response to low- and high-frequency electroacupuncture. J Neurosci Res. 2012;90(7):1464–73.

61. Jiang Y, Liu J, Liu J, Han J, Wang X, Cui C. Cerebral blood flow-based evidence for mechanisms of low- versus high-frequency transcutaneous electric acupoint stimulation analgesia: a perfusion fMRI study in humans. Neuroscience. 2014;268C:180–93.

62. Xiang XH, Chen YM, Zhang JM, Tian JH, Han JS, Cui CL. Low- and high-frequency transcutaneous electrical acupoint stimulation induces different effects on cerebral μ-opioid receptor availability in rhesus monkeys. J Neurosci Res. 2014;92(5):555–63.

Scutellaria barbata flavonoids alleviate memory deficits and neuronal injuries induced by composited Aβ in rats

Xiao G. Wu[1], Shu S. Wang[2], Hong Miao[1], Jian J. Cheng[1], Shu F. Zhang[1] and Ya Z. Shang[1*]

Abstract

Background: The aim of the present study was to investigate the effects of *Scutellaria barbata* flavonoids (SBF) on memory impairment and neuronal injury induced by amyloid beta protein 25–35 in combination with aluminum trichloride (AlCl3) and recombinant human transforming growth factor-β1 (RHTGF-β1) (composited Aβ) in rats.

Methods: The composited Aβ-treated model of Alzheimer's disease (AD)-like memory impairment and neuronal injury was established in male rats by right intracerebroventricular injection of composited Aβ, and the effects of SBF were assessed using this rat model. Spatial learning and memory of rats were assessed in the Morris water maze, and neuronal injury was assessed by light and electron microscopy with hematoxylin-eosin or uranyl acetate and lead nitrate-sodium citrate staining, respectively.

Results: In the Morris water maze, memory impairment was observed in 94.7% of the composited Aβ-treated rats. The composited Aβ-treated rats took longer than sham-operated rats to find the hidden platform during position navigation and reversal learning trials. They also spent less time swimming in the target quadrant in the probe trial. Optical and electron microscopic observations showed significant neuropathological changes including neuron loss or pyknosis in hippocampus, typical colliquative necrosis in cerebral cortex, mitochondrial swelling and cristae fragmentation and a large number of lipofuscin deposits in the cytoplasm. Treatment with SBF (35–140 mg/kg) reduced the memory impairment and neuronal injury induced by composited Aβ.

Conclusion: SBF-mediated improvement of composited Aβ-induced memory impairment and neuronal injury in rats provides an appropriate rationale for evaluating SBF as a promising agent for treatment of AD.

Keywords: *Scutellaria barbata* flavonoids, Aβ 25-35, AlCl3, RHTGF-β1, Memory, Neuronal injuries

Background

Alzheimer's disease (AD) is a chronic and progressive neurodegenerative disease in the elderly, and it is accompanied by gradual memory loss. In general, atrophy of the nervous system, loss of neurons and synapses, as well as disorders of subcellular structure and function are closely associated with the occurrence and development of AD [1, 2]. In particular, extracellular senile plaques (SP), which are primarily composed of aggregated beta-amyloid (Aβ), and intracellular neurofibrillary tangles (NFT), which are composed of insoluble aggregates of hyperphosphorylated tau protein in the brain, are considered the most important histopathogenic traits in AD. Multiple neurotoxic events in the brain, such as Aβ aggregation, tau protein hyperphosphorylation, disruption of calcium homeostasis, and production of reactive oxygen species, have been shown to occur when animals were intraventricularly injected with Aβ [3]. The deposited Aβ may result in massive SP and NFT formation, and the combined effects of deposited Aβ and hyperphosphorylated tau protein exacerbate neurotoxicity and advance dementia [4]. An animal model of AD was

*Correspondence: 973358769@qq.com
[1] Hebei Province Key Research Office of Traditional Chinese Medicine Against Dementia/Institute of Traditional Chinese Medicine, Chengde Medical College/Hebei Province Key Laboratory of Traditional Chinese Medicine Research and Development, Chengde, Hebei 067000, China
Full list of author information is available at the end of the article

established using Aβ25–35 in combination with aluminum trichloride (AlCl3) and recombinant human transforming growth factor-β1 (RHTGF-β1) injected into the lateral cerebral ventricle (composited Aβ-treated rat). This model provides a comprehensive simulation of human histopathogenic traits [5]. Aluminum can prevent conversion of sedimentary Aβ into soluble Aβ, and RHTGF-β1 can enhance sedimentary Aβ formation and accelerate occurrence of AD [6]. Thus, several composited Aβ-induced neuronal dysfunctions are relevant to AD, and an intervention that can decrease composited Aβ-mediated neuronal injury may be useful in the treatment of AD.

Scutellaria barbata flavonoids (SBF), which are isolated from the aerial parts of *S. barbata* D. Don, have been shown to alleviate fever, inflammation, peroxidation, as well as improve memory deficits and neuroendocrine and abnormal free radical changes in ovariectomized rats [7–9]. However, the effects of SBF on impaired learning and memory and neuronal damage induced by composited Aβ in rats has not been reported. In the present study, the effects of SBF were assessed using a composited Aβ-treated rat model of AD-like memory impairment and brain injury, which was established by intracerebroventricular injection of Aβ25–35 in combination with AlCl3 and RHTGF-β1.

Materials
Animals
Four-month-old male Sprague–Dawley rats were purchased from the Experimental Animal Center of Hebei Medical University (Clean grade, Certification No. scxk (Ji) 2010-1-003). Rats were housed in groups of four or five per cage with free access to food and water under controlled laboratory conditions with a 12-h light–dark cycle and an ambient temperature of 22–24 °C. Before the operation, the rats were allowed to acclimatize to the laboratory environment for 1 week. All animal procedures were carried out in accordance with the Regulations of Experimental Animal Administration issued by the State Committee of Science and Technology of China on Oct. 31, 1988 [10]. All efforts were made to minimize the animal number and their discomfort.

Drug and reagents
SBF was prepared by the Phytochemistry Laboratory, Institute of Traditional Chinese Medicine, Chengde Medical College, Chengde City, China. One kg of dried aerial parts of *S. barbata* D. Don was boiled twice for 1 h with 80% alcohol, and the extract was filtered with filter paper. The filtration was performed, and the extract was evaporated under reduced pressure until no alcohol remained. The concentrated solution was adjusted to pH

2 by adding 1 N HCl and was maintained at room temperature for 24 h until the sediment completely formed. The sediment was SBF, and the flavonoid was not less than 85%. Scutellarein was the major ingredient as shown by high performance liquid chromatography assay [11]. Aβ25-35, AlCl3 and RHTGF-β1 were purchased from Shanghai Qiangyao Bioabiotechnology Co., Ltd (Shanghai, China), Tianjin Beichen Reagent Company Inc (Tianjin, China) and Prospect Biosystems (Newark, NJ, USA), respectively. Other reagents were AR grade and were supplied by commercial sources.

Methods
Surgical procedure
One hundred male Sprague–Dawley rats (300–350 g, 4 months of age) were used in the experiments. Eighty rats were microinjected with composited Aβ into the right lateral cerebral ventricle and designated as composited Aβ-treated rats. Twenty rats were subjected to a sham operation. The rats were anaesthetized with 10% chloral hydrate (300 mg/kg, intraperitoneal) and restrained in a brain stereotaxic apparatus (RWD, Shenzhen, China). On the first day of the operation, as shown in Additional files 1 and 2, 1 μL of RHTGF-β1 (10 ng) was microinjected into the lateral cerebral ventricle area [posterior (P): 1.0 mm to the bregma, lateral (L): 1.4 mm to the midline, and ventral (V): 4.6 mm to the skull]. A catheter was inserted into the lateral cerebral ventricle area [posterior (P): 1.2 mm to the bregma, lateral (L): 2.0 mm to the midline, and ventral (V): 4.6 mm to the skull] [12]. On the second day of operation, 4 μg (1 μL) Aβ25–35 and 3 μL AlCl3 (1%) were microinjected daily for 14 days in the morning and 5 days in the afternoon, respectively. The sham-operated group was subjected to the same operation and received a saline microinjection. Seventy-six composited Aβ-treated rats survived, the success rate of the operation was 95%. Eighteen sham-operated rats survived, the success rate of the operation was 90%.

Experimental design
The entire experiment took 86 days and Fig. 1 showed the timeline of experimental design. All rats were allowed to recover for 45 days after the operation. The Morris water maze was used to screen rats for learning deficits and to assess their spatial memory. The rats underwent 4 consecutive days of water maze training with 2 trials per day. Composited Aβ-treated rats that displayed a learning deficit on day 4 of training in the Morris Water Maze were randomly divided into 4 groups: composited Aβ-treated group or 3 drug-treated groups (3 doses). Rats in the drug-treated groups were administered 35, 70 and 140 mg/kg (oral) of SBF daily for 38 days. The sham-operated rats were given saline. The rats' spatial

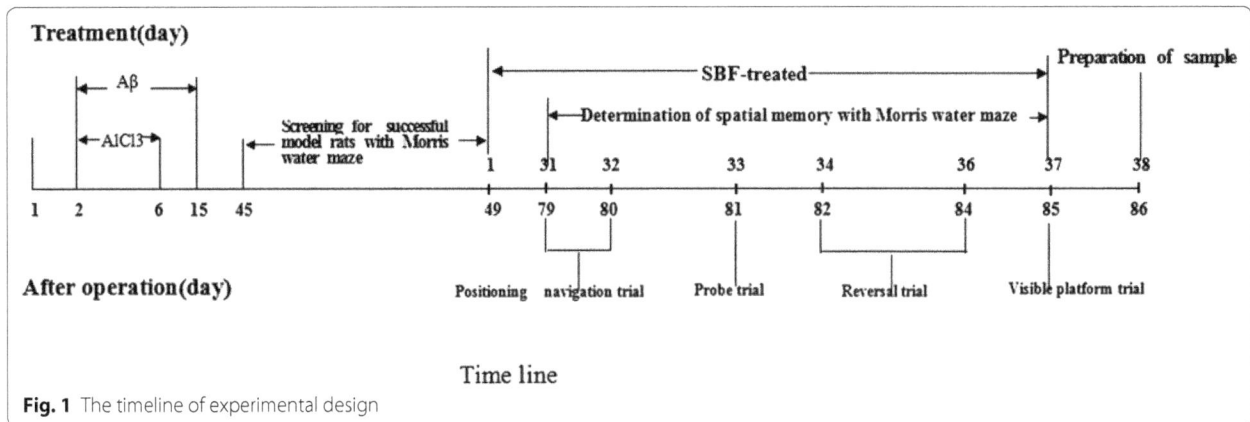

Fig. 1 The timeline of experimental design

memory was tested in the Morris water maze over 7 consecutive days, from day 31 to day 37 of SBF administration (namely, day 79 to day 85 after the operation). The medication lasted throughout the Morris water maze test period. All the rats were killed by decapitation 60 min after the last administration of SBF or saline on day 38 of administration.

Screening for successful model rats and assessment of behavior in the Morris Water Maze

The Morris water maze was used to assess learning and memory and screen for successful model rats [13]. The Morris water maze was a stainless steel circular pool with a diameter of 120 cm and a depth of 50 cm. It was purchased from the Institute of Materia Medica, Chinese Academy of Medical Science and Peking Union Medical College (Beijing, China). When the water maze test was performed, the pool water was blackened with several drops of ink. The water depth was 31.5 cm, and the temperature was maintained at 23 ± 1 °C. A circular transparent plexiglass platform was set 1.5 cm below the water surface. Each spatial signal around the maze was invariable during all water maze tests. For descriptive data collection, the pool was subdivided into four equal quadrants formed by imaginary lines. The hidden platform was placed in the first quadrant (Q1). All swimming behaviors (measured by latency or trajectory) of rats were captured by a video camera linked to computer-based graphics analytic software (Institute of Materia Medica, Chinese Academy of Medical Science and Peking Union Medical College).

Screening for successful memory impairment of composited Aβ-treated rats

On day 45 after the operation, all rats underwent four consecutive days of Morris water maze training to screen for memory impairment (screening for successful

composited Aβ-treated rats) (Fig. 1). The screening ratio (SR) was calculated from the average latency to find the hidden platform on day 4 of water maze training for each composited Aβ-treated rat and sham-operated rats. The average latency to find the hidden platform on day 4 of water maze training for each composited Aβ-treated rat was "A", and the average latency of sham-operated rats was "B". Then, SR = (A − B)/B. When SR was larger than 0.2 for a composited Aβ-treated rat, it was considered a successful composited Aβ-treated rat with impaired memory [14].

Determination of spatial memory

Spatial memory was assessed for seven consecutive days with two trials per day using the Morris water maze. The time spent finding the hidden platform was recorded, and an average value was calculated from the data of two trials to determine intraday memory performance. The water maze test procedure was designed such that the rats were allowed to swim and search for the hidden platform within 60 s. If a rat missed the hidden platform within 60 s, the experimenter then placed the rat on the platform. When a rat reached the hidden platform (independently or assisted), the rat was allowed to remain there for 20 s, and then the rat was removed from the pool. Each rat was allowed a 10 s recovery time between the two trials. Memory measurement was divided into four parts: 2 days of positioning navigation trial, 1 day of probe trial, 3 days of reversal trial, and finally 1 day of visible platform trial [15].

Positioning navigation trial

The positioning navigation trial was used to evaluate memory acquisition on days 1 and 2 in the Morris water maze. This was performed on days 31 and 32 after initiation of treatment with SBF, which corresponded to days 79 and 80 after the operation (Fig. 1). The location of the hidden platform was the same as during screening of the composited Aβ-treated rats (Q1). The average value of latency over 2 trials was taken as the intraday memory acquisition score.

Probe trial

The probe trial was used to evaluate memory retention on day 3 of the Morris water maze test, which was conducted on day 33 after initiation of treatment with SBF and day 81 after the operation (Fig. 1). The platform was removed from the pool, and the rats were allowed to swim 60 s and search for the target quadrant (Q1) where the platform was located during the positioning navigation trial. Swimming time in the target quadrant (Q1) was recorded for 60 s and taken as the memory retention score.

Reversal trial

The reversal trial was used to evaluate re-learning for three consecutive days on days 4, 5, and 6 of the Morris water maze test, which corresponded to day 34, 35 and 36 of SBF treatment and day 82, 83 and 84 after the operation (Fig. 1). The platform was placed on the opposite side of the target quadrant (Q3). The average latency over two trials was taken as the rats' intraday re-learning achievement.

Visible platform trial

The visible platform trial was used to evaluate swimming speed on day 7 of the Morris water maze test. The aim was to exclude the influence of motivational or sensorimotor factors upon learning and memory performance. All rats were subjected to a 1 day visible platform trial on day 37 after initiation of SBF treatment, which corresponded to day 85 after the operation (Fig. 1). The platform was elevated 2 cm above the water surface. The swimming speed of all rats in the pool was recorded.

Detection of neuronal injury

Under ether anesthesia, the rats were killed by decapitation 60 min after the last administration of SBF or saline on day 38 of treatment (Fig. 1). For three rats from each group, the right hemisphere was gently separated on ice and then routinely processed as previously described [16]. Coronal sections, approximately 4 µm-thick, were cut and stained with hematoxylin-eosin (HE). Stained neurons were visualized and photographed at a magnification of 4× or 400× using an Olympus VANOX microscope from Olympus Optical Co. Ltd. (Tokyo, Japan). An investigator blinded to the experimental design counted neurons per 0.125 mm in the CA1 region of the hippocampus and per 0.0352 mm^2 of the cerebral cortex at 400×. Three subfields of the hippocampal CA1 region

and cerebral cortex were selected from each rat brain. The average number of normal neurons was determined in each group at a magnification of 400×. Neurons were identified as normal if they appeared undamaged with round or oval cell bodies, which distinguished them from glial cells. In addition, hippocampi of the left hemisphere were double-fixed with 2.5% glutaraldehyde and 1% osmic acid and then sectioned with an ultramicrotome. The sections were placed on a 200-mesh copper grid and stained with uranyl acetate and lead nitrate-sodium citrate as described previously [17]. The ultrastructure of cells was observed with a JEOL 100CX II transmission electron microscope and photographed at a magnification of 10,000–35,000×.

Statistical analysis

Data are presented as mean ± SEM. Statistical analysis was performed using a SAS/STAT Microsoft package obtained from SAS, USA. Two-way analysis of variance (ANOVA) with repeated measures was used to analyze group differences in latency to reach the platform in the Morris water maze test, and one-way ANOVA followed by Duncan's multiple-range test was used to analyze group differences in the probe trial and the number of neurons. Differences with P values <0.05 were considered statistically significant.

Results

Screening AD model rats using the Morris water maze test

In recording adaptive swimming, we found that the sham-operated rats always swam freely, and the composited Aβ-treated rats always swam around the pool perimeter (Fig. 2a). Over the 4 days of testing model rats in the Morris water maze, the time to find the hidden platform (latency) progressively declined in all animals. When the screening ratio (SR), which was based on the latency to find the hidden platform on day 4 for composited Aβ-treated and sham-operated rats, was more than 0.2, this animal was considered as a successful model rat. The percentage of successful model rats was 94.7% (Fig. 2b).

Effect of SBF on rat memory acquisition in the Morris water maze test

The positioning navigation trial was used to evaluate rat memory acquisition on day 1 and 2 of the Morris water maze test. During the 2 days memory acquisition trial, the latency to find the hidden platform progressively declined in all rats. However, as shown in Fig. 3, the latency of the composited Aβ-treated group was 540% and 454% [F (1, 6) = 187.37, P < 0.01] greater than that of the sham-operated group on days 1 and 2, respectively. The prolonged latency of the composited Aβ-treated group was significantly shortened by treatment with SBF

a

b

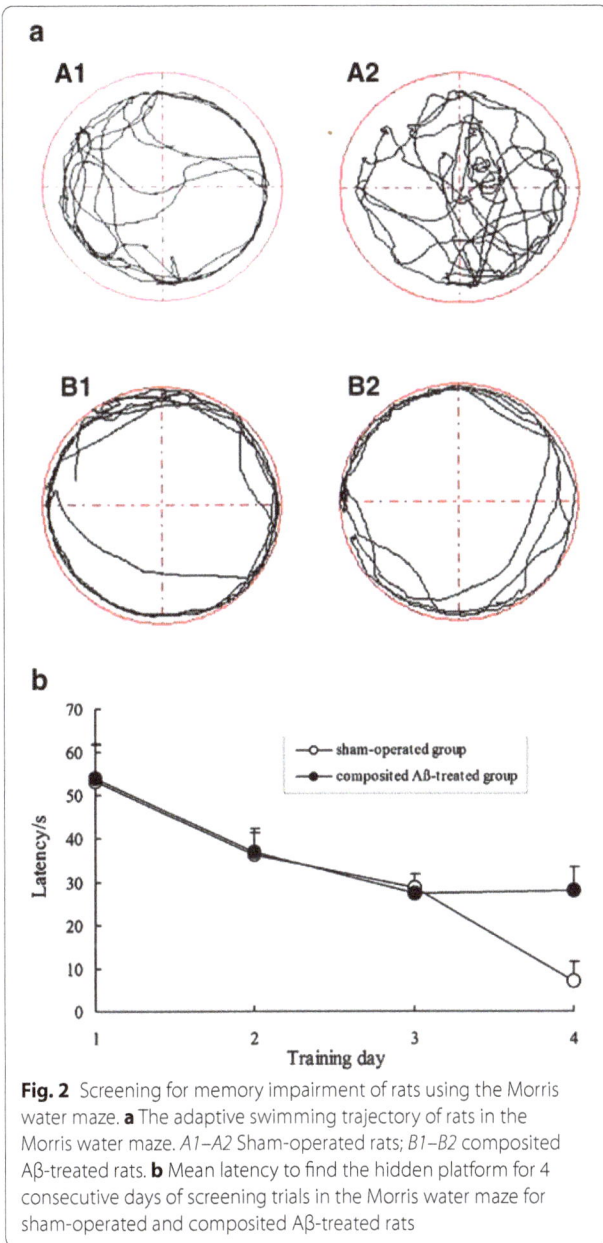

Fig. 2 Screening for memory impairment of rats using the Morris water maze. **a** The adaptive swimming trajectory of rats in the Morris water maze. *A1–A2* Sham-operated rats; *B1–B2* composited Aβ-treated rats. **b** Mean latency to find the hidden platform for 4 consecutive days of screening trials in the Morris water maze for sham-operated and composited Aβ-treated rats

at doses of 35 mg/kg [$F (1, 6) = 5.71, P < 0.05$], 70 mg/kg [$F (1, 6) = 17.51, P < 0.01$], and 140 mg/kg [$F (1, 6) = 79.67, P < 0.01$].

Effect of SBF on rat memory retention in the Morris water maze test

The probe trial was used to evaluate rat memory retention on day 3 of the Morris water maze test. As shown in Fig. 4a and b, the time that composited Aβ-treated rats swam in the target quadrant (Q1) decreased by 32.14% within 60 s compared with sham control rats [$F (1, 6) = 7.16, P < 0.05$]. The reduced swimming time of the

composited Aβ-treated group was differently attenuated by 3 doses of SBF, which increased swimming time 4.63% in response to 35 mg/kg SBF, 8.40% in response to 70 mg/kg SBF, and 25.26% in response to 140 mg/kg SBF [$F (1, 6) = 3.82, P < 0.05$].

Effect of SBF on rat memory re-learning in the Morris water maze test

The reversal trial was used to evaluate rat memory re-learning on days 4, 5, and 6 of the Morris water maze test. Figure 3 shows that the composited Aβ-treated rats took 113, 521, and 652% longer to find the hidden platform than the sham control rats [$F (1, 6) = 26.55, P < 0.01$]. It is interesting that on days 4, 5, and 6 of the Morris water maze test, the 3 doses of SBF differentially shortened the longer latencies, which decreased 20.43, 31.24, and 55.53% in response to 35 mg/kg SBF [$F (1, 6) = 7.23, P < 0.05$], 51.77, 50.11, and 61.08% in response to 70 mg/kg SBF [$F (1, 6) = 17.51, P < 0.01$], and 74.04, 61.5, and 80.51% in response to 140 mg/kg SBF [$F (1, 6) = 79.67, P < 0.01$].

Effect of SBF on rat swimming speed in the Morris water maze test

The visible platform trial was used to evaluate rat swimming speed on day 7 of training in the Morris water maze test. The times spent finding the visible platform for rats in each group were not significantly different [$F (4, 30) = 0.79, P > 0.05$]. Therefore, individual differences in rat swimming speed could be excluded, which indicated that motivation and motor skills were essentially intact.

Effect of SBF on rat neuronal injuries induced by composited Aβ-treatment

Three rats from each group were decapitated 60 min after the last administration of SBF or saline on day 38 of drug treatment. In several composited Aβ-treated rats, visual inspection revealed a yellow surface, and a thin or collapsed cerebral cortex. Optical microscopy of HE stained brains from the composited Aβ-treated group showed marked pathological changes in neurons of the hippocampus and cerebral cortex, such as neurofibrillary degeneration, neuronophagia, nuclear pyknosis, and nuclear margination (Fig. 5aB1, B2), as compared with the sham-operated group (Fig. 5aA1, A2, A3). In addition, neurons in part of the cerebral cortex of composited Aβ-treated rats showed typical colliquative necrosis, which was characterized by disrupted cell membranes, fragmented nuclei, and extensive infiltration of inflammatory cells in the necrotic region (Fig. 5aB3). However, in composited Aβ-treated rats that had been treated with SBF for 38 d, neuronal injuries in the hippocampus

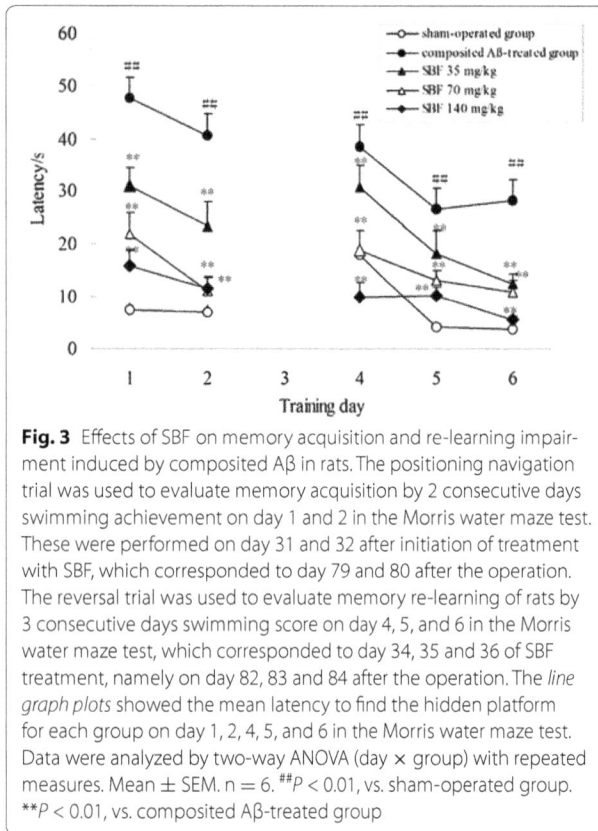

Fig. 3 Effects of SBF on memory acquisition and re-learning impairment induced by composited Aβ in rats. The positioning navigation trial was used to evaluate memory acquisition by 2 consecutive days swimming achievement on day 1 and 2 in the Morris water maze test. These were performed on day 31 and 32 after initiation of treatment with SBF, which corresponded to day 79 and 80 after the operation. The reversal trial was used to evaluate memory re-learning of rats by 3 consecutive days swimming score on day 4, 5, and 6 in the Morris water maze test, which corresponded to day 34, 35 and 36 of SBF treatment, namely on day 82, 83 and 84 after the operation. The *line graph plots* showed the mean latency to find the hidden platform for each group on day 1, 2, 4, 5, and 6 in the Morris water maze test. Data were analyzed by two-way ANOVA (day × group) with repeated measures. Mean ± SEM. n = 6. ##$P < 0.01$, vs. sham-operated group. **$P < 0.01$, vs. composited Aβ-treated group

and cerebral cortex were markedly attenuated in a dose-dependent manner (Fig. 5aC1–E1, C2–E2, C3–E3).

In addition to pathological changes, the number of neurons was significantly reduced in the brains of composited Aβ-treated rats, as compared with those of the sham-operated group. The neuron count was $63.86 \pm 4.35\%$ ($P < 0.01$) lower than that of the sham-operated group in 0.125 mm sections of the hippocampal CA1 area and $55.46 \pm 5.48\%$ ($P < 0.01$) lower in 0.0352 mm^2 sections of the cerebral cortex (Fig. 6a). It is noteworthy that the decreased neuron count in composited Aβ-treated rats was dramatically reversed by treatment with SBF for 38 days. The number of neurons was increased 18.98% by 35 mg/kg ($P < 0.05$), 47.36% by 70 mg/kg ($P < 0.01$), and by 140 mg/kg 106.81% ($P < 0.01$) in the hippocampus CA1 subfield and 14.24% by 35 mg/kg ($P < 0.05$), 59.33% by 70 mg/kg ($P < 0.01$), and 85.63% by 140 mg/kg ($P < 0.01$) in the cerebral cortex subfield (Fig. 6a).

The ultrastructure of neurons was examined with electron microscopy. Compared with the sham-operated group (Fig. 6cA), neurons in the composited Aβ-treated group were severely damaged, showing mitochondrial swelling and cristae fragmentation, increased mitochondrial electron density, dilation of the rough endoplasmic

reticulum, depolymerization of polyribosomes and polymicrotubules, smaller postsynaptic density (PSD), production of secondary lysosomes, and a large number of lipofuscin deposits in the cytoplasm. The nuclear membrane appeared rough and sunken, euchromatin was condensed and denatured, myelin sheath layers were loose or attenuated, and internal axons and fibers were degenerated (Fig. 6cB). However, 140 mg/kg SBF administered for 38 days dramatically attenuated these neuronal pathological changes induced by composited Aβ, and damage to neuronal subcellular structure was reduced (Fig. 6bC).

Discussion

It is well known that the loss of learning and memory is the major clinical symptom in AD patients [18]. In the present study, the Morris water maze was used to assess memory impairment in the AD-like model rat. We found that the percentage of successful model rats was 94.70%, which indicated that the established method for screening model rats injected with Aβ25–35 in combination with AlCl3 and RHTGF-β1 was credible. These successful model rats were used to measure the effects of SBF. On day 1 and 2 of the positioning navigation trial, the rats in the composited Aβ-treated group took longer to find the hidden platform than the sham-operated group, which demonstrated impaired spatial memory acquisition in the composited Aβ-treated rats. On day 3 of the probe trial, the rats in the composited Aβ-treated group spent less time swimming in the target quadrant, which indicated decreased memory retention in composited Aβ-treated rats. On day 4, 5, and 6 of the memory re-learning trial, the rats in the composited Aβ-treated group required more time to find the hidden platform compared with rats in the sham-operated group. This result suggests that the composited Aβ can impair memory re-learning. However, when the composited Aβ-treated rats were treated with 35, 70 or 140 mg/kg SBF for 37 d, composited Aβ-induced impairment of memory acquisition, memory retention, and re-learning was reversed, which suggests that SBF has potential value for treatment of AD.

In the present study, light and electron microscopic observation showed that the rats microinjected with composited Aβ displayed dramatic neuropathological changes, including loss of neurons, nuclear pyknosis, neurofibrillary degeneration, neuronophagia, a significant infiltration of inflammatory cells, and disrupted subcellular structures. However, when rats injected with composited Aβ were treated with SBF for 38 d, the neuropathological changes were ameliorated. These results support our previous studies [8, 9, 19–21] and suggest that the effect of SBF on memory deficits induced by composited Aβ may be derived primarily from improving neuron survival.

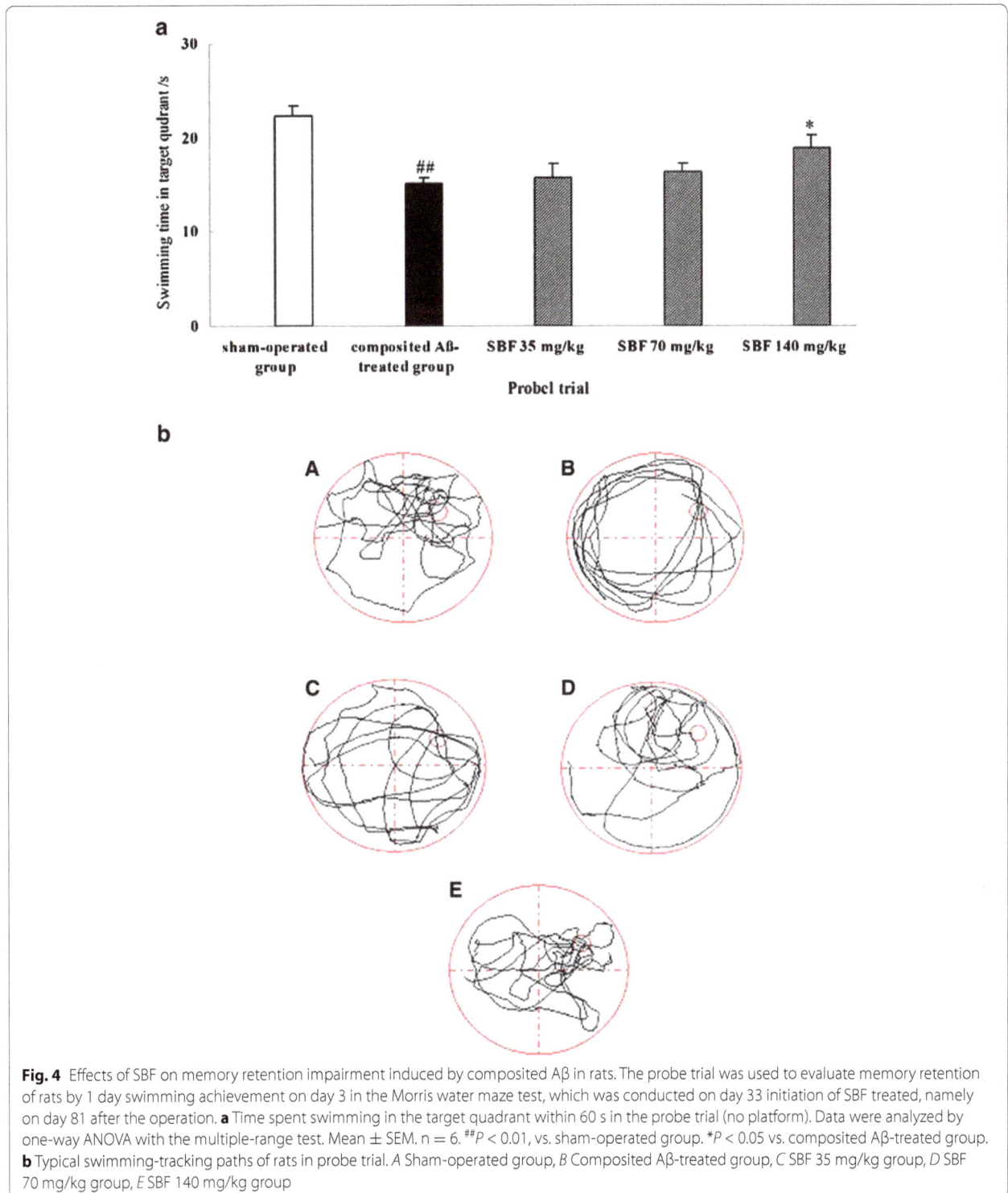

Fig. 4 Effects of SBF on memory retention impairment induced by composited Aβ in rats. The probe trial was used to evaluate memory retention of rats by 1 day swimming achievement on day 3 in the Morris water maze test, which was conducted on day 33 initiation of SBF treated, namely on day 81 after the operation. **a** Time spent swimming in the target quadrant within 60 s in the probe trial (no platform). Data were analyzed by one-way ANOVA with the multiple-range test. Mean ± SEM. n = 6. ##$P < 0.01$, vs. sham-operated group. *$P < 0.05$ vs. composited Aβ-treated group. **b** Typical swimming-tracking paths of rats in probe trial. A Sham-operated group, B Composited Aβ-treated group, C SBF 35 mg/kg group, D SBF 70 mg/kg group, E SBF 140 mg/kg group

Conclusion

In summary, the current findings show that SBF can improve composited Aβ-induced memory deficits and neurodegeneration, which suggests that SBF may be particularly useful in the treatment of neurodegenerative diseases such as AD.

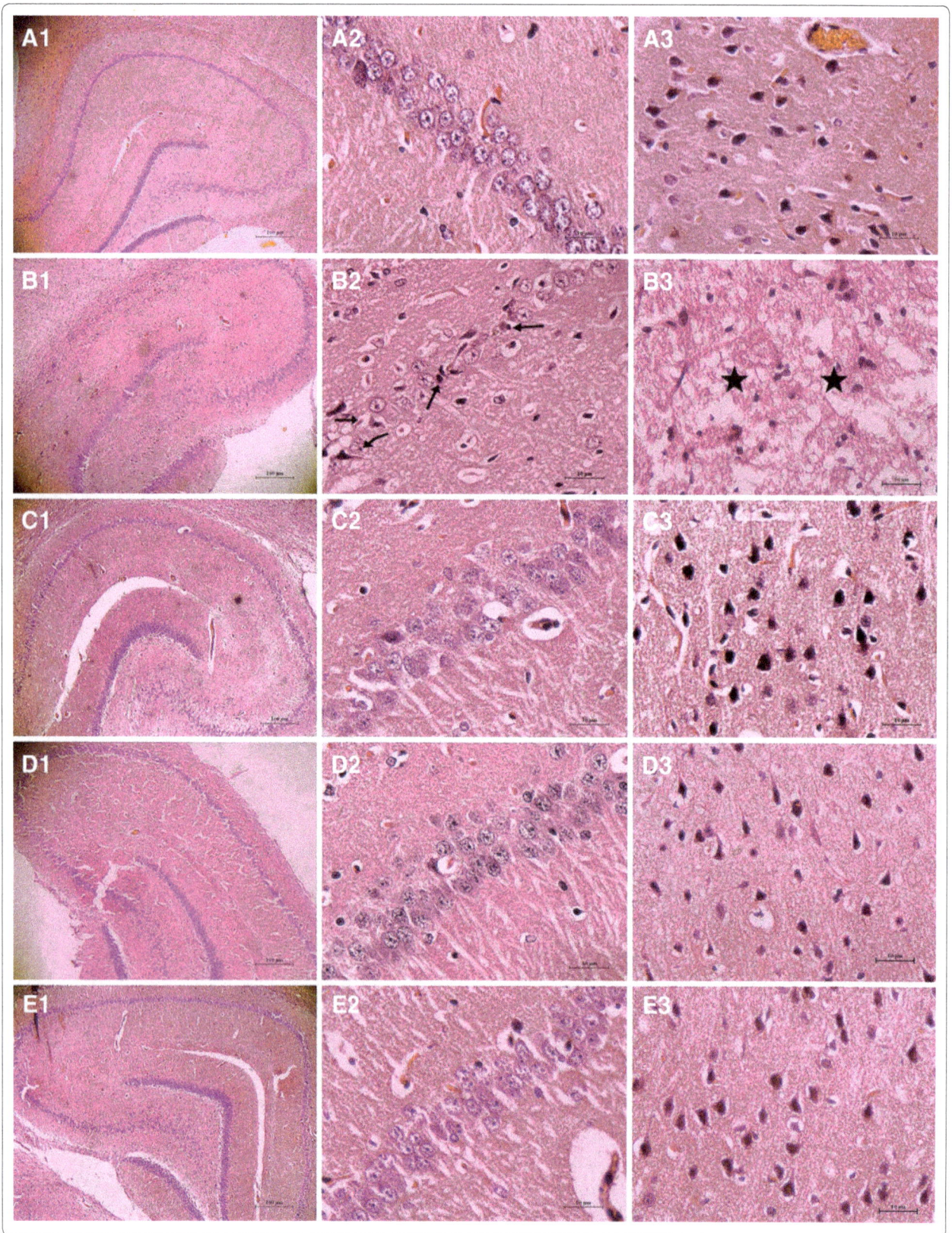

(See figure on previous page.)

Fig. 5 Effects of SBF on pathological changes in the hippocampus and cerebral cortex induced by composited Aβ in rats. Representative images of hippocampal and cerebral cortical neurons stained with HE. *A1–E1* Hippocampus ×40; *A2–E2* Hippocampus CA1 ×400; *A3–E3* Cerebral cortex ×400. *A1–A3* Sham-operated group; *B1–B3* Composited Aβ-treated group; showing loss of neurons, neurofibrillary degeneration (→), neuronophagia (←), nuclear pyknosis (↗), nuclear margination (↙), colliquative necrosis (★)with disrupted cellular membranes. Nuclei were fragmented, and large numbers of inflammatory cells infiltrated regions of the cerebral cortex in composited Aβ-treated rats. *C1–C3* SBF 35 mg/kg group; *D1–D3* SBF 70 mg/kg group; *E1–E3* SBF 140 mg/kg group. *Scale bar* 10 or 100 μm

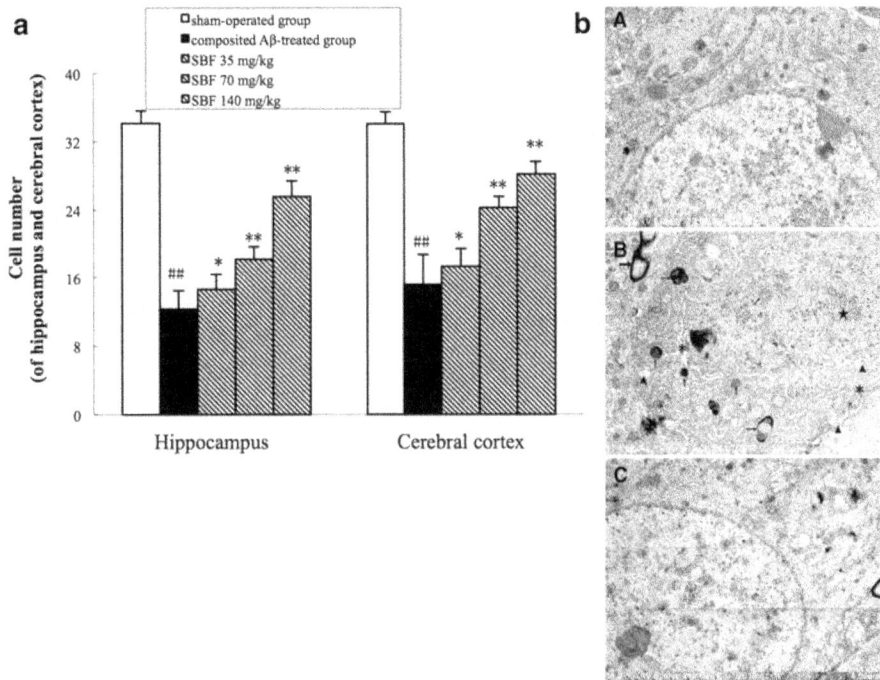

Fig. 6 a Numbers of neurons in the hippocampus and cerebral cortex, which were counted under a light microscope (×400). Each volume represents mean ± SEM from nine visual fields of three independent samples (n = 3). ##$P < 0.01$, vs. sham control. *$P < 0.05$, **$P < 0.01$, vs. composited Aβ-treated. **b** Subcellular structure of hippocampal neurons assessed by electron microscopic observation. *A* Sham-operated group ×12,000, *scale bar* 4 μm; *B* Composited Aβ-treated group; showing mitochondrial swelling, cristae fragmentation, and increased electron density (▲), rough endoplasmic reticulum dilation (.), polyribosome and polymicrotubule depolymerization, secondary lysosome (↑) production, a large number of lipofuscin (→) deposits in the cytoplasm, rough and curved nuclear membranes, condensed and denatured euchromatin (★), loose or attenuated myelin sheath layers, internal axon and fiber degeneration, and almost normal golgiosomes. ×10,000, *scale bar* 5 μm; *C* SBF 140 mg/kg group, ×12,000, *scale bar* 4 μm

Abbreviations

Aβ: beta-amyloid; AlCl3: aluminum trichloride; RHTGF-β1: recombinant human transforming growth factor-β1; Composited Aβ: amyloid beta protein 25–35 in combination with aluminum trichloride and recombinant human transforming growth factor-β1; AD: Alzheimer's disease; SP: senile plaques; NFT: intracellular neurofibrillary tangles; SBF: *Scutellaria barbata* flavonoids; SR: screening ratio; HE: hematoxylin-eosin; ANOVA: analysis of variance; PSD: postsynaptic density.

Authors' contributions

XGW and HM performed the Morris water maze test. SSW and JJC contributed the neuropathology measured. SFZ contributed to the data analysis and technical support. YZS conceived and designed the study. All authors read and approved the final manuscript.

Author details

[1] Hebei Province Key Research Office of Traditional Chinese Medicine Against Dementia/Institute of Traditional Chinese Medicine, Chengde Medical College/Hebei Province Key Laboratory of Traditional Chinese Medicine Research and Development, Chengde, Hebei 067000, China. [2] Hebei Research Institute for Family Planning, Shijiazhuang, Hebei 050000, China.

Acknowledgements

Authors thank to Yang Gao, Shuai Ma and Xiaojing Wang for technical supported.

Competing interests

The authors declare that they have no competing interests.

Funding
The project was supported by Hebei Provincial Natural Science Foundation (No. C2009001007, H2014406048) and Hebei Provincial Administration of Traditional Chinese Medicine (Nos. 05027, 2014062) of China.

References
1. Ruan Z, Zhang HY. Advances in studies of drugs treatment of Alzheimer's disease. Chin New Drugs Clin Rem. 2012;31:175–87.
2. Ma YX, Yu ZW. Contemporary Dementia Medicine. 2007, 1st ed, Beijing: Science and Technology Literature Press; pp 597–520.
3. Haass C, Selkoe DJ. Soluble protein oligomers in neurodegeneration: lessons from the Alzheimer's amyloid beta-peptide. Nat Rev Mol Cell Biol. 2007;8:101–12.
4. Perl DP. Neuropathology of Alzheimer's disease. Mt Sinai J Med. 2010;77:32–42.
5. Fang F, Yan Y, Feng ZH, Liu XQ, Wen M, Huang H. Study of Alzheimer's disease model induced multiple factors. Chongqing Med. 2007;36:146–51.
6. Guo K, Wu XG, Miao H, Cheng JJ, Cui YD, Shang YZ. Regulation and mechanism of *Scutellaria barbata* flavonoids on apoptosis of cortical neurons and cytochondriome induced by composited Aβ. Chin Hosp Pharm J. 2015;35:1994–9.
7. Dong YC, Shang YZ. Advances of *Scutellaria Barbata* in pharmacology. J Chengde Med Coll. 2009;26:98–100.
8. Xi YL, Liu MH, Zhang XF, Li M, Dong YC, Miao H, Shang YZ. Improvement of *Scutellaria Barbata* flavonoid on impaired memory of ovariectomy rats. Chin J Gerontol. 2011;31:242–5.
9. Xi YL, Zhang SF, Miao H, Shang YZ. Changes of MDA level, GSH-Px activity and NO content in ovariectomized rats and the interventional effect exerted by flavonoids from *Scutellaria Barbata*. Chin J Hosp Pharma J. 2011;31:1996–8.
10. The Ministry of Science and Technology of the People's Republic of China. Regulations for the administration of affairs concerning experimental animals. 1988-10-31.
11. Xi YL, Miao H, Shang YZ. Measurement of *Scutellaria Barbata* flavonoid concentration with ultraviolet spectrophotometry. J Chengde Med Col. 2009;26:66–7.
12. Paxinos G, Watson C, Carrive P, Kirkcaldie M, Ashwell Ken WS. Chemo-architectonic atlas of the rat forebrain. Chemoarchitectonic atlas of the rat brain. 2008, 2nd ed. New York: Academic Press; pp 275–80.
13. Morris R. Developments of a water-maze procedure for studying spatial learning in the rats. J Neurosic Methods. 1984;11:47–60.
14. Zhao XL, Fang XB, Li DP. Establishing vascular dementia model in rats. J Chin Med Univ. 2002;31(166–7):176.
15. Yu JC, Liu CZ, Zhang XZ, Han JX. Acupuncture improved cognitive impairment caused by multi-infarct dementia in rats. Physiol Behav. 2005;86:434–41.
16. Shang YZ, Miao H, Cheng JJ, Qi JM. Effects of amelioration of total flavonoids from stems and leaves of Scutellaria baicalensis Georgi on cognitive deficits, neuronal damage and free radicals disorder induced by cerebral ischemia in rats. Biol Pharm Bull. 2006;29:805–10.
17. Song HR, Cheng JJ, Miao HJ, Shang YZ. Scutellaria flavonoid supplementation reverses ageing-related cognitive impairment and neuronal changes in aged rats. Brain Inj. 2009;23:146–53.
18. Ubhi K, Masliah E. Alzheimer's disease: recent advances and future perspectives. J Alzheimers Dis. 2013;33(S1):85–94.
19. Yin XX, Zhang SF, Xi YL, Miao H, Shang YZ. Effect of flavonoids from *Scutellaria barbata* on protein expression of apoptotic genes in the brain of ovariectomized rats. Chin J New Drugs. 2010;19:1255–9.
20. Fan Y, Wu XG, Zhao HX, Shang YZ. Effects of *Scutellaria barbata* flavonoids on abnormal expression of NOS, HSP70 and apoE induced by Aβ25-35 in rat astrocytes. Chin J Pathophysiol. 2014;30(359–63):379.
21. Zhao HX, Guo K, Cui YD, Wu XG, Shang YZ. Effect of *Scutellaria barbata* flavonoids on abnormal changes of Bcl-2, Bax, Bcl-xL and Bak protein expression in mitochondrial membrane induced by composite Aβ25-35. Chin J Pathophysiol. 2014;30:2262–6.

16

BDNF DNA methylation changes as a biomarker of psychiatric disorders

Galina Y. Zheleznyakova[1,2]*, Hao Cao[1] and Helgi B. Schiöth[1]

Abstract

Brain-derived neurotrophic factor (BDNF) plays an important role in nervous system development and function and it is well established that BDNF is involved in the pathogenesis of a wide range of psychiatric disorders. Recently, numerous studies have associated the DNA methylation level of *BDNF* promoters with certain psychiatric phenotypes. In this review, we summarize data from current literature as well as from our own analysis with respect to the correlation of *BDNF* methylation changes with psychiatric disorders and address questions about whether DNA methylation related to the *BDNF* can be useful as biomarker for specific neuropsychiatric disorders.

Keywords: *BDNF*, DNA methylation, Biomarkers, Psychiatric disorders

Background

Brain-derived neurotrophic factor (BDNF) is a member of the neurotrophin family which plays an important role in neural differentiation, survival of nerve cells, neurite outgrowth, and synaptic plasticity. BDNF has been shown to regulate the development, plasticity and survival of dopaminergic, cholinergic and serotonergic neurons. Also, it regulates glutamatergic neurotransmitter release and promotes the development of GABAergic neurons. BDNF is widely expressed throughout the mammalian brain, including the cerebral cortex, hippocampus, basal forebrain, striatum, hypothalamus, brainstem, limbic structures and cerebellum [1]. This makes BDNF a key factor in learning and memory, reward-related processes, cognitive function and circuit formation.

The human *BDNF* has a complex gene structure, consisting of 11 exons (I–V, Vh, VI-VIII, VIIIh, IX), 9 of which (exon I–VII, IX) contain functional promoters. Exons II, III, IV, V, Vh, VI, and VIIIh do not have a translation start site so translation of these exons starts from the ATG of exon IX. All *BDNF* mRNAs contain the sequence for the pro-BDNF protein, encoded by exon IX. The use of translation start sites in exons I, VII, and VIII can lead to the pre-proBDNF proteins with longer N-termini. Alternative splice sites are situated in exons II, V, VI and in exon IX. In addition exon IX contains two alternative polyadenylation sites [2]. The use of different splice sites leads to the formation of numerous *BDNF* transcripts variants that determine a tissue-specific *BDNF* expression regulation as well as the regulation in responses to environmental stimuli and signaling events [2, 3]. mRNAs transcribed from the non-protein-coding anti*BDNF* gene and forming duplexes with *BDNF* mRNAs may play an important role in the regulation of *BDNF* expression [2]. Additionally, *BDNF* expression is regulated at the posttranscriptional level by enzymatic cleavage of the pro-BDNF protein into a mature BDNF protein. Pro-BDNF and BDNF can interact with two distinct transmembrane receptors, the p75 neurotropin receptor (p75NTR) and the tropomyosin-related kinase receptor B (TrkB). While pro-BDNF binds preferentially to p75NTR, inducing neuronal apoptosis and long-term depression, mature BDNF binds to TrkB and promotes a downstream signal cascade, leading to neuronal differentiation and survival, neurite outgrowth as well as synaptic plasticity [3, 4].

The BDNF protein has been extensively studied as an important factor involved in the pathogenesis of a wide

*Correspondence: galina.zheleznyakova@ki.se
[2] Department of Clinical Neuroscience, Karolinska Institute, Karolinska University Hospital, CMM L8:04, 17176 Stockholm, Sweden
Full list of author information is available at the end of the article

range of psychiatric disorders, such as major depression, schizophrenia and bipolar disorders. The use of several animal models have also implicated BDNF in anxiety-like behaviors and have shown a decreased *BDNF* expression in response to different types of stressors [5, 6]. A Val66Met polymorphism (rs6265) of *BDNF* has been associated with different psychiatric conditions. This polymorphism is related to intracellular traffic, synaptic location, secretion of BDNF as well as poorer working memory performance, reduced cerebellar and hippocampal volumes, and cognitive ability [7, 8]. The polymorphism has been demonstrated to modulate a range of clinical features in schizophrenia patients. Higher frequency of the Met allele has also been associated with depression, anxiety, anorexia, bulimia nervosa and suicidal behavior [9, 10].

Numerous studies have addressed the association between psychological disturbances and levels of BDNF protein in serum or plasma. There are several sources of BDNF in blood: BDNF might be secreted by platelets, immune and vascular endothelial cells [11, 12]. BDNF is also able to overcome the blood–brain barrier [13]. With the correlations reported between BDNF levels in the brain and blood, altered BDNF levels has been established as characteristic for several psychological disorders. Low serum BDNF protein levels have been found in patients with depression, schizophrenia, anxiety and borderline personality disorder [14–17]. While certain treatments with antidepressants increased levels of BDNF in serum [14], a pre-treated level of BDNF has been shown to possibly predict the response to antidepressant treatment and has been correlated with depression rating improvements during therapy [18]. However, such clinical parameters as age of onset, the severity of symptoms as well as clinical effectiveness of the treatment were not reflected by BDNF levels in blood [14]. Additionally, proBDNF and the mature BDNF form cannot be discriminated by measurement in blood although they affect neuronal cells differently [16]. Since alterations of BDNF levels in blood associate with several psychological disorders, it cannot be considered as a specific biomarker for certain disease.

Epigenetic alterations as DNA methylation, histone modifications and non-coding RNAs are considered to be strongly associated with pathogenesis of psychiatric disorders (reviewed in [19, 20]) with a large number of studies having examined the association between the *BDNF* methylation level and certain psychological diagnoses. Epigenetic mechanisms have been shown to be very important for *BDNF* expression regulation [3, 4, 21, 22]. DNA methylation-related chromatin remodeling of *BDNF* regulatory regions may play critical roles in regulating gene transcription in response to neuronal activity

[23, 24]. Epigenetic modifications, on the other hand, may potentially provide robust and stable biomarkers of disease activity. In this review, we have summarized the information about individual CpG sites and CpG regions previously tested in *BDNF* promoters and shown to be connected to psychiatric disorders. Using open access databases, we have analyzed the DNA methylation level of *BDNF* promoters in brain samples of individuals with psychiatric disorders. This review addresses the question of whether *BDNF* methylation changes might be regarded as suitable biomarkers of a specific disorder.

A role of DNA methylation in gene expression

Epigenetic changes are gene expression and phenotype alterations heritable through cell division that are not caused by modifications in DNA sequences [25]. The main epigenetic mechanisms include DNA methylation, histone modifications and non-coding RNAs. DNA methylation is the first described and the most studied epigenetic modification [26]. Mammalian DNA methylation occurs predominantly in the nucleotide sequence $5'CpG3'$. There are about 28 million CpG sites in the haploid human genome. CpG islands are defined as those sequences that have a length greater than 200 bp, a CpG content of at least 50 % and a CpG frequency greater than 0.6 of observed number to the expected number of CpGs [27]. The promoter regions of 60–70 % of all human genes contain CpG islands [26]. Traditionally high density CpG islands have been considered mostly hypomethylated [27, 28], however more recent studies have shown that dense CpG islands, depending on cell type, might be predominately hypermethylated [29]. A DNA methylation pattern is established and maintained by DNA methyltransferases (DNMT) namely de novo DNMT3A and DNMT3B and the maintenance DNMT1 [26]. DNA methylation affects gene expression, involving multiple mechanisms. Gene expression silencing is mediated by methylated DNA by attracting transcriptionally repressive methyl-CpG-binding proteins (MBPs). In turn, these proteins recruit histone deacytelases (HDACs) and chromatin-remodeling complexes, such as an NCoR-SMRT complex (nuclear receptor corepressor and silencing mediator for retinoid and thyroid hormone receptors), a NuRD (Nucleosome Remodeling Deacetylase) complex, which results in gene repression. The DNA methylation of a gene enhancer may also lead to gene repression. On the other hand, unmethylated CpG sites are bound by methyl-sensitive transcription factors, CXXC domain-containing activator complexes, thereby contributing to gene expression (reviewed in [30]). Unmethylated CpG sites might also serve as transcriptional factors "landing lights", marking gene promoter regions which distinguishes them from the transcriptionally irrelevant intergenic chromatin [27]. Gene body DNA methylation may have a positive influence on gene transcription [31] and intragenic DNA methylation may affect alternative gene splicing [32]. Other interesting findings are the correlation between the density of gene-body DNA methylation and replication timing [30], and the influence of 5′UTR and 3′UTR DNA methylation on the elongation and termination of transcription [33].

Initially DNA methylation has been associated with prevention of particular gene expression. However, recent studies have introduced a more complicated impact of DNA methylation on gene expression regulation with several studies having identified a poor correlation between methylation levels of some genes and their expression level [27]. Differential DNA methylation of CpG islands associated with repressed genes has been found between somatic cells [27] which might imply stochastic DNA methylation of repressed genes. A few studies indicated that binding of transcription factors may precede DNA methylation changes in the enhancer, suggesting an inactive role of DNA methylation in enhancer activity [34]. Thus, DNA methylation is a complex epigenetic modification, which does not always determine gene expression activity. Several studies align with the idea that DNA methylation changes might be triggered by an antisense transcription, changes in histone modification and chromatin protein activity and thus might be a consequence rather than a reason for gene regulation [34–36].

Dynamic changes in DNA methylation are considered important mechanisms in the developmental regulation of gene expression. Embryonic stem cells are pluripotent and characterized by hypomethylation of CpG islands. During differentiation, genes essential for cell specification remain unmethylated while opposite genes, specific for other cell line development, are kept methylated. According to this notion, somatic cells demonstrate different DNA methylation patterns of a number of genes. A genome-wide analysis, comparing the DNA methylation profile across brain and blood, reveals highly tissue-specific differences in DNA methylation between different cortical regions, cerebellum and blood. It has also been shown that tissue-specific differentially methylated regions (TS-DMR) across the cerebellum and frontal cortex are associated with stable gene expression differences [37]. One of most interesting findings was an over-representation of intragenic CpG islands and an under-representation of promoter-associated CpG islands among TS-DMR. Low density CpG promoters were characterized by widespread tissue-specific DNA methylation across brain regions and blood, in comparison with CpG-rich promoters [37]. An intriguing recent study has also demonstrated a significant underrepresentation

of promoter regions and an overrepresentation of CpG shores and shelves, gene bodies, as well as underrepresentation of CpG-rich promoters among fetal brain DMRs [38]. Another whole genome DNA methylation study has shown that similar pathways are affected in the brain and blood of Parkinson's patients. Differently methylated regions between the blood and brain have been predominately presented in high-methylation fractions which are associated with gene bodies and intragenic regions [39].

5-hydroxymethylcytosine (5hmC), derived from oxidation of 5-methylcytosine (5mC) by the Ten-Eleven Translocation (TET) enzymes, is now considered a new epigenetic DNA modification with relevant roles in regulating DNA demethylation and transcription. 5hmC is generally associated with transcribed genes promoters and bodies, positively correlated with transcription levels and detected in the mammalian genome in all cell types, with the highest content present in the brain [40].

The role of DNA methylation in the regulation of *Bdnf* expression was actively investigated by Martinowich and colleagues [23]. The authors found a three-four times higher level of the *Bdnf* exon IV transcript in Dmnt1 mutant mice in comparison with controls. It was also demonstrated that the activation of *Bdnf* transcription is regulated by neuronal activity. Enhanced transcription of the *Bdnf* exon IV promoter was observed in mouse embryonic cortical cells treated with 50 mM KCL, which is known to simulate neuronal activity by activation of voltage-sensitive calcium channels leading to calcium influx and membrane depolarization. More importantly, the authors identified that the region upstream of the *Bdnf* promoter IV transcriptional start site contains Ca^{2+}-responsive elements, namely the calcium-responsive element 1 (CaRE1), an upstream stimulatory factor-binding site (E-box) and a cyclic adenosine monophosphate (cAMP) response element (CRE), which overlap with several CpG sites. A site-specific DNA methylation in combination with a luciferase activity test showed that DNA methylation of some of these CpG sites can significantly inhibit the *Bdnf* promoter IV activity induced previously by membrane depolarization. Further experiments showed that the methylation level of several CpG sites in the *Bdnf* exon IV was significantly lower in KCl-treated culture of mouse E14 cortical cells compared with control culture. This confirms that the methylation level of the *Bdnf* promoter IV can be changed upon depolarization. Subsequent chromatin immunoprecipitation analysis revealed that methyl-CpG-binding protein MeCP2 (transcription repressor) is more tightly associated with methylated DNA within the *Bdnf* exon IV than CRE-binding protein (transcription activator). Coimmunoprecipitation assay demonstrated that the histone deacytelase HDAC1 and corepressor mSin3A also associated with the *Bdnf* promoter. All three proteins dissociated from the promoter upon membrane depolarization suggesting that *Bdnf* expression activation requires the dissociation of the MeCP2-HDAC-mSin3A repression complex. All together, these findings indicated that *Bdnf* expression level is determined by the DNA methylation pattern and chromatin modifications which, in turn, can be regulated by membrane depolarization. In a latter study, the regulation of human *BDNF* transcription by membrane depolarization was confirmed [41]. The authors indicated that neuronal activity-regulated transcription of human *BDNF* promoter I depends primarily on the novel asymmetric E-box-like element, PasRE (basic helix-loop-helix (bHLH)-PAS transcription factor response element), which is bound by the bHLH-PAS transcription factors ARNT2 (aryl hydrocarbon receptor nuclear translocator 2) and NPAS4 (neuronal PAS domain protein 4). While neuronal activity-regulated transcription of the *BDNF* promoter IV is regulated predominately by CRE, PasRE elements and the upstream stimulatory factor binding element (UBE). The CRE and PasRE elements overlap with CpG sites (Fig. 1), however a separate study is necessary to investigate if DNA methylation of these CpG sites can influence transcription of the *BDNF* promoters following membrane depolarization.

Several studies in rats have demonstrated that stressful environment conditions, such as an early-life adverse experience or maltreatment, may induce long-lasting changes in the methylation level of the *Bdnf* promoter IV which is associated with the lower *Bdnf* expression level in prefrontal cortex. Moreover, the offspring derived from maltreated-females showed hypermethylation of the *Bdnf* in the prefrontal cortex and hippocampus, suggesting that DNA methylation modifications might be inherited across generations [42, 43].

DNA methylation of *BDNF* in psychiatric disorders

DNA methylation alterations of *BDNF*, in connection to various psychiatric disorders, have been extensively studied in last several years (Table 1). Firstly, *BDNF* was studied by applying the enrichment microarray analysis; Mill and colleagues [44] tested the methylation level of several *BDNF* regions. They did not reveal any difference in the methylation level in patients with schizophrenia and bipolar disorders in comparison with controls. However, they identified an influence of rs6265 genotype, situated in exon IX on the methylation level of the surrounding region. Depending on the allele (C or T) of the rs6265, an additional CpG site can emerge in the region. CC (Val homozygotes) genotype carriers demonstrated a significant increase in methylation levels of four nearby CpG

sites in comparison with CT and TT (Met homozygotes) genotype carriers. This is especially interesting, as several studies have shown the opposite effect of the Val/Val and Met/Met genotype on the schizophrenic and non-psychotic psychiatric disease phenotype [9]. In the recent study of Chagnon and colleagues, a significantly higher methylation level of one *BDNF* region (exon VI, 3 CpG sites) was observed in older women with anxiety and/or depression compared with controls [45]. This difference was more pronounced in CT genotype carriers of rs6265 in comparison with the CC genotype carriers. TT carriers were not found among both patients and controls. The higher DNA methylation in women with anxiety/depression compared with healthy controls was confirmed in a second small CT genotype carriers' cohort (eight subjects). No difference was detected for CC and TT carriers. A comprehensive study assessing the whole *BDNF* methylation levels in a large cohort of CC, CT and TT carriers will be necessary to elucidate the impact of rs6265 on the methylation level of distal *BDNF* regions.

Keller and colleagues were the first to investigate the *BDNF* DNA methylation changes in suicide victims in comparison with controls [46]. Using bisulfite pyrosequencing and direct bisulfite sequencing, EpiTYPER as a confirmation analyses, these authors analyzed the methylation levels of CpG sites at *BDNF* promoter/exon IV in the Wernicke area of the brain. A significant increase of the average methylation level of 4 CpG sites located downstream of TSS (+10, +16, +25, +28) (Fig. 1b) and methylation levels of two separate CpG sites (+10, +25) was found in suicide completers. Moreover, they also indicated an association between the average methylation level of these 4 CpG sites and the *BDNF* transcript IV levels.

Fuchikami and colleagues were the first to examine the possibility of DNA methylation changes as a biomarker of major depression. Applying the EpiTYPER technique, these authors determined the methylation level of two CpG islands associated with promoter I and promoter IV of *BDNF* in major depressive disorder (MDD) patients in comparison with healthy individuals. The methylation levels of 29 out of 35 CpG sites inside of promoter I (Fig. 1a) were significantly different between patients and controls, although different CpG sites demonstrated multidirectional methylation changes. 21 CpG sites showed increased methylation levels in controls, while the other 8 CpG sites showed increased methylation levels in depression patients [47].

In a study of major depressed patients with suicidal behavior, higher *BDNF* promoter VI methylation levels were found to be strongly associated with a previous history of suicidal attempts, suicidal ideation and less improvement during antidepressant treatment,

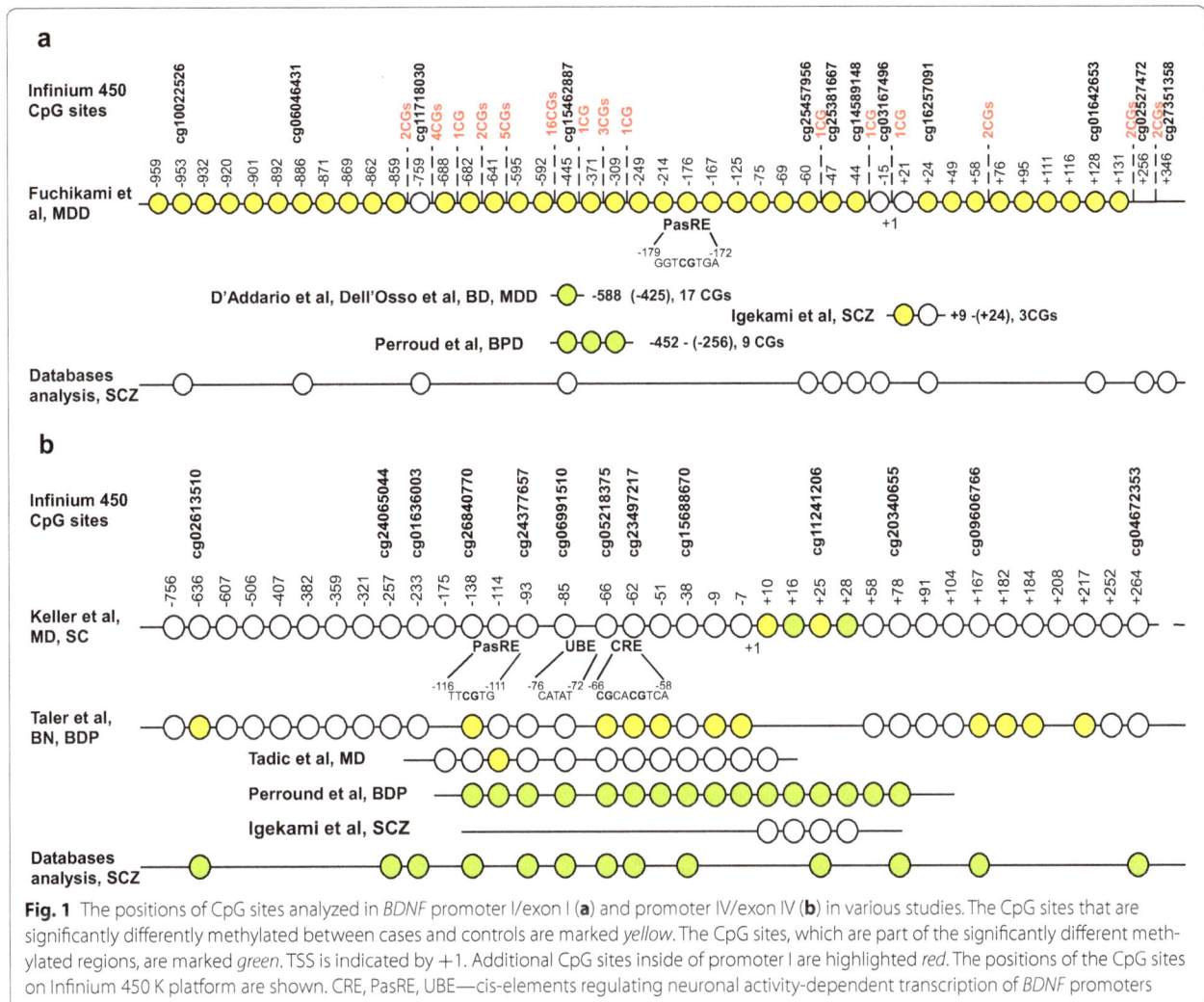

Fig. 1 The positions of CpG sites analyzed in *BDNF* promoter I/exon I (**a**) and promoter IV/exon IV (**b**) in various studies. The CpG sites that are significantly differently methylated between cases and controls are marked *yellow*. The CpG sites, which are part of the significantly different methylated regions, are marked *green*. TSS is indicated by +1. Additional CpG sites inside of promoter I are highlighted *red*. The positions of the CpG sites on Infinium 450 K platform are shown. CRE, PasRE, UBE—cis-elements regulating neuronal activity-dependent transcription of *BDNF* promoters

independent of the antidepressant type [48]. As *BDNF* methylation status was not measured after the treatment in this study, it is not possible to conclude if treatment outcomes might be reflected by DNA methylation status. In two subsequent studies, authors found a significant association between the *BDNF* promoter VI methylation levels and late-life depression [49] as well as depression related to breast cancer [50]. It is worth mentioning, that both studies did not reveal any association between the methylation level of the analyzed region and rs6265 genotype.

Kleimann and colleagues, for the first time, examined an effect of electroconvulsive therapy (ECT) on DNA methylation of *BDNF* [51] in treatment-resistant major depressive patients. The difference in the methylation level of *BDNF* promoter I was presented between remitters/responders and non-remitters/non-responders over the whole series of ECT treatment. It is difficult to say if the found difference was conditioned by only ECT since

there was no information about *BDNF* methylation level before ECT and most patients were previously treated by antidepressants and/or antipsychotics.

By means of bisulfite pyrosequencing, Igekame and colleagues found a significant increase (about 1 %) of the methylation level of one CpG site in the promoter I of *BDNF* in schizophrenia patients compared with controls [52] (Fig. 1a). Only in the male group of patients the additional CpG site was approximately 2 % higher methylated. It should be noted that the differences were not significant after multiple corrections and the sample size is not large enough to estimate a methylation level difference as low as 1–2 %. Authors did not reveal any difference in the methylation level of *BDNF* promoter IV.

On the contrary, Kordi-Tamandani and colleagues revealed that the methylated allele frequency of the *BDNF* promoter IV was lower in the schizophrenia patients, than in controls. According to the methylation

Table 1 Summary of human studies of the *BDNF* promoters' DNA methylation in psychiatric disorders

Reference	Year	*BDNF* region	Chromosomal position (hg19)	Phenotype	Tissue	Samples	Method	Statistical power
Fuchikami et al.	2011	Promoter I Promoter IV	chr11:27743473–27744564 chr11:27722840–27723980	Major depression (MDD)	Peripheral blood	20 MDD, 18 CT	EpiTYPER	CpG8,9—75.7% CpG76—54.3% CpG80,81—79.1% For rest CpGs—>80%
D'Addario et al.	2012	Promoter I	chr11:27744031–27744193	Bipolar disorder I, II (BDI, BDII)	Peripheral blood	49 BD I, 45 BD II, 52 CT	Methylation-specific real-time PCR	BDII vs CT—62.5% Antidep. vs antidep-free—93%
D'Addario et al.	2013	Promoter I	chr11:27744031–27744193	Major depression	Peripheral blood	41 MDD, 44 CT	Methylation-specific real-time PCR	Methylation level —83.1% Expression level—65.9%
Ikegame et al.	2013	Promoter I Promoter IV	chr11:27743390–27743763 chr11:27722994–27723372	Schizophrenia (SCZ)	Peripheral blood	100 SCZ, 100 CT	Bisulfite pyrosequencing	CpG72—52.4%
Perroud et al.	2013	Promoter I Promoter IV	chr11:27743862–27744057 chr11:27723057–27723293	Borderline personality disorder (BPD)	Peripheral blood	115 BPD, 52 CT	High resolution melt analysis	BPD vs CT—100%
Dell'Osso et al.	2014	Promoter I	chr11:27744031–27744194	Bipolar disorder I, II, major depression	Peripheral blood	43MDD, 61 BD I, 50 BD II, 44 CT	Methylation-specific real-time PCR	MDD, BDII vs BDI and CT—100%
Kleimann et al.	2015	Promoter I Promoter IV Promoter VI	chr11:27743416–27744782 (3 regions) chr11:27723103–27723511 chr11:27722216–27722863 (2 regions)	Treatment-resistant major depression (electroconvulsive therapy)	Peripheral blood	11MDD	Direct bisulfite sequencing	Remit. vs non-remit. 4 treatment sessions: 91–100%
Chagnon et al.	2015	Promoter I Exon III Promoter VI/Exon VI	NS	Anxiety/major depression	Saliva	19 MDD, 24 CT	Bisulfite pyrosequencing	MDD vs CT—86.3% CT gen. MDD vs CT gen. CT—88.3%
Keller et al.	2010	Promoter IV	chr11:27723126–277231144 (4 CpG sites)	Major depression, suicide	Brain (Wernicke area)	44 SU, 33 CT	Bisulfite pyrosequencing, direct bisulfite sequencing, EpiTYPER	CpG1—98.1% CpG3—96.3% Average level—98.3%
Kordi-Tamandani et al.	2012	Promoter IV	NS	Schizophrenia	Peripheral blood	80 SCZ, 71 CT	Methylation-specific PCR	Methylation level—99% Expression level—94%
Tadic et al.	2014	Promoter IV	chr11:27723103–27723380	Major depression (antidepressant treatment)	Peripheral blood	39 MDD	Direct bisulfite sequencing	NA
Thaler et al.	2014	Promoter IV	chr11:27722840–27723980	Bulimic nervosa (BN), Borderline personality disorder	Peripheral blood	64 BN(F), 32 CT	EpiTYPER	BN vs CT—in average for all CpG sites—99.8%
Kang et al.	2013	Promoter VI	chr11:27721688–27721823	Major depressive, suicidal behavior (antidepressant treatment)	Peripheral blood	108 MDD	Bisulfite pyrosequencing	Previous suicidal attempt—76.7% Suicidal ideation during treatment—83.6 and 96.6%
Kang et al.	2015a	Promoter VI	chr11:27721688–27721823	Depression related to breast cancer	Peripheral blood	74 D, 235 CT	Bisulfite pyrosequencing	D vs CT within 1 week and 1 year in average—81.2%
Kang et al.	2015b	Promoter VI	chr11:27721688–27721823	Late-life depression	Peripheral blood	101 D, 631 CT	Bisulfite pyrosequencing	D vs CT at baseline and after 2 years in average—97.7%

Table 1 continued

Reference	Year	*BDNF* region	Chromosomal position (hg19)	Phenotype	Tissue	Samples	Method	Statistical power
Unternaehrer et al.	2015	Exon VI	chr11:27721543– 277221857	Low maternal care (LC) vs. high maternal care (HC)	Peripheral blood	45 LC, 40 HC	EpiTYPER	NA
Mill et al.	2008	Promoter IX	chr11:27679911–27680006	Schizophrenia, bipolar disorder	Brain (frontal cortex)	35 SZ, 35 BD, 35 CT	Enriched unmethylated DNA microarray, bisulfite pyrosequencing	Val homozygotes (78) vs Met carries (27)—100 %

data, the relative expression level of *BDNF* was significantly higher in schizophrenia patients than in controls [53].

In the study of D'Addario, a 7 % increase of DNA methylation at the region of *BDNF* promoter I (Fig. 1a) was observed in bipolar disorder (BD) II patients, but not BD I, compared with controls [54]. This was in correlation with the significantly decreased *BDNF* expression in BD II subjects. It should be taken in account that these data do not reflect the initial DNA methylation levels of BD patients, since part of the patients enrolled in the study were maintained on a diverse antidepressant treatment for at least 1 month. Interestingly, the authors showed, that BD patients on antidepressant treatment revealed a higher *BDNF* methylation level compared with antidepressants-free patients. However, the patients treated by valproate and lithium demonstrated a significantly decreased *BDNF* methylation level, in comparison with the control level.

In the subsequent study, these authors extended the *BDNF* promoter I methylation level analysis to the group of patients with major depression on stable pharmacologic treatment in comparison with healthy individuals [55]. In concordance with the previous study, a significantly increased methylation level of the analyzed region inside of *BDNF* promoter I was observed in MDD patients together with a significant reduction of *BDNF* expression. These authors also showed that MDD patients treated only by antidepressant drugs (i.e., selective serotonin and selective norepinephrine reuptake inhibitors) had a 10 % higher methylation level of the *BDNF* promoter in comparison with patients treated by combinatory therapy of antidepressants and mood stabilizers [55].

However, in a further study which was performed on a larger cohort of MDD, BD I and BD II patients, these authors were not able to show the effect of mood stabilizers on DNA methylation [56]. Patients treated by lithium and valproate tend to demonstrate *BDNF* methylation levels close to controls in comparison with patients treated by other antidepressant agents such as selective serotonin reuptake inhibitors, serotonin norepinephrine reuptake inhibitors and atypical antipsychotics. MDD subjects and BD II patients showed a significantly higher methylation level of the analyzed region in comparison with BD I subjects [56].

In the absence of an initial DNA methylation status for the patients, the results of these studies are difficult to interpret. It is not possible to discriminate if these described changes in the methylation level among different diagnostic groups are associated with disease status or whether they are connected with various pharmacological treatments. It was noted that BD I patients were mostly treated by mood stabilizers, while inside of the BD II and MDD groups, patients obtained a different therapy [56]. Thus, the *BDNF* promoter methylation analysis in drug-naive MDD, BD patients is necessary in order to make a reliable conclusion about whether this parameter might be used as biomarker.

Interesting results have been obtained in a study by Tadic and colleagues where the correlation between DNA methylation of *BDNF* promoter IV (Fig. 1b) in major depressive patients and antidepressant treatment response was assessed [57]. Of the 12 analyzed CpG sites, the methylation level of one CpG site was about 2 % lower in non-responders compared to responders. Following this, in vitro experiments showed a decreased luciferase expression of a vector containing an unmethylated fragment of *BDNF* promoter IV, in response to both SSRI and the SNRI treatment. These findings were connected with the ability of antidepressants to phosphorylate MeCP2, which leads to its dissociation from a promoter and consequently to the activation of expression. Moreover, these authors suggested that the DNA methylation status may play a significant role in the binding of MeCP2 to the promoter region and described that the mechanism of antidepressant action on *BDNF* can only be active in carriers of methylated allele at the specific CpG site. However, it is difficult to say that this conclusion was supported by experimental in vivo data, as both responders and non-responders demonstrated a strongly hypomethylated (4–6 %) status of the analyzed region.

DNA methylation levels of the *BDNF* promoter I and promoter IV (Fig. 1) were studied in patients with borderline personality disorder (BDP), whose disease phenotype is closely related to the depression and suicide phenotype. Using the high resolution melt (HRM) analysis, Perround and colleagues observed that regions in the *BDNF* promoter I and promoter IV had an almost 8 and 18 % higher methylation level respectively for BDP patients [58]. Moreover, a larger number of childhood maltreatment was significantly associated with a higher methylation status of *BDNF* promoters (mean percentage at both regions). Another very interesting result of this study is that during the intensive dialectical behavior therapy (I-DBT) non-responders showed increased *BDNF* methylation levels, while responders showed a decrease in *BDNF* methylation status, in some cases comparable to the methylation level of controls. This suggests that *BDNF* methylation changes might be relevant for treatment response prediction. The limitation of this study is that most of the subjects were on antidepressant treatment before I-DBT, that way the determined methylation level of BDP patients before treatment does not directly reflect a baseline methylation level of such patients.

An additional study of the influence of childhood maternal care on *BDNF* methylation level was performed by Unternaehrer and colleagues [59]. Authors showed greater whole blood DNA methylation in the low versus high maternal care group in a CpG island situated within the *BDNF* exon VI. More importantly, authors investigated differential blood cell distribution as a potential factor in connection with maternal care and DNA methylation of *BDNF*. It should be considered as an example of a standard experimental set up for such types of studies due to the blood cell specific DNA methylation pattern.

Thaler and colleagues explored DNA methylation changes of the *BDNF* promoter IV (Fig. 1b) in women with bulimic eating syndromes [60]. These women displayed increases in the methylation level at specific CpG sites, especially in cases when the bulimic syndromes were complicated by borderline personality disorder or history of severe childhood abuse. It is interesting that majority of found CpG sites were binding sites for various transcriptional factors. As no multiple corrections were applied, additional studies will be required to confirm the obtained differences.

Open access study analysis
Material
Four databases from the ArrayExpress Archive of Functional Genomics Data (http://www.ebi.ac.uk/array-express) have been included in the analysis. Detailed information about each database can be found in Table 2.

Method
In the databases, the DNA methylation level was assessed at over 485,000 CpG sites using the Illumina Infinium Human Methylation450 Bead Chip. 25 probes corresponding to 12 CpG sites situated in the *BDNF* promoter I/exon I (Fig. 1a) and to 13 CpG sites situated in the *BDNF* promoter IV/exon IV were included in the

analysis (Fig. 1b). The methylation level of each promoter was calculated by averaging the methylation levels of the corresponding CpG sites. Distribution normality for all variables was checked using Kolmogorov–Smirnov test. Because of non-Gaussian distribution, statistical comparisons of methylation levels between patients and controls were performed using the non-parametric Mann–Whitney test, although in the text and in the tables values are presented as mean ± SEM. A Bonferroni correction was used to adjust for multiple comparisons. Statistical analyses were performed using GraphPad Prism5 (GraphPad) and the statistical software R (http://www.r-project.org). A significance level of a = 0.05 or less was considered significant. The statistical power analysis for the described studies and the open access databases was performed with a web browser program "Post-hoc Power Calculator" (http://clincalc.com/Stats/Power.aspx#1).

Results
According to results of previous studies both promoter I and IV of *BDNF* demonstrated strongly hypomethylated levels in all analyzed cohorts (Table 3). Frontal cortex methylation levels of both promoters I and IV were lower in schizophrenia subjects compared to controls (E-GEOD-61431, E-GEOD-61380, E-GEOD-61107 databases). Cerebellum methylation levels of promoter IV were lower in schizophrenia patients, at the same time cerebellum methylation levels of promoter I were similar in patients and controls. After applying multiple corrections, a significant difference in the methylation level of *BDNF* promoter I (p = 0.0023, Mann–Whitney test; E-GEOD-61380 database,) and of *BDNF* promoter IV (p = 0.0015, Mann–Whitney test; E-GEOD-61107 database) was found between schizophrenia patients and healthy individuals (Table 3). However, the power analysis indicated that the E-GEOD-61380 database is not

Table 2 Open access analyzed databases

Database	Phenotype	Brain region	Groups	Age (years: mean ± SD)
E-GEOD-61107	Schizophrenia	Frontal cortex	23 SCZ: 7F, 16M	51.61 ± 21.55
			24 CT: 5F, 19M	71.29 ± 9.76
E-GEOD-61380	Schizophrenia	Frontal cortex	18 SCZ: 3F, 15M	45.5 ± 16.61
			15 CT: 2F, 13M	42.2 ± 14.85
E-GEOD-61431	Schizophrenia	Frontal cortex	20 SCZ: 9F, 11M	62.05 ± 15.87
			23 CT: 6F,17M	62.04 ± 18.74
E-GEOD-61431	Schizophrenia	Cerebellum	21 SCZ: 10F, 11M	61.76 ± 16.61
			23 CT: 6F, 17M	61.39 ± 19.25
E-GEOD-41826	Major depression	Frontal cortex: Split glial and neuronal cells	29 MDD: 15F, 14M	32 ± 15.92
			29 CT: 15F, 14M	32.1 ± 16.06

Table 3 Methylation levels of *BDNF* promoters I and IV assessed in patients from open access databases

	Patients		Controls		p value	Statistical power
	Mean	SEM	Mean	SEM		
Database E-GEOD-61107 (Schizophrenia, frontal cortex)						
Promoter I	0.093	0.0026	0.099	0.002	0.09	
Promoter IV	0.113	0.0028	0.126	0.003	0.0015*	90.6 %
Database E-GEOD-61380 (Schizophrenia, frontal cortex)						
Promoter I	0.105	0.0009	0.108	0.002	0.0023*	30.4 %
Promoter IV	0.119	0.0012	0.12	0.0016	0.61	
Database E-GEOD-61431 (Schizophrenia, frontal cortex)						
Promoter I	0.123	0.0016	0.128	0.0017	0.13	
Promoter IV	0.157	0.0018	0.161	0.002	0.22	
Database E-GEOD-61431 (Schizophrenia, cerebellum)						
Promoter I	0.119	0.0027	0.117	0.0018	0.98	
Promoter IV	0.141	0.003	0.148	0.0029	0.0345	40 %
Database E-GEOD-41826 (MDD, frontal cortex, neurons)						
Promoter I	0.094	0.0007	0.093	0.0008	0.24	
Promoter IV	0.126	0.0009	0.125	0.001	0.39	
Database E-GEOD-41826 (MDD, frontal cortex, glia)						
Promoter I	0.106	0.001	0.107	0.001	0.30	
Promoter IV	0.125	0.001	0.126	0.001	0.32	

* Significant after multiple correction

powerful enough to determine a 0.3 % methylation level difference.

We did not observe any difference between MDD patients and controls in the methylation levels of *BDNF* promoters I and IV in the frontal cortex neuronal and glial cells (E-GEOD-41826). We separately analyzed several CpG sites which were determined as significantly differently methylated in previous studies (Fig. 1). The difference was found in the methylation level of cg14589148 (p = 0.0147, Mann–Whitney test; E-GEOD-61380 database), cg25457956 and cg10022526 (p = 0.0396 and p = 0.0227, Mann–Whitney test; E-GEOD-61431 database, cerebellum), however these data did not remain significant after multiple corrections.

Discussion

The variety and complexity of psychiatric disorders is very high and biomarkers able to reliably differentiate characteristics of certain similar disorders, determine severity and treatment efficiency which could be very valuable. Taking into the consideration the inaccessibility of the target tissue—the brain—in psychiatric disorders, an ideal biomarker should be easily peripherally measured but at the same time it should reflect disease-associated alterations in the target tissue. DNA methylation is a stable and heritable modification and can be reliably measured from a small amount of material regardless of the storage conditions. These remarkable characteristics

make DNA methylation a robust biomarker of disease activity. Numerous cancer studies have proven that DNA methylation changes allow manifestations of different pathological stages of disease and monitoring of treatment efficiency (reviewed in [61]).

At present, a growing body of data has associated *BDNF* promoters' methylation level with development of various neuropsychiatric disorders. Most of the studies have analyzed different regions within promoter I and promoter IV. As it is demonstrated in Fig. 1a, the promoter I region is differently methylated in major depression and bipolar disorders patients in the studies done by D'Addario. These partly overlap with the region differently methylated in BPD patients of the Perroud's study and with one CpG site differently methylated in major depression patients of the Fuchikami's study. Similarly, within promoter IV, the CpG sites are differently methylated in suicide completers of Keller's study, in patients with BDP and BN of the Taler's study, and in major depressive patients in Tadic's study, which partially overlap with the differently methylated region in BPD patients in Perroud' study (Fig. 1b). These overlapping regions within *BDNF* promoter I and promoter IV may be of special interest as possible biomarker of psychiatric diseases, taking into consideration that several independent studies reported about the differences in the methylation level of these regions. Although the methylation levels' alteration of these regions associated with multiple disorders do not allow the consideration of these methylation changes as reliable biomarkers for certain psychiatric disturbances.

Most of the studies have been performed using peripheral blood cells. The main question which appears is to what extent DNA methylation changes in blood can reflect the changes in the target tissue—the brain; a highly tissue-specified *BDNF* expression implies variation of *BDNF* promoter methylation level in various tissues. However, it has been reported that there might not be an exact correlation between gene DNA methylation and its expression level [27]. Moreover, all studies were concentrated on the methylation levels of *BDNF* promoters, which are CpG rich. It is well established that differently methylated regions across the brain and blood are primarily located in intragenic regions and are underrepresented in promoter and regulatory gene regions. CpG rich promoters were characterized by less tissue-specific DNA methylation across brain regions and blood [37, 39]. Recently, a strong correlation between the ventral prefrontal cortex and quadriceps for the methylation levels of *BDNF* promoter I has been found [62]. Similar epigenetic changes, particularly DNA methylation, in the brain and peripheral tissues in connection to psychiatric disorders might be initiated by environmental factors such as maternal stress or diet during early prenatal development or even have an inherited character. In the postnatal period, mothering behavior, early life traumas, environmental stressors factors and hormone dissonance may be responsible for the widespread epigenetic alterations associated with the psychiatric phenotype [19, 42, 43]. Keller and colleagues demonstrated that *BDNF* promoters' DNA methylation changes in brain are associated with major depression and suicide. In one of the brain open-access databases, we revealed a significant but minor (1.3 %) difference in the average methylation level of *BDNF* promoter IV in schizophrenia patients.

Most of the changes found in the *BDNF* methylation levels between patients and healthy individuals are very subtle. The question about whether these differences may initiate changes in the *BDNF* expression levels has been partly addressed in previous studies. Thus, Keller and colleagues indicated much lower *BDNF* transcript IV levels in samples showing 20 to 30 % methylation of 4 CpG sites in *BDNF* promoter IV compared with samples showing 3 to 5 % methylation [46]. In the study of D'Addario and colleagues, a 9 % alteration in the *BDNF* promoter I methylation level between BDII patients and controls was matched with changes in the *BDNF* expression level in the blood cells [54]. It may suggest that the 9–15 % difference of the *BDNF* methylation level is functionally relevant and can induce changes in the *BDNF* transcripts level. In turn, Perroud and colleagues were not able to find any correlation between the *BDNF* promoters' methylation and BDNF protein levels, although an 8 and 18 % methylation level difference was found respectively in *BDNF* promoter I and promoter IV between BDP patients and controls [58]. The discordance, in the association of the BDNF protein level with the DNA methylation level, might be conditioned by other regulators of *BDNF* expression: particularly histone modifications, miRNAs, antiBDNF transcripts, formation of dsRNA duplexes with *BDNF* transcripts, alternative splicing, and posttranscriptional cleavage. Recent studies have introduced the idea that DNA methylation may not even have an active influence on gene expression, but instead it might reflect gene expression regulation, mediated by histone modifications or chromatin structure [34]. Additionally, DNA hydroxymethylation, which cannot be distinguished from DNA methylation by bisulfite treatment, can impact *BDNF* expression in a manner opposite to DNA methylation. Therefore, a complex analysis of several factors determining *BDNF* expression is necessary to make the conclusion of whether the small changes in the *BDNF* methylation level may affect the *BDNF* expression changes both on transcript and protein levels.

Despite a relatively large number of studies, the use of the *BDNF* methylation level as a biomarker of psychiatric disorders still needs considerable further research to become reality. The main reason is the lack of confirmatory research for each particular disease. Another factor is the use of a variety of techniques for methylation level determination (Table 1), which hampers the analysis of different areas within the *BDNF* promoters without providing a correct comparison of the results of different studies for the same disorder. Although, methylation-specific real-time PCR and high resolution melt analysis are very sensitive methods with the ability to detect as little as 0.1–1 % of methylated DNA [63, 64], they cannot provide individual CpG sites' resolution, allowing the determination of the average methylation level of a whole region. Primer design, PCR bias or the presence of too many CpG sites in the analyzed region might affect the obtained results. The bisulfite sequencing-based techniques widely applied in the studies differ also in their coverage and sensitivity. Direct bisulfite sequencing can accurately detect an intermediate difference ($\geq$20 %) in methylation level while with pyrosequencing a minor difference of 5 % can be reliably detected while the resolution of cloning bisulfite sequencing is dependent on the number of sequenced clones [65, 66]. Furthermore, the inclusion of medicated and treated patients in the studies does not allow for specification of whether the observed DNA methylation changes are related to the specific disease phenotype or are a consequence of medical or psychiatric treatment. It is known that certain agents, applied for psychiatric therapy, cause epigenetic modifications [67]. Insufficient attention has been paid to *BDNF* methylation level investigations in the brain. So far only Keller's study and our analysis indicate a partial correlation of the *BDNF* methylation level in the brain to the development of psychiatric disorders. However, we did not find any difference in the methylation level of the CpG site (cg11241206), differently methylated between controls and suicide completers in Keller's study. Measured methylation levels of others CpG sites (Fig. 1), previously described as differently methylated in the studies, using blood cells did not show any correlation after multiple corrections. The restrictions of the method did not allow us to completely assess the methylation level of the regions analyzed in previous studies using brain samples as Infinium HumanMethylation450 BeadChip Kit covers far from all CpG sites in *BDNF* promoter I and IV (Fig. 1). A detailed analysis in the brain with a method, determining the methylation levels of all CpG sites, is required. Both Keller's and our study covered only certain brain areas (frontal cortex, cerebellum, Wernicke area), while *BDNF* DNA methylation changes in such brain regions as hippocampus, nucleus accumbens, amygdala [3, 68, 69] may be essential for psychiatric disorders development.

Conclusions

Summing up the results of this research provides a good reason to believe that the methylation levels of certain regions within *BDNF* promoters can be considered as biomarker of specific diseases. Several independent studies on different patients' cohorts with a standardized method for the methylation level analysis are necessary to confirm this suggestion. Applying the most modern approaches for the analysis of methylation will allow highlighting of the role of both DNA methylation and DNA hydroxymethylation (primarily occurring in the neuronal cells) with regard to the development of mental illnesses. Considering the easy accessibility of blood samples, it is the DNA methylation level of blood cells that might be used in clinical practice for accurate disease diagnosis and treatment-efficacy monitoring. The question of DNA methylation discrepancy within various blood cell lines [70] and possible differences of cell composition between psychiatric patients and healthy individuals [71] should also be taken in account. Modern techniques of cell sorting and counting will help to smooth over such differences. Considering the fact that most changes in DNA methylation linked to mental illness are fairly small in terms of percentage, it is necessary to use a high-resolution method that can reliably detect small differences. We suggest that through further investigations, an unequivocal answer if the *BDNF* DNA methylation level is a suitable psychiatric disorder biomarker may be provided.

Abbreviations
ARNT2: aryl hydrocarbon receptor nuclear translocator 2; BD: bipolar disorder; BDNF: brain-derived neurotrophic factor; BDP: borderline personality disorder; CaRE1: calcium-responsive element 1; CRE: cAMP response element; DNMT: DNA methyltransferase; ECT: electroconvulsive therapy; HDACs: histone deacytelases; HRM: high resolution melt; I-DBT: dialectical behavior therapy; MBPs: methyl-CpG-binding proteins; MDD: major depressive disorder; MSP: methylation-specific real-time PCR; NCoR: nuclear receptor corepressor; NPAS4: neuronal PAS domain protein 4; NuRD: nucleosome remodeling deacetylase; p75NTR: p75 neurotropin receptor; PasRE: basic helix-loop-helix transcription factor response element; SMRT: silencing mediator for retinoid and thyroid hormone receptors; SNRIs: serotonin norepinephrine reuptake inhibitors; SSRIs: selective serotonin reuptake inhibitors; TET: ten-eleven translocation enzymes; TrkB: tropomyosin-related kinase receptor B; TS-DMR: tissue-specific differentially methylated region; UBE: upstream stimulatory factor binding element.

Authors' contributions
GYZ and HBS conceived this review. GYZ drafted the manuscript, performed analyses, interpreted data. HC participated in data analyses. HBS provided critical revision of the manuscript. All authors read and approved the final manuscript.

Author details
[1] Department of Neuroscience, Uppsala University, Husargatan 3, BMC, 75124 Uppsala, Sweden. [2] Department of Clinical Neuroscience, Karolinska Institute, Karolinska University Hospital, CMM L8:04, 17176 Stockholm, Sweden.

Acknowledgements
We are grateful to Christina Zhukovsky for proofreading the article.

Competing interests
The authors declare that they have no competing interests.

Funding
HS was supported by the Swedish Research Council and the Swedish Brain Foundation. Hao Cao was supported by the China Research Council. The funders had no role in the design of the study and collection, analysis, and interpretation of data and in writing the manuscript.

References
1. Murer MG, Yan Q, Raisman-Vozari R. Brain-derived neurotrophic factor in the control human brain, and in Alzheimer's disease and Parkinson's disease. Prog Neurobiol. 2001;63(1):71–124.
2. Pruunsild P, et al. Dissecting the human *BDNF* locus: bidirectional transcription, complex splicing, and multiple promoters. Genomics. 2007;90(3):397–406.
3. Boulle F, et al. Epigenetic regulation of the *BDNF* gene: implications for psychiatric disorders. Mol Psychiatry. 2012;17(6):584–96.
4. Mitchelmore C, Gede L. Brain derived neurotrophic factor: epigenetic regulation in psychiatric disorders. Brain Res. 2014;1586:162–72.
5. Tsankova NM, et al. Sustained hippocampal chromatin regulation in a mouse model of depression and antidepressant action. Nat Neurosci. 2006;9(4):519–25.
6. Jha S, et al. Enriched environment treatment reverses depression-like behavior and restores reduced hippocampal neurogenesis and protein levels of brain-derived neurotrophic factor in mice lacking its expression through promoter IV. Transl Psychiatry. 2011;1:e40. doi:10.1038/tp.2011.33.

7. Lee Y, et al. Association between the BDNF Val66Met polymorphism and chronicity of depression. Psychiatry Investig. 2013;10(1):56–61.

8. Brooks SJ, et al. BDNF polymorphisms are linked to poorer working memory performance, reduced cerebellar and hippocampal volumes and differences in prefrontal cortex in a Swedish elderly population. PLoS ONE. 2014;9(1):e82707. doi:10.1371/journal.pone.0082707.

9. Notaras M, et al. A role for the BDNF gene Val66Met polymorphism in schizophrenia? A comprehensive review. Neurosci Biobehav Rev. 2015;51:15–30.

10. Sarchiapone M, et al. Association of polymorphism (Val66Met) of brain-derived neurotrophic factor with suicide attempts in depressed patients. Neuropsychobiology. 2008;57(3):139–45.

11. Rosenfeld RD, et al. Purification and identification of brain-derived neurotrophic factor from human serum. Protein Expr Purif. 1995;6(4):465–71.

12. Kerschensteiner M, et al. Activated human T cells, B cells, and monocytes produce brain-derived neurotrophic factor in vitro and in inflammatory brain lesions: a neuroprotective role of inflammation? J Exp Med. 1999;189(5):865–70.

13. Pan W, Banks WA, Fasold MB, Bluth J, Kastin AJ. Transport of brain-derived neurotrophic factor across the blood-brain barrier. Neuropharmacology. 1998;37(12):1553–61.

14. Molendijk ML, et al. Serum levels of brain-derived neurotrophic factor in major depressive disorder: state-trait issues, clinical features and pharmacological treatment. Mol Psychiatry. 2011;16(11):1088–95.

15. Nurjono M, et al. A review of brain-derived neurotrophic factor as a candidate biomarker in Schizophrenia. Clin Psychopharmacol Neurosci. 2012;10(2):61–70.

16. Suliman S, et al. Brain-derived neurotrophic factor (BDNF) protein levels in anxiety disorders: systematic review and meta-regression analysis. Front Integr Neurosci. 2013;7:55.

17. Koenigsberg HW, et al. Platelet protein kinase C and brain-derived neurotrophic factor levels in borderline personality disorder patients. Psychiatry Res. 2012;199(2):92–7.

18. Wolkowitz OM, et al. Serum BDNF levels before treatment predict SSRI response in depression. Prog Neuropsychopharmacol Biol Psychiatry. 2011;35(7):1623–30.

19. Guintivano J, Kaminsky ZA. Role of epigenetic factors in the development of mental illness throughout life. Neurosci Res. 2016;102:56–66.

20. Pishva E, et al. The epigenome and postnatal environmental influences in psychotic disorders. Soc Psychiatry Psychiatr Epidemiol. 2014;49(3):337–48.

21. Varendi K, et al. miR-1, miR-10b, miR-155, and miR-191 are novel regulators of BDNF. Cell Mol Life Sci CMLS. 2014;71(22):4443–56.

22. Ikegame T, et al. DNA methylation of the BDNF gene and its relevance to psychiatric disorders. J Hum Genet. 2013;58(7):434–8.

23. Martinowich K, et al. DNA methylation-related chromatin remodeling in activity-dependent BDNF gene regulation. Science. 2003;302(5646):890–3.

24. Vialou V, et al. Epigenetic mechanisms of depression and antidepressant action. Annu Rev Pharmacol Toxicol. 2013;53:59–87.

25. Egger G, et al. Epigenetics in human disease and prospects for epigenetic therapy. Nature. 2004;429(6990):457–63.

26. Allis CD, Jenuwein T, Reinberg D. Epigenetics. CSHL Press; 2007

27. Illingworth RS, Bird AP. CpG islands–'a rough guide'. FEBS Lett. 2009;583(11):1713–20.

28. Weber M, et al. Distribution, silencing potential and evolutionary impact of promoter DNA methylation in the human genome. Nat Genet. 2007;39(4):457–66.

29. Zhang Y, et al. DNA methylation analysis of chromosome 21 gene promoters at single base pair and single allele resolution. PLoS Genet. 2009;5(3):e1000438. doi:10.1371/journal.pgen.1000438.

30. Spruijt CG, Vermeulen M. DNA methylation: old dog, new tricks? Nat Struct Mol Biol. 2014;21(11):949–54.

31. Ball MP, et al. Targeted and genome-scale strategies reveal gene-body methylation signatures in human cells. Nat Biotechnol. 2009;27(4):361–8.

32. Maunakea AK, et al. Intragenic DNA methylation modulates alternative splicing by recruiting MeCP2 to promote exon recognition. Cell Res. 2013;23(11):1256–69.

33. Choi JK, et al. Nucleosome deposition and DNA methylation at coding region boundaries. Genome Biol. 2009;10(9):R89. doi:10.1186/gb-2009-10-9-r89.

34. Schübeler D. Epigenetic Islands in a genetic ocean. Science. 2012;338(6108):756–7.

35. Tufarelli C, et al. Transcription of antisense RNA leading to gene silencing and methylation as a novel cause of human genetic disease. Nat Genet. 2003;34(2):157–65.

36. Lehnertz B, et al. Suv39 h-mediated histone H3 lysine 9 methylation directs DNA methylation to major satellite repeats at pericentric heterochromatin. Curr Biol CB. 2003;13(14):1192–200.

37. Davies MN, et al. Functional annotation of the human brain methylome identifies tissue-specific epigenetic variation across brain and blood. Genome Biol. 2012;13(6):R43. doi:10.1186/gb-2012-13-6-r43.

38. Spiers H, et al. Methylomic trajectories across human fetal brain development. Genome Res. 2015;25:338. doi:10.1101/gr.180273.114.

39. Masliah E, et al. Distinctive patterns of DNA methylation associated with Parkinson disease: identification of concordant epigenetic changes in brain and peripheral blood leukocytes. Epigenetics. 2013;8(10):1030–8.

40. Wen L, et al. Whole-genome analysis of 5-hydroxymethylcytosine and 5-methylcytosine at base resolution in the human brain. Genome Biol. 2014;15(3):R49. doi:10.1186/gb-2014-15-3-r49.

41. Pruunsild P, et al. Identification of cis-elements and transcription factors regulating neuronal activity-dependent transcription of human BDNF gene. J Neurosci. 2011;31(9):3295–308.

42. Roth TL, et al. Lasting epigenetic influence of early-life adversity on the BDNF gene. Biol Psychiatry. 2009;65(9):760–9.

43. Roth TL, Sweatt JD. Epigenetic marking of the BDNF gene by early-life adverse experiences. Horm Behav. 2011;59(3):315–20.

44. Mill J, et al. Epigenomic profiling reveals DNA-methylation changes associated with major psychosis. Am J Hum Genet. 2008;82(3):696–711.

45. Chagnon YC, et al. DNA methylation and single nucleotide variants in the brain-derived neurotrophic factor (BDNF) and oxytocin receptor (OXTR) genes are associated with anxiety/depression in older women. Genet Aging. 2015;6:230.

46. Keller S, et al. Increased BDNF promoter methylation in the Wernicke area of suicide subjects. Arch Gen Psychiatry. 2010;67(3):258–67.

47. Fuchikami M, et al. DNA methylation profiles of the brain-derived neurotrophic factor (BDNF) gene as a potent diagnostic biomarker in major depression. PLoS ONE. 2011;6(8):e23881. doi:10.1371/journal.pone.0023881.

48. Kang H-J, et al. BDNF promoter methylation and suicidal behavior in depressive patients. J Affect Disord. 2013;151(2):679–85.

49. Kang HJ, et al. Longitudinal associations between BDNF promoter methylation and late-life depression. Neurobiol Aging. 2015;36(4):1764. doi:10.1016/j.neurobiolaging.2014.12.035.

50. Kang H-J, et al. A longitudinal study of BDNF promoter methylation and depression in breast cancer. Psychiatry Investig. 2015;12(4):523–31.

51. Kleimann A, et al. BDNF serum levels and promoter methylation of BDNF exon I, IV and VI in depressed patients receiving electroconvulsive therapy. J Neural Transm. 2014;122(6):925–8.

52. Ikegame T, et al. DNA methylation analysis of BDNF gene promoters in peripheral blood cells of schizophrenia patients. Neurosci Res. 2013;77(4):208–14.

53. Kordi-Tamandani DM, et al. DNA methylation and expression profiles of the brain-derived neurotrophic factor (BDNF) and dopamine transporter (DAT1) genes in patients with schizophrenia. Mol Biol Rep. 2012;39(12):10889–93.

54. D'Addario C, et al. Selective DNA methylation of BDNF promoter in bipolar disorder: differences among patients with BDI and BDII. Neuropsychopharmacol. 2012;37(7):1647–55.

55. D'Addario C, et al. Epigenetic modulation of BDNF gene in patients with major depressive disorder. Biol Psychiatry. 2013;73(2):e6–7. doi:10.1016/j.biopsych.2012.07.009.

56. Dell'Osso B, et al. Epigenetic modulation of BDNF gene: differences in DNA methylation between unipolar and bipolar patients. J Affect Disord. 2014;166:330–3.

57. Tadić A, et al. Methylation of the promoter of brain-derived neurotrophic factor exon IV and antidepressant response in major depression. Mol Psychiatry. 2014;19(3):281–3.

58. Perroud N, et al. Response to psychotherapy in borderline personality disorder and methylation status of the BDNF gene. Transl Psychiatry. 2013;3:e207. doi:10.1038/tp.2012.140.

59. Unternaehrer E, et al. Childhood maternal care is associated with DNA methylation of the genes for brain-derived neurotrophic factor (BDNF)

and oxytocin receptor (OXTR) in peripheral blood cells in adult men and women. Stress. 2015;18(4):451–61.

60. Thaler L, et al. Methylation of BDNF in women with bulimic eating syndromes: associations with childhood abuse and borderline personality disorder. Prog Neuropsychopharmacol Biol Psychiatry. 2014;54:43–9.

61. Mikeska T, Craig JM. DNA methylation biomarkers: cancer and beyond. Genes. 2014;5(3):821–64.

62. Stenz L, et al. BDNF promoter I methylation correlates between postmortem human peripheral and brain tissues. Neurosci Res. 2015;91:1–7.

63. Wojdacz TK, Dobrovic A. Methylation-sensitive high resolution melting (MS-HRM): a new approach for sensitive and high-throughput assessment of methylation. Nucleic Acids Res. 2007;35(6):e41. doi:10.1093/nar/gkm013.

64. Shen L, Waterland RA. Methods of DNA methylation analysis. Curr Opin Clin Nutr Metab Care. 2007;10(5):576–81.

65. Lewin J, et al. Quantitative DNA methylation analysis based on four-dye trace data from direct sequencing of PCR amplificates. Bioinformatics. 2004;20(17):3005–12.

66. Uhlmann K, et al. Evaluation of a potential epigenetic biomarker by quantitative methyl-single nucleotide polymorphism analysis. Electrophoresis. 2002;23(24):4072–9.

67. Milutinovic S, et al. Valproate induces widespread epigenetic reprogramming which involves demethylation of specific genes. Carcinogenesis. 2007;28(3):560–71.

68. Deltheil T, et al. Behavioral and serotonergic consequences of decreasing or increasing hippocampus brain-derived neurotrophic factor protein levels in mice. Neuropharmacology. 2008;55(6):1006–14.

69. Berton O, et al. Essential role of BDNF in the mesolimbic dopamine pathway in social defeat stress. Science. 2006;311(5762):864–8.

70. Reinius LE, et al. Differential DNA methylation in purified human blood cells: implications for cell lineage and studies on disease susceptibility. PLoS ONE. 2012;7(7):e41361. doi:10.1371/journal.pone.0041361.

71. Maes M, et al. Evidence for a systemic immune activation during depression: results of leukocyte enumeration by flow cytometry in conjunction with monoclonal antibody staining. Psychol Med. 1992;22(1):45–53.

17

Interaction between cytochrome P450 2A6 and Catechol-*O*-Methyltransferase genes and their association with smoking risk in young men

Wei-Chih Ou[1†], Yi-Chin Huang[5†], Chih-Ling Huang[2], Min-Hsuan Lin[3], Yi-Chun Chen[3], Yi-Ju Chen[4], Chen-Nu Liu[1], Mei-Chih Chen[1], Ching-Shan Huang[3*‡] and Pei-Lain Chen[1*‡] (ORCID)

Abstract

Background: Although some effects of gene–gene interactions on nicotine–dopamine metabolism for smoking behavior have been reported, polymorphisms of cytochrome P450 (CYP) 2A6 and catechol-*O*-methyltransferase (COMT) have not been studied together to determine their effects on smokers. The aim of this study was to investigate the effects of the interaction between the *CYP* 2A6 and *COMT* genes on smoking behavior in young Taiwanese men.

Results: A self-report questionnaire regarding smoking status was administered to 500 young men. Polymorphisms of the *CYP* 2A6 and *COMT* genes as well as urinary nicotine and urinary cotinine levels were determined. The odds ratio for starting smoking was significantly lower in subjects carrying a *CYP2A6* low activity/variant *COMT* rs4680 genotype than in those possessing a *CYP2A6* wild-type/variant *COMT* rs4680 genotype (0.44, 95% confidence interval = 0.19–0.98, P = 0.043). Comparisons of Fagerstrom Test for Nicotine Dependence (FTND), Physiological Cigarette Dependence Scale (PCDS), and Cigarette Withdrawal symptoms (CWS-21) among the smokers with different *CYP2A6/COMT* polymorphisms were not significantly different. The adjusted urinary nicotine concentrations were not significantly different between the two groups carrying different genotypes. The adjusted urinary cotinine level was significantly different between the *COMT* rs4680 wild-type group and *COMT* rs4680 variant group [92.46 ng/µL vs. 118.24 ng/µL (median value), P = 0.041] and between the *COMT* rs4680 wild-type/*COMT* rs165599 variant group and *COMT* rs4680 variant/*COMT* rs165599 variant group (97.10 ng/µL vs. 122.18 ng/µL, P = 0.022).

Conclusions: These findings suggest that a single nucleotide polymorphism (rs4680) of the *COMT* gene and the interaction between the *CYP* 2A6 and *COMT* genes affect smoking status in young Taiwanese men.

Keywords: Catechol-*O*-methyltransferase, Cotinine, Cytochrome P450 2A6, Nicotine, Smoking status

Background

Tobacco smoking is a multi-factorial behavior with both genetic and environmental determinants [1]. Genetic factors have a greater influence on smoking cessation than do environmental factors [2]. Genetic factors are responsible for 30–50% of the variance in the risk of withdrawal symptoms, 40–75% of the variation in smoking initiation, 50% of the variance in cessation success, and 70–80% of the variation in smoking maintenance [1]. Genetic risk information enhances the motivation for smoking cessation [3]. Therefore, assessment of genetic background could be a promising tool to understand smoking risk and to guide the selection of the most effective cessation treatment for an individual smoker.

*Correspondence: ching.shan.h@gmail.com; plchen@ctust.edu.tw
†Wei-Chih Ou and Yi-Chin Huang contributed equally to this work
‡Ching-Shan Huang and Pei-Lain Chen contributed equally to this work
[1] Department of Medical Laboratory Science and Biotechnology, Central Taiwan University of Science and Technology, No. 666 Buzih Road, Beitun District, Taichung City 40601, Taiwan
[3] Administration Center for Research and Education, Changhua Christian Hospital, Changhua, Taiwan
Full list of author information is available at the end of the article

Nicotine is the major psychoactive ingredient in tobacco, and it modulates dopamine activity in the midbrain, which contributes to the development and maintenance of rewarding behaviors such as smoking [4]. Smokers modulate their smoking to maintain brain nicotine levels within a certain concentration range, and factors that alter nicotine clearance affect smoking behavior [4]. Individuals who eliminate nicotine rapidly are less likely to achieve low craving scores even after smoking freely [4]. Consequently, genetic polymorphisms in both nicotine metabolism and dopamine catabolism genes influence smoking status, interact with each other to result in risk modulation, and affect smoking cessation therapies.

The cytochrome P450 (CYP) 2A6 gene, located on chromosome 19q12-q13.2, consists of nine exons. It is involved in producing a 494-amino-acid protein that oxidizes coumarin, nicotine, and tobacco-specific nitrosamines [5]. CYP2A6 is the primary human enzyme involved in nicotine metabolism [4]. CYP2A6 catalyzes the C-oxidation of nicotine to the inactive metabolite cotinine and the subsequent conversion of cotinine into trans-3′-hydroxycotinine [4]. CYP2A6 is the most studied enzyme involved in both adult and adolescent smokers [6]. The results of studies among Taiwanese individuals indicate that the variant status of CYP2A6 is different from that among other ethnic groups [7]. Therefore, we hypothesized that, for Taiwanese individuals, polymorphisms in the CYP2A6 gene that affect smoking status could be different from those in other ethnic groups.

The catechol-O-methyltransferase (COMT) gene is located on chromosome 22q11.21, has eight exons, and produces a 271-amino-acid protein that metabolizes catecholamines [8]. Low enzyme activity of the Met allele at codon 108/158 (in the rs4680 polymorphism) of the COMT gene, which encodes a key enzyme involved in the metabolic inactivation of dopamine, has been associated with nicotine dependence [9]. Another polymorphism of COMT, rs165599, has been related to the response to bupropion therapy for smoking cessation [10]. However, those associations have been inconsistent among ethnic groups [10, 11]. Thus, it seems necessary to perform a genetic study of smoking status for each ethnicity.

Smoking addiction is currently a significant social problem in Taiwan [12]. Nonetheless, very few genetic investigations of nicotine–dopamine metabolism and smoking status among Taiwanese individuals have been performed. Recently, for Taiwanese smokers in a group of methadone maintenance patients, polymorphisms of the μ-opioid receptor gene were associated with the plasma concentration of cotinine [13]. Very recently, our team reported that the interaction of the dopamine D2 receptor (DRD2) TaqIB and monoamine oxidase A (MAOA)

affected smoking intensity in young men [14]. Those findings encouraged us to perform more genetic studies of Taiwanese smokers. In relation to nicotine–dopamine metabolism, smoking status has been reported to correlate better with some gene–gene interactions than with a single gene only. These interactions include COMT and MAOA [15, 16], MAOA and CYP2A6 [17], CYP2A6 and the nicotine acetylcholine receptor gene [18, 19], and CYP 2A6 and DRD2 TaqIA [20]. However, the effects of CYP2A6 and COMT together have not been explored, and we hypothesized that a single polymorphism as well as an interaction of the two genes could be involved in smoking status.

In women not using oral contraceptives, nicotine and cotinine clearance is 13 and 24% higher, respectively, than in men [6]. Sex differences exist for cravings, affect, and preference for immediate smoking after cue exposure [21]. Because Taiwanese men smoke significantly more cigarettes than Taiwanese women [12, 22], only men were invited to participate in our study. In this study, the polymorphisms CYP2A6*1A (wild-type), CYP 2A6*1B (polymorphism of faster nicotine clearance) [23], CYP2A6*4C (the most studied polymorphism of decreased nicotine metabolism) [24], COMT Val/Met (rs4680) [9], and COMT rs165599 [10] were determined. Our objectives were to investigate the effects of the interaction between the CYP 2A6 and COMT genes and their association with smoking risk in young Taiwanese men.

Methods
Participants and procedures
This cross-sectional study was advertised to all students at both Chang Jung Christian University and Central Taiwan University of Science and Technology. The volunteers contacted the authors of the study, and convenience samples were then screened for eligibility at the health centers of the two universities. All study subjects provided written, informed consent at the beginning of study, and the study was approved by the review board of Chang Jung Christian University (CJCU-99004) and Central Taiwan University of Science and Technology (CTUST-99016). The study was conducted in accordance with Good Clinical Practice procedures and the Declaration of Helsinki.

We administered a self-report questionnaire to all of the study subjects [25–27]. The questionnaire included demographic data, smoking background and status. In addition, the questionnaire included the fagerstrom test for nicotine dependence (six-item FTND) [25], the 15-item short form of the Physiological Cigarette Dependence Scale (PCDS) derived from the 30-item PCDS [27], and the Withdrawal Symptoms Scale (Cigarette Withdrawal Scale, CWS-21) [26, 27]. These questionnaires used biomarkers (nicotine and cotinine concentrations) as validation, with no over- or under-exaggeration. Never smokers were defined as persons who had never smoked in their lifetime. Current smoking was defined as ever smoking cigarettes on 1 or more days of the past 30 days. Ever smokers were defined as persons who smoked at one time, had quit, and were not currently smoking. The current smokers were divided into two groups according to their intensity of cigarette smoking: light smokers and heavy smokers, depending on number of cigarettes per day lower than or equal to (or higher than) the average value of all the smokers, respectively. The exclusion criteria were (1) a history of diagnosed mental health disease or cancer, (2) alcoholism or drug abuse, (3) severe communication problems, or (4) terminal illness. When the survey was completed, blood and urine samples were obtained at a university center by trained research assistants (licensed nurses or medical technologists).

Determination of CYP2A6 and COMT polymorphisms

In this study, to determine the genotypes of the variants of interest, total genomic DNA was isolated from blood cells using a blood DNA isolation kit (Favorgen, Ping-Tung, Taiwan). Five milliliters of whole blood with EDTA as an anticoagulant were required. Approximately 40 alleles of the *CYP2A6* gene have been identified [28]. However, only the wild-type (*CYP2A6**1A) and two highly prevalent (>10%) variants of *CYP2A6**1B (approximately 45%) [29] and *CYP2A6**4C (approximately 15%) [30], which have been observed in Chinese individuals, were determined in this project.

The polymorphisms of *CYP2A6* were identified using polymerase chain reaction-restriction fragment length polymorphism (PCR–RFLP) [31]. We designed the forward primer 5′-CACCGAAGTGTTCCCTATG CTG-3′ and reverse primer 5′-TGTAAAATGGGCATG AACGCCC-3′ according to the GenBank accession system. PCR was performed with a thermal cycler (Bio-Rad, Carlsbad, CA, USA). The PCR conditions were as follows: first cycle, denaturation at 94 °C for 3 min; cycles 2–31, denaturation at 94 °C for 1 min, annealing at 55 °C for 1 min, and elongation at 72 °C for 2 min, with a final extension for 7 min at 72 °C. We detected a 1332-base pair (bp) fragment on a 1% agarose gel after electrophoresis at 100 V for 60 min. Using *BstU-I* as the restriction enzyme, one (1332-bp) and two (291 and 1041-bp) fragments were obtained for *CYP2A6**1A and *CYP2A6**non-1A, respectively. Using the restriction enzyme *Bsu36-I*, three fragments (104, 437, and 792-bp) were observed for *CYP2A6**1A or *CYP2A6**1B. Four fragments (64, 104, 437, and 728-bp) were found for *CYP2A6**4C. Positive controls were run for each of the genotyping

assays. The DNAs of *CYP2A6**1A/*1A, *CYP2A6**1A/*1B, *CYP2A6**1B/*1B, *CYP2A6**1A/*4C, and *CYP2A6**1B/*4C, which have been found in Taiwanese and Chinese populations, were identified by DNA sequencing [29, 30]. Additional file 1: Table S1 lists the result.

For *COMT* rs4680, the forward primer 5′-CTGTGGCT ACTCAGCTGTG-3′ and reverse primer 5′-CCTT TTTCCAGGTCTGACAA-3′ were used to amplify a 169-bp fragment [10]. Using *N1a III* as the restriction enzyme, three (114, 32, and 23-bp), four (96, 32, 23, and 18-bp), and five (114, 96, 32, 23, and 18-bp) fragments were obtained for the G/G, A/A, and G/A genotypes, respectively [10]. For COMT rs165599, the forward primer 5′-CATTCAAAGCTCCCCTTGAC-3′ and reverse primer 5′-GGGAGTAGG-GAAGGAGATGC-3′ were utilized to amplify a 301-bp fragment [32]. Using *Msp I* as the restriction enzyme, one (301-bp), two (166 and 135-bp), and three (301, 166, and 135-bp) fragments were obtained from the A/A, G/G, and A/G genotypes, respectively [32].

Determination of urinary nicotine and cotinine

To evaluate the effects of genetic polymorphisms on the metabolism of nicotine and cotinine, urinary nicotine and cotinine levels of smokers were measured. Gas chromatography–mass spectrometry (GC/MS) was performed as previously described [33], with the following difference: GC–MS analyses were performed on a ThermoElectron DSQII quadrupole mass spectrometer connected directly to a ThermoElectron focus gas chromatograph and an autosampler AS 3000 (Thermo Electron Corporation, Dreieich, Germany). All urine samples were stored at −20 °C before analysis. All of the analyses were performed in duplicate and repeated if values differed by >10%. Tobacco cigarettes currently smoked in Taiwan contain 0.57–0.64 mg of nicotine per cigarette on average [12]. The nicotine and cotinine concentrations in the urine of each subject were divided by the number of daily cigarettes smoked and defined as the adjusted nicotine and adjusted cotinine concentration.

The effects of gene polymorphism interactions on smoking behaviors

The *CYP2A6* genotypes consisted of wild-type (*1A/*1A), high -activity (*1A/*1B and *1B/*1B), and low-activity (*1A/*4C, *1B/*4C, and *4C/*4C) genotypes. The *COMT* rs4680 genotypes consisted of wild-type (G/G) and variant (G/A and A/A). The *COMT* rs165599 genotypes consisted of wild-type (A/A) and variant (A/G and G/G) genotypes. To assess the interaction between the effects of *CYP2A6* and *COMT* gene polymorphisms on smoking behaviors, multiple models were used to analyze the *CYP2A6*, *COMT* rs4680, and *COMT* rs165599 data: (1)

single gene (model 1: *CYP2A6*) or single SNP (model 2: *COMT* rs4680, *COMT* rs165599, respectively); (2) 2 SNPs (model 3: *COMT* rs4680 and *COMT* rs165599); and (3) multiple genes (models 4–7). We evaluated the effect of the interactions between different gene combinations on smoking status (Table 2), smoking intensity (Additional file 2: Table S2), nicotine dependence (FTND), physiological cigarette dependence (PCDS), nicotine toxicity and withdrawal symptoms (CWS-21) (Additional file 3: Table S3), and urine nicotine/cotinine concentration (Table 3) in young men.

Statistical analysis

To evaluate the effect of the genetic variants on smoking status and smoking intensity, this study assigned an odds ratio (OR) as 1 to subjects carrying the wild-type. The Mantel–Haenszel Chi square test was utilized to calculate the ORs and their 95% confidence intervals (CIs) (Table 2; Additional file 2: Table S2). To compare the significance of FTND, PCDS, and CWS-21 and to compare the urinary nicotine and cotinine clearance among subjects carrying different *CYP2A6* and *COMT* polymorphisms, Student's *t* test or analysis of variance (ANOVA), as appropriate, was applied to compare quantitative data. A P value of <0.05 was defined as statistically significant for each analysis (Additional file 3: Table S3). When the result of ANOVA was statistically significant, multiple comparisons were followed by application of Scheffé's post hoc test. However, if the data in any group did not

fit a normal distribution, the Mann–Whitney U test with Bonferroni adjustment was utilized to compare the data between the two groups (Table 3). All data were analyzed using SPSS (version 18.0 software for Windows, SPSS Inc., Chicago, IL).

Results

We recruited a total of 500 men aged 20–25 years. Analysis of the questionnaires revealed that there were 219 never smokers, 261 current smokers, and 20 ever smokers. Due to the small sample size (moderate power analysis in general, $\alpha = 0.05$ and 80% power requires 200 samples), the 20 ever smokers were excluded from further study. Mean age did not differ between the 261 current smokers and the 219 never smokers (22.6 ± 1.69 vs. 22.4 ± 1.42, $t = 1.371$, P = 0.176, data not shown).

The distributions of *CYP2A6* and *COMT* polymorphisms are shown in Table 1. Using the frequencies of *CYP2A6**1A/*1A, *CYP2A6**1A/*1B, and *CYP2A6**1B/*1B as examples, the distributions of *CYP2A6* genotypes agreed with Hardy–Weinberg equilibrium: P = 0.713 and 0.332 for current smokers and never smokers, respectively. The distribution of *COMT* rs165599 genotypes also agreed with Hardy–Weinberg equilibrium: P = 0.966 and 0.668 for current smokers and never smokers, respectively. The distribution of *COMT* rs4680 genotypes did not agree with Hardy–Weinberg equilibrium: P = 0.003 and 0.012 for current smokers and never smokers, respectively.

Table 1 Distribution of CYP2A6 and COMT polymorphisms

Genotypes	Current smokers [n = 261 (n%)]	Hardy–Weinberg equilibrium	Never smokers [n = 219 (n%)]	Hardy–Weinberg equilibrium
CYP2A6		P[a] = 0.713		P[a] = 0.332
1A/1A	63 (24.1)		46 (21.0)	
1A/1B	100 (38.3)		88 (40.2)	
1B/1B	44 (16.9)		31 (14.2)	
1A/4C	24 (9.2)		25 (11.4)	
4C/4C	4 (1.5)		3 (1.37)	
1B/4C	26 (10.0)		26 (11.9)	
COMT rs4680		P[b] = 0.003		P[b] = 0.012
G/G	147 (56.3)		113 (51.6)	
G/A	73 (28.0)		69 (31.5)	
A/A	41 (15.7)		37 (16.9)	
COMTrs165599		P[c] = 0.966		P[c] = 0.668
A/A	61 (23.4)		45 (20.6)	
A/G	130 (49.8)		112 (51.1)	
G/G	70 (26.8)		62 (28.3)	

[a] For CYP2A6 1A/1A, 1A/1B, 1B/1B

[b] For COMT rs4680

[c] For COMT rs165599

Table 2 Odds ratios for the effects of *CYP2A6* and *COMT* polymorphisms on smoking status

Genotypes interaction	Current smokers N = 261	Never smokers N = 219	OR (95% CI)	P[a]
Model 1				
CYP2A6				
Wild type	63	46	1.0	
High activity	144	119	0.88 (0.56–1.39)	0.591
Low activity	54	54	0.73 (0.43–1.25)	0.249
Model 2				
COMT				
COMT rs4680				
Wild type	147	113	1.0	
Variant	114	106	0.83 (0.58–1.19)	0.301
COMT rs165599				
Wild type	61	45	1.0	
Variant	200	174	0.85 (0.55–1.31)	0.458
Model 3				
COMT rs4680/COMT rs165599				
Wild type/wild type	27	13	1.0	
Wild type/variant	120	100	0.58 (0.28–1.18)	0.128
Variant/wild type	34	32	0.51 (0.23–1.16)	0.107
Variant/variant	80	74	0.52 (0.25–1.08)	0.078
Model 4				
COMT rs4680 wild type				
CYP2A6 wild type	35	25	1.0	
CYP2A6 high activity	76	65	0.84 (0.45–1.54)	0.563
CYP2A6 low activity	36	23	1.12 (0.54–2.33)	0.765
Model 5				
COMT rs4680 variant				
CYP2A6 wild type	28	21	1.0	
CYP2A6 high activity	68	54	0.94 (0.48–1.84)	0.867
CYP2A6 low activity	18	31	0.44 (0.19–0.98)	0.043
Model 6				
COMT rs165599 wild type				
CYP2A6 wild type	15	8	1.0	
CYP2A6 high activity	33	30	0.59 (0.22–1.58)	0.289
CYP2A6 low activity	13	7	0.99 (0.28–3.48)	0.988
Model 7				
COMT rs165599 variant				
CYP2A6 wild type	48	38	1.0	
CYP2A6 high activity	111	89	0.99 (0.59–1.64)	0.961
CYP2A6 low activity	41	47	0.69 (0.38–1.26)	0.224

[a] Mantel–Haenszel Chi square test

The genotypes of (1) CYP2A6: wild-type (*1A/*1A), high activity (*1A/*1B and *1B/*1B), low activity (*1A/*4C, *1B/*4C, and *4C/*4C); (2) COMT rs4680: wild-type (G/G), variant (G/A and A/A); and (3) COMT rs165599: wild-type (A/A), variant (A/G and G/G)

As shown in Table 2, after using never smokers as the reference group, the OR was significantly lower in the subjects carrying the genotype of *CYP2A6* low activity/variant *COMT* rs4680 than in those possessing the genotype of *CYP2A6* wild-type/variant *COMT* rs4680 (0.44, 95% CI 0.19–0.98, P = 0.043). The other 14 ORs were not statistically significant (P = 0.078–0.988).

The average number of cigarettes per day among the 261 current smokers was 10. There were 127 heavy smokers and 131 light smokers (data for three smokers were missing). With light smokers as the reference group, 15 ORs for heavy smoking were not statistically significant (P = 0.061–0.112, data in Additional file 2: Table S2).

Table 3 Comparisons of adjusted urinary nicotine concentration and adjusted urinary cotinine concentration among subjects (N = 122) carrying different CYP2A6 and COMT polymorphisms

	N	Adjusted urinary nicotine, ng/μL median (min–max)	Adjusted urinary cotinine, ng/μL median (min–max)
Model 1			
CYP2A6			
Wild type	17	86.23 (6.14–296.36)	120.90 (20.39–485.32)
High activity	76	70.45 (6.28–1117.87)	111.08 (8.34–822.11)
Low activity	29	61.59 (15.28–456.87)	75.87 (10.87–266.44)
P[a]		NS	NS
Model 2			
COMT			
COMT rs4680			
Wild type	66	63.86 (6.28–646.38)	92.46 (8.34–506.97)
Variant	56	67.87 (6.14–1117.87)	118.24 (13.59–822.11)
P[a]		NS	0.041
COMT rs165599			
Wild type	27	68.10 (12.42–212.74)	89.42 (23.06–218.62)
Variant	95	64.11 (6.14–1117.87)	107.24 (8.34–822.11)
P[a]		NS	NS
Model 3			
COMT rs4680/COMT rs165599			
Wild type/wild type	13	89.29 (12.42–212.74)	79.37 (23.06–218.62)
Wild type/variant	53	63.61 (6.28–646.38)	97.10 (8.34–506.97)*
Variant/wild type	14	67.87 (15.28–177.61)	95.86 (32.18–202.0)
Variant/variant	42	69.46 (6.14–1117.87)	122.18 (13.59–822.11)*
P[a]		NS	
Model 4			
COMT rs4680 wild type			
CYP2A6 wild type	9	95.04 (25.04–296.36)	105.70 (53.48–485.32)
CYP2A6 high activity	39	72.99 (6.28–646.38)	97.45 (8.34–506.97)
CYP2A6 low activity	18	42.54 (19.38–371.29)	60.20 (10.87–266.44)
P[a]		NS	NS
Model 5			
COMT rs4680 variant			
CYP2A6 wild type	8	74.91 (6.14–217.41)	141.53 (20.39–228.68)
CYP2A6 high activity	37	68.10 (17.68–1117.87)	115.78 (13.59–822.11)
CYP2A6 low activity	11	66.13 (15.28–456.87)	161.65 (39.19–224.53)
P[a]		NS	NS
Model 6			
COMT rs165599 wild type			
CYP2A6 wild type	3	95.04 (62.36–188.57)	102.30 (79.37–120.90)
CYP2A6 high activity	17	67.64 (12.42–212.74)	89.42 (32.18–218.62)
CYP2A6 low activity	7	78.05 (15.28–177.61)	63.55 (23.06–202.00)
P[a]		NS	NS

For the 261 current smokers, FTND, PCDS, and CWS-21 were analyzed for 181, 227, and 210 subjects, respectively, because of missing data. Each of the eight comparisons for FTND, PCDS, and CWS-21 among the groups with different *CYP2A6/COMT* polymorphisms was not significantly different (P = 0.224–0.911, 0.054–0.700, and 0.075–0.836, respectively) (data in Additional file 3: Table S3).

Of the 261 current smokers, 122 subjects provided urine samples for the determination of nicotine and

Table 3 continued

	N	Adjusted urinary nicotine, ng/µL median (min–max)	Adjusted urinary cotinine, ng/µL median (min–max)
Model 7			
COMT rs165599 variant			
CYP2A6 wild type	14	74.92 (6.14–296.36)	141.53 (20.39–485.32)
CYP2A6 high activity	59	72.99 (6.28–1117.87)	111.09 (8.34–822.11)
CYP2A6 low activity	22	59.62 (19.38–456.87)	81.66 (10.87–266.44)
P[a]		NS	NS

NS not statistically significant

[a] Mann–Whitney U test or Kruskal–Wallis test with Bonferroni adjustment

* Significantly different from the (COMT rs4680 wild-type/COMT rs165599 variant) group versus the (COMT rs4680 variant/COMT rs165599 variant) group by Scheffe's Post hoc test, P value = 0.022

cotinine levels by GC/MS. The values for adjusted nicotine concentration and adjusted cotinine concentration were not normally distributed in either genotype group. The SD was too high: near the mean value or even greater than the mean value. Therefore, the Mann–Whitney U test or Kruskal–Wallis test with Bonferroni adjustment was used for comparison of the values of adjusted nicotine concentration and adjusted cotinine concentration between groups carrying different genotypes. As shown in Table 3, the adjusted urinary nicotine concentration did not differ significantly in any of the comparisons. The median adjusted urinary cotinine concentration differed between the *COMT* rs4680 wild-type group and the *COMT* rs4680 variant group (92.46 ng/µL vs. 118.24 ng/µL, P = 0.041) and between the *COMT* rs4680 wild-type/*COMT* rs165599 variant group and the *COMT* rs4680 variant/*COMT* rs165599 variant group (97.10 ng/µL vs. 122.18 ng/µL, P = 0.022). The other comparisons were not statistically significant.

Discussion

All subjects in this study were young adult university students. Alcohol and drug abusers were excluded. Therefore, the effects of age, education status and alcohol and drug interactions on smoking were absent.

Our results show that the distribution of *COMT* rs4680 does not agree with Hardy–Weinberg equilibrium, consistent with reports that Asiatic individuals have Hardy–Weinberg disequilibrium of the *COMT* rs4680 polymorphism [8]. The main finding of this study is that among adult males with variant *COMT* rs4680, the subjects carrying the low-activity genotype of *CYP2A6* have a 0.44-fold lower risk of starting smoking than those possessing the wild-type genotype of *CYP2A6*. In other words, the OR is 2.27-fold higher in subjects carrying the *CYP2A6* wild-type/variant *COMT* rs4680 genotype than in those possessing the *CYP2A6* low activity/variant

COMT rs4680 genotype. The *CYP2A6* and *COMT* genes were reported to be associated with smoking status. *CYP2A6**4C is a whole-deletion type, decreased nicotine metabolism polymorphism [34]. In Japanese adults and young Japanese students, the frequency of the *CYP2A6**4C gene was significantly higher among non-smokers than smokers [34, 35]. Among Chinese males, participants with the *CYP2A6**4C genotype had a lower risk of smoking initiation and smoking persistence than those with the *CYP2A6**1/*CYP2A6**1 genotype [17]. For people living in southern China, reduced metabolic function of *CYP2A6* in smokers appears to be associated with fewer cigarettes smoked, later initiation of smoking regularly, shorter smoking duration, and lower likelihood of smoking cessation [36]. For Caucasian individuals, the *CYP2A6* slow inactivator genotype increased the risk of nicotine dependence when smoking was initiated during adolescence. However, it reduced the risk of smoking initiation, lowered cigarette consumption, and decreased the duration of smoking among adult dependent smokers [37]. The continued effect of slow metabolism on reducing cigarette consumption, throughout the smoking history of people with *CYP2A6* slow inactivators, may affect tolerance and withdrawal mechanisms among these individuals [37]. Smokers with *CYP2A6* slow inactivators smoke fewer cigarettes and tend to be less dependent on nicotine than smokers with normal activity alleles [38]. With respect to smoking initiation, adolescents with slower activity alleles may progress to nicotine dependence more slowly than normal metabolizers [38]. Very recently, researchers reported that *CYP2A6* slow metabolism was associated with increased adolescent smoking cessation in Caucasian individuals [39]. The ORs for current smoking are reportedly higher in *COMT* rs4680 G/G (the high activity allele) carriers than in those possessing the *COMT* rs4680 variant among healthy Caucasian men of Croatian origin [40], Americans of European ancestry [41], and Japanese men [15]. On the other hand, the *COMT* rs4680 variation (G/A or A/A, the low-activity alleles) was associated with nicotine dependence in men and women of African-American and European-American descent [9], smoking severity among Chinese male smokers [42], heaviness of smoking in Caucasian pregnant women [43], and susceptibility to cigarette smoking among Thai males [11]. Our results demonstrate for the first time that the combination of the low-activity *CYP2A6* genotype and low-activity *COMT* genotype is associated with the risk of starting smoking.

We also found that the adjusted urinary cotinine concentration was higher in subjects with low-activity *COMT* genes than in those with high-activity *COMT* genes. Additionally, it was higher in subjects with the *COMT* rs4680 variant/*COMT* rs165599 variant than in those with the *COMT* rs4680 wild-type/*COMT* rs165599 variant. The urinary cotinine concentration is a reliable easy-to-use marker for plasma levels of cotinine and the sum of nicotine metabolites in smokers [44]. Therefore, our findings indicate that cotinine and the sum of nicotine metabolites are metabolized more slowly in subjects carrying the low-activity genotype than in those possessing the high-activity genotype. However, such a difference did not affect FTND, PCDS, or CWS-21 scores, and it was not related to the risk of heavier smoking. The smoking intensity of the university students was lower (average cigarettes/day = 10 and average FTND score = 3.7) than that of Taiwanese adult smokers, e.g., average cigarettes/day = 24 and average FTND score = 7.1 for Chinese adults [42]. This finding may be the reason, at least in part, that the low activity genotypes of *CYP2A6* and *COMT* were associated with high nicotine dependence scores and heavier smoking, as we reported in this study. For Taiwanese university students, the primary reason for the first contact with smoking was curiosity. Anxiety, avoiding stress, and the difficulties of smoking cessation explained continuing smoking behavior among university students [45]. The environmental factors may be more predominant than certain genetic factors (e.g., polymorphisms of *CYP2A6* and *COMT* genes) among Taiwanese smokers in the university setting.

There are several limitations to our study. The percentage of female smokers in the Taiwanese population is low, only 4.4%, and they are difficult to recruit as participants. In our report, study participation was restricted to young male Taiwanese smokers. Although the total number of study subjects was relatively large, the numbers of individuals with some of the genotypes were too small to reach statistically significant power. Therefore, further studies with a larger sample size and that include female smokers are needed.

Conclusions

A single nucleotide polymorphism (rs4680) in the *COMT* gene and the interaction between the *CYP2A6* and *COMT* genes affect smoking status in young Taiwanese men. Effective smoking prevention and cessation intervention programs are required to reduce smoking among university students [46]. We found that the interaction of the low-activity *CYP2A6* genotype and low-activity *COMT* genotype is associated with the risk of starting smoking. In addition, interaction of the *DRD2* TaqIB and *MAOA* genes also affects smoking intensity in Taiwanese young men [14]. This knowledge is useful for developing an approach to reducing smoking among Taiwanese university students. A clearer understanding of the relative roles of genetic and non-genetic factors in the initiation of smoking could have implications for the design of smoking prevention programs [47].

Abbreviations
CYP2A6: cytochrome P450 2A6; COMT: catechol-*O*-methyltransferase; FTND: Fagerstrom Test for Nicotine Dependence; PCDS: Physiological Cigarette Dependence Scale; CWS: Cigarette Withdrawal Symptoms Scale.

Authors' contributions
Conceived and designed the experiments: WCO, PLC, CSH. Performed the experiments: WCO, PLC, MHL, YJC, CNL, and MCC. Analyzed the data: CLH, YCC,YCH. Wrote the paper: CSH, PLC, YCH. All authors read and approved the final manuscript.

Author details
[1] Department of Medical Laboratory Science and Biotechnology, Central Taiwan University of Science and Technology, No. 666 Buzih Road, Beitun District, Taichung City 40601, Taiwan. [2] Department of Nursing, Chang Jung Christian University, Tainan, Taiwan. [3] Administration Center for Research and Education, Changhua Christian Hospital, Changhua, Taiwan. [4] Company Limited of Ditech Enterprise, Taipei, Taiwan. [5] Division of Infectious Diseases, Jen-Ai Hospital, Taichung, Taiwan.

Acknowledgements
We express our deep appreciation to the National Science Council of Taiwan (Grant NSC–100–2320–B–371–001), Changhua Christian Hospital, Taiwan (Grant CCH–ICO10008).

Competing interests
The authors declared that they have no competing interests.

Funding
This study was financially supported by Central Taiwan University of Science and Technology (Grant CTU103–P–20, CTU103-P-21).

References
1. Quaak M, van Schayck CP, Knaapen AM, van Schooten FJ. Genetic variation as a predictor of smoking cessation success. A promising preventive and intervention tool for chronic respiratory diseases? Eur Respir J. 2009;33:468–80.
2. Kim YS, Ko H, Yoon C, Lee DH, Sung J. Social determinants of smoking behavior: the healthy twin study, Korea. J Prev Med Public Health. 2012;45:29–36.
3. Wright AJ, French DP, Weinman J, Marteau TM. Can genetic risk information enhance motivation for smoking cessation? An analogue study. Health Psychol. 2006;25:740–52.

4. Tsuang MT, Francis T, Minor K, Thomas A, Stone WS. Genetics of smoking and depression. Hum Genet. 2012;131:905–15.

5. Di YM, Chow VD, Yang LP, Zhou SF. Structure, function, regulation and polymorphism of human cytochrome P450 2A6. Curr Drug Metab. 2009;10:754–80.

6. Benowitz NL, Hukkanen J, Jacob P. 3rd. Nicotine chemistry, metabolism, kinetics and biomarkers. Handb Exp Pharmacol. 2009;192:29–60.

7. Mwenifumbo JC, Myers MG, Wall TL, Lin SK, Sellers EM, Tyndale RF. Ethnic variation in CYP2A6*7, CYP2A6*8 and CYP2A6*10 as assessed with a novel haplotyping method. Pharmacogenetics Genom. 2005;15:189–92.

8. Jimenez-Jimenez FJ, Alonso-Navarro H, Garcia-Martin E, Agundez JA. COMT gene and risk for Parkinson's disease: a systematic review and meta-analysis. Pharmacogenetics Genom. 2014;24:331–9.

9. Beuten J, Payne TJ, Ma JZ, Li MD. Significant association of catechol-O-methyltransferase (COMT) haplotypes with nicotine dependence in male and female smokers of two ethnic populations. Neuropsychopharmacology. 2006;31:675–84.

10. Berrettini WH, Wileyto EP, Epstein L, Restine S, Hawk L, Shields P, Niaura R, Lerman C. Catechol-O-methyltransferase (COMT) gene variants predict response to bupropion therapy for tobacco dependence. Biol Psychiatry. 2007;61:111–8.

11. Suriyaprom K, Tungtrongchitr R, Harnroongroj T. Impact of COMT Val 108/158 Met and DRD2 Taq1B gene polymorphisms on vulnerability to cigarette smoking of Thai males. J Mol Neurosci. 2013;49:544–9.

12. Health Promotion Administration. Taiwan tobacco control: annual report 2012. 2013. http://health99.hpa.gov.tw/media/public/zip/21747.zip. Accessed 24 Apr 2016.

13. Chen YT, Tsou HH, Kuo HW, Fang CP, Wang SC, Ho IK, Chang YS, Chen CH, Hsiao CF, Wu HY, et al. OPRM1 genetic polymorphisms are associated with the plasma nicotine metabolite cotinine concentration in methadone maintenance patients: a cross sectional study. J Hum Genet. 2013;58:84–90.

14. Huang CL, Ou WC, Chen PL, Liu CN, Chen MC, Lu CC, Chen YC, Lin MH, Huang CS. Effects of interaction between dopamine D2 receptor and monoamine oxidase a genes on smoking status in young men. Biol Res Nurs. 2015;17:422–8.

15. Tochigi M, Suzuki K, Kato C, Otowa T, Hibino H, Umekage T, Kato N, Sasaki T. Association study of monoamine oxidase and catechol-O-methyltransferase genes with smoking behavior. Pharmacogenetics Genom. 2007;17:867–72.

16. Shiels MS, Huang HY, Hoffman SC, Shugart YY, Bolton JH, Platz EA, Helzlsouer KJ, Alberg AJ. A community-based study of cigarette smoking behavior in relation to variation in three genes involved in dopamine metabolism: Catechol-O-methyltransferase (COMT), dopamine beta-hydroxylase (DBH) and monoamine oxidase-A (MAO-A). Prev Med. 2008;47:116–22.

17. Tang X, Guo S, Sun H, Song X, Jiang Z, Sheng L, Zhou D, Hu Y, Chen D. Gene-gene interactions of CYP2A6 and MAOA polymorphisms on smoking behavior in Chinese male population. Pharmacogenetics Genom. 2009;19:345–52.

18. Rodriguez S, Cook DG, Gaunt TR, Nightingale CM, Whincup PH, Day IN. Combined analysis of CHRNA5, CHRNA3 and CYP2A6 in relation to adolescent smoking behaviour. J Psychopharmacol. 2011;25:915–23.

19. Wassenaar CA, Dong Q, Wei Q, Amos CI, Spitz MR, Tyndale RF. Relationship between CYP2A6 and CHRNA5-CHRNA3-CHRNB4 variation and smoking behaviors and lung cancer risk. J Natl Cancer Inst. 2011;103:1342–6.

20. Ohmoto M, Takahashi T, Kubota Y, Kobayashi S, Mitsumoto Y. Genetic influence of dopamine receptor, dopamine transporter, and nicotine metabolism on smoking cessation and nicotine dependence in a Japanese population. BMC Genet. 2014;15:151.

21. Doran N. Sex differences in smoking cue reactivity: craving, negative affect, and preference for immediate smoking. Am J Addict. 2014;23:211–7.

22. Huang CL, Cheng CP, Huang HW. The development of a Chinese-language instrument to measure social smoking motives among male Taiwanese smokers. J Transcult Nurs. 2013;24:371–7.

23. Mwenifumbo JC, Lessov-Schlaggar CN, Zhou Q, Krasnow RE, Swan GE, Benowitz NL, Tyndale RF. Identification of novel CYP2A6*1B variants: the CYP2A6*1B allele is associated with faster in vivo nicotine metabolism. Clin Pharmacol Ther. 2008;83:115–21.

24. Schoedel KA, Hoffmann EB, Rao Y, Sellers EM, Tyndale RF. Ethnic variation in CYP2A6 and association of genetically slow nicotine metabolism and smoking in adult Caucasians. Pharmacogenetics. 2004;14:615–26.

25. Huang CL, Lin HH, Wang HH. The psychometric properties of the Chinese version of the fagerstrom test for nicotine dependence. Addict Behav. 2006;31:2324–7.

26. Lu CC, Lin HH, Chen CJ, Huang CL. Psychometric testing of the Chinese version of the dimensions of Tobacco Dependence Scale. J Clin Nurs. 2009;18:2470–7.

27. Huang CL, Lin HH, Wang HH. Cigarette dependence questionnaire: development and psychometric testing with male smokers. J Adv Nurs. 2010;66:2341–9.

28. Raunio H, Rahnasto-Rilla M. CYP2A6: genetics, structure, regulation, and function. Drug Metabol Drug Interact. 2012;27:73–88.

29. Nurfadhlina M, Foong K, Teh LK, Tan SC, Mohd Zaki S, Ismail R. CYP2A6 polymorphisms in Malays, Chinese and Indians. Xenobiotica. 2006;36:684–92.

30. Oscarson M, McLellan RA, Gullsten H, Yue QY, Lang MA, Bernal ML, Sinues B, Hirvonen A, Raunio H, Pelkonen O, Ingelman-Sundberg M. Characterisation and PCR-based detection of a CYP2A6 gene deletion found at a high frequency in a Chinese population. FEBS Lett. 1999;448:105–10.

31. Chiang CT. The polymorphisms of CYP2A6 among Taiwanese lung cancer patients. Master's thesis. Chunghua University (Tainan, Taiwan). 2006. http://handle.ncl.edu.tw/11296/ndltd/29131916603407156420. Accessed 24 Apr 2016.

32. Chan RC, Chen RY, Chen EY, Hui TC, Cheung EF, Cheung HK, Sham P, Li T, Collier D. The differential clinical and neurocognitive profiles of COMT SNP rs165599 genotypes in schizophrenia. J Int Neuropsychol Soc. 2005;11:202–4.

33. Dempsey D, Tutka P, Jacob P 3rd, Allen F, Schoedel K, Tyndale RF, Benowitz NL. Nicotine metabolite ratio as an index of cytochrome P450 2A6 metabolic activity. Clin Pharmacol Ther. 2004;76:64–72.

34. Iwahashi K, Waga C, Takimoto T. Whole deletion of CYP2A6 gene (CYP2A6AST;4C) and smoking behavior. Neuropsychobiology. 2004;49:101–4.

35. Waga C, Iwahashi K. CYP2A6 gene polymorphism and personality traits for NEO-FFI on the smoking behavior of youths. Drug Chem Toxicol. 2007;30:343–9.

36. Liu T, David SP, Tyndale RF, Wang H, Zhou Q, Ding P, He YH, Yu XQ, Chen W, Crump C, et al. Associations of CYP2A6 genotype with smoking behaviors in southern China. Addiction. 2011;106:985–94.

37. O'Loughlin J, Paradis G, Kim W, DiFranza J, Meshefedjian G, McMillan-Davey E, Wong S, Hanley J, Tyndale RF. Genetically decreased CYP2A6 and the risk of tobacco dependence: a prospective study of novice smokers. Tob Control. 2004;13:422–8.

38. Gold AB, Lerman C. Pharmacogenetics of smoking cessation: role of nicotine target and metabolism genes. Hum genet. 2012;131(6):857–76.

39. Chenoweth MJ, O'Loughlin J, Sylvestre MP, Tyndale RF. CYP2A6 slow nicotine metabolism is associated with increased quitting by adolescent smokers. Pharmacogenetics Genom. 2013;23:232–5.

40. Nedic G, Nikolac M, Borovecki F, Hajnsek S, Muck-Seler D, Pivac N. Association study of a functional catechol-O-methyltransferase polymorphism and smoking in healthy Caucasian subjects. Neurosci Lett. 2010;473:216–9.

41. Redden DT, Shields PG, Epstein L, Wileyto EP, Zakharkin SO, Allison DB, Lerman C. Catechol-O-methyl-transferase functional polymorphism and nicotine dependence: an evaluation of non replicated results. Cancer Epidemiol Biomark Prev. 2005;14:1384–9.

42. Guo S, da Chen F, Zhou DF, Sun HQ, Wu GY, Haile CN, Kosten TA, Kosten TR, Zhang XY. Association of functional catechol O-methyl transferase (COMT) Val108Met polymorphism with smoking severity and age of smoking initiation in Chinese male smokers. Psychopharmacology. 2007;190:449–56.

43. Munafo MR, Freathy RM, Ring SM, St Pourcain B, Smith GD. Association of COMT Val(108/158)Met genotype and cigarette smoking in pregnant women. Nicotine Tob Res. 2011;13:55–63.

44. Nagano T, Shimizu M, Kiyotani K, Kamataki T, Takano R, Murayama N, Shono F, Yamazaki H. Biomonitoring of urinary cotinine concentrations associated with plasma levels of nicotine metabolites after daily cigarette smoking in a male Japanese population. Int J Environ Res Public Health. 2010;7:2953–64.

A novel approach to emotion recognition using local subset feature selection and modified Dempster-Shafer theory

Morteza Zangeneh Soroush[1], Keivan Maghooli[1*], Seyed Kamaledin Setarehdan[2] and Ali Motie Nasrabadi[3]

Abstract

Background: Emotion recognition is an increasingly important field of research in brain computer interactions.

Introduction: With the advance of technology, automatic emotion recognition systems no longer seem far-fetched. Be that as it may, detecting neural correlates of emotion has remained a substantial bottleneck. Settling this issue will be a breakthrough of significance in the literature.

Methods: The current study aims to identify the correlations between different emotions and brain regions with the help of suitable electrodes. Initially, independent component analysis algorithm is employed to remove artifacts and extract the independent components. The informative channels are then selected based on the thresholded average activity value for obtained components. Afterwards, effective features are extracted from selected channels common between all emotion classes. Features are reduced using the local subset feature selection method and then fed to a new classification model using modified Dempster-Shafer theory of evidence.

Results: The presented method is employed to DEAP dataset and the results are compared to those of previous studies, which highlights the significant ability of this method to recognize emotions through electroencephalography, by the accuracy of about 91%. Finally, the obtained results are discussed and new aspects are introduced.

Conclusions: The present study addresses the long-standing challenge of finding neural correlates between human emotions and the activated brain regions. Also, we managed to solve uncertainty problem in emotion classification which is one of the most challenging issues in this field. The proposed method could be employed in other practical applications in future.

Keywords: Emotion identification, Local subset feature selection, Machine learning methods, Independent component analysis, Dempster Shafer theory, Brain computer interactions

Introduction

A fundamental controversy that has been driving extensive research in phycology and neuroscience today concerns what emotion really is. Though seemingly simple, the definition of emotion has in fact remained as an area of little consensus. Most often, the term emotion refers to a psycho-physiological process triggered by conscious and unconscious perception of an object or situation and is commonly associated with mood, temperament, personality, disposition, and motivation. Emotion is central to almost any interpersonal communication and is generally expressed through both verbal and nonverbal cues. Quite undeniably, emotions pervade every aspect of human life, having profound influences on our actions as well as our perceptions. This has led to the development of systems that attempt to recognize and interpret human affects to establish affective human–computer interactions (HCI). However, as yet most human–computer interaction systems are far from being emotionally intelligent and thus, tend to fail to distinguish and discriminate emotional states and decide upon following proper

---

*Correspondence: k_maghooli@srbiau.ac.ir
[1] Department of Biomedical Engineering, Science and Research Branch, Islamic Azad University, Tehran, Iran
Full list of author information is available at the end of the article

actions. Therefore, affective computing, as a growing field, sets its goal to bridge this gap by identifying emotional states using the exhibited cues and generating proper responses [1].

Over the past few years, the studies on emotion recognition through EEG have received increasing attention and are now extending into interdisciplinary fields that range from psychology to different branches of engineering. They typically include preliminary researches on emotion theories and applications to affective BCIs [2, 3], which allow for identifying, analyzing and responding to user's affective states based on physiological signals.

Emotion recognition is a key step towards emotional intelligence in advanced human–machine interaction. It is mainly served through analyzing either emotional expressions or physiological signals. The former refers to any observable emotional cues that communicates emotion, while the latter, which has so far received little attention, includes information that lies in signals originating from the central and peripheral nervous system such as blood pressure, respiration, skin conductivity, pupil dilation, heart rate, and so forth. In the field of affective computing, different signals have been drawn into focus to study emotion recognition. For a comprehensive review of emotion recognition methods, one can refer to Calvo and D'Mello [4].

EEG is largely employed to investigate the brain activity associated to emotion since it allows for the identification of immediate responses to emotional stimuli and could potentially reflect emotional states in a relatively cost-and computation-effective manner. Nevertheless, emotion recognition based on EEG could come across as challenging, factoring in the fuzzy boundaries and individual differences related to emotions. Furthermore, it seems theoretically unlikely to obtain the correct category for an EEG that corresponds to different emotional states since emotion is generally regarded as a function of various variables such as time, culture, and race [5].

With the rapid growth of micro-nano technologies and embedded systems, it is no longer far-fetched to have BCI systems ported from a laboratory demonstration to real-life applications. Thanks to new advances in materials and integrated electronic systems technologies, a new generation of dry electrodes and embedded systems have been developed to fulfill the basic needs for increased practicability, wearability, and portability of BCI systems in real-world environments [6, 7].

Recently, an increasing number of affective computing researches have been conducted with the aim of building computational models that employ EEG features to estimate emotional states. A review of such models can be found in [8], the work of Kim et al. Affective neuroscience seeks, among other goals, to study the neural associations between human emotions and the obtained brain activity, particularly such EEG signatures of emotion that are more likely to be shared across individuals. Researches in the literature suggest that while processing modules for particular emotions appear to be non-existent, finding neural signatures of emotions, signified by a distributed pattern of brain activity [9], seem theoretically and practically possible. Mauss and Robinson [10] came to the conclusion that the emotional state tends to involve circuits as opposed to any isolated brain region. Furthermore, it is widely believed that identifying neural patterns which are common across individuals and are also stable across sessions can contribute significantly to EEG-based emotion recognition. On the other hand, cortical activity following emotional cues is attributed to the lateralization effect. Schmidt and Trainor [11] discovered that valence and intensity could be identified by the pattern of asymmetrical frontal EEG activity and the overall frontal EEG activity, respectively. Muller et al. noticed a correlation between gamma power and a negative valence over the left temporal region [12]. Bringing into attention the relation between frontal EEG asymmetry and approach and withdrawal emotions, Davidson and Fox [13] and Davidson [14] demonstrated that the left frontal activity mirrors heightened approach tendencies, while withdrawal tendencies are reflected in the right frontal activity. Nie et al. in [15] noted the prevalence of the subject-independent features attributed to positive and negative emotions in the right occipital lobe and parietal lobe for the alpha band, the central site for the beta band, and the left frontal lobe and right temporal lobe for the gamma band. Balconi et al. suggested that valence and arousal rating affect frequency band modulations such that high arousal and negative or positive stimuli can trigger an increased response [16].

Despite all earlier efforts, the lack of recognizable neural signatures of emotion has continued to be a major barrier. Finding such a strategy to settle this issue will be a breakthrough of substantive significance, paving the way for several subsequent developments in psychology, cognitive sciences, and other relevant fields. Therefore, the current study, through combining novel approaches and proposing a new structure, aims to identify the active regions using suitable electrodes with acceptable level of accuracy.

According to the Circumplex Model, emotions are distributed in a two-dimensional circular space where the vertical and horizontal axes represent arousal and valence dimensions respectively. The two axes intersect at one point, dividing the space into four main quadrants which are used in labeling data in this research. The current study aims to manage the novel methods, and propose a structure for active neural structures associated with specific emotions and to present an optimal strategy for applying these approaches to achieve an accurate classification of emotions. The proposed structure makes use of novel and optimized algorithms for extracting emotions in an effective and organized manner to bring about the best possible results. Using EEG channels, this study attempts to identify brain regions that are active when experiencing a specific emotion. To this end, ICA algorithm is employed to remove artifacts and extract the independent components. Then, based on the extracted mapping, channels will receive a corresponding value.

In this setting, the absolute values of active and inactive regions will be obtained. The normalized value as well as the average value of each channel are then calculated and compared to a threshold value, which leads to the selection of active channels that are suited to our task. The process is repeated for each of the four classes of emotions, choosing the informative channels. The channels that are common in all classes would further be selected

to allow for extraction of the proposed features. The proposed method would proceed to implement the feature selection along the arousal and valence dimensions. In the end, emotions are classified using the optimized Dempster Shafer method. Figure 1 illustrates the block diagram of the presents approach.

Materials and methods
Dataset used
The database contains all recorded signal data, frontal face video for a group of the participants, subjective ratings from the participants as well as the subjective ratings from the initial online subjective annotation and the list of 120 videos used. Koelstra et al. built the DEAP database aiming at examining spontaneous human affective states that are specifically induced by music videos [1]. The dataset contains 32 healthy participants half males and half females, with the age range of 19 to 37 (mean = 26.9). For each participant, 40 videos

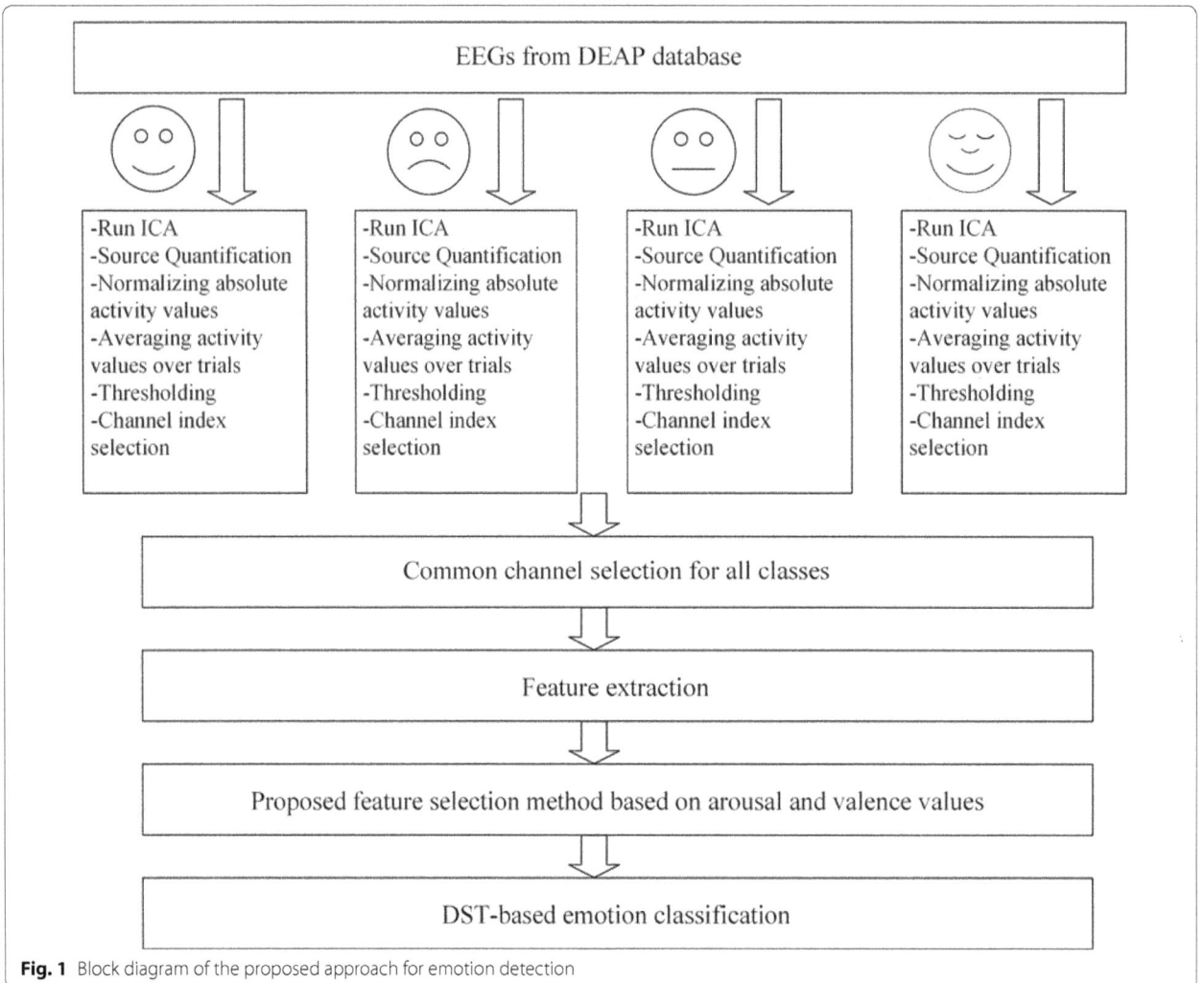

Fig. 1 Block diagram of the proposed approach for emotion detection

were separately presented in 40 trials with the EEG and peripheral physiological signals simultaneously recorded. In each of them, the index of the current trial was first displayed for 2-s; and a consecutive 5-s recording proceeded as the baseline condition; then the music video was shown for 1 min; finally, the subjective-ratings on arousal, valence, liking and dominance scales were collected.

Channel selection

In this section, we propose a method to select most active channels associated with different states of emotions. As mentioned before, emotions can be described through the arousal-valence plane which allows considering four different regions as emotional states. Figure 2 shows the arousal-valence plane as well as the emotional states. Here, we have simply named these four quarters as: Quarter 1 (Q1), Quarter 2 (Q2), Quarter 3 (Q3) and Quarter 4 (Q4).

Arousal and valence distribution in DEAP dataset is also represented in such plane. 1280 samples (32 individuals, each 40 trials) are almost uniformly distributed in arousal-valence plane indicating that there are adequate numbers of samples in each class. This section aims to determine neural correlates between each emotional state, i.e. class, and the registered EEG signals and thus selecting the EEG channels that display appreciable higher activity.

EEG activity can be demonstrated using blind source separation (BSS) methods like ICA. The current study applies Runica as well as second order blind identification (SOBI), JADE and COMBI which are believed to be the best BSS methods for EEG signal processing applications in several surveys such as [17, 18]. EEGs for each class are first fed into BSS methods to get sources separated. 32 EEG sources (i.e. independent components) are estimated and reconstructed in each BSS method. Based on the surveys, we employed the mentioned BSS methods to evaluate and compare them in terms of emotion recognition and emotion-related neural activity.

It should be noted that, EEGs in DEAP database have been preprocessed before and it has been observed that no noticeable artifacts or noises exist which means all extracted sources are correspondent to neural activity. Neural activity is estimated for each component and then averaged over samples in each emotional class to have the average activity maps for each emotional state. Figures 3, 4 depict the average activity mapping for 32 channels in Q1–Q4 emotional states, respectively.

EEG source separation and topographic mapping are carried out using EEGLAB in this study. Activity values are then normalized with respect to minimum and maximum activity in the dataset. All normalized activity

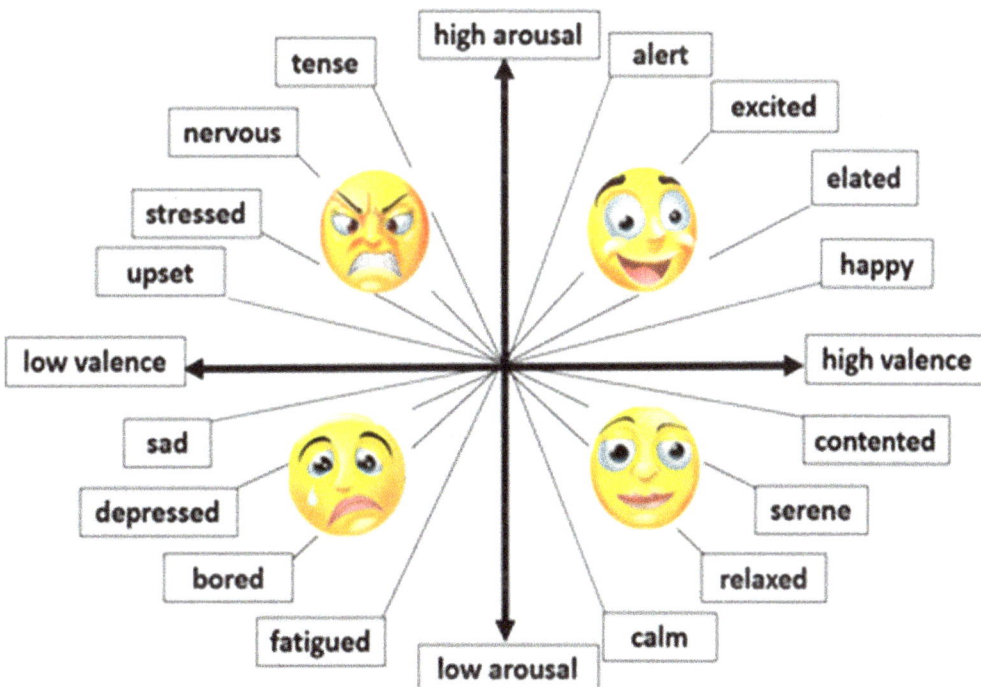

Fig. 2 Arousal-valence plane and label distribution for DEAP dataset

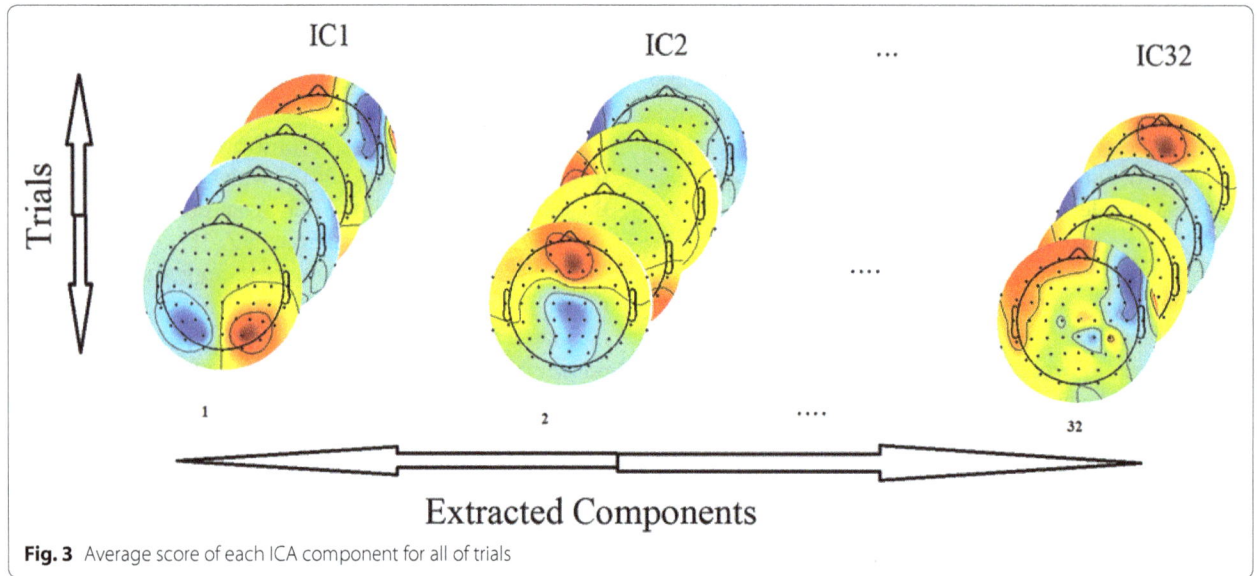

Fig. 3 Average score of each ICA component for all of trials

values vary in the range of $[-1, 1]$. Since both active and inactive regions (i.e. channels) are of importance, we focus on the absolute value of neural activity to find most active and significant channels in emotional changes.

Channels with activity values being higher than a specific threshold are considered as "Emotional Channels" in each class. This threshold is determined based on a trial and error procedure to achieve best classification performance.

Since only the selected channels are taken to the next step, this method holds promise to be less time-consuming and more accurate. Channel indices for each emotional state are determined with respect to channel activity and only common channels among all four classes are considered to be processed in the rest of the proposed method.

Feature extraction

Prior to classification of samples, effective features are extracted from selected channels. Several studies like [19–34] have applied different features while working on DEAP database. This study makes use of features that have been previously proposed as well as nonlinear features which are believed to be effective in emotion recognition. These features are estimated from the entire 1-min selected EEG channels which were explained in the previous section. Since we concentrate on nonlinear features which are mostly extracted from the signal phase space, we need longer windows (e.g. 1 or 2 min at sampling frequency of 256 or 128 Hz) to reconstruct the EEG phase space. Moreover, some features such as different kinds of entropies need at least 4000 samples to be estimated correctly and precisely.

Table 1 lists the proposed features and the abbreviations.

For reasons of space, we avoid explaining these well-known features here. For more information, refer to the mentioned references.

Local subset feature selection

This section focuses on feature selection algorithm. Taking a close look at labels in this dataset, i.e. arousal and valence, we can select a number of informative features simply by considering these values. To this end, the current study benefits form one of the recent and successful feature selection methods called Bandit [42–47] where features are selected based on defined regions in the feature space. Turning the problem of feature selection into a sequential decision-making problem, this method applies the concept of feature tree, as a developed model of decision trees, to divide the sample space into a few localities and assign features to each of them. In addition to splitting and leaf nodes in a typical decision tree, a feature tree includes another type of node named 'feature node', which shows a feature that is attributed to all of its decedents and can have no more than one child. A Compound Locality further refers to a sub-tree corresponding to a set of neighbor localities. This representation simplifies the selection of similar features since neighbor localities are more likely to share mutual features, which will be factored together in the parent feature node. Figure 5 depicts a sample feature tree where the feature nodes are represented by a circle with a single feature inside, a splitting node by a rectangle containing a feature and a threshold, and localities by leaves. In order for the localities to be dependent on a limited number of features, it

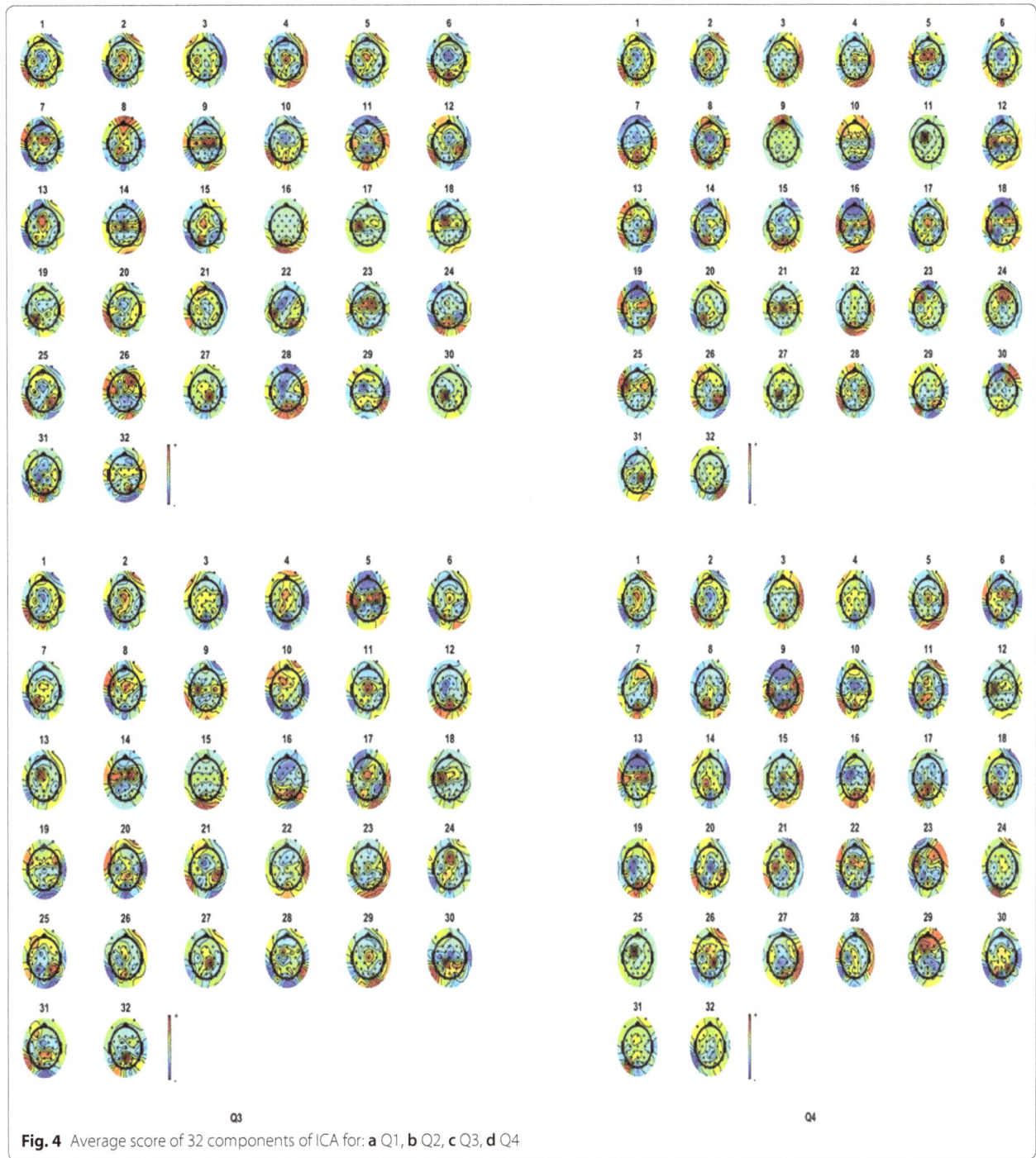

Fig. 4 Average score of 32 components of ICA for: **a** Q1, **b** Q2, **c** Q3, **d** Q4

has been assuming that partitioning can be represented using a univariate binary decision tree [42].

Feature trees assign a sample, either training or test, to a descendant in the root repeatedly, based on the value of the corresponding feature, until it is assigned to a unique leaf. Accordingly, a subset of training samples and a subset of features, that is the set of feature nodes

from the leaf to the root, are accumulated in each locality as the process precedes. For a test sample classification, it is first assigned to a locality according to the feature tree and is then classified in the locality through the corresponding features and training samples. To ensure an effective local feature selection, we employ a criterion which helps us compare different feature

Table 1 Most common features in emotion recognition through EEG

#	Feature description	Abbreviation	Explained in
1	Correlation dimension	CD	[22, 37, 38]
2	Fractal dimension	FD	[40, 41, 49]
3	Largest Lyapunov exponent	LLE	[37, 40, 41]
4	Sample entropy	SpEn	[33, 36]
5	Recurrence rate	RR	[35, 39]
6	Determinism	DET	[35, 39]
7	Average diagonal line length	L	[35, 39]
8	Entropy	ENT	[35, 39]
9	Differential entropy	DeEn	[19, 27]

trees. We expect that the sample of different classes be separable in the new space formed by the selected features. With that in mind, S and ft are assumed to be the training set and the feature tree, respectively. Given ft and a random sample x, we can find the subset of S that belongs to the same locality as x. Let $s \subset L(x, s, ft, k)$ be the k-nearest neighbors of x among the members of this subset. The score of ft with respect to the training set S is computed as:

$$SCORE(ft) = \frac{1}{K \cdot |S|} \sum_{x \in s} \sum_{y \in L(x,s,ft,k)} \begin{cases} 1 \text{ label } (y) = \text{label } (x) \\ 0 \text{ otherwise} \end{cases} \quad (1)$$

where label $(\cdot)$ signifies the class of a sample.

In another perspective, each node of a feature tree is regarded as an equivalent of a state in the Reinforcement Learning (RL) machine, consisting of a sequence of nodes from the root to the current node. The RL agent selects an action for each state, which in this setting, means choosing the node type and the corresponding feature index. Accordingly, the set of all possible actions in each state is Actions $= \{f1, f2, .., Ff, S1, S2, ..., SF, T\}$ with F being the number of features, fi and si showing a feature node and a splitting node respectively, and T being the terminating action, which finishes feature selection in the current node, leaving it as a leaf [42].

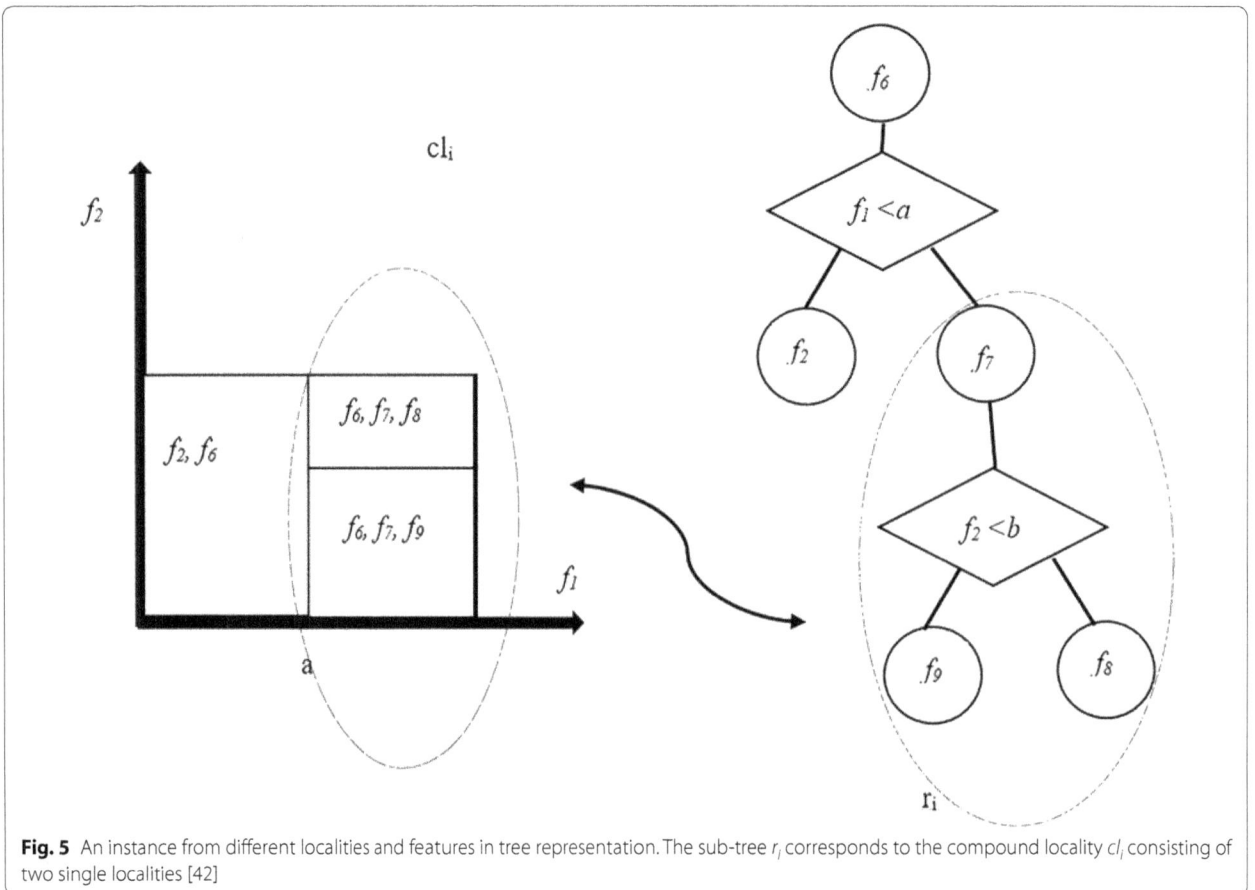

Fig. 5 An instance from different localities and features in tree representation. The sub-tree r_i corresponds to the compound locality cl_i consisting of two single localities [42]

Classification

Since emotions are described by arousal and valence values, we can consider four emotional quarters, i.e. Q1–Q4 classes, in two independent binary classifications. Q1, denotes samples with high valence-high arousal (HVHA). Similarly, Q2, Q3 and Q4 classes mark samples with low valence-high arousal (LVHA), low valence-low arousal (LVLA) and high valence-low arousal (HVLA), respectively. In this paper, we classify samples based on two feature subsets by two separate and independent multi-layer perceptron (MLP) neural networks. MLP is among the most popular classifiers in pattern recognition problems. This classification model works in two main steps: training and testing. In the training phase, weights are adjusted to achieve the least training error. Then, the test samples will be made use of to evaluate the classifier in the testing phase. Numerous studies have employed MLP to identify emotions [48–54].

As the feature selection procedure returns two different subsets as the output, we propose to employ Dempster-Shafer theory (DST) of evidence to combine two MLPs trained by two different feature subsets. DST is reported to be one of the most commonly used methods to reduce uncertainty and increase classification accuracy [38].

Introduced by Dempster and then modified by Shafer, DST is a widely used, theoretical framework which offers a way to handle imprecise, uncertain and partial information. In addition, this theory is applied to fuse different information sources and feature subsets [55]. Therefore, fusion of classifiers can also be performed with the help of this framework. Posterior probability values can be combined using DST and final decision could be made. This theory can reduce uncertainty and incompleteness and lead to a higher accuracy of classification by applying a combination rule for belief functions (Bel) of different information sources. These sources could be some experts or classification models trained by subsets of features. Different classifiers can be combined through this theory. Combination of classification models yields considerably better classification results. DST is explained as follows.

Let us suppose $\varphi = \{s_1, s_1, \ldots, s_m\}$. The number of all possible subsets or hypothesis is $2^\varphi = \{s_1, s_2, \{s_1, s_2\}, \ldots, \{s_1, s_2, \ldots, s_m\}\}$. Bels (or mass values) could be defined for each subset. A mass value determines the degree of belief which is assigned to a specific subset. A Bel should satisfy the following conditions:

$$m(\phi) = 0 \tag{2}$$

$$m(S) \geq 0, \quad \forall_{S \subseteq \varphi} \tag{3}$$

$$\sum_{S \subseteq \varphi} m(S) = 1 \tag{4}$$

With some assumption, we can consider posterior probabilities of classifiers as mass values. As it is mentioned, mass values have some characteristics. There are some methods to transfer the output of a classifier into mass functions [29]. In the current study, we have used softmax operator [38] which is defined as following:

$$m_i(\{s_j\}) = \frac{exp(R_{ji})}{\sum_{j=1}^{C} R_{ji}} \quad j = 1, \ldots, C \tag{5}$$

In which R_{ji} is the jth posterior probability value of i th classifier. C signifies the number of classes and m indicates the mass value. Also the combination of mass values assigned by n different independent sources can be performed through Dempster's combination rule as follows:

$$m(S) = \frac{\sum_{S_1 \cap \ldots \cap S_n = S} \prod_{i=1}^{n} m_i(S_i)}{1 - K} \tag{6}$$

$$K = \sum_{S_1 \cap \ldots \cap S_n = \phi} \prod_{i=1}^{n} m_i(S_i) \tag{7}$$

where K is the normalization factor or the degree of conflict. Final decision can be made through several ways such as choosing a hypothesis with the maximum value of mass, belief or plausibility. In this paper, we decide to go for the maximum value of mass function. For the sake of simplicity, maximum Bel is chosen to determine selected hypothesis [29–31].

To clarify more, it should be noted that in the training phase relabeling should be done in order to put the problem into DST framework. Relabeling is carried out based on what is suggested in [53]. The Euclidian distance between each class prototype and each training sample is calculated. Then a membership function is defined based on the distance which determines the level of ambiguity in the data. Membership values for each training sample is thresholded. A training sample might be assigned to a specific class or a set of classes based on the membership values and the considered threshold. Figure 6 shows the classification procedure in this study.

In testing phase, samples are classified through trained MLPs and the output is normalized using the softmax operator to follow belief function properties. For more information about combining MLPs using DST refer to [55].

In the present paper, two different feature subsets are extracted. Relabeling is carried out for each subset and then two MLPs are trained. In testing phase, MLP

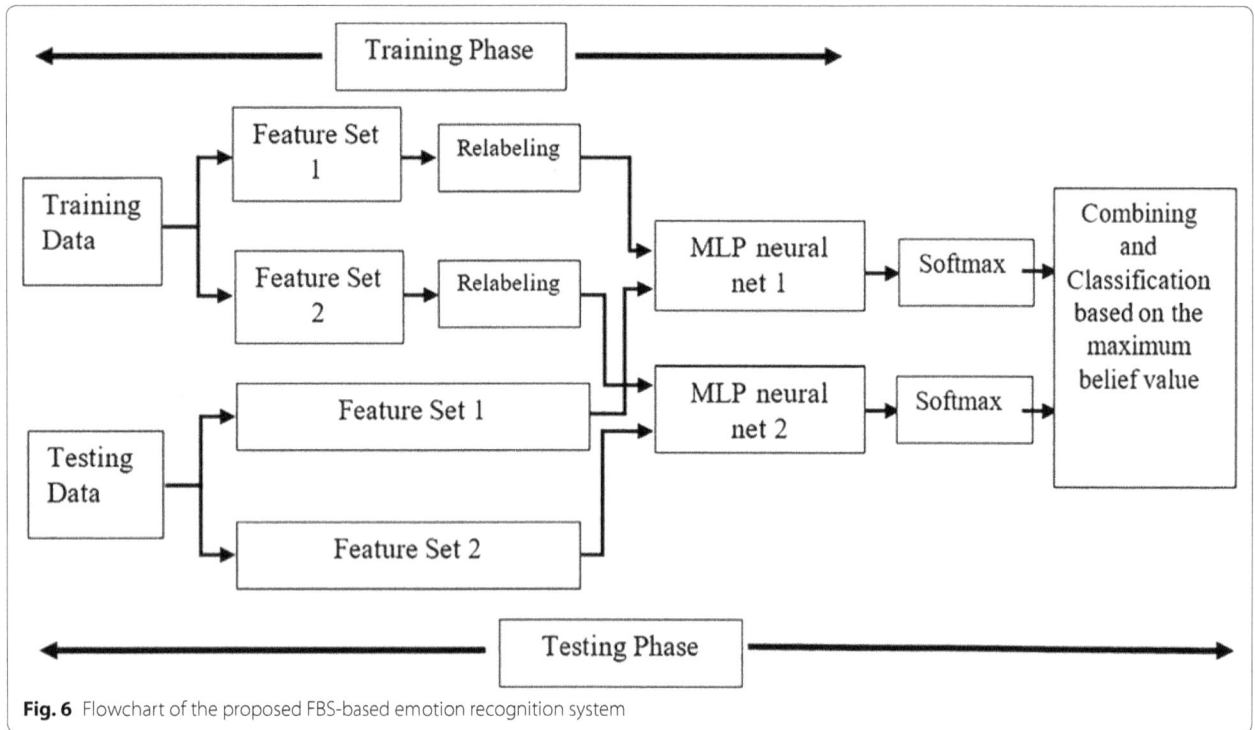

Fig. 6 Flowchart of the proposed FBS-based emotion recognition system

outputs are normalized using softmax operator to have belief functions. Based on DST, belief functions are combined and final decision for each test sample is made.

Evaluation

Classification accuracy, that is the ratio of correctly classified instances to the total number of test samples, as well as confusion and confidence matrices were taken into account to appraise the proposed method. Confusion matrix is a table layout that allows visualization of the classification performance. Each row of the matrix demonstrates the test samples in a predicted class while each column denotes the test instances in an actual class, or the other way around.

Confidence matrix

There are several evaluation methods to ensure acceptable and reliable classification results. One of the most widely-used methods is K-fold cross validation where the data set is divided into 10 subsets, with one subset being retained as the test set and the remaining k-1 being used as training data. In most of the literature, K is chosen as 10 according to the size of the data set.

Results

We present a new method to determine neural activity related to each emotion class which results in EEG emotion-related channel selection. For each BSS method, 32

EEG sources and consequently neural activity maps are reconstructed and then averaged over all samples in each emotional state. Common channels over four emotion classes are considered for the next step. All mentioned features in Table 1 are extracted from the selected EEG channels for all samples. The same features are extracted for each emotion class. These feature have been claimed to be effective in emotion recognition based on the previous studies. The proposed method of feature selection determines features representing and describing arousal and valence values the best. The main idea of this method is to formulate the problem of local feature subset selection as a sequential decision making problem in which we look for a series of good splitting actions. We suggest a sequential decision making process to create feature trees. In other words, the suggested method partitions the sample space into localities and select features for them. The partitions and the corresponding local features are represented using a novel notion of feature tree. As mentioned before, arousal and valence are two major quantities which describe emotions and emotional states. Taking this in mind, we divide the sample space into two main parts and finally we achieve two localities (i.e. arousal and valence) and consequently two subsets of features. Ten most significant features in each subset are selected and finally these features (for train and test samples) are fed into MLPs and DST in order to classify emotions.

Table 2 demonstrates classification methods with respect to different classifiers and algorithms. All implementations are performed using MATLAB (release R2016a) running on Windows 7 Laptop PC with Intel(R) Core (TM) 2 Duo 2.0 GHz processor with 4 GB RAM. As it can be seen, four well-known BSS methods, four most common classifiers and the proposed method are employed and the results are presented in Table 2. For each BSS method and classifier, accuracy and processing time are reported. Besides, statistical analysis using one way ANOVA test is carried out and p-values are represented. Significant differences are in the bold face for each BSS method as well as each classification model. Taking a closer look, we can easily conclude that the proposed Classification method and SOBI are the best combination. Moreover, the proposed features are almost successful in all classification schemes. This suggests that nonlinear features can describe emotions appropriately.

The results suggest that the modified Dempster Shafer method can significantly separate different classes of emotions when second order blind identification (SOBI) algorithm is applied. On the other hand, ranking the channels led to presenting the corresponding channels for each emotion. Having implemented the selecting threshold, the more considerably active channels associated with each emotion were eventually selected, and presented in Table 3.

Afterwards, the intersection between the selected channels was computed. According to the results, the number of selected channels is much lower in other methods indicating that activated regions are approximately constant in each emotion (regardless of the source separations methods).

As Table 3 signifies, temporal areas are prominently more active when experiencing happiness, whereas central and frontal areas play a more significant role in Class 4 emotion, i.e. sadness.

According to Table 2, the modified Dempster Shafer method produces better performance results in comparison with other blind source separation algorithms. Therefore, confusion and confidence matrices are computed to evaluate the errors of the presented method. As shown in Table 4, the desired label value for each class and decided class are defined and at the end, CCR value is reported as 0.9054, which is more appropriate. It should be noted that Q1 to Q4 refer to four different emotion classes according to the arousal–valance plane containing 458, 296, 260 and 266 samples (total $= 1280$), respectively.

$$CCR = \frac{\sum_{i=1}^{4} Q_{ii}}{\sum_{j=1}^{4} \sum_{i=1}^{4} Qji} \tag{8}$$

As mentioned earlier, identifying the correlations between different emotions and brain regions has

Table 2 A comparison among source separation algorithms with respect to different classifiers

Index channels	Runica 14	SOBI 16	COMBI 17	JADE 15	p-value –
MLP					
Accuracy (%)	77.16	79.57	76.33	80.28	0.0646
Time (min)	118.46	120.78	116.89	113.45	
KNN					
Accuracy (%)	79.11	81.46	77.16	73.28	0.0894
Time (min)	112.56	110.32	118.96	103.52	
Bayes					
Accuracy (%)	82.57	84.65	78.24	79.67	0.0743
Time (min)	121.32	122.85	119.65	118.45	
SVM					
Accuracy (%)	84.65	86.78	85.96	83.13	0.0531
Time (min)	115.43	112.47	108.75	111.65	
Modified DST					
Accuracy (%)	88.49	*90.54*	86.72	89.32	*0.0417*
Time (min)	122.25	120.82	123.67	126.95	
p-value	0.0631	*0.0301*	*0.0472*	0.0787	

Table 3 A comparison among the values of the selected electrodes in each quarter with respect to source separation algorithms

	Q1	Q2	Q3	Q4	Intersection
Runica	Fp1, Fp2, Fz, F4, F3, F8, Cz, C4, C3, Pz, P3, T4	Pz, P4, P3, F4 O1, T4, F3	T3, T4, C3, T6, P3, T5, P4, F4, O1	P3, T4, F4, Pz, P4, O1, O2, T6, T5, F3	F3, F4, O1, T4
SOBI	Fp1, Fz, F4, F3, F8, Cz, P4, Cz, Pz, P3, O2	Pz, P4, P3, O2, Cz, F3	F3, T4, C3, T6, P3, T5, Cz, O2	P3, Cz Pz, P4, O1, O2, T6, T5, F3	Cz, O2, F3
COMBI	Fp1, Fp2, Fz, F4, O1, F8, Cz, C4, C3, Pz, P3, T4	Pz, P4, P3, O1, T4, F3, FP1	T3, T4, C3, T6, P3, T5, P4, O1, Fp1	P3, Fp1, Pz, P4, O1, O2, T4, T5, F3	O1, Fp1, T4
JADE	F3, Fp2, Fz, F4, F3, F8, Cz, C4, C3, Pz, P3, O1, T4	Pz, P4, P3, O1, T4, F3	T3, T4, C3, T6, P3, T5, F4, F3, O1,	P3, F4, Pz, P4, O1, O2, T4, T5, F3	F3, O1, T4

Table 4 Confusion and confidence matrices of the proposed method

	Target			
	Q1	Q2	Q3	Q4
Decision				
Q1	407	8	9	10
	88.86%	2.70%	3.46%	3.75%
Q2	23	268	8	3
	5.02%	90.54%	3.07%	1.12%
Q3	17	13	236	5
	3.71%	4.39%	90.76%	1.87%
Q4	11	7	7	248
	2.40%	2.36%	2.69%	93.23%

The upper value in each cell represents the number of samples correctly classified through the proposed method

remained a major challenge in the field of emotion recognition. According to the proposed structure, which includes averaging the corresponding values of active regions through various trials, this study introduces average activation within brain regions for each class of emotion. Figure 7 reports average activation in brain regions for 320 trials in various emotions. The most striking results to emerge from the data analysis is that the frontal region is particularly activated when experiencing emotions in Q1 quarter, also, temporal and occipital regions activation evidently correlate with experiencing emotions in Q2 and Q4 quarters, respectively.

Discussion

As mentioned, detection of brain regions that associate with an emotion is a matter of leading importance in the field of BCI and cognitive sciences. The current study has been able to successfully identify these regions through applying novel methods of feature extraction, selection of emotion-related features, and implementation of Dempster Shafer method as well as upgrading the classic methods. Moreover, this research has made use of blocks containing novel approaches in emotion detection, each of which has the capacity to have improved the results on its own. As one of the novelties, this work uses each of these fully-automated blocks to serve the purpose.

Dempster-Shafer theory is quite well-known in pattern recognition while the classification problem contains uncertainty. In emotion recognition, previous studies such as [54] have employed DST in order to identify emotions through facial expression. It shows that emotion classification is quite subject-oriented and includes imperfect data with uncertain labels. Based on the results of the current study and [54], DST seems to be an effective method of classification in both facial and EEG-based emotion recognition. Since in several samples, individuals did not reflect a specific emotion, DST should be used to decrease the uncertainty.

Some studies such as [56] have tried to classify emotions into four quadrants like what has been done in this work. Emotions are mostly described by arousal and valence which result in arousal-valence plane with four quadrants. In [56] three EEG channels (Fz, Cz and Pz) are claimed to be the most important information sources in emotion recognition. This proves the findings in Table 3 and Fig. 7. Although they have tried to develop a real-time system by means of processing event related potential (ERP), the classification performance is still low.

DEAP dataset has been known as a reliable and rich dataset in emotion recognition. Also, it is noted in numerous studies like [57–60] that visual emotion elicitation has more influential effects. Those mentioned studies, like us, have used DEAP EEG signals. These signals can be considered information sources whereby we can classify emotions. Among these sources EEG has very

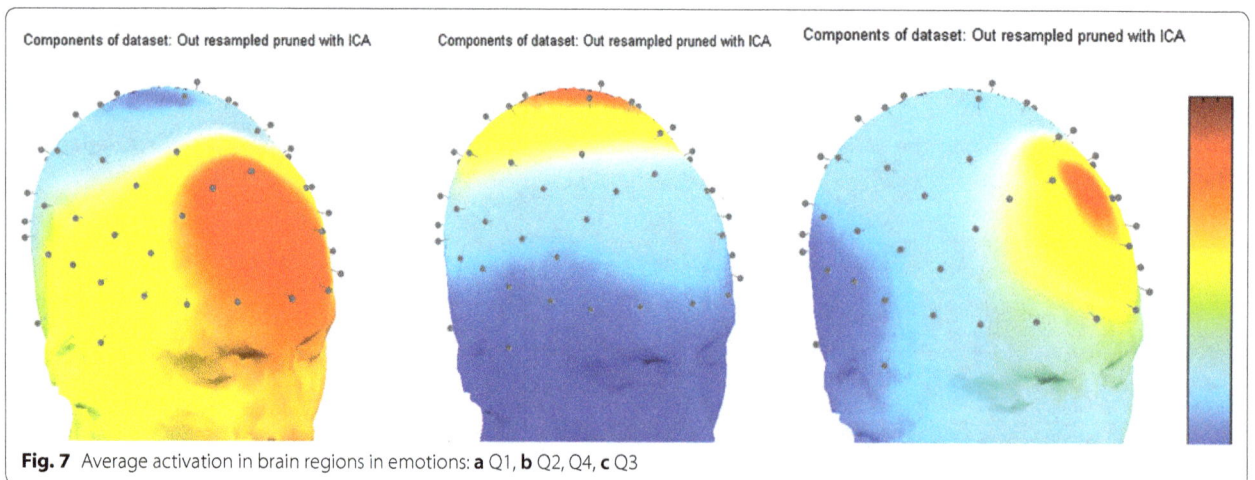

Fig. 7 Average activation in brain regions in emotions: **a** Q1, **b** Q2, Q4, **c** Q3

high spatial and temporal resolution. In addition EEG signals are easily available and price effective.

Most emotion assessment methods consist of three main steps including the biological signal which is processed, extracted features and the classification model. Extracted feature may come from traditional approaches or modern ones which are more related to nonlinear analysis. For example [59–62] employed discrete wavelet transform (DWT) to extract EEG bands and classify emotions while it should be mentioned that DWT cannot exactly and efficiently extract and separate EEG bands since it totally depends on the wavelet kernel [56–59] report that EEG spectral analysis can solve the problem and results in a higher recognition performance while those approaches seem to be still limited and unsuccessful in comparison with the recent methods which apply nonlinear analysis. We can see that both traditional and modern processing approaches have been employed to classify emotions. But common traditional methods which focus on time domain statics, frequency or frequency-scale domain are mostly useful for analyzing linear signals with specific mathematical characteristics such as linear, stationary and Gaussian distributed [63]. However, it is obvious that biological systems such as brain are inherently complex, non-Gaussian, nonlinear, and non-stationary [64]. That is the reason why nonlinear analysis has gained a lot of attention as a novel methodology over the past years. Nonlinear analysis makes it possible to extract more meaningful information and features

from the recordings of brain activity [65]. In this study, we focus on EEG nonlinear analysis by extracting features mostly related to signal phase space. Results show that the proposed features are effective.

This research also contributes to the existing literature through organizing the recently proposed approaches.

Identifying active regions for each emotion not only extends our knowledge and ability in the field of BCI, but also comes in particularly useful in diagnosis and treatment applications for mental diseases such as depression, autism etc. Studies in the literature review suggest [19–24] that several emotions at Q1 originate from temporal region, which is near auditory region, this can aid in mental illness treatments. Also, correlations between the active brain regions and emotions in Q3 quarter reveals that, from a psychological perspective, it would be enough to expose the aforementioned regions to electromagnetic waveforms to change the brain mode.

The current study also provides considerable insight into the distribution of activated brain regions associated with different emotional states.

Figure 8 provides a comparison of the share of activation of each brain region while experiencing different classes of emotion. As illustrated, emotions do not originate from a single, specific region but rather from interconnected regions. However, this should not be taken to mean that each region will be equally activated. With that in mind, a strong point of the current study lies in identifying the dominant regions with respect to each class of emotions.

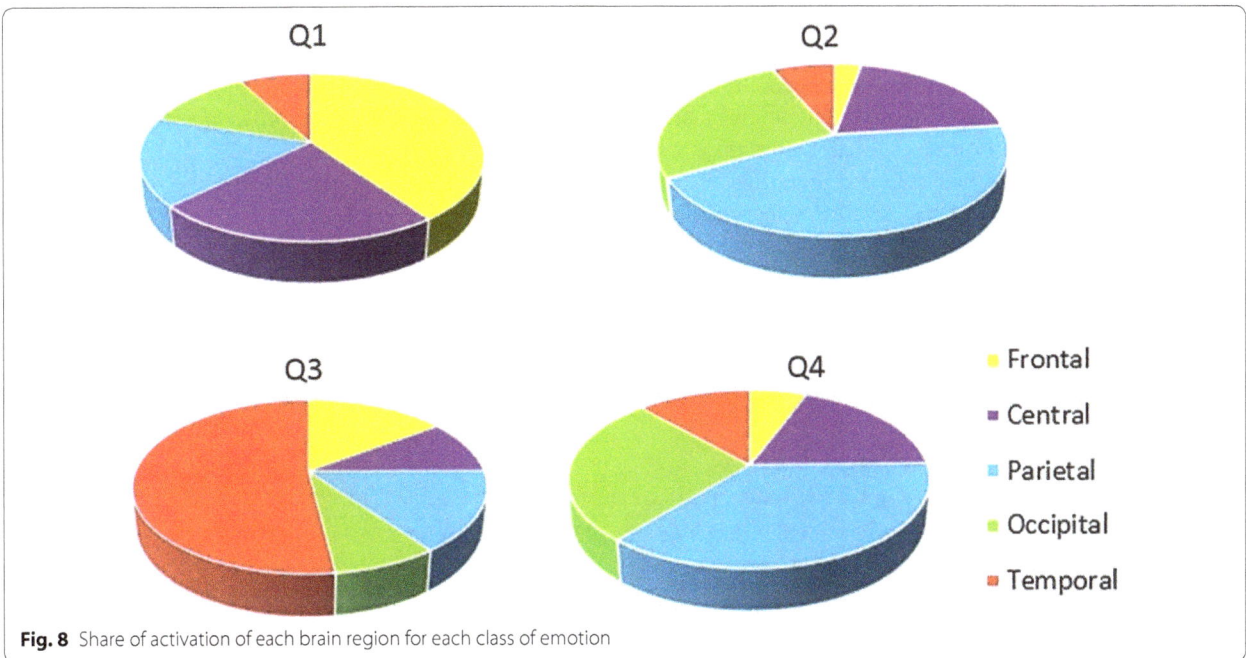

Fig. 8 Share of activation of each brain region for each class of emotion

Table 5 A comparison of the provided methods in other papers and the proposed method for Emotion Recognition

Authors	Year	Method	Classification accuracy (%)
Fan and Chou [66]	2018	Recurrence quantification analysis, logistic regression	75.7%
Zhong et al. [33]	2017	Spectral and time features, multiple-fusion-layer based ensemble classifier of stacked autoencoder (MESAE)	77.19% (arousal accuracy), 76.17% (valence accuracy)
Atkinson and Campos [22]	2016	Statistical and spectral features, Hjorth parameters, fractal dimension, minimum-Redundancy-Maximum-Relevance, support vector machine	62.39% (valence), 60.72% (arousal)
Xu and Plataniotis [32]	2016	Power spectral density, stacked denoising autoencoders, deep belief network	85.86% (arousal accuracy of SDAE), 84.77% (valence accuracy of SDAE), 88.33% (arousal accuracy of DBN), 88.59% (valence accuracy of DBN)
Jie et al. [67]	2014	Sample entropy, support vector machine	79.11%
Yin et al. [33]	2017	Spectral and time features, multiple-fusion-layer based ensemble classifier of stacked autoencoder	77.19% (arousal accuracy) 76.17% (valence accuracy)
Tripathi et al. [21]	2017	Convolutional neural networks, deep neural network	58.44% (valence, DNN), 55.70% (arousal, DNN), 66.79% (valence, CNN), 57.58% (arousal, CNN)
Alam et al. [29]	2016	Convolutional neural networks	81.17%
Kumar et al. [25]	2016	Bispectrum, least square support vector machine, radial basis function, linear neural network	64.86% (arousal), 61.17% (valence)
Our work	2018	The proposed method	90.54%

Table 5 enables comparison among available methods in the literature and the proposed approach.

Like every single study, our work has some limitations. The proposed method has different steps and it can be problematic while dealing with datasets such as DEAP containing large number of instances and features. The long processing time could be one of the disadvantages. One proposal to resolve this problem is to select effective EEG channels (like what is carried out in this study) in order to consider just the dominant channels and brain regions related to emotions. Active brain regions and EEG channels related to emotions can be determined through other methods such as connectivity analysis which is more complex and time consuming. Although BSS methods have some shortcomings such as initial criteria and assumptions, they are quite simple and fast to implement. In addition, other evaluation functions can be employed for the wrapper step and therefore, we will have faster convergence of the feature selection algorithm. Using a Monte Carlo scheme for searching, the suggested method is likely to be stable with respect to the changes in the feature subset. But it is noteworthy that the proposed method can be unstable for other datasets and evaluation functions.

Conclusion

The present study has sought to address the long-standing challenge of finding neural correlates between human emotions and the activated brain regions. It has been stressed that all the regions interconnect and none of them is the sole responsible for any specific emotional state. However, some contribute more than others to certain classes of emotion.

The findings presented in this paper can significantly add to the growing body of literature on emotion recognition. Nevertheless, accurate determination of active regions would not conclude here and is still in need of further investigation. One of the methods which seems to be more appropriate among recent studies is the use of two or more modalities. Since each modality shows a different approach from its own aspect, it is expected that combining modalities would produce better results. Future research can explore fusion of EEG and MEG recordings or EEG-fMRI. Since different emotions have different effects on metabolic behavior of blood in capillaries and electrical activity of neurons, it is recommended to assess adding another modality as well as fusion of various modalities.

Authors' contributions
MZS and KM conceived of the presented idea. MZS developed the theory and performed the computations. AMN and SKS verified the analytical methods. MZS wrote the manuscript with support from KM. All authors provided critical feedback and helped shape the research, analysis and manuscript. KM supervised the project. All authors read and approved the final manuscript.

Author details
[1] Department of Biomedical Engineering, Science and Research Branch, Islamic Azad University, Tehran, Iran. [2] Control and Intelligent Processing Centre of Excellence, School of Electrical and Computer Engineering, College of Engineering, University of Tehran, Tehran, Iran. [3] Department of Biomedical Engineering, Faculty of Engineering, Shahed University, Tehran, Iran.

Acknowledgements
Authors would thank science and research branch, islamic azad university for their support.

Competing interests
The authors declare that they have no competing interests.

Funding
This research did not receive any specific grant from funding agencies in the public, commercial, or not-for-profit sectors.

References
1. Koelstra S, Muhl C, Soleymani M, Lee JS, Yazdani A, Ebrahimi T, Patras I. Deap: a database for emotion analysis; using physiological signals. IEEE Trans Affect Comput. 2012;3(1):18–31.
2. Yazdani A, Lee JS, Ebrahimi T. Implicit emotional tagging of multimedia using EEG signals and brain computer interface. In: Proceedings of the first SIGMM workshop on Social media. New York: ACM; 2009. p. 81–88.
3. Ekman P, Friesen WV, O'sullivan M, Chan A, Diacoyanni-Tarlatzis I, Heider K, Scherer K. Universals and cultural differences in the judgments of facial expressions of emotion. J Pers Soc Psychol. 1987;53(4):712.
4. Calvo RA, D'Mello S. Affect detection: an interdisciplinary review of models, methods, and their applications. IEEE Trans Affect Comput. 2010;1(1):18–37.
5. Kim J, André E. Emotion recognition based on physiological changes in music listening. IEEE Trans Pattern Anal Mach Intell. 2008;30(12):2067–83.
6. Lin CT, Liao LD, Liu YH, Wang IJ, Lin BS, Chang JY. Novel dry polymer foam electrodes for long-term EEG measurement. IEEE Trans Biomed Eng. 2011;58(5):1200–7.
7. Grozea C, Voinescu CD, Fazli S. Bristle-sensors—low-cost flexible passive dry EEG electrodes for neurofeedback and BCI applications. J Neural Eng. 2011;8(2):025008.
8. Kim M-K, Kim M, Oh E, Kim S-P. A review on the computational methods for emotional state estimation from the human EEG. Comput Math Methods Med. 2013;2013:573734. https://doi.org/10.1155/2013/573734.
9. Kassam KS, Markey AR, Cherkassky VL, Loewenstein G, Just MA. Identifying emotions on the basis of neural activation. PLoS ONE. 2013;8(6):e66032.
10. Mauss IB, Robinson MD. Measures of emotion: a review. Cogn Emot. 2009;23(2):209–37.
11. Schmidt LA, Trainor LJ. Frontal brain electrical activity (EEG) distinguishes valence and intensity of musical emotions. Cogn Emot. 2001;15(4):487–500.
12. Müller MM, Keil A, Gruber T, Elbert T. Processing of affective pictures modulates right-hemispheric gamma band EEG activity. Clin Neurophysiol. 1999;110(11):1913–20.
13. Davidson RJ, Fox NA. Asymmetrical brain activity discriminates between positive and negative affective stimuli in human infants. Science. 1982;218(4578):1235–7.
14. Davidson RJ. Anterior cerebral asymmetry and the nature of emotion. Brain Cogn. 1992;20(1):125–51.
15. Nie D, Wang XW, Shi LC, Lu BL. EEG-based emotion recognition during watching movies. In: 5th international IEEE/EMBS conference on Neural Engineering (NER), 2011. Piscataway: IEEE; 2011. p. 667–70.
16. Balconi M, Brambilla E, Falbo L. Appetitive vs. defensive responses to emotional cues. Autonomic measures and brain oscillation modulation. Brain Res. 2009;1296:72–84.
17. Vázquez RR, Velez-Perez H, Ranta R, Dorr VL, Maquin D, Maillard L. Blind source separation, wavelet denoising and discriminant analysis for EEG artefacts and noise cancelling. Biomed Signal Process Control. 2012;7(4):389–400.
18. Klemm M, Haueisen J, Ivanova G. Independent component analysis: comparison of algorithms for the investigation of surface electrical brain activity. Med Biol Eng Compu. 2009;47(4):413–23.
19. Liu W, Zheng WL, Lu BL. Multimodal emotion recognition using multimodal deep learning. 2016. arXiv preprint arXiv:1602.08225.
20. Du C, Du C, Li J, Zheng WL, Lu BL, He H. Semi-supervised Bayesian Deep multi-modal emotion recognition. 2017. arXiv preprint arXiv:1704.07548.
21. Tripathi S, Acharya S, Sharma RD, Mittal S, Bhattacharya S. Using deep and convolutional neural networks for accurate emotion classification on DEAP Dataset. In: AAAI. 2017. p. 4746–4752.
22. Atkinson J, Campos D. Improving BCI-based emotion recognition by combining EEG feature selection and kernel classifiers. Expert Syst Appl. 2016;47:35–41.
23. Srinivas MV, Rama MV, Rao CR. Wavelet based emotion recognition using RBF algorithm. Int J Innovative Res Electr Electron Instrum Control Eng. 2016. https://doi.org/10.17148/IJIREEICE.2016.4507.
24. Jadhav N, Manthalkar R, Joshi Y. Electroencephalography-based emotion recognition using gray-level co-occurrence matrix features. In: Proceedings of international conference on computer vision and image processing. Singapore: Springer. 2017. p. 335–43.
25. Kumar N, Khaund K, Hazarika SM. Bispectral analysis of EEG for emotion recognition. Procedia Comput Sci. 2016;84:31–5.
26. Ebrahimzadeh E, Alavi SM, Samsami KF. Implementation and designing of line-detection system based on electroencephalography (EEG). 2013.
27. Liu W, Zheng WL, Lu BL. Emotion recognition using multimodal deep learning. In: International conference on neural information processing. 2016; Cham: Springer; p. 521–9.
28. Liu W, Zhang L, Tao D, Cheng J. Reinforcement online learning for emotion prediction by using physiological signals. Pattern Recogn Lett. 2017. https://doi.org/10.1016/j.patrec.2017.06.004.
29. Alam MGR, Abedin SF, Moon SI, Kim SH, Talukder A, Bairagi AK, Hong CS. Deep Learning based emotion recognition through biosensor observations. 한국정보과학회 학술발표논문집. 2016;1231–2.
30. Shin HC, Roth HR, Gao M, Lu L, Xu Z, Nogues I, Summers RM. Deep convolutional neural networks for computer-aided detection: CNN architectures, dataset characteristics and transfer learning. IEEE Trans Med Imaging. 2016;35(5):1285–98.
31. Nikravan M, Ebrahimzadeh E, Izadi MR, Mikaeili M. Toward a computer aided diagnosis system for lumbar disc herniation disease based on MR images analysis. Biomed Eng Appl Basis Commun. 2016;28(06):1650042.
32. Xu H, Plataniotis KN. Affective states classification using EEG and semi-supervised deep learning approaches. In: IEEE 18th international workshop on multimedia signal processing (MMSP), 2016. Piscataway: IEEE; 2016. p. 1–6.
33. Yin Z, Zhao M, Wang Y, Yang J, Zhang J. Recognition of emotions using multimodal physiological signals and an ensemble deep learning model. Comput Methods Programs Biomed. 2017;140:93–110.
34. W.-L. Zheng, J.-Y. Zhu, and B.-L. Lu, "Identifying stable patterns over time for emotion recognition from eeg," IEEE Transactions on Affective Computing, 2017. 10.1109/TAFFC.2017.2712143.
35. Marwan N, Romano MC, Thiel M, Kurths J. Recurrence plots for the analysis of complex systems. Phys Rep. 2007;438(5–6):237–329.
36. Sharma R, Pachori RB, Acharya UR. Application of entropy measures on intrinsic mode functions for the automated identification of focal electroencephalogram signals. Entropy. 2015;17(2):669–91.
37. Shayegh F, Sadri S, Amirfattahi R, Ansari-Asl K. A model-based method for computation of correlation dimension, Lyapunov exponents and synchronization from depth-EEG signals. Comput Methods Programs Biomed. 2014;113(1):323–37.
38. Hoseingholizade S, Golpaygani MRH, Monfared AS. Studying emotion through nonlinear processing of EEG. Procedia Soc Behav Sci. 2012;32:163–9.
39. Abdossalehi M, Nasrabadi AM, Firoozabadi M. Combining independent component analysis with chaotic quantifiers for the recognition of positive, negative and neutral emotions using EEG signals. Indian J Sci Res. 2014;5(1):432–7.
40. Naji M, Firoozabadi M, Azadfallah P. Emotion classification during music listening from forehead biosignals. SIViP. 2015;9(6):1365–75.
41. Naji M, Firoozabadi M, Azadfallah P. Classification of music-induced emotions based on information fusion of forehead biosignals and electrocardiogram. Cognit Comput. 2014;6(2):241–52.
42. Ebrahimzadeh E, Manuchehri MS, Amoozegar S, et al. A time local subset feature selection for prediction of sudden cardiac death from ECG signal. Med Biol Eng Comput. 2018;56(7):1253. https://doi.org/10.1007/s11517-017-1764-1.
43. Ebrahimzadeh E, Fayaz F, Ahmadi F, Nikravan M. A machine learning-based method in order to diagnose lumbar disc herniation disease by MR image processing. MedLife Open Access. 2018;1(1):1.
44. Ebrahimzadeh E, Kalantari M, Joulani M, Shahraki RS, Fayaz F, Ahmadi F. Prediction of paroxysmal Atrial Fibrillation: a machine learning based approach using combined feature vector and mixture of expert classification on HRV signal. Comput Methods Programs Biomed. 2018;165(10):53–67.

45. Ashtiani MHZ, Ahmadabadi MN, Araabi BN. Bandit-based local feature subset selection. Neurocomputing. 2014;138:371–82.

46. Ebrahimzadeh E, Najjar AB. A novel approach to predict sudden cardiac death using local feature selection and mixture of experts. Comput Intell Electr Eng. 2016;7(3):15–32.

47. Ebrahimzadeh E, Alavi SM, Bijar A, Pakkhesal A. A novel approach for detection of deception using Smoothed Pseudo Wigner-Ville Distribution (SPWVD). J Biomed Sci Eng. 2013;6(01):8.

48. Ebrahimzadeh E, Pooyan M, Jahani S, Bijar A, Setaredan SK. ECG signals noise removal: selection and optimization of the best adaptive filtering algorithm based on various algorithms comparison. Biomed Eng Appl Basis Commun. 2015;27(04):1550038.

49. Ebrahimzadeh E, Pooyan M. Early detection of sudden cardiac death by using classical linear techniques and time-frequency methods on electrocardiogram signals. J Biomed Sci Eng. 2011;4(11):699.

50. Ebrahimzadeh E, Pooyan M. Prediction of sudden cardiac death (SCD) using time-frequency analysis of ECG signals. Comput Intell Electr Eng. 2013;3(4):15–26.

51. Ebrahimzadeh E, Pooyan M, Bijar A. A novel approach to predict sudden cardiac death (SCD) using nonlinear and time-frequency analyses from HRV signals. PLoS ONE. 2014;9(2):e81896.

52. Ebrahimzadeh E, Fayaz F, Ahmadi F, Dolatabad MJR. Linear and nonlinear analyses for detection of sudden cardiac death (SCD) using ECG and HRV signals. Trends Res. 2018;1(01):1–8.

53. Amoozegar S, Pooyan M, Ebrahimzadeh E. Classification of brain signals in normal subjects and patients with epilepsy using mixture of experts. Comput Intell Electr Eng. 2013;4(1):1–8.

54. Shoyaib M, Abdullah-Al-Wadud M, Chae O. A skin detection approach based on the Dempster-Shafer theory of evidence. Int J Approx Reason. 2012;53(4):636–59.

55. Tabassian M, Ghaderi R, Ebrahimpour R. Combining neural networks based on Dempster-Shafer theory for classifying data with imperfect labels. In: Mexican international conference on artificial intelligence. Berlin: Springer; 2010; p. 233–44.

56. Singh MI, Singh M. Development of a real-time emotion classifier based on evoked EEG. Biocybern Biomed Eng. 2017;37(3):498–509.

57. Zhuang N, Zeng Y, Tong L, Zhang C, Zhang H, Yan B. Emotion recognition from EEG signals using multidimensional information in EMD domain. BioMed Res Int. 2017;2017:8317357. https://doi.org/10.1155/2017/83173 57.

58. Li Y, Huang J, Zhou H, Zhong N. Human emotion recognition with electroencephalographic multidimensional features by hybrid deep neural networks. Appl Sci. 2017;7(10):1060.

59. Ang AQ, Yeong YQ, Wee W. Emotion classification from EEG signals using time-frequency-DWT features and ANN. J Comput Commun. 2017;5(03):75.

60. Mangala Gowri SG, Cyril Prasanna Raj P. Energy density feature extraction using different wavelets for emotion detection. Int J Appl Eng Res. 2018;13(1):520–7.

61. Tonoyan Y, Chanwimalueang T, Mandic DP, Van Hulle MM. Discrimination of emotional states from scalp-and intracranial EEG using multiscale Rényi entropy. PLoS ONE. 2017;12(11):e0186916.

62. Murugappan M. Human emotion classification using wavelet transform and KNN. In: international conference on pattern analysis and intelligent robotics (ICPAIR), 2011. Piscataway: IEEE; 2011. vol 1, p. 148–53.

63. Verma GK, Tiwary US. Multimodal fusion framework: a multiresolution approach for emotion classification and recognition from physiological signals. NeuroImage. 2014;102:162–72.

64. Paraschiv-Ionescu A, Aminian K. Nonlinear analysis of physiological time series. In: Nait-Ali A, editor. Advanced biosignal processing. Berlin: Springer; 2009. p. 307–34.

65. Stam CJ. Nonlinear dynamical analysis of EEG and MEG: review of an emerging field. Clin Neurophysiol. 2005;116:2266–301.

66. Fan M, Chou CA. Recognizing affective state patterns using regularized learning with nonlinear dynamical features of EEG. In: IEEE EMBS international conference on biomedical & health informatics (BHI), 2018. Piscataway: IEEE; 2018. p. 137–40.

67. Jie X, Cao R, Li L. Emotion recognition based on the sample entropy of EEG. Bio-Med Mater Eng. 2014;24(1):1185–92.

Interaction of basolateral amygdala, ventral hippocampus and medial prefrontal cortex regulates the consolidation and extinction of social fear

Chu-Chu Qi[1], Qing-Jun Wang[3], Xue-zhu Ma[1], Hai-Chao Chen[3], Li-Ping Gao[3], Jie Yin[1] and Yu-Hong Jing[1,2]*

Abstract

Background: Following a social defeat, the balanced establishment and extinction of aversive information is a beneficial strategy for individual survival. Abnormal establishment or extinction is implicated in the development of mental disorders. This study investigated the time course of the establishment and extinction of aversive information from acute social defeat and the temporal responsiveness of the basolateral amygdala (BLA), ventral hippocampus (vHIP) and medial prefrontal cortex (mPFC) in this process.

Methods: Mouse models of acute social defeat were established by using the resident–intruder paradigm. To evaluate the engram of social defeat, the intruder mice were placed into the novel context at designated time to test the social behavior. Furthermore, responses of BLA, vHIP and mPFC were investigated by analyzing the expression of immediate early genes, such as zif268, arc, and c-fos.

Results: The results showed after an aggressive attack, aversive memory was maintained for approximately 7 days before gradually diminishing. The establishment and maintenance of aversive stimulation were consistently accompanied by BLA activity. By contrast, vHIP and mPFC response was inhibited from this process. Additionally, injecting muscimol (Mus), a GABA receptor agonist, into the BLA alleviated the freezing behavior and social fear and avoidance. Simultaneously, Mus treatment decreased the zif268 and arc expression in BLA, but it increased their expression in vHIP.

Conclusion: Our data support and extend earlier findings that implicate BLA, vHIP and mPFC in social defeat. The time courses of the establishment and extinction of social defeat are particularly consistent with the contrasting BLA and vHIP responses involved in this process.

Keywords: Social defeat, Information extinction, Basolateral amygdala, Ventral hippocampus, Medial prefrontal cortex

*Correspondence: jingyh@lzu.edu.cn
[1] Institute of Anatomy and Histology & Embryology, Neuroscience, School of Basic Medical Sciences, Lanzhou University, No. 199 of Donggang West Road, Lanzhou 730000, Gansu, People's Republic of China
Full list of author information is available at the end of the article

Background

World Health Organization has identified mood disorders as a major cause of mortality, morbidity and disability worldwide [1, 2]. Social defeat is a critical phenotype of mood disorders, including severe depression, anxiety, bipolar disorder, autism and schizophrenia. Also social defeat is manifested by symptoms such as social fear, social avoidance and social withdrawal [3–5]. Overcoming social defeat is the primary determinant of the efficacy of drugs and therapeutic methods on mental disorders. However, the etiology and mechanisms of social defeat remain poorly understood.

Social defeat is induced by physical and psychological stresses, and implicates the cerebral cortex and multiple brain regions of the limbic system [6–8]. Among these regions, the basolateral amygdala (BLA) establishes and consolidates conditioned fears and harmful stimulations. The establishment of conditioned defeat is impaired by infusing the BLA with anisomycin to inhibit protein synthesis. The consolidation of conditioned defeat is enhanced by overexpressing the cyclic adenosine monophosphate (cAMP) response element binding protein in the BLA through a viral vector [9–11]. Therefore, fear consolidation involves a new type of protein synthesis and the formation of neural microcircuit in the BLA. The medial prefrontal cortex (mPFC) is associated with the motivation and the integration in the development of depression and autism. On the one hand, stress stimulation inhibits the mPFC. On the other hand, mPFC activity caused by optogenetics or deep brain stimulation alleviates the symptoms of depression, and which partially contributes to fear extinction through unclear mechanisms [12, 13]. The hippocampus plays pivotal roles in regulating social behavior. Significant evidence indicates that the dorsal and ventral hippocampus (vHIP) play different roles in processing fear and harmful information from context and conditional stimulation [14]. The bidirectional neural circuit between the vHIP and the hypothalamus integrates harmful information and then determines the vulnerability or resilience toward stress stimulation [15].

The severity of social defeat is determined by the strength and duration of the stimuli. Although different parameters have been considered in establishing rodent models of social defeat, the key criteria are based on common symptoms, including social avoidance, social fear and social withdrawal [16–18]. Social defeat is established in adult rodent through one or more harmful stimulation, followed by gradual recovery through stress removal. The appropriate social strategy is selected according to past experience and learning ability, involving the acquisition, consolidation, retrieval and extinction of social information under specific conditions.

Nevertheless, the duration of social defeat is determined by different behavioral paradigms. The changes in the behavior and responses of brain regions are difficult to correlate with one another. Literature has focused on the formation of social defeat and its mechanisms. Few studies have investigated the process of social defeat from establishment to extinction. Our work aims to explore the time characteristics of the consolidation and extinction of acute social defeat and the simultaneous responses of BLA, vHIP, and mPFC. We utilized the resident–intruder paradigm to establish an animal model of acute social defeat. The duration of the consolidation and extinction of social defeat were evaluated. The temporal features of the responses of BLA, vHIP, and mPFC to acute social defeat were also investigated by quantifying the expression of immediate early genes (IEGs), namely, zif268, arc, and c-fos, which are indicators of neural activity.

Methods

Materials

Muscimol (Mus, cat. G019–5 Mg) and rabbit polyclonal anti-c-fos (cat. HPA018531) were obtained from Sigma (St. Louis, MO, USA). Mouse monoclonal anti-c-fos (cat. Sc8047) and GAPDH (cat. Sc-69778) were obtained from Santa Cruz (Santa Cruz, CA, USA). Rabbit polyclonal anti-parvalbumin antibody (cat. bs-1299R) was purchased from Bioss (Bioss technology company, Beijing, China). Based on the sequences retrieved from a gene bank, Mouse zif268 (accession: NM007913) and arc (accession: NM001276684) primers were designed and produced by Takara Biotechnological Company (Takara Biotech, Co., Ltd., Dalian, China). Kits (cat. 9108) for total RNA extraction were purchased from Takara Biotechnological Company (Takara Biotech, Co., Ltd., Dalian, China). SYBR Green PCR Master Kits (cat. A6001) were purchased from promega (Promega Corporation, USA).

Animals

Male C57BL/6 mice weighing approximately 20–22 g and male Kunming (KM) mice weighing approximately 35–40 g were obtained from the Experimental Center of Lanzhou University. Animals were reared in a clean house under a 12-h light/dark cycle, temperature of 22–25 °C, and humidity of 50–60%. Mice were fed with regular diet and purified water ad libtum. All experiments were conducted in accordance with the guidelines of the Policies Governing the Use of Live Vertebrate Animals of the Lanzhou University.

Social defeat

One KM mouse raised alone in a cage for 2 weeks was designated as the resident. The C57BL/6 mice were randomly assigned to a control without the social attack (n = 12) and social defeat with the social attack according to the previous methods [19]. In brief, a C57BL/6 mouse was introduced as the intruder. For 10 min, the C57BL/6 mouse was exposed to the cage with the KM mouse. The aggressive attack was stopped using a perforated plastic barrier, which allows for continued visual, auditory and olfactory contact. After 6 h, the barrier was removed and physical contact was allowed for 10 min. After the second attack, the C57BL/6 mouse was placed back in its home cage. Cumulated frequency of attack is about 40 times per mouse. Mice in social defeat were divided into subgroups on the basis of the designated time at which the animals were sacrificed after social aggression (1, 3, 7, and 15 days; n = 12 per subgroup).

Stereotactic injections

C57BL/6 mice were anesthetized with isoflurane after the completion of social aggression. Mus (40 ng/0.25 μl) or an equal volume of saline was bilaterally injected into the BLA (bregma coordinates: AP − 1.7 mm; ML ±3.3 mm; DV − 3.8 mm from the brain surface). After 3 days, mice were sacrificed following behavioral examination.

Open field test

While exploring a 50 cm × 50 cm open-field arena, the behavior of the mice was assessed during a 5-min test. Locomotor activity and freezing time were measured by a video-tracking system (TM-vision, Chengdu Techman Software Co., Ltd., Chengdu, China).

Social interaction

Social fear and avoidance were assessed using the modified open-field system [20]. Briefly, two 9 cm × 9 cm mesh enclosures were placed at the opposite sides of the open field. One enclosure contained a novel KM mouse as the social target, and another enclosure did not contain a mouse as the social un-target. The experimental mouse was allowed to freely explore a 50 cm × 50 cm arena containing the target and un-target enclosures. The time spent on the social interaction zone (14 cm × 26 cm) surrounding the target enclosure and the reference zones (14 cm × 26 cm) surrounding the un-target enclosure was measured using a video tracking system (TM-vision, Chengdu Techman Software Co., Ltd., Chengdu, China).

Sucrose preference

This test consisted of a 2-bottle procedure in which mice were given the choice between consuming water or a 1% sucrose solution according to previously described method with modification [21]. In brief, animals were singly housed in a cage that had two drinking bottles. One of the bottles had water, while the other bottle had a 1% sucrose solution. Water and sucrose consumption was measured the following day (8:00 A.M.). The position of the sucrose bottle was counterbalanced (left versus right) across the different cages to control for potential side-preference bias.

Marble-burying test

The marble-burying test was performed according to previously described methods with minor modifications [22]. Briefly, the apparatus consisted of a plastic box (15 × 10 × 10 cm) and 9 clean glass marbles (10 mm diameter) that were evenly spaced (4 cm apart) on sawdust (2 cm deep). The number of marbles that were at least 2/3 buried after 5 min was recorded.

Histology

Following behavioral testing, mice were returned to their home cages. After 2 h, mice were deeply anesthetized with isoflurane and transcardially perfused with 20 ml of heparinized saline solution and then with 30 ml of 4% paraformaldehyde in 0.1 M phosphate buffer (PB) at pH 7.4 and 4 °C. Brains were harvested and stored in the same fixative for 90 min at 4 °C followed by at least 24 h of immersion in 20% sucrose solution in 0.1 M PB with 4% paraformaldehyde. Coronal Sects. (30 μm thickness) were obtained using a cryostat microtome. Sections containing the BLA were mounted onto glass slides and counterstained with Cresyl Violet to precisely locate the microinjection site under light microscopy. The remaining sections were used for immunohistochemistry.

Immunohistochemistry

c-Fos immunolabelling was performed using a rabbit polyclonal c-Fos antibody. In brief, sections were quenched in 0.3% hydrogen peroxide (H_2O_2) for 20 min to remove endogenous peroxidase activity. After serial washing in 0.01 M phosphate- buffered saline (PBS), sections were incubated in phosphate-buffered saline containing rabbit anti c-fos antibody (1:200), 0.3% Triton X, and 0.1% bovine serum albumin (BSA) for 24 h at 4 °C. The incubated sections were then washed and incubated for 90 min in biotinylated goat-anti-rabbit antisera (1:200), followed by washing in 0.01 M PBS. Sections were then incubated in Strep-avidin–biotin–peroxidase complex (ABC) (1:200) for 90 min and then immersed in 0.02% 3,3-diaminobenzidine (DAB) containing 0.01% H_2O_2 in 0.01 M PBS until a brown reaction product developed.

Quantification of immunohistochemical staining

Photomicrographs were taken with an Olympus microscope BX3 and Olympus DP73 digital camera. Regions of interest were defined in accordance with the mouse brain atlas based on specific landmarks that comprise cellular groups. The anterior–posterior (AP) level from the bregma of the analyzed regions was as follows: BLA (AP: -0.6 mm to -0.26 mm), vHIP (AP: -2.8 mm to -3.8 mm) and mPFC (AP: 2.34 mm–1.34 mm). c-Fos immunoreactive profiles were captured from a fixed area under $200 \times$ magnification in at least 3 sections per region per mouse and quantified using ImageJ software (NIH, Bethseda, MD). Given that c-Fos expression levels did not differ between the left and right sides regions in response to any of the experimental procedures, counts were averaged to yield the mean number of c-fos-positive profiles per region per animal.

RNA extraction and quantitative real-time PCR

Following behavioral testing, mice were returned to their home cages. After 2 h, mice were deeply anesthetized with isoflurane and sacrificed. The mouse skull was opened and whole brain was removed. Fresh tissues of BLA, vHIP and mPFC were isolated from the corresponding coronal sections under the stereomicroscope. Total RNA was extracted from the BLA, vHIP or mPFC using RNAiso plus reagent (Takara Biotech, Co., Ltd., Dalian, China) in accordance with the manufacturer's instructions. DNA contamination was removed with RNase-free DNase. cDNA was synthesized from 1 μg of RNA with M-MuLV reverse transcriptase and random hexamer following the manufacturer's instructions (Fermentas, Burlington, Canada). Quantitative real-time PCR (Q-RT-PCR) was performed using PIKoREAl96 detector (Thermo Scientific, USA). The mRNA levels of zif268 and arc in triplicate samples of reverse-transcribed cDNA were checked with SYBR Green PCR Master Kit (Promega Corporation, USA) in accordance with the manufacturer's instructions. The primers for mouse zif268 were 5′-CGAACAACCCTATGAGCACCTG-3′ (forward) and 5′-GGCTGGGATAACTCGTCTCCAC-3′ (reverse). The primers for mouse arc were 5′-GCCAAAC-CCAATGTGATCCTG-3′ (forward) and 5′-CTGCTTG-GACACTTCGGTCAAC-3′ (reverse). The mouse gapdh primers were 5′-GCGAGACCCCACTAACATCAA-3′ (forward) and 5′-GTGGTTCACACCCATCACAAA-3′ (reverse). The assays were initiated for 5 min at 95 °C, 40 cycles of 15 s at 94 °C, and 1 min at 60 °C. The threshold cycles of the target gene and gapdh were calculated. The amplification of zif268 and arc cDNA was normalized to the expression of gapdh. The relative mRNA expression levels of zif268 and arc were calculated using the $2^{\Delta CT}$ method.

Protein extraction and Western blot analysis

Following behavioral testing, mice were returned to their home cages. After 2 h, mice were deeply anesthetized with isoflurane and sacrificed. The mouse skull was opened and whole brain was removed. Fresh tissues

of BLA, vHIP and mPFC were isolated from the corresponding coronal sections under the stereomicroscope. Total proteins were extracted from BLA, vHIP or mPFC samples using RIPA buffer that contained protease inhibitors. The extracted proteins (50 g) were fractionated on 10% sodium dodecyl sulfate polyacrylamide gel, and then transferred onto polyvinylidene fluoride membranes. The membranes were blotted with anti-c-Fos (1:1000), anti-GAPDH (1:5000), and horseradish peroxidase-conjugated second antibodies (1:5000). Immunoreactive protein bands were visualized by enhanced chemiluminescence using the Bioanalytical imaging system (Azure Biosystems, INC, USA).

Statistical analysis

The data were expressed the mean $\pm$ SEM. Statistical analysis was performed using SPSS statistical program, version 17.0. The difference between the two groups was analyzed by Student's t test, whereas that among three or more groups was analyzed by one-way analysis of variance with least significant difference test. A difference with $p < 0.05$ was considered statistically significant.

Results

Behavioral changes after acute aggressive stimulation

Spontaneous exploration behavior was examined using the open-field test. As shown in Fig. 1c, the freezing time of the intruder mice increased dramatically at days 1 and 3 after stimulation compared with the control mice ($F = 4.46$, $p < 0.01$). At day 7 after stimulation, the freezing time of the intruder mice was shorter than that at day 1 after stimulation ($F = 4.46$, $p < 0.05$) but was longer than that of the control mice ($F = 4.46$, $p < 0.05$). The freezing time of the intruder mice at day 15 after social stimulation was the same as that of the control mice ($F = 4.46$, $p > 0.05$). The above data suggests that aversive information from acute stimulation is maintained at least for 7 days before gradually diminishing. The intruder mice recovered their exploratory behavior at 15 days after social defeat. The time spent on the social interaction zone is shown in Fig. 1b, d. At day 1 and day 3 after social aggression, intruder mice spent less time on the interaction zone compared with the control mice ($F = 8.98$, $p < 0.01$). On day 7 after stimulation, intruder mice spent more time on the interaction zone than on days 1 and 3 ($F = 8.98$, $p < 0.05$) but still spent less on the interaction zone than control mice ($F = 8.98$, $p < 0.05$). On day 15 after stimulation, the intruder mice spent the same time on the interaction zone as control mice ($F = 8.98$, $p > 0.05$). These data suggest that information for social defeat stress from acute social aggression is maintained for 7 days before diminishing.

Response of the BLA to social defeat stress

Immediate early genes, including zif268, arc and c-fos were used as indices for the evaluation of neural activity. We detected the expression levels of these genes through Q-RT-PCR, Western blotting, and immunohistochemistry. First, we analyzed the mRNA levels of zif268 and arc by using Q-RT-PCR. As shown in Fig. 2a ($F = 21.5$), b ($F = 26.7$), the mRNA levels of zif268 and arc in intruder mice gradually increased at day 1, peaked at day 3, decreased at day 7, and were the same as those in control mice at day 15 after stimulation. Second, we examined c-Fos protein levels by using Western blotting. As shown in Fig. 2c, d ($F = 5.6$), c-Fos expression in intruder mice dramatically increased at day 3 and then slightly decreased at day 7. c-Fos protein levels in intruder mice on days 3 and 7 after stimulation were higher than those in control mice. c-Fos positive cells were labeled and counted as described in "Methods" section. As shown in Fig. 2e, f ($F = 16.357$), the number of c-Fos positive cells dramatically increased at day 3 after stimulation and then decreased. The above data suggests that aggressive stimulation facilitates BLA activation at the beginning of the stimulus (from day 1 to day 7). This response then diminished during the later stages of the stimulus (from day 7 to day 15).

Response of vHIP to social defeat stress

zif268, arc mRNA were analyzed by Q-RT-PCR. As shown in Fig. 3a ($F = 22.233$), b ($F = 23.655$), the levels of these genes decreased on days 1 and 3 after stimulation and increased at days 7 and 15 after stimulation. We also analyzed the expression of c-Fos protein. Similar to those of zif268 and arc, the expression of c-Fos protein decreased at day 3 and increased at day 15 after stimulation (Fig. 3c, d, $F = 4.73$). c-Fos-positive cells were labeled and counted as described in "Methods" section. As shown in Fig. 3e, f ($F = 5.287$), the number of c-Fos-positive cells in intruder mice decreased significantly at days 3 and 7 after stimulation compared with those in the control mice, and then increased to the same levels as those in the control mice at day 15 after stimulation. These results suggest that vHIP is inhibited by aggressive stimulation at the beginning of aggression (from day 1 to day 3), and then gradually recovered (from day 7 to day 15).

Response of mPFC to social defeat stress

Levels of zif268 and arc mRNA were analyzed by Q-RT-PCR. As shown in Fig. 4a ($F = 99.345$), b ($F = 43.18$), the levels of these genes decreased on days 1, 3, 7 and 15 after stimulation. The expression of c-Fos protein decreased at days 1 and 3 and increased at day 7 after stimulation (Fig. 4c, d, $F = 11.4$). c-Fos positive cells were labeled and counted as described in "Methods" section. As shown in

Fig. 4e, f ($F = 23.965$), the number of c-Fos-positive cells in intruder mice decreased significantly at days 3 and 7 after stimulation compared with those in the control mice, and then increased to the same levels as those in the control mice at day 15 after stimulation.

Effects of Mus microinjection to the BLA on social behavior

Mus, as $GABA_A$ receptor agonist were microinjected to BLA immediately after social aggression. Interestingly, on day 3 after microinjection with Mus or saline, the freezing time of the mice in the Mus-group was lower than that of the mice in the saline-group (Fig. 5c, $p < 0.01$). Also, the mice in the Mus-group spent more time on the interaction zone than the mice in the saline-group (Fig. 5b, d, $p < 0.05$). To identify whether social defeat accompanied depression or anxiety, sucrose preference and marble burying test were performed before test of social interaction. The results showed Mus injection increased sucrose preference (Fig. 5e, $p < 0.05$), but no significant effects on marble burying (Fig. 5f, $p > 0.05$), which suggested social defeat induced by acute social aggression accompanied depression-like behavior, but not anxiety.

Effects of Mus microinjection to the BLA on IEGs expression

Mus were microinjected to BLA immediately after social aggression. At day 3 after social aggression, animals were sacrificed at 2 h after social interaction test. We quantified the expression levels of zif268 and arc in the BLA, vHIP and mPFC. As shown in Fig. 6a, b, the expression levels of zif268 and arc significantly decreased in the BLA and increased in the vHIP of the Mus-group compared with those in the saline-group ($p < 0.05$). In mPFC, no difference was observed between Mus-treated group and saline-treated group. c-Fos immunochemistry was performed to evaluated neural activity following social interaction test. In vHIP, numbers of c-Fos-positive cells increased in Mus-treated group compared with the saline-treated group (Fig. 6c, d, $p < 0.05$). In mPFC, numbers of c-Fos-positive cell also increased in Mus-treated group compared with the saline-treated group (Fig. 6e, f, $p < 0.05$).

Discussion

We found that social defeat induced by acute aggression is characterized by social fear and avoidance, and is accompanied by a depression-like behavior. Behavioral test revealed that social fear was severe on days 1 and 3 and gradually diminished on days 7 and 15 after aggression. On days 1 and 3 after aggression, the expression of IEGs (including zif268, arc, and c-Fos) increased in the BLA but decreased in the vHIP and mPFC. On days 7 and 15 after aggression, the expression of IEGs decreased in the BLA but increased in the vHIP. Thus, BLA played

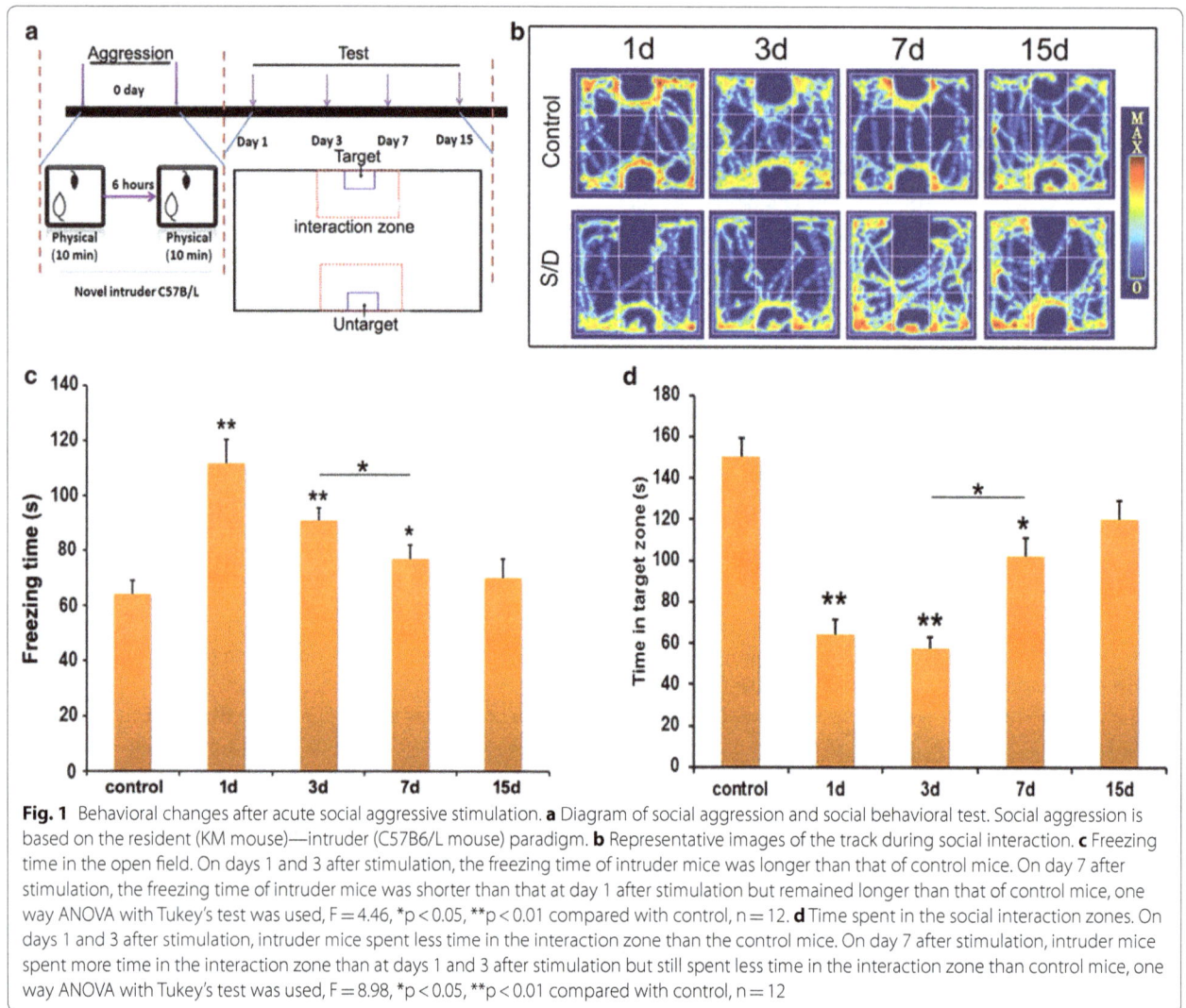

Fig. 1 Behavioral changes after acute social aggressive stimulation. **a** Diagram of social aggression and social behavioral test. Social aggression is based on the resident (KM mouse)—intruder (C57B6/L mouse) paradigm. **b** Representative images of the track during social interaction. **c** Freezing time in the open field. On days 1 and 3 after stimulation, the freezing time of intruder mice was longer than that of control mice. On day 7 after stimulation, the freezing time of intruder mice was shorter than that at day 1 after stimulation but remained longer than that of control mice, one way ANOVA with Tukey's test was used, F = 4.46, *p < 0.05, **p < 0.01 compared with control, n = 12. **d** Time spent in the social interaction zones. On days 1 and 3 after stimulation, intruder mice spent less time in the interaction zone than the control mice. On day 7 after stimulation, intruder mice spent more time in the interaction zone than at days 1 and 3 after stimulation but still spent less time in the interaction zone than control mice, one way ANOVA with Tukey's test was used, F = 8.98, *p < 0.05, **p < 0.01 compared with control, n = 12

an important role in establishing social defeat. Equal volumes of Mus and saline were microinjected into the bilateral BLA immediately after aggression to verify this hypothesis. On day 3 after aggression, social fear and freezing behavior were more significantly ameliorated by Mus treatment than by saline treatment. In addition, Mus treatment reduced the expression of IEGs in the BLA but increased that in the vHIP. The amygdala is critical in mediating fear- and anxiety-related behavior and is the key site for the acquisition and storage of fear memory. The plasticity of the sensory inputs from the thalamus and the cortical areas to the projection neurons in the BLA is the core mechanism underlying Pavlovian fear conditioning [23–25]. The associations between conditioned and unconditioned stimuli are formed through this mechanism. According to the neural circuit model of the amygdala function, fear output is

generated by the associative information conveyed from the BLA by internuclear excitatory projections from the basal and basomedial nuclei to the medial region of the central amygdala. This passive information transfer model is currently being challenged because growing evidence indicates that the BLA and central amygdala can independently mediate parallel or additional associative functions under aversive conditioning [26, 27]. Another emerging evidence is that fear acquisition is controlled by the plasticity of the inhibitory synapses and the interneurons in the amygdala [28]. On the one hand, regulating the inhibition in the BLA and the specific inhibitory synapses on principal neurons in the BLA is associated with the behavioral suppression of fear following the extinction of learning. On the other hand, the activity of local GABAergic neurons is regulated by the plasticity of their excitatory inputs in the BLA and the central lateral

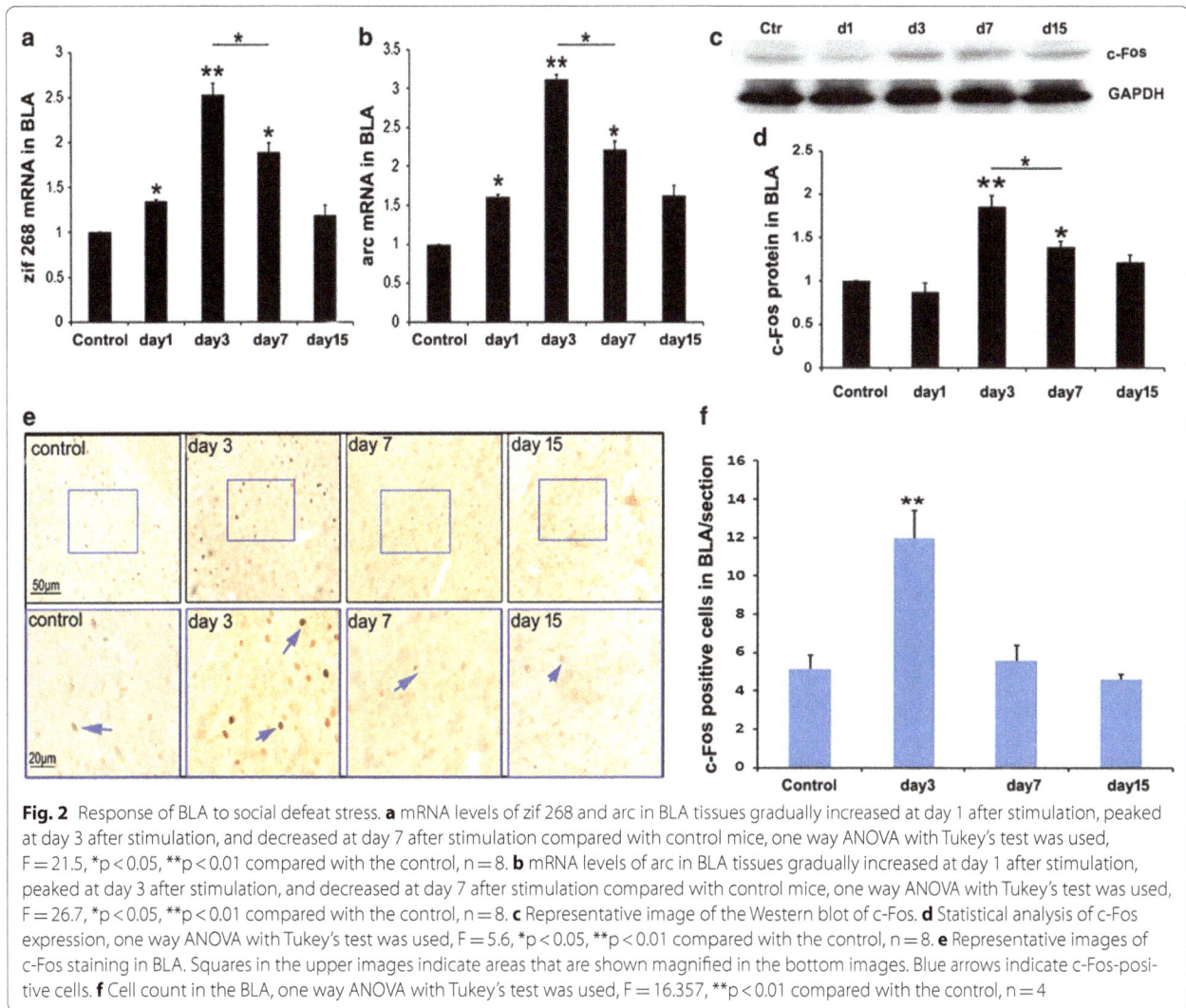

Fig. 2 Response of BLA to social defeat stress. **a** mRNA levels of zif 268 and arc in BLA tissues gradually increased at day 1 after stimulation, peaked at day 3 after stimulation, and decreased at day 7 after stimulation compared with control mice, one way ANOVA with Tukey's test was used, $F = 21.5$, *$p < 0.05$, **$p < 0.01$ compared with the control, $n = 8$. **b** mRNA levels of arc in BLA tissues gradually increased at day 1 after stimulation, peaked at day 3 after stimulation, and decreased at day 7 after stimulation compared with control mice, one way ANOVA with Tukey's test was used, $F = 26.7$, *$p < 0.05$, **$p < 0.01$ compared with the control, $n = 8$. **c** Representative image of the Western blot of c-Fos. **d** Statistical analysis of c-Fos expression, one way ANOVA with Tukey's test was used, $F = 5.6$, *$p < 0.05$, **$p < 0.01$ compared with the control, $n = 8$. **e** Representative images of c-Fos staining in BLA. Squares in the upper images indicate areas that are shown magnified in the bottom images. Blue arrows indicate c-Fos-positive cells. **f** Cell count in the BLA, one way ANOVA with Tukey's test was used, $F = 16.357$, **$p < 0.01$ compared with the control, $n = 4$

amygdala [29]. A recent study revealed that specific local interneurons in the BLA were differentially recruited during conditioned and un-conditioned stimulation associations, thereby mediating the inhibition and disinhibition of distinct subcellular domains for controlling fear learning. Therefore, multiple plastic systems, particularly those integrating GABAergic neurons, can collectively encode aspects of the stimulus associations in the amygdala. The local interneurons in the BLA are heterogeneous interneurons displaying different morphological, electrophysiological, and neurochemical characteristics. Parvalbumin positive interneurons constitute approximately 40% of these interneurons and exert robust perisomatic inhibitory effects on the projection neurons [30, 31]. We found that the ratio of c-Fos to parvalbumin double labeled cells in the BLA was approximately 20% of the total c-Fos immunopositive cells on day 3 after social

aggression (Additional file 1: Figure S1). These findings suggested that the interneurons in BLA are involved in the regulation of social defeat.

The extinction of fear memory is one treatment method for post-traumatic stress disorder, because the establishment of a novel social interaction is accompanied by the extinction of previous social fear. In this study, the recovery due to social interaction was observed on day 15 after aggression, suggesting that the previous aversive stimulation was gradually diminished. Researchers have recently used a condition stimulus memory retrieval–extinction procedure to prevent fear recovery after extinction in rats and humans [32–35]. Consolidation refers to the process wherein memories are retained after their retrieval and destabilization. Destabilization refers to the return of a memory to a labile phase after memory retrieval. Researchers have inferred that

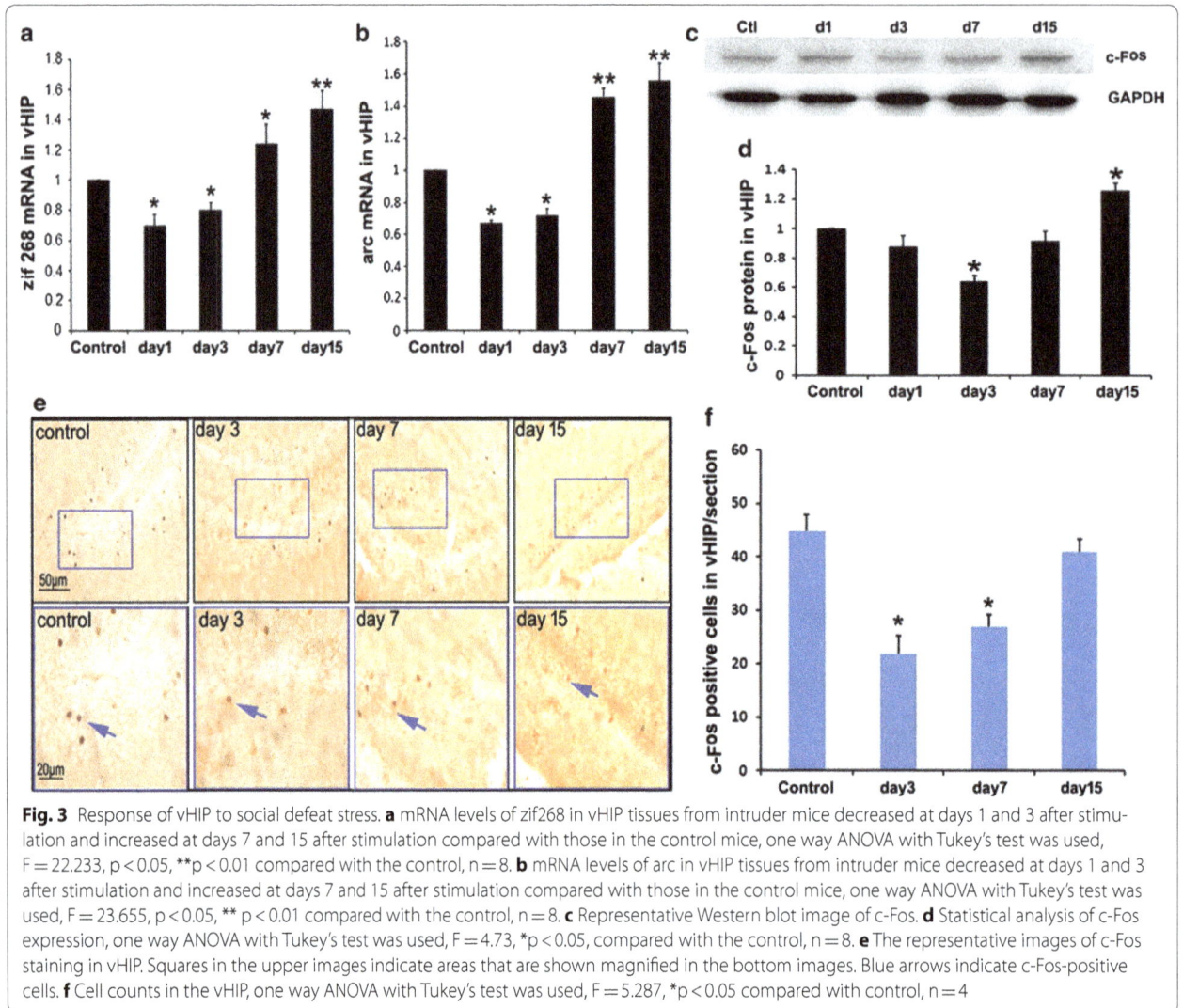

Fig. 3 Response of vHIP to social defeat stress. **a** mRNA levels of zif268 in vHIP tissues from intruder mice decreased at days 1 and 3 after stimulation and increased at days 7 and 15 after stimulation compared with those in the control mice, one way ANOVA with Tukey's test was used, $F = 22.233$, $p < 0.05$, **$p < 0.01$ compared with the control, $n = 8$. **b** mRNA levels of arc in vHIP tissues from intruder mice decreased at days 1 and 3 after stimulation and increased at days 7 and 15 after stimulation compared with those in the control mice, one way ANOVA with Tukey's test was used, $F = 23.655$, $p < 0.05$, ** $p < 0.01$ compared with the control, $n = 8$. **c** Representative Western blot image of c-Fos. **d** Statistical analysis of c-Fos expression, one way ANOVA with Tukey's test was used, $F = 4.73$, *$p < 0.05$, compared with the control, $n = 8$. **e** The representative images of c-Fos staining in vHIP. Squares in the upper images indicate areas that are shown magnified in the bottom images. Blue arrows indicate c-Fos-positive cells. **f** Cell counts in the vHIP, one way ANOVA with Tukey's test was used, $F = 5.287$, *$p < 0.05$ compared with control, $n = 4$

memory consolidation is hampered when the expression of the conditioned responses is disrupted by post-retrieval neural pharmacological manipulations within a specific time interval (i.e., a "reconsolidation window" of up to 2 h post retrieval. This strategy effectively promoted the extinction of aversive memory, which aided in ameliorating the symptoms of mood disorders [36–38]. Our results suggested that aversive memory became extinct after 15 days without additional social defeat. Once the aversive information is forgotten, the learning ability for a novel stimulation is recovered. Another recent study found that autism is associated with genetic variation and the copy number deletion of P-Rex1, which encodes the phosphatidylinositol-3,4,5-trisphosphate-dependent Rac exchange factor1. The genetic deletion or knockdown of P-Rex1 in the CA1 region of the mouse hippocampus produced autism-like behaviors, such as

impaired social interactions, reversal learning deficits in the water maze, and extinction-resistant memory of fear conditioning [39, 40]. These behavioral changes were possibly due to impaired active forgetting or, in a general sense, the failure to update memories. Context recognition involves hippocampal function. The inhibition of the vHIP induced by social aggression disturbs the recognition of novel context and social objects at an early stage (on days 1 and 3 after social defeat). The hippocampal response to novel stimulation resulted in the recovery of the learning ability at a later stage (on days 7 and 15 after social defeat).

The mPFC is associated with motivation as the center of emotion integration. A previous study posited that the activation of mPFC diminished social defeat [41]. Deep brain stimulation in the mPFC ameliorated the symptoms of patients suffering from severe depression [42].

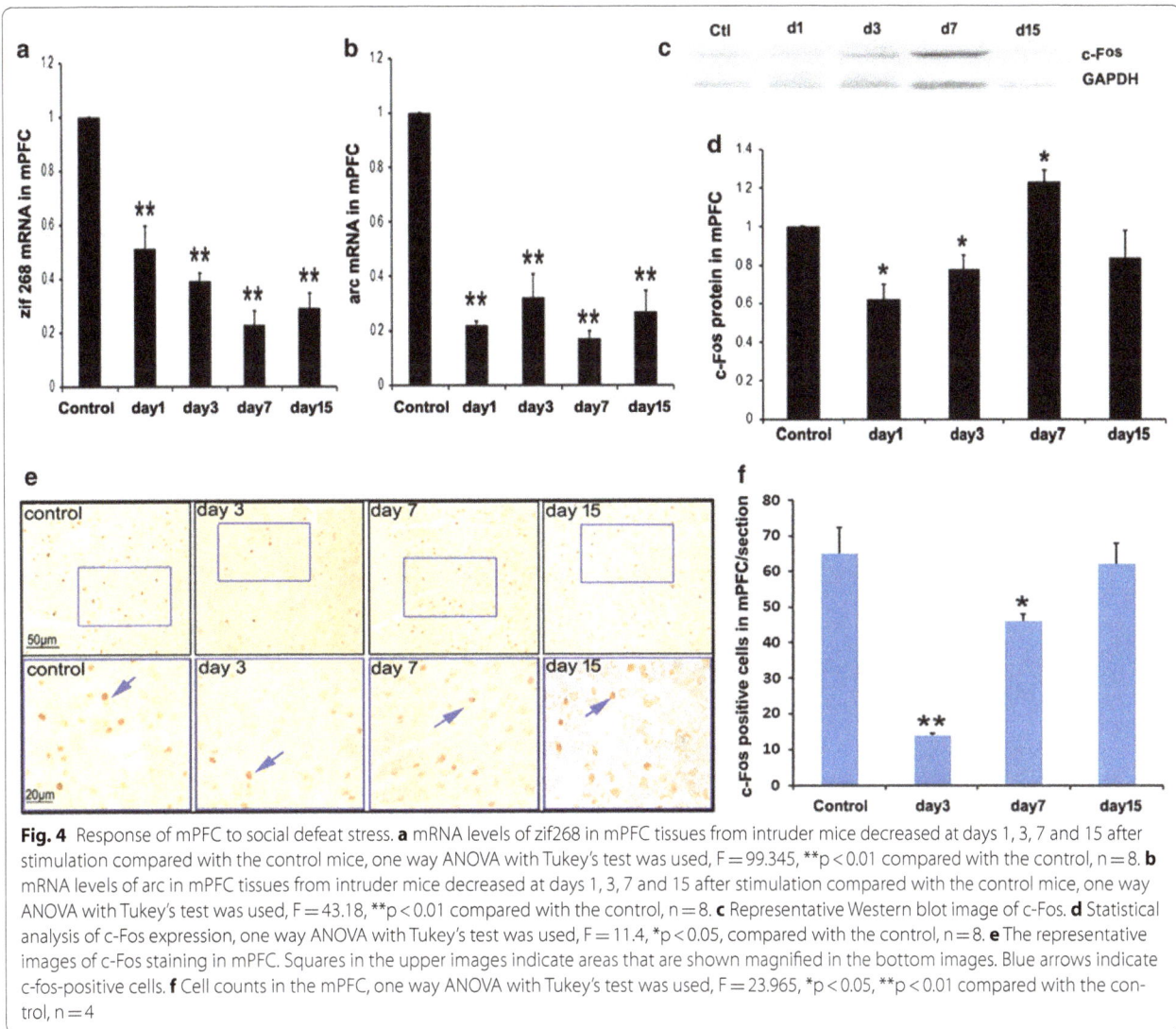

Fig. 4 Response of mPFC to social defeat stress. **a** mRNA levels of zif268 in mPFC tissues from intruder mice decreased at days 1, 3, 7 and 15 after stimulation compared with the control mice, one way ANOVA with Tukey's test was used, $F = 99.345$, **$p < 0.01$ compared with the control, $n = 8$. **b** mRNA levels of arc in mPFC tissues from intruder mice decreased at days 1, 3, 7 and 15 after stimulation compared with the control mice, one way ANOVA with Tukey's test was used, $F = 43.18$, **$p < 0.01$ compared with the control, $n = 8$. **c** Representative Western blot image of c-Fos. **d** Statistical analysis of c-Fos expression, one way ANOVA with Tukey's test was used, $F = 11.4$, *$p < 0.05$, compared with the control, $n = 8$. **e** The representative images of c-Fos staining in mPFC. Squares in the upper images indicate areas that are shown magnified in the bottom images. Blue arrows indicate c-fos-positive cells. **f** Cell counts in the mPFC, one way ANOVA with Tukey's test was used, $F = 23.965$, *$p < 0.05$, **$p < 0.01$ compared with the control, $n = 4$

The social avoidance of the intruder mice reduced the expression of IEGs in the mPFC for novel contexts and social objects at an early stage of social defeat. The social interaction of the control mice led to the high expression of IEGs in the mPFC for novel social objects. The inhibition of the BLA by Mus treatment increased the social interaction and exploration time for novel contexts, suggesting that BLA establishes and consolidates social information. Stress recovery was aided by inhibiting the function of BLA after an aversive stimulation at an early stage. Disturbances at critical times affect the efficacy of the consolidation or extinction of the aversive stimulation. Consolidation and extinction are based on synaptic plasticity and new protein synthesis, both of which are dependent on the duration of the neural activity. Therefore, the time window of a treatment is important. Salinas

reported that training-related IGF-II-dependent memory enhancement is restricted to a temporal window of less than a day. However, the enhancing effect re-emerges at a later time if IGF-II is combined with memory retrieval, which reactivates the memory and induces reconsolidation. The IGF-II effect following retrieval is also temporally limited and restricted to a temporal window that overlaps with the reconsolidation-sensitive period of inhibition avoidance [43]. For the retrieval-induced memory fragility and the IGF-II-dependent enhancement, both of them require new protein synthesis, but in different brain regions, such as the amygdala in the former and the hippocampus in the latter. Therefore, social fear memory was in a sensitive period during the first 3 days after aggression. When activated, this memory could either be significantly weakened or enhanced.

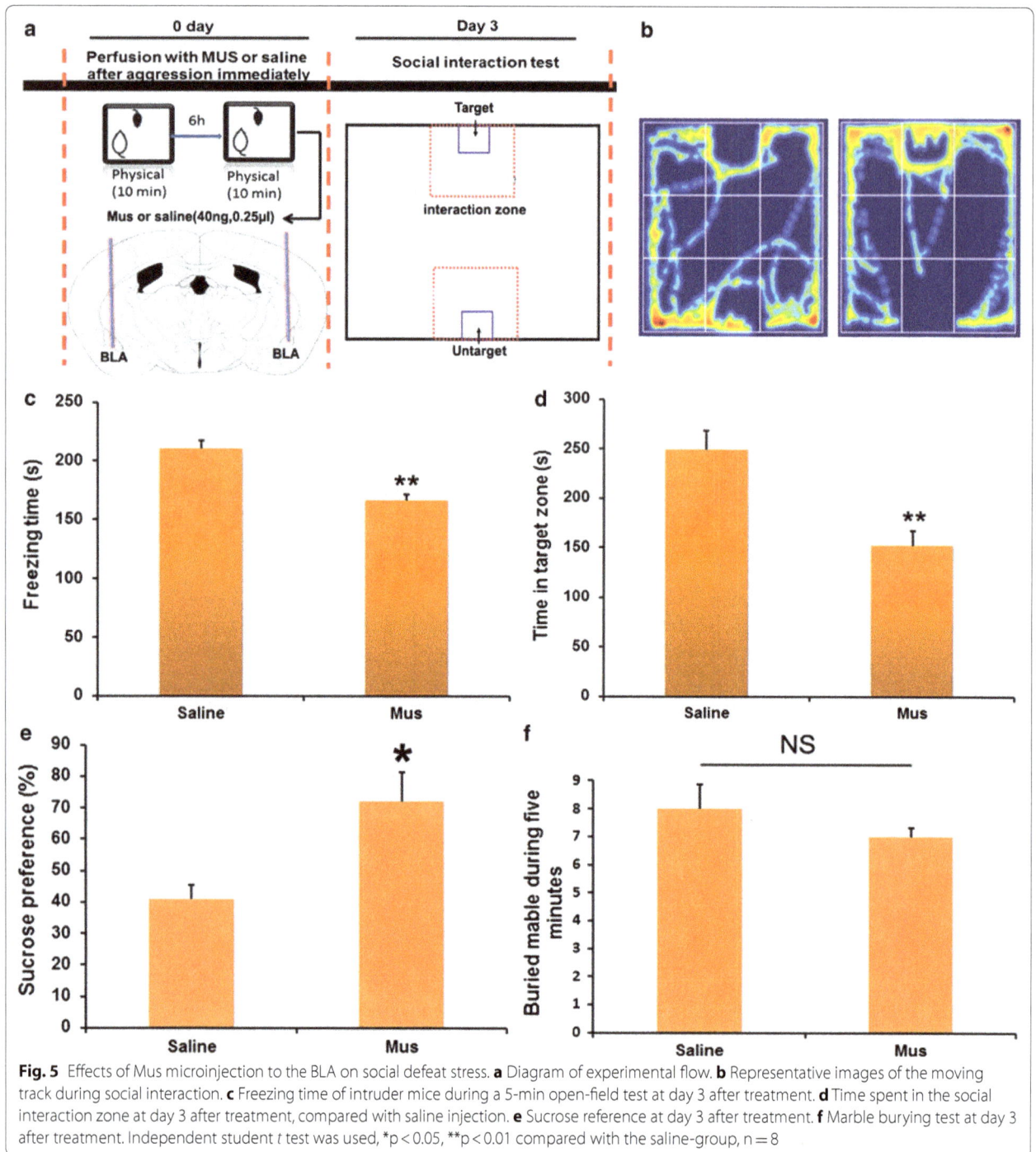

Fig. 5 Effects of Mus microinjection to the BLA on social defeat stress. **a** Diagram of experimental flow. **b** Representative images of the moving track during social interaction. **c** Freezing time of intruder mice during a 5-min open-field test at day 3 after treatment. **d** Time spent in the social interaction zone at day 3 after treatment, compared with saline injection. **e** Sucrose reference at day 3 after treatment. **f** Marble burying test at day 3 after treatment. Independent student t test was used, *p < 0.05, **p < 0.01 compared with the saline-group, n = 8

These findings suggested that reconsolidation is a lingering consolidation process [44, 45].

Although the methodology was limited, our data revealed the duration of social defeat from consolidation to extinction after an acute social aggression. In the future, we will explore the relationship between the responses of the BLA and the vHIP toward social defeat, particularly the functions of the neural circuit between the BLA and the vHIP in recognizing social contexts and objects. We aim to use extinction training and noninvasive treatment to alleviate social defeat and explore the mechanisms underlying the temporal windows of consolidation and extinction.

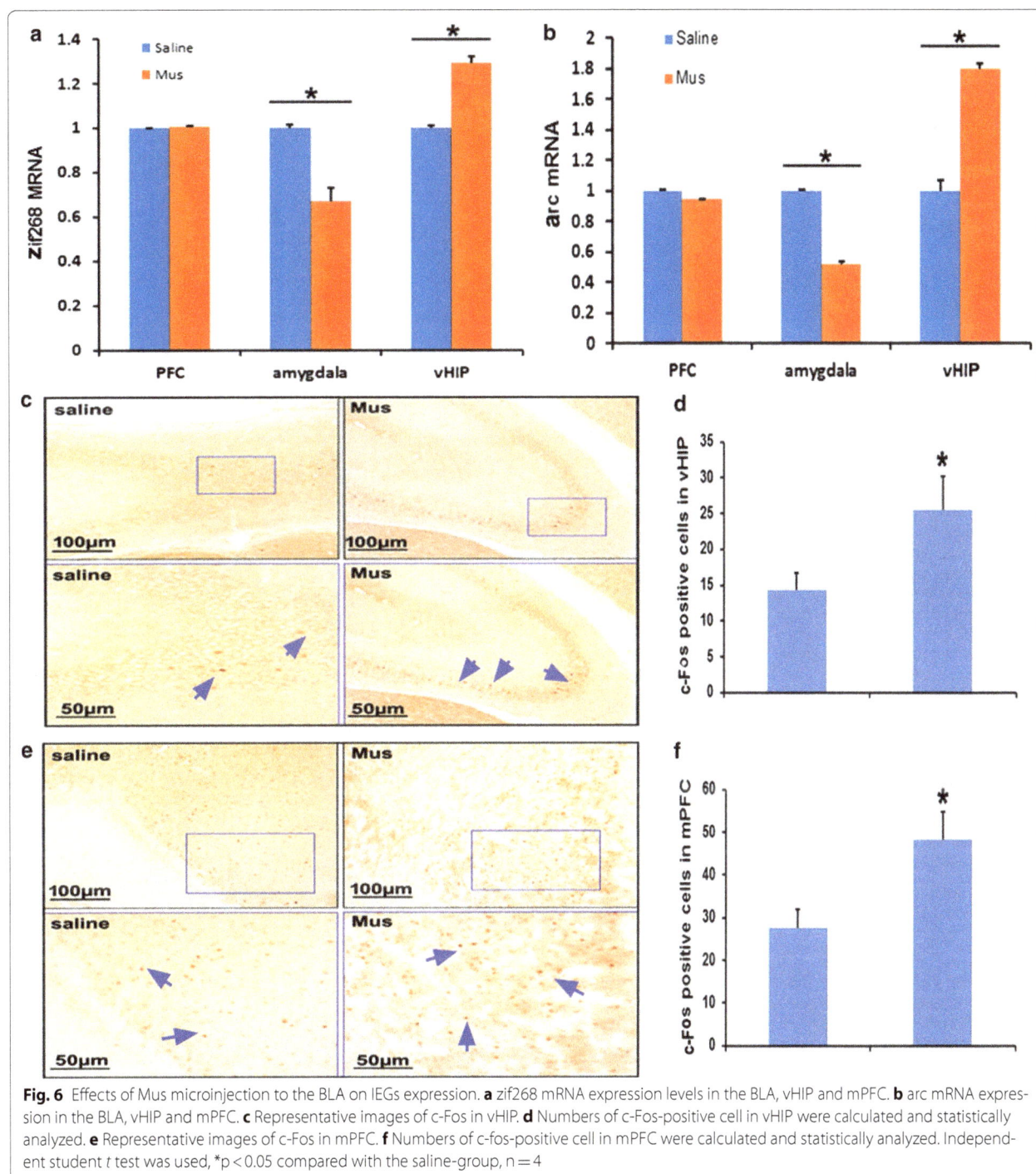

Fig. 6 Effects of Mus microinjection to the BLA on IEGs expression. **a** zif268 mRNA expression levels in the BLA, vHIP and mPFC. **b** arc mRNA expression in the BLA, vHIP and mPFC. **c** Representative images of c-Fos in vHIP. **d** Numbers of c-Fos-positive cell in vHIP were calculated and statistically analyzed. **e** Representative images of c-Fos in mPFC. **f** Numbers of c-fos-positive cell in mPFC were calculated and statistically analyzed. Independent student t test was used, *p < 0.05 compared with the saline-group, n = 4

Conclusion

Acute social defeat was induced by using a social aggressive attack according to the intruder–resident paradigm. The social behavior of the intruder mice toward novel contexts and objects was measured on days 1, 3, 7, and 15 after aggression. The expression of IEGs in the BLA, vHIP, and mPFC was analyzed at 2 h after behavioral

test. The results indicated that social fear and avoidance were significant on days 1–3 after aggression and were accompanied by a high expression of IEGs in the BLA and a low expression of IEGs in the vHIP and mPFC. On days 7–15 after aggression, the social interaction gradually increased and was accompanied by a low expression of IEGs in the BLA and a high expression of IEGs in the vHIP. Inhibiting the function of BLA after aggression ameliorated social defeat, which suggested that BLA consolidates social fear. This study posited that social defeat can be treated by suppressing the consolidation or prompting the extinction of aversive stimulations.

Additional file

Additional file 1: Figure S1. To double-label BLA with c-fos and parvalbumin, BLA sections were stained with parvalbumin and developed with DAB. c-Fos was labeled and developed with DAB-nickel ammonium sulfate. Representative images of c-Fos and parvalbumin double labeling, blue arrows indicate the double labelling cells; black arrows indicate the single labelling cells.

Authors' contributions
Y-HJ and C-CQ planned experiments, interpreted data, and approved the version to be published. C-CQ performed most of the experiments and analyzed data and Y-HJ wrote the paper. Q-JW and X-ZM participated in the behavioral test. H-CC, L-PG and JY participated in acquisition of the study specimens. All authors read and approved the final manuscript.

Author details
[1] Institute of Anatomy and Histology & Embryology, Neuroscience, School of Basic Medical Sciences, Lanzhou University, No. 199 of Donggang West Road, Lanzhou 730000, Gansu, People's Republic of China. [2] Key Laboratory of Preclinical Study for New Drugs of Gansu Province, Lanzhou University, No. 199 of Donggang West Road, Lanzhou 730000, Gansu, People's Republic of China. [3] Institute of Biochemistry and Molecular Biology, School of Basic Medical Sciences, Lanzhou University, No. 199 of Donggang West Road, Lanzhou 730000, Gansu, People's Republic of China.

Acknowledgements
This work is partly supported by National Natural Science Foundation of China (Nos. 81370448 and 81570725) to Jing Yu Hong.

Competing interests
The authors declare that they have no competing interests.

Funding
National Natural Science Foundation of China (Nos. 81370448 and 81570725).

References
1. Kessler RC, Akiskal HS, Ames M, Birnbaum H, Greenberg P, Hirschfeld RM, et al. Prevalence and effects of mood disorders on work performance in a nationally representative sample of U.S. workers. Am J Psychiatry. 2006;163(9):1561–8.
2. Han B, Compton WM, Blanco C, Colpe LJ. Prevalence, treatment, and unmet treatment needs of US adults with mental health and substance use disorders. Health Aff. 2017;36(10):1739–47.
3. Toyoda A. Social defeat models in animal science: what we have learned from rodent models. Anim Sci J. 2017;88(7):944–52.
4. Blanchard DC, Griebel G, Blanchard RJ. Conditioning and residual emotionality effects of predator stimuli: some reflections on stress and emotion. Prog Neuropsychopharmacol Biol Psychiatry. 2003;27(8):1177–85.
5. Treit D, Pinel JP, Fibiger HC. Conditioned defensive burying: a new paradigm for the study of anxiolytic agents. Pharmacol Biochem Behav. 1981;15(4):619–26.
6. Dabrowska J, Hazra R, Ahern TH, Guo JD, McDonald AJ, Mascagni F, et al. Neuroanatomical evidence for reciprocal regulation of the corticotrophin-releasing factor and oxytocin systems in the hypothalamus and the bed nucleus of the stria terminalis of the rat: implications for balancing stress and affect. Psychoneuroendocrinology. 2011;36(9):1312–26.
7. Cooper MA, McIntyre KE, Huhman KL. Activation of 5-HT1A autoreceptors in the dorsal raphe nucleus reduces the behavioral consequences of social defeat. Psychoneuroendocrinology. 2008;33(9):1236–47.
8. Markham CM, Taylor SL, Huhman KL. Role of amygdala and hippocampus in the neural circuit subserving conditioned defeat in Syrian hamsters. Learn Mem. 2010;17(2):109–16.
9. Jasnow AM, Shi C, Israel JE, Davis M, Huhman KL. Memory of social defeat is facilitated by cAMP response element-binding protein overexpression in the amygdala. Behav Neurosci. 2005;119(4):1125–30.
10. Taylor SL, Stanek LM, Ressler KJ, Huhman KL. Differential brain-derived neurotrophic factor expression in limbic brain regions following social defeat or territorial aggression. Behav Neurosci. 2011;125(6):911–20.
11. Bader LR, Carboni JD, Burleson CA, Cooper MA. 5-HT1A receptor activation reduces fear-related behavior following social defeat in Syrian hamsters. Pharmacol Biochem Behav. 2014;122:182–90.
12. Klavir O, Prigge M, Sarel A, Paz R, Yizhar O. Manipulating fear associations via optogenetic modulation of amygdala inputs to prefrontal cortex. Nat Neurosci. 2017;20(6):836–44.
13. Parthoens J, Verhaeghe J, Stroobants S, Staelens S. Deep brain stimulation of the prelimbic medial prefrontal cortex: quantification of the effect on glucose metabolism in the rat brain using [(18) F]FDG microPET. Mol Imaging Biol. 2014;16(6):838–45.
14. Czerniawski J, Ree F, Chia C, Ramamoorthi K, Kumata Y, Otto TA. The importance of having Arc: expression of the immediate-early gene Arc is required for hippocampus-dependent fear conditioning and blocked by NMDA receptor antagonism. J Neurosci. 2011;31(31):11200–7.
15. McDonald AJ. Cortical pathways to the mammalian amygdala. Prog Neurobiol. 1998;55(3):257–332.
16. Green MR, Barnes B, McCormick CM. Social instability stress in adolescence increases anxiety and reduces social interactions in adulthood in male Long-Evans rats. Dev Psychobiol. 2013;55(8):849–59.
17. Razzoli M, Carboni L, Andreoli M, Ballottari A, Arban R. Different susceptibility to social defeat stress of BalbC and C57BL6/J mice. Behav Brain Res. 2011;216(1):100–8.
18. Venzala E, Garcia-Garcia AL, Elizalde N, Tordera RM. Social vs. environmental stress models of depression from a behavioural and neurochemical approach. Eur Neuropsychopharmacol. 2013;23(7):697–708.
19. Beiderbeck DI, Neumann ID, Veenema AH. Differences in intermale aggression are accompanied by opposite vasopressin release patterns within the septum in rats bred for low and high anxiety. Eur J Neurosci. 2007;26(12):3597–605.
20. Filiano AJ, Martens LH, Young AH, Warmus BA, Zhou P, Diaz-Ramirez G, et al. Dissociation of frontotemporal dementia-related deficits and neuroinflammation in progranulin haploinsufficient mice. J Neurosci. 2013;33(12):5352–61.
21. Iniguez SD, Riggs LM, Nieto SJ, Dayrit G, Zamora NN, Shawhan KL, et al. Social defeat stress induces a depression-like phenotype in adolescent male c57BL/6 mice. Stress. 2014;17(3):247–55.
22. Mouri A, Ukai M, Uchida M, Hasegawa S, Taniguchi M, Ito T, et al. Juvenile social defeat stress exposure persistently impairs social behaviors and neurogenesis. Neuropharmacology. 2018;133:23–37.
23. An B, Kim J, Park K, Lee S. Amount of fear extinction changes its underlying mechanisms. Elife. 2017;03:6.
24. Bocchio M, Nabavi S, Capogna M. Synaptic plasticity, engrams, and network oscillations in amygdala circuits for storage and retrieval of emotional memories. Neuron. 2017;94(4):731–43.
25. Moscarello JM, LeDoux JE. Active avoidance learning requires prefrontal suppression of amygdala-mediated defensive reactions. J Neurosci. 2013;33(9):3815–23.
26. Jimenez SA, Maren S. Nuclear disconnection within the amygdala reveals a direct pathway to fear. Learn Mem. 2009;16(12):766–8.
27. Trouche S, Sasaki JM, Tu T, Reijmers LG. Fear extinction causes target-specific remodeling of perisomatic inhibitory synapses. Neuron. 2013;80(4):1054–65.
28. Polepalli JS, Wu H, Goswami D, Halpern CH, Sudhof TC, Malenka RC. Modulation of excitation on parvalbumin interneurons by neuroligin-3 regulates the hippocampal network. Nat Neurosci. 2017;20(2):219–29.
29. McDonald AJ, Betette RL. Parvalbumin-containing neurons in the rat basolateral amygdala: morphology and co-localization of Calbindin-D (28 k). Neuroscience. 2001;102(2):413–25.
30. Lucas EK, Jegarl AM, Morishita H, Clem RL. Multimodal and site-specific plasticity of amygdala parvalbumin interneurons after fear learning. Neuron. 2016;91(3):629–43.

31. Wolff SB, Grundemann J, Tovote P, Krabbe S, Jacobson GA, Muller C, et al. Amygdala interneuron subtypes control fear learning through disinhibition. Nature. 2014;509(7501):453–8.

32. Monfils MH, Cowansage KK, Klann E, LeDoux JE. Extinction-reconsolidation boundaries: key to persistent attenuation of fear memories. Science. 2009;324(5929):951–5.

33. Clem RL, Huganir RL. Calcium-permeable AMPA receptor dynamics mediate fear memory erasure. Science. 2010;330(6007):1108–12.

34. Schiller D, Monfils MH, Raio CM, Johnson DC, Ledoux JE, Phelps EA. Preventing the return of fear in humans using reconsolidation update mechanisms. Nature. 2010;463(7277):49–53.

35. Schiller D, Kanen JW, LeDoux JE, Monfils MH, Phelps EA. Extinction during reconsolidation of threat memory diminishes prefrontal cortex involvement. Proc Natl Acad Sci USA. 2013;110(50):20040–5.

36. Milton AL, Everitt BJ. The psychological and neurochemical mechanisms of drug memory reconsolidation: implications for the treatment of addiction. Eur J Neurosci. 2010;31(12):2308–19.

37. Nader K, Schafe GE, Le Doux JE. Fear memories require protein synthesis in the amygdala for reconsolidation after retrieval. Nature. 2000;406(6797):722–6.

38. Alberini CM. Mechanisms of memory stabilization: are consolidation and reconsolidation similar or distinct processes? Trends Neurosci. 2005;28(1):51–6.

39. Shuai Y, Lu B, Hu Y, Wang L, Sun K, Zhong Y. Forgetting is regulated through Rac activity in Drosophila. Cell. 2010;140(4):579–89.

40. Davis RL, Zhong Y. The biology of forgetting—a perspective. Neuron. 2017;95(3):490–503.

41. Chaudhury D, Walsh JJ, Friedman AK, Juarez B, Ku SM, Koo JW, et al. Rapid regulation of depression-related behaviours by control of midbrain dopamine neurons. Nature. 2013;493(7433):532–6.

42. Accolla EA, Aust S, Merkl A, Schneider GH, Kuhn AA, Bajbouj M, et al. Deep brain stimulation of the posterior gyrus rectus region for treatment resistant depression. J Affect Disord. 2016;194:33–7.

43. Chen DY, Stern SA, Garcia-Osta A, Saunier-Rebori B, Pollonini G, Bambah-Mukku D, et al. A critical role for IGF-II in memory consolidation and enhancement. Nature. 2011;469(7331):491–7.

44. Alberini CM, Milekic MH, Tronel S. Mechanisms of memory stabilization and de-stabilization. Cell Mol Life Sci CMLS. 2006;63(9):999–1008.

45. Taubenfeld SM, Milekic MH, Monti B, Alberini CM. The consolidation of new but not reactivated memory requires hippocampal C/EBPbeta. Nat Neurosci. 2001;4(8):813–8.

Assessing ADHD symptoms in children and adults: evaluating the role of objective measures

Theresa S. Emser[1,2]*, Blair A. Johnston[3], J. Douglas Steele[4], Sandra Kooij[5], Lisa Thorell[6] and Hanna Christiansen[1]

Abstract

Background: Diagnostic guidelines recommend using a variety of methods to assess and diagnose ADHD. Applying subjective measures always incorporates risks such as informant biases or large differences between ratings obtained from diverse sources. Furthermore, it has been demonstrated that ratings and tests seem to assess somewhat different constructs. The use of objective measures might thus yield valuable information for diagnosing ADHD. This study aims at evaluating the role of objective measures when trying to distinguish between individuals with ADHD and controls. Our sample consisted of children (n = 60) and adults (n = 76) diagnosed with ADHD and matched controls who completed self- and observer ratings as well as objective tasks. Diagnosis was primarily based on clinical interviews. A popular pattern recognition approach, support vector machines, was used to predict the diagnosis.

Results: We observed relatively high accuracy of 79% (adults) and 78% (children) applying solely objective measures. Predicting an ADHD diagnosis using both subjective and objective measures exceeded the accuracy of objective measures for both adults (89.5%) and children (86.7%), with the subjective variables proving to be the most relevant.

Conclusions: We argue that objective measures are more robust against rater bias and errors inherent in subjective measures and may be more replicable. Considering the high accuracy of objective measures only, we found in our study, we think that they should be incorporated in diagnostic procedures for assessing ADHD.

Keywords: ADHD, Children/adults, Objective assessment, Classification, Support vector machines

Background

Attention deficit/hyperactivity disorder (ADHD) is characterized by a combination of age-inappropriate levels of inattention, impulsive behavior and hyperactivity. Symptoms must become apparent before the age of 12 years and cause significant impairments in more than one setting, e.g., at school or work, or with family and peers [1]. The diagnostic and statistical manual of mental disorders (DSM V; [1]) distinguishes three subtypes of ADHD, the predominantly inattentive type (IA), the predominantly hyperactive/impulsive type (HI) and the combined type (C). Children of the IA type show more than six out of the nine relevant symptoms specified as inattentive

behavior and less than six out of the nine relevant symptoms specified as hyperactive/impulsive behavior. The predominantly HI type is characterized by more than six HI symptoms and less than six IA symptoms, whereas children of the C type show more than six symptoms in both areas. Although ADHD was long regarded solely as a childhood disorder, it is now agreed that the disorder persists into adulthood (e.g., [2, 3]), and even into old age [4, 5]. Estimations of adulthood ADHD's prevalence rates range from 2.5 to 5% [6–12], slightly smaller than those reported for children and youths that range from 5.0 to 7.1% [13, 14].

Assessment of ADHD using ratings and tests

Most diagnostic guidelines (e.g., [15–17]) require that ADHD be assessed and diagnosed by relying on information provided via a variety of methods (e.g., clinical

---
*Correspondence: Emser_T@ukw.de
[2] Clinic for Child and Adolescent Psychiatry, University Clinic Würzburg, Margarete-Höppel-Platz 1, 97080 Würzburg, Germany
Full list of author information is available at the end of the article

interviews, observations and ratings) and collected from multiple sources (e.g., parents and teachers). However, using subjective measures always incorporates the risk of informant biases [18] and clinicians are often confronted with great inconsistencies between ratings obtained from different sources [19, 20]. Although the discrepancies between different informants can be of clinical relevance [21], the use of objective measures in addition to subjective ratings might yield valuable information facilitating the diagnosis of ADHD. In the present study, we therefore aimed to investigate the role of *objective* measures when trying to distinguish between individuals with ADHD and controls. We also aimed to investigate how objective measures are related to subjective measures by investigating how well we could discriminate between ADHD and controls when using the combination of these two types of measures. The combination of objective and subjective measures may provide additional information than objective measures alone as it has been argued that tests and ratings may capture at least partly different constructs [22, 23] and should not be used interchangeably. Toplak and colleagues [23] argue that one important difference between ratings and tests is that the former measure typical performance (i.e., how an individual normally performs), whereas tests usually capture optimal performance (i.e., how well an individual performs under relatively optimal conditions). Thus, objective measures assess performance free of influences of the different situations. However, this study primarily investigated whether only objective measures would be sufficient to develop a statistical model as the bias and inter-operator error inherent in subjective measures are not well suited to developing a robust and objective classifier. Whilst the value of including subjective measures in a classifier alongside objective measures has been explored, developing an objective statistical method using only subjective data would not be expected to produce a robust classifier that would generalize to corresponding data acquired by other operators.

The relative importance of individual variables towards a diagnosis of ADHD is an issue that has not been empirically examined, at least not in studies employing statistical methods that can handle numerous variables to make an objective prediction. Similarly, few studies focus on objective measurements of ADHD symptom levels rather than constructs (such as executive functioning deficits) that are known to be associated with ADHD.

Objective measures
Test battery of attention
In Germany, where this study was conducted, a frequently used neuropsychological test is the test battery of attention for adolescents and adults (TAP; [24]) or for children aged 6–11 (KiTAP; [25]). The various subtests enable the assessment of aspects of two of the three core symptoms of ADHD, namely inattention and impulsivity. A detailed description of the tasks is provided in the method section. One study using the TAP in a sample of children with ADHD and healthy controls demonstrated that two test measures (reaction time variability of the Go/NoGo task, number of errors of the reaction change task) were needed to classify 90% of the children correctly [26]. Drechsler et al. [27] detected significant group differences between children with and without ADHD in four of the KiTAP's six subtests. Nevertheless, they did not recommend using it for diagnostic purposes due to its weak specificity. Another study on the psychometric properties of the KiTAP reported values for split-half reliability of .55–.96 for children aged 8–12 [25] and .32–.72 for children aged 6–7 years [28]. The psychometric properties of the TAP/KiTAP are thus not fully satisfactory, and norm references are missing for some age groups. An alternative is the Quantified Behavior Test, a neuropsychological test becoming increasingly important in ADHD diagnostics.

The Quantified Behavior Test
The Quantified Behavior Test for children aged 6–12 (QbTest 6–12; [29]) and the Quantified Behavior Test Plus for subjects 12 years and older (Qb+©; [30]) are computerized neuropsychological tests that assess the three core symptoms of ADHD using a continuous performance test (CPT). One great advantage of these tests is that in addition to providing estimates of the participant's performance (e.g., omission and commission errors), they also measure head movements via a motion tracking system. For example, the system generates measures of the time the subject has moved more than 1 cm/s, as well as the distance they traveled during the test or the surface covered through their movements. Reh et al. [31] reported promising results determining the QbTest 6–12's factorial and discriminant validity with a three-factor solution corresponding to the three areas of ADHD impairment. These explained 76% of the total variance and reliability estimates ranging from $\alpha = .60$ (impulsivity) to $\alpha = .95$ (hyperactivity) for these factors. Findings have been less consistent regarding the QbTest 6–12's convergent and discriminant validity. One study exhibited significant differences between children with ADHD, their siblings, and healthy controls, and the authors identified the factor of hyperactivity as a possible "intermediate phenotype" [32]. Hult et al. [33] examined the diagnostic validity of the QbTest 6–12 applying ROC curves in a clinical sample of children diagnosed with ADHD and a clinical control group of individuals with primarily autism spectrum disorder, observing moderate

sensitivity (47–67%) and specificity values (72–84%). In a third study, multi-trait, multi-method analyses comparing self- and observer ratings (Conners 3 rating scales) with objective measures provided support for the convergent validity of the QbTest 6–12 especially for the variables assessing inattention, but discriminant validity was not supported [34]. However, discrimination analyses based on the QbTest 6–12 also achieved 73.8% accuracy in predicting whether a child had an ADHD diagnosis (all subtypes) or not with the variables measuring activity revealing the greatest impact. There are studies of the Qb+$^{©}$, the version used for adolescents and adults, demonstrating high sensitivity (86%) and specificity (83%) when trying to differentiate between subjects with and without ADHD [35, 36]. However, sensitivity dropped substantially when trying to differentiate between individuals with ADHD and other clinical groups such as bipolar II disorder (36%) or borderline personality disorder (41%; [35]). However, in another study, with a large sample of patients that came in for ADHD assessment, we were able to differentiate patients for which an ADHD diagnosis was confirmed (66% of 773 subjects) versus patients that had symptoms of inattention, impulsivity or hyperactivity due to other disorders (34% of 773 subjects). All individuals performed the QbTest, the objective measure also used in this study. Of those individuals predicted not to have an ADHD diagnosis based on the QbTest, 67% actually had no diagnosis; of those individuals predicted to have an ADHD diagnosis, 79% actually had a diagnosis. In the whole sample, the correct classification rate was 76.4%, sensitivity was 90%, and specificity was just 45% [37]. Another study reported satisfactory overall classification rates (87.8% correctly identified ADHD patients), but lower correct prediction rates regarding the area under the curve (AUC) range for sensitivity (36.5–58.5%) and specificity (80–100%; [38]). Hirsch and Christiansen [37] verified the three factorial structure of the Qb+$^{©}$ and provided support for convergent validity using multi-trait, multi-method analyses, but the discriminant validity of this instrument was only partially supported. The measure of impulsivity has been shown to be the least sensitive symptom with regard to discriminating between adults with and without ADHD as well as between patients with ADHD or other psychiatric disorders [35, 36, 39].

Aim of the present study

In summary, there are several studies reporting promising results regarding the ability of the QbTest 6–12 and the Qb+$^{©}$ to differentiate between patients with and without ADHD. Nevertheless, findings are inconsistent, and often suggest using neuropsychological tests only as an additional resource within a comprehensive assessment strategy incorporating a variety of methods [27]. In the clinical community there is a high controversy about the usefulness of objective measures for diagnostic purposes as problems regarding sensitivity, specificity and ecological validity have been reported [40]. In light of the evidence that ratings and tests seem to assess partly different constructs, objective and subjective measures could be seen as complementing each other. The diagnostic value of objective tests becomes all the more important when the potential risks of subjective measures are taken into account, informant bias being the most important thereof. There is lack of studies evaluating the differential contributions of objective and subjective measures for correctly classifying ADHD. Whilst the study investigates the relative contribution of subjective measures in a classifier, the diagnostic accuracy using objective measurements only is considered more generalisable due to the inherent inter-operator variability in subjective measures. In contrast to most previous studies using neuropsychological measures and ratings to differentiate between patients with ADHD and healthy controls, we used machine learning rather than discriminant function analysis or logistic regression analysis. The advantage of the former is that it is data-driven and less sensitive to outliers [41]. Furthermore, it is a multivariate approach, as it does not rely on summary scores, but considers every single item. The risk of losing information is therefore reduced [41]. More specifically, the present study used support vector machine (SVM). This machine-learning approach is known to be very robust and capable of translating well in studies using imaging data [42]. However, it has been predominantly implemented in studies using neuroimaging data to diagnostically classify clinical populations [43, 44] and not in studies using standard clinical assessments as recommended by the various ADHD diagnostic guidelines outlined above.

The first aim of this study was thus to investigate the accuracy of employing only variables from the objective measures to reveal their specific potential contribution free from the potential confound of subjective measures. We further aimed to investigate how objective measures are related to subjective measures by investigating how well we could discriminate between ADHD and controls when using the combination of these two types of measures. In contrast to previous research, we used a machine-learning technique (SVM) to analyze the data.

Methods
Participants and procedure

Thirty children with ADHD and thirty controls matched at group level according to age and gender were enrolled in the childhood ADHD prediction. Thirty-eight adults with ADHD and thirty-eight age and gender-matched controls were enrolled in the adulthood ADHD prediction resulting in a total sample of N = 136. All children and adults with ADHD were recruited through an ADHD outpatient clinic within the university. Control children were recruited through local schools and children who participated in the study were given a movie voucher. Control adults were recruited at the university and via advertisements; they also received movie vouchers for study participation. No established or suspected ADHD diagnosis, or family history of ADHD were allowed for the individuals in the control groups.

Clinically-referred children were included in the study if they met the DSM-IV [45] criteria for ADHD (either combined, predominantly inattentive or predominantly hyperactive/impulsive subtype) and had an IQ-score ≥ 80 (short version of the Wechsler Intelligence Scale for Children IV [46]: block-design, similarities, digit span, information and picture arrangement; [47]). The exclusion criteria were symptoms of inattention, hyperactivity or impulsivity due to other medical conditions such as hyperthyroidism, autism, epilepsy, brain disorders and any genetic or medical disorder associated with externalizing behavior. Comorbid disorders like oppositional defiance disorder (ODD) or conduct disorder (CD) did not constitute an exclusion criterion as they are prevalent in about 30–50% of the population [48]. Other comorbid disorders (e.g. learning disorders, anxiety or depression) also did not result in exclusion as long as ADHD was the primary diagnosis. Participants were allowed to take medication but were asked to stop taking it 2 days before the objective tests were applied. Similar inclusion and exclusion criteria applied to adults with the exception that IQ was not assessed. Adult patients were recruited from a specialized outpatient clinic whose standard diagnostic procedure does not include extensive testing of cognitive abilities. Instead, achieved schooling and current job position are gathered. According to that, none of the patients were estimated to score below IQ of 80 as all of them have at least completed middle school. ADHD diagnoses were based on a DSM-IV-oriented clinical interview conducted by an experienced clinician, as this is known to be a highly reliable method for making an ADHD diagnosis [49–51]. For the children, we conducted the Schedule for Affective Disorders and Schizophrenia for School-Age Children-Present and Lifetime Version interview (K-SADS-PL; [52]) with a parent. Its inter-rater reliability ranges from .93 to 1.0 [53]. The adult patients completed the Wender Reimherr Interview (WRI; [54]), which has inter-rater reliability ranging from .45–.95 [55]. Rating scales were completed at home and the objective tests were instructed by clinicians or research assistants.

In the child sample, the male-to-female ratio was 21/9 (ADHD) and 19/11 (controls). The ADHD group's mean age was 8.9 years (SD = 1.4, range 7.0–11.0 years) and the controls' 8.7 years (SD = 1.2, range 6.9–10.8 years). A percentage of 26.7 of the children diagnosed with ADHD were predominantly inattentive, 3.3% were predominantly hyperactive-impulsive and 60% fulfilled the diagnostic criteria for the combined subtype. Unfortunately, for 10% of the children the subtype information was not available. The adult ADHD group's mean age was 35.1 years (SD = 11.7, range 19–63 years); and the controls' 32.2 years (SD = 9.6, range 21–56 years). Both adult groups had a male-to-female ratio of 25/13. A percentage of 10.5 of the adults diagnosed with ADHD were predominantly inattentive, 2.6% were predominantly hyperactive-impulsive and 81.6% fulfilled the diagnostic criteria for the combined subtype. Unfortunately, for 5.3% of the adults the subtype information was not available.

Children with ADHD had a significantly lower IQ than the controls (t (58) = −4.49, p < .001), a factor known to be typical of this population (e.g., [56, 57]). In their twin-study, Kuntsi et al. [58] found that the association between ADHD and lower IQ is based predominantly on genetic influences rather than environmental effects. Controlling for IQ would therefore not have affected the composition of our ADHD-population. We thus decided against controlling for IQ as a possible confound because that can bias classification results. The high mean IQ of our ADHD (M = 113.1; SD = 11.6) and control groups (M = 125.8; SD = 10.8) is most likely due to the high percentage of children from academic families in a small university town (80.000 inhabitants of which 27.000 are students and ~ 10.000 academics working at the university with a further ~ 10.000 working in related academic institutions). Considering IQ's high rate of heritability (one that even rises with age [59]) and the additional role of the socio-economic status of those with a high IQ in particular [60], our sample's IQ values are not that surprising. For details on demographics, please see Table 1. Furthermore, Table 3 shows correlations between IQ and the subjective and objective variables.

Measures

The standard diagnostic procedure for ADHD at the outpatient clinic from which our participants were recruited incorporates a variety of measures like clinical interviews, self- and observer ratings and neuropsychological tests. Instruments used for our SVM analyses are described in greater detail below.

Table 1 Demographic characteristics of the sample

	Adults		Children	
	ADHD	Controls	ADHD	Controls
n	38	38	30	30
Mean age (SD)	35.1 (11.7)	32.2 (9.6)	8.9 (1.4)	8.7 (1.2)
Gender				
Male (%)	25 (65.8)	29 (65.8)	21 (70)	19 (63.3)
Female (%)	13 (34.2)	16 (34.2)	9 (30)	11 (36.7)
Mean IQ (SD)	N/A	N/A	113.1 (11.6)	125.8 (10.8)

SD standard deviation, *N/A* not available

Conners ADHD rating scales self- and observer rating long version (CAARS-L: S/O)

The CAARS-L: S [61] is a self-rating instrument that assesses ADHD symptoms in adults aged 18 years and above. The long version consists of 66 items rated on a 4-point Likert-type scale ranging from 0 (*not at all/ never*) to 3 (*very much/very frequently*). Factor analyses for the original and the German version have supported a four-factor structure consisting of inattention/memory problems, hyperactivity/restlessness, impulsivity/ emotional lability, and problems with self-concept [62, 63]. The internal consistency of each of these subscales ranges between .82 and .85, and all four subscales reveal high sensitivity and specificity [63]. The CAARS-L: S thus represents a reliable and cross-culturally valid measure of current ADHD symptoms in adults [64]. The observer version CAARS-L: O also assesses ADHD symptoms using the same items and rating scale as the CAARS-L: S, but symptoms are rated by someone who has a close relationship with the subject under examination [65]. Observer ratings were performed by a person with a close relationship to the participant. In most cases, their partner or spouse was selected but it was sometimes a parent or close friend. This version's factorial validity has been confirmed and its psychometric properties proved to be satisfactory. In our study the internal consistency of the CAARS-L: S/O ranged from $\alpha = .90/.89$ to $\alpha = .95/.94$.

Conners-3 parent/teacher ratings

The Conners-3 parent/teacher ratings [66] are two questionnaires assessing ADHD symptoms and associated problems like oppositional behavior or learning problems in children and adolescents aged 6–18 years. The long version contains 105/111 items (parent/teacher) rated on a 4-point Likert-scale from 0 (*not at all/never*) to 3 (*very much/very frequently*). The Conners 3 incorporates the following ten scales:

inattention, hyperactivity/impulsivity, learning problems, executive functions, aggression, peer relations (content scales); DSM IV-inattention, DSM IV-hyperactivity/impulsivity, DSM IV-conduct disorder, DSM IV-oppositional defiant disorder (symptom scales); ADHD index, Global index. The German version has revealed good to very good internal consistency (Cronbach's $\alpha = .74–.96$). Also, confirmatory factor analyses of the Conners 3 German version confirmed the factor structure for the content scales in the original American version [67]. In our sample we found a Cronbach's alpha of .85 for the content scales and $\alpha = .79$ for the symptom scales of the Conners 3 parent rating scale.

Quantified Behavior Test for adolescents and adults (Qb+©)

The Qb+© [30] is a continuous performance task (CPT) measuring sustained attention combined with a simultaneous high resolution motion tracking system that takes 20 min to complete. Presented stimuli are a blue circle, a blue square, a red circle, and a red square. A response key is to be pressed when two identical stimuli are shown in succession. The target/non-target ratio is 25/75. During performance, the participant's head movements are recorded with an infrared camera tracking a reflective marker attached to the headband the participant is wearing. One thus obtains data from a total of nine parameters that measure each of the three core ADHD symptoms. Activity is measured by five parameters: time active (i.e., time the subject has moved more than 1 cm/s in percentage of the task's entire duration), Distance (i.e., distance traveled by the reflective headband marker in m), area (i.e., surface covered by the headband reflector during the test in cm^2), microevents (i.e., small movements exceeding 1 mm), and motion simplicity (i.e., complexity of the motion pattern in %). Inattention is measured by the following parameters: reaction time (RT), RT variability (i.e., standard deviation of RT in ms), and omission errors. The third ADHD domain, impulsivity, is assessed by commission errors. Psychometric properties of the Qb+© are described in the introduction.

Quantified Behavior Test for children aged 6–12 (QbTest)

Similar to the Qb+©, the QbTest [29] consists of a standard CPT and a parallel registration of the participants' movements with an infrared camera following a reflective marker attached to a headband. Stimuli are either a gray circle (target) or a gray circle with a cross (non-target) in random order of appearance. These are presented for 100 ms at an inter-stimuli-interval of 1900 ms. The target/non-target ratio is 50/50. The task is to press a button as quickly as possible when the target appears. The same parameters measuring the three core ADHD symptoms in the Qb+© are also included in the childhood version (see descriptions above). In addition to these nine parameters, inattention also includes normalized variability in reaction time (i.e., RTVar divided by RT) and the impulsivity factor contains anticipatory reactions (i.e., reactions < 150 ms are considered coincidental). The QbTest's psychometric properties are described in the introduction.

Test battery of attention for adolescents and adults and for children aged 6–11 (TAP/KiTAP)

The TAP's [24] and KiTAP's [25] three subtests below were used for our assessment of both age groups: Go/NoGo, divided attention and sustained attention. The Go/NoGo task assesses selective attention and in it, participants are instructed to press a button ("go") when a target stimulus appears. For example, in the TAP an "×" and a "+" are presented and participants have to press the button when the "×" appears, but not when the "+" appears. In the divided-attention subtest, a visual and auditory task have to be processed simultaneously. In the sustained attention task, one has to be attentive for a period of about 15 min. The KiTAP's tasks are embedded in a story about a haunted castle. In the divided-attention task, children look at an owl that shuts its eyes from time to time while they hear a low or high sound. Their task is to press the button either when the owl shuts its eyes or when they hear the same sound twice in a row. In the sustained-attention task on the other hand, ghosts in different colors are presented and children have to press a button if the same-colored ghost appears twice in a row. Psychometric properties are described in the introduction.

Analyses

Analyses apply feature selection to identify those variables most relevant to the diagnosis, and we took a popular pattern recognition approach (SVM) to make the diagnosis prediction. To ensure each prediction was made based on data that was novel to the classifier, as would occur in routine clinical practice, we used cross-validation. Due to the differences in measures for childhood and adulthood ADHD diagnoses, we carried out two separate but identical analyses for each age group.

Variable preparation

As the first step, the variables were standardized to reduce errors due to scaling. This involved subtracting the mean value of each variable and dividing by the standard deviation. Standardization aims to ensure that the automated selection of variables is based on their predictive value, rather than on their relative variability or magnitude.

Individual scan classification

All analyses were performed in Matlab 2012a (The Mathworks Inc.) and Matlab-based calculations used the SVM toolbox [68] and custom Matlab scripts. To investigate which variables predicted ADHD diagnosis, we applied a linear support vector machine (SVM; [69, 70]) pattern-recognition method to each dataset, with standard leave-one-out cross validation (LOOCV). The advantages and technical details of SVM and pattern-recognition approaches in general are described in more detail elsewhere [43, 71]. Put simply, one subject is removed from the data set and the aim is to identify the set of variables that best separate the N-1 subjects into patients and controls. The optimal set of variables is then used to predict whether the subject that was removed belongs to the patient or control group. This process is repeated until all subjects have been classified.

To identify which variables are most important to the prediction we employed feature selection. This technique involves ranking the variables from largest to smallest absolute differences between groups within each training set (excluding the subject left out to ensure it is novel to the classifier). Potential thresholds were explored over a wide range, whereby all variables with differences between the groups above the threshold are included in the classification. The threshold that yielded the highest training stage accuracy (the accuracy obtained during the second [inner] LOOCV procedure—which does not include the novel data) was used in the final prediction. This approach has been described in greater detail elsewhere [72]. Notably, as feature selection took place for each training set (each combination of N-1 subjects), a different combination of variables can be selected for each subject's prediction. This approach optimized the number of variables required to classify the data. We calculated the classification accuracy, sensitivity, and specificity at each stage. In addition to the approach including all variables, we investigated the feasibility of predicting applying the objective QbTest and TAP scores only (versions for both children and adults) to see whether they could independently predict diagnosis without relying on the subjective Conners' scores.

Results

Our child datasets included age, gender, Conners-3 parent/teacher ratings, QbTest 6–12 and the KiTAP scores; the adult datasets age, gender, CAARS-L: S/O, QbTest+© and TAP. IQ and medication history were not included in the prediction for reasons as outlined above. Tables 2 and 3 show correlations between age, IQ (child sample), the symptom scales of the subjective measures and objective variables.

Table 2 Correlations between age, the symptom scales of the CAARS: S/O, variables of the TAP and the Qb+© factors for the adult sample

	1	2	3	4	5	6	7	8	9	10	11	12	13	14	15	16	17	18	19	20
1 age	–																			
2 CAARS: S DSM IA	.04	–																		
3 CAARS: S DSM HY/Imp	.16	.03	–																	
4 CAARS: S DSM ADHD	.16	.50**	.88**	–																
5 CAARS: O DSM IA	−.02	.41**	.10	.29*	–															
6 CAARS: O DSM HY/Imp	.16	.02	.53**	.47**	−.00	–														
7 CAARS: O DSM ADHD	.16	.12	.54**	.52**	.24*	.97**	–													
8 TAP1 reaction time	.22	.21	.14	.22	.17	−.06	−.05	–												
9 TAP1 RT SD	−.08	.15	.09	.15	.33**	−.13	−.05	.43**	–											
10 TAP1 errors	−.21	.05	−.04	−.02	.18	.15	.19	−.28*	.13	–										
11 TAP1 omission errors	−.19	.09	.12	.15	.24*	.10	.15	.14	.43**	.12	–									
12 TAP2 errors	−.08	−.13	.04	−.03	.14	.06	.09	.15	.36**	.21	−.01	–								
13 TAP2 omission errors	.09	.25*	.14	.24*	.34**	.07	.15	.25*	.19	.11	.25*	.10	–							
14 TAP3 reaction time	.33**	.10	.02	.06	.18	.03	.07	.55**	.25*	−.03	.06	.10	.17	–						
15 TAP3 RT SD	.09	.03	−.01	.01	.13	.03.	.06	.11	.34**	.03	.15	.05	.12	.43**	–					
16 TAP3 errors	−.03	−.02	.19	.16	.13	−.03	.01	.00	.13	.18	.27*	.22	.09	−.15	.05	–				
17 TAP3 omission errors	.10	.29*	.18	.30**	.48**	.06	.18	.20	.28*	.12	.35**	.11	.39**	.41**	.33**	.26*	–			
18 Qb activity	−.02	.20	.18	.25*	.38**	−.07	.02	.26*	.29*	.06	.21	.17	.10	.33**	.16	.15	.43**	–		
19 Qb impulsivity	.13	.12	.01	.07	.26*	.15	.21	−.09	.13	.36**	.39**	.22	.38**	−.06	.15	.51**	.37**	.05	–	
20 Qb inattention	.26*	.14	.11	.17	.32**	.07	.15	.50**	.29*	.19	.11	.29*	.20	.65**	.39**	.11	.53**	.45**	.13	–

CAARS: S CAARS self rating, *CAARS: O* CAARS observer rating, *IA* inattention, *HY/Imp* hyperactivity/impulsivity, *TAP1* Go/Nogo task of the test battery of attention, *TAP2* selective attention task, *TAP3* sustained attention task, *RT* reaction time in ms, *SD* standard deviation

* p < .05 level (two-tailed) ** p < .01 level (two-tailed)

Table 3 Correlations between age, IQ, the symptom scales of the Conners-3 parent ratings, variables of the KiTAP and the QbTest factors for the child sample

	1	2	3	4	5	6	7	8	9	10	11	12	13	14	15	16	17	18	19	20
1 age	–																			
2 IQ	.01	–																		
3 CP DSM inattention	–.15	–.41**	–																	
4 CP DSM HY/Imp	–.31*	–.18	.70**	–																
5 CP ADHD index	–.27*	–.38*	.89**	.82**	–															
6 KiTAP1 RT	–.21	–.10	.19	.21	.22	–														
7 KiTAP1 RT SD	–.02	–.23	.04	.09	.13	.44**	–													
8 KiTAP1 errors	–.11	–.01	–.21	–.21	–.20	–.40**	.04	–												
9 KiTAP1 omission errors	–.02	.11	–.14	–.04	–.17	.01	.12	.14	–											
10 KiTAP2 RT	–.29*	–.15	.24	.22	.25	.53**	.23	–.01	–.11	–										
11 KiTAP2 RT SD	–.11	–.09	–.07	–.12	–.02	–.03	.20	.20	–.06	.14	–									
12 KiTAP2 errors	–.16	–.25	–.04	–.06	–.07	–.09	.25	.26*	–.05	.09	.32*	–								
13 KiTAP2 omission errors	–.18	–.18	.13	.04	.15	.02	.15	–.01	–.05	.07	.39**	.54**	–							
14 KiTAP3 RT	–.33*	–.10	–.09	.03	.05	.58**	.32*	–.11	.03	.50**	.06	.09	.17	–						
15 KiTAP3 RT SD	–.15	–.27*	.05	.04	.10	.35**	.32*	–.17	.04	.26*	.10	.17	.14	.44**	–					
16 KiTAP3 errors	–.00	–.11	.23	.18	.22	–.01	.21	.30*	–.04	–.09	.01	.13	.06	–.01	.30*	–				
17 KiTAP3 omission errors	–.26*	–.26*	.19	.20	.35**	.21	.51**	.15	.03	.23	.27*	.30*	.37**	.36**	.44**	.26*	–			
18 Qb activity	.03	–.33*	–.02	.05	.01	.00	.04	.05	.11	.03	–.12	.06	.12	.20	.14	.23	–.04	–		
19 Qb impulsivity	.01	–.30*	.15	.08	.21	–.26*	.11	.37**	–.09	–.10	.36**	.18	.10	–.20	–.00	.47**	.01	.18	–	
20 Qb inattention	.27*	–.35**	.13	–.03	.12	.17	.23	–.02	.14	.25	.13	–.05	.19	.31*	.27*	.25*	.23	.41**	.22	–

CP Conners' parents scale, *HY/Imp* hyperactivity/impulsivity, *KiTAP1* Go/Nogo task of the test battery of attention for children, *KiTAP2* selective attention task, *KiTAP3* sustained attention task, *RT* reaction time in ms, *SD* standard deviation

* p < .05 level (two-tailed) ** p < .01 level (two-tailed)

As expected, we found significant negative correlations between IQ, the Conners' symptom scale for inattention and the ADHD index as well as the Qb factors. Furthermore, there were significant positive correlations between corresponding variables of the different TAP/KiTAP tasks. Regarding the adult sample, the Qb factor for impulsivity correlated significantly positive with the number of errors of most of the TAP tasks, indicating that patients who produced a lot of errors in the TAP also scored high on the impulsivity factor of the Qb+©. Additionally, the Qb factor inattention correlated significantly positive with the inattention symptom scale of the CAARS observer scale as well as with the TAP variables reaction time and reaction time variance (RT SD). Finally, there were significant correlations between the number of omission errors in the TAP tasks and the ADHD and inattention symptom scales of the CAARS. Regarding the child sample, we also found positive correlations between the Qb impulsivity factor and the number of errors in the KiTAP tasks Go/Nogo and sustained attention. Furthermore, there were positive correlations between the Qb inattention factor and the reaction time and reaction time variance of the sustained attention task. In general, there were only few significant correlations between the subjective and the objective variables, a fact already shown in previous studies [31, 37].

Prediction of ADHD diagnosis in adults

Using a linear SVM and feature selection on the adult dataset, we were able to predict an ADHD diagnosis with 89.5% accuracy (sensitivity = .90, specificity = .90, $\chi^2 = 44.26$, p < .0001). The majority of the variables relevant to the classification were selected from the CAARS scores. Many of the scores from the self-ratings were especially predictive, with each of the 51 variables selected in 36.20% of the predictions on average. Similarly, the observer-rated scores contained many predictive variables, with each variable selected in 20% of the cross-validated classifiers on average. This was expected, as symptom severity scores are likely to readily distinguish patients from controls.

We did not find the test battery of attention scores to be particularly predictive of ADHD diagnosis. Of the 28 variables included in the calculation, each variable was selected in 2.96% of the predictions on average. The 16 QbTest+© variables entered into the classifier were selected in 8.96% of the predictions on average.

The variables selected in all of the predictions were questions from the self- and observer-rated CAARS. From the self-ratings, we found the following items to be relevant to all predictions: *"I have trouble keeping my attention focused when working"*, *"I feel restless inside even if I am sitting still"*, *"Things I hear or see distract me*

from what I'm doing", and *"I am restless or overactive".* Similarly, three items from the observer-rated questionnaire were used in all predictions: *"is easily frustrated"*, *"is distracted by sights or sounds when trying to concentrate"*, and *"can't keep his/her mind on something unless it's really interesting".*

In addition, although not used in all the predictions, a number of self-rated CAARS items were selected in over 75% of predictions: *"Many things set me off easily"*, *"My moods are unpredictable"*, *"Sometimes my attention narrows so much that I'm oblivious to everything else; other times it's so broad that everything distracts me"*, *"I can't keep my mind on something unless it's really interesting"*, *"I am distracted when things are going on around me".*

When including only objective measures (the output from the QbTest+© and TAP tasks), we predicted an ADHD diagnosis with 79% accuracy (sensitivity = .82, specificity = .76, $\chi^2 = 23.28$, p < .0001). The following variables were used in over 85% of predictions: overall omission errors made at the subtest sustained attention in the TAP; QbTest+©: omission errors, error rate, normalized reaction time variance, normalized reaction time variance without outliers, and the ability of the patient to distinguish between target and non-target.

Prediction of ADHD diagnosis in children

By applying the same technique used to predict diagnosis in the adult population to 30 children with ADHD and 30 controls, we were able to predict diagnosis with 86.7% accuracy (sensitivity = .83, specificity = .90, $\chi^2 = 29.53$, p < .0001). As in the adult study, the Conners' scores proved to be the most predictive of an ADHD diagnosis. Only 12 parent-rated scores were entered into the classification procedure, and those variables were selected in 36.53% of the predictions on average. The Conners' parent subscores relating to executive function, inattention DSM-IV ratings and the ADHD index were selected in all predictions, and the general inattention score was selected in 75% of the predictions. None of the variables taken from the KiTAP were selected in any of the predictions, while the 15 QbTest 6–12 variables entered into the classifier were selected in only 1.11% of the predictions on average.

When using only the output from the QbTest 6–12 and KiTAP tasks, it was possible to predict an ADHD diagnosis with 78% accuracy (sensitivity = .80, specificity = .77, $\chi^2 = 17.09$, p < .0001). The following variables were used in over 98% of predictions: KiTAP: sustained attention—number of omission errors, GoNogo—median of reaction time and number of errors; QbTest 6–12: distance participant moved during testing, area covered by the patient during testing, micro movements exceeding 1 mm, complexity of movement-pattern, multiple pressing of the

Table 4 Prediction results

	Adult prediction		Child prediction	
	All variables	Objective variables	All variables	Objective variables
Accuracy (%)	89.5	79.0	86.7	78.0
Sensitivity	.90	.82	.83	.80
Specificity	.90	.76	.90	.77

test button, reaction time variance without outliers, normalized reaction time variance without outliers, anticipatory, reactions < 150 ms that are considered accidental. All prediction results are summarized in Table 4.

Discussion

In this study we aimed to determine the accuracy with which objective and subjective measures can predict the diagnosis in individuals with and without ADHD. Based on the fact that questionnaire data suffer from rater bias and that diverse methods seem to assess partly different constructs, we wanted to examine both the combined effect of subjective and objective measures as well as the unique effects of the objective measures obtained from the QbTest 6–12, Qb+©, KiTAP or TAP.

ADHD assessment in adults

Our results demonstrate that using both subjective and objective measures in adults, it was possible to predict an ADHD diagnosis with an accuracy of 89.5%, with self-rated scores being the most predictive ones (selected in an average of 36.20% predictions) followed by the observer-rated scores (selected on average in 20%). Variables of both the Qb+© and TAP were less relevant to predicting an ADHD diagnosis than were the self- and observer-ratings. Nevertheless, prediction was still possible using only these objective measures with an accuracy of 79%.

Regarding the TAP, the variable omission errors from the subtest "sustained attention" was selected in more than 85% of the predictions; the same accounts for the Qb+© variables omission errors, error rate, reaction time variance, and the participant's ability to distinguish between target and non-target. This finding is in line with previous findings, as a review of 33 studies on the neuropsychology of adults with ADHD identified omission errors and reaction time variance as variables well able to discriminate between adults with ADHD and controls [73]. This is further supported by our analysis that revealed some significant correlations between the number of omission errors in the TAP, the overall ADHD and inattention symptom scales of the CAARS. These two variables are generally considered to be indicative

of inattention, which has been supported in previous factor analyses [38]. Our findings thus reveal those variables indicative of inattention as the most predictive ones for diagnosing ADHD in adults. This is in line with research suggesting that inattention is the ADHD symptom domain most likely to persist through lifetime, while hyperactivity and impulsivity seem to decline to a greater extent [74]. It is unlikely that these results are due to our sample having a higher proportion of the inattentive subtype as those were only 10.5%, but 81.6% of the participants had the combined subtype. Furthermore, our findings demonstrate high accuracy rates when the prediction was based on objective measures only, thus supporting their diagnostic value independently of subjective measures, removing a significant source of variability and thus increase the likelihood that the classification accuracy obtained would be able to be independently replicated. This is important, as in clinical practice we do not just want to know whether patients are inattentive in daily life (due to several potential reasons besides a primary attention deficit), but also whether they are inattentive in structured situations such as when completing a neuropsychological task. Thus, as emphasized by Toplak et al. [23], ratings and tests capture at least partly different constructs and should therefore be seen as complementing one another. This is further supported by our findings that showed rather low and non-significant correlations between subjective and objective measures. Furthermore, an objective assessment of a patient's impairment might be especially relevant in cases where observer-ratings are unavailable [75], when self-ratings might be questionable due to the potential faking of results (e.g., [76, 77]), or when answers are considered biased [18]. Recent studies have provided additional support for the value of objective assessments. For example, Hirsch and Christiansen [78] showed that inattention as measured with the Qb+© was indicative of overall impairment, adding key supplemental information. Another study demonstrated that the Qb+© is sensitive to medication effects, showing an improvement in 54% of patients who reported no changes in the subjective measure [79].

ADHD assessment in children

We were able to predict an ADHD diagnosis in children based on all of the variables with 86.7% accuracy. Here, no self-ratings were used, but the sub-scores "executive functioning", "DSM IV inattention" and the "ADHD index" of the parent-ratings were selected in all predictions demonstrating their diagnostic value. The prediction using the objective measures did not produce as accurate a classifier as the combined objective and subjective measures in our child sample. However, predicting an ADHD diagnosis using only the objective measures was still significant with 78% accuracy.

Similar to the adult sample, the variable omission errors of the subtest "sustained attention" of the KiTAP was selected in more than 98% of the predictions, as was the median of the reaction time and number of errors in the "Go/NoGo" subtest. This is in line with previous research showing that children with ADHD commit both more omission errors and commission errors than healthy controls [80–82]. Looking at the QbTest 6–12, the most important variables for the prediction differ from those of the adult sample, as the variables assessing hyperactivity were predominantly selected, namely the distance moved and the area covered by the participant, micro-movements, complexity of movement patterns, as well as multiple pressing of the button, reaction time variance, and reaction times < 150 ms. This reflects the findings on the development of ADHD symptoms from childhood to adulthood, demonstrating that hyperactivity is more observable in children than in adults [14, 83, 84]. Adults, in contrast, report more feelings of restlessness or being driven by an internal motor than overtly exhibiting hyperactive behavior. Furthermore, it is interesting that for the QbTest, the variables assessing hyperactivity were most often selected for the prediction, whereas for the Conners-3 parent ratings the subscore assessing inattention seemed to be more important. Hyperactive behavior thus appears to be evaluated better applying objective measures rather than subjective reports. A likely reason for this finding is that the QbTest can capture tiny movements that the patient alone might not even notice. Including objective measures thus resulted in high accuracy for the children. Regarding hyperactivity, the objective measures even outperformed the ratings. These findings support the inclusion of objective measures in ADHD diagnostics.

We found significant negative correlations between IQ, the Conners' symptoms scale of inattention and the ADHD index, two of the KiTAP variables indicative for inattention (reaction time variance and omission errors) and the Qb factors. This is not surprising as the children with ADHD had lower IQ, which is known to be typical for this population [56, 57]. The fact that we found these correlations not only for the objective measures but also for some of the subjective variables underlines that the performance in the objective tasks was not only due to the lower IQ, but also influenced by the deficits these children present.

Limitations and future research

According to the DSM-criteria [1] for ADHD, impairment should be established in multiple settings. It would therefore have been valuable to also include teacher ratings in the present study. Unfortunately, there was too much missing data for the teacher ratings to be absorbed in our analyses. This is a problem we confront constantly during our daily diagnostic routine. Here, objective measures are given additional weight, as they have the potential to add valuable information not otherwise obtainable.

Another limitation of our study is the relatively small number of participants in each group (adults ADHD/controls: 38; children ADHD/controls: 30). As we aimed to be able to make reliable claims regarding the diagnostic accuracy of the instruments assessed, we focused on having gender- and age-matched groups. This resulted in relatively small group sizes, but the total number of participants ($N = 136$) can be regarded as satisfactory.

Future research should preferably include a clinical control sample, as it is highly relevant for clinicians to be able to distinguish between patients with ADHD and those exhibiting similar symptoms due to another underlying disorder (e.g., inattention is also common in patients with depression).

Conclusions

In conclusion, we took a sophisticated statistical approach in this study to examine the diagnostic contributions of various measures assessing ADHD and to assess their classification accuracy. The present findings are highly relevant for clinicians, and can help to improve the workup for diagnosing ADHD. Our investigation's findings demonstrate that when using both subjective and objective measures, an ADHD diagnosis can be accurately predicted with high sensitivity (adults: .90, children and adolescents: .83) and specificity (adults: .90, children and adolescents: .90). Whilst the combination of objective and subjective measures produced more accurate results than the classification based on objective measures only, the latter was still highly satisfactory and removes a potential source of error. The core symptom of hyperactivity is captured especially well in children via objective measures. Considering the evidence that ratings and tests seem to assess at least partly different constructs [23], objective measures always add unique information. Considering that our study revealed only objective measures to be highly accurate, the fact that subjective measures are always influenced by rater bias, and that teachers' appraisals are not made routinely available to clinicians, we recommend that objective measures be included in ADHD diagnostics not only to supplement ratings, but as an integral element thereof.

Authors' contributions
TE was a major contributor in writing the manuscript; provided the data; discussed the results. BJ was a major contributor in writing the manuscript; analyzed the data and provided the results. DS gave valuable input regarding the analyses. SK provided expertise in adult ADHD and was a contributor in writing. LT provided expertise regarding assessment of ADHD and was a

contributor in writing the manuscript. HC provided expertise in the theoretical background and was a contributor in writing the manuscript. All authors read and approved the final manuscript.

Author details
[1] Clinical Child and Adolescent Psychology, Department of Psychology, Philipps University Marburg, Gutenbergstr. 18, 35037 Marburg, Germany. [2] Clinic for Child and Adolescent Psychiatry, University Clinic Würzburg, Margarete-Höppel-Platz 1, 97080 Würzburg, Germany. [3] Division of Neuroscience, Medical Research Institute, Ninewells Hospital and Medical School, University of Dundee, Dundee DD1 9SY, UK. [4] School of Medicine (Neuroscience), University of Dundee, Dundee DD1 9SY, UK. [5] PsyQ, Psycho-medical Programs, Expertise Center Adult ADHD, Jan van Nassaustraat 125, 2596 BS The Hague, The Netherlands. [6] Department of Clinical Neuroscience, Karolinska Institutet, Tomtebodavägen 18A, 5th floor, 171 77 Stockholm, Sweden.

Acknowledgements
Not applicable.

Competing interests
The authors declare that they have no competing interests.

Funding
Not applicable.

References
1. APA. Diagnostic and statistical manual of mental disorders-fifth edition (DSM-5). Arlington: American Psychiatric Publishing, Inc.; 2013.
2. Fischer M, Barkley RA. The persistence of ADHD into adulthood: (once again) it depends on whom you ask. ADHD Rep. 2007;15:7–16.
3. Steinhausen HC, Drechsler R, Foldenyi M, Imhof K, Brandeis D. Clinical course of attention-deficit/hyperactivity disorder from childhood toward early adolescence. J Am Acad Child Adolesc Psychiatry. 2003;42:1085–92.
4. Michielsen M, Semeijn E, Comijs HC, van de Ven P, Beekman AT, Deeg DJ, et al. Prevalence of attention-deficit hyperactivity disorder in older adults in The Netherlands. Br J Psychiatry. 2012;201:298–305.
5. Thorell LB, Holst Y, Christiansen H, Kooij JJS, Bijlenga D, Sjöwall D. Neuropsychological deficits in adults age 60 and above with attention deficit hyperactivity disorder. Eur Psychiatry. 2017. https://doi.org/10.1016/j.eurpsy.2017.06.005.
6. Bell AS. A critical review of ADHD diagnostic criteria: what to address in the DSM-V. J Atten Disord. 2011;15:3–10.
7. Davidson MA. ADHD in adults: a review of the literature. J Atten Disord. 2008;11:628–41.
8. de Zwaan M, Gruss B, Muller A, Graap H, Martin A, Glaesmer H, et al. The estimated prevalence and correlates of adult ADHD in a German community sample. Eur Arch Psychiatry Clin Neurosci. 2012;262:79–86.
9. Kessler RC, Adler L, Ames M, Barkley RA, Birnbaum H, Greenberg P, et al. The prevalence and effects of adult attention deficit/hyperactivity disorder on work performance in a nationally representative sample of workers. J Occup Environ Med. 2005;47:565–72.
10. Kessler RC, Adler L, Barkley R, Biederman J, Conners CK, Demler O, et al. The prevalence and correlates of adult ADHD in the United States: results from the National Comorbidity Survey Replication. Am J Psychiatry. 2006;163:716–23.
11. Polanczyk GV, Willcutt EG, Salum GA, Kieling C, Rohde LA. ADHD prevalence estimates across three decades: an updated systematic review and meta-regression analysis. Int J Epidemiol. 2014;43:434–42.
12. Simon V, Czobor P, Balint S, Meszaros A, Bitter I. Prevalence and correlates of adult attention-deficit hyperactivity disorder: meta-analysis. Br J Psychiatry. 2009;194:204–11.
13. Polanczyk G, de Lima MS, Horta BL, Biederman J, Rohde LA. The worldwide prevalence of ADHD: a systematic review and metaregression analysis. Am J Psychiatry. 2007;164:942–8.
14. Willcutt EG. The prevalence of DSM-IV attention-deficit/hyperactivity disorder: a meta-analytic review. Neurotherapeutics. 2012;9:490–9.
15. National Institute for Health and Care Excellence. Attention deficit hyperactivity disorder: diagnosis and management, clinical guideline. 2018. https://www.nice.org.uk/guidance/NG87. Accessed 11 May 2018.
16. American Association of Pediatrics. Clinical practice guideline: diagnosis and evaluation of the child with attention-deficit/hyperactivity disorder. Pediatrics. 2000;105:1158–70.
17. Taylor E, Dopfner M, Sergeant J, Asherson P, Banaschewski T, Buitelaar J, et al. European clinical guidelines for hyperkinetic disorder—first upgrade. Eur Child Adolesc Psychiatry. 2004;13(Suppl 1):I7–30.
18. Edwards M, Gardner E, Chelonis J, Schulz E, Flake R, Diaz P. Estimates of the validity and utility of the Conners' continuous performance test in the assessment of inattentive and/or hyperactive-impulsive behaviors in children. J Abnorm Child Psychol. 2007;35:393–404.
19. Achenbach TM, McConaughy SH, Howell CT. Child/adolescent behavioral and emotional problems: implications of cross-informant correlations for situational specificity. Psychol Bull. 1987;101:213–32.
20. van der Ende J, Verhulst FC. Informant, gender and age differences in ratings of adolescent problem behaviour. Eur Child Adolesc Psychiatry. 2005;14:117–26.
21. De Los Reyes A, Augenstein TM, Wang M, Thomas SA, Drabick DA, Burgers DE, et al. The validity of the multi-informant approach to assessing child and adolescent mental health. Psychol Bull. 2015;141:858–900.
22. Toplak ME, Bucciarelli SM, Jain U, Tannock R. Executive functions: performance-based measures and the behavior rating inventory of executive function (BRIEF) in adolescents with attention deficit/hyperactivity disorder (ADHD). Child Neuropsychol. 2009;15:53–72.
23. Toplak ME, West RF, Stanovich KE. Practitioner review: do performance-based measures and ratings of executive function assess the same construct? J Child Psychol Psychiatry. 2013;54:131–43.
24. Zimmermann P, Fimm B. Testbatterie zur Aufmerksamkeitsprüfung. Herzogenrath: Psytest; 2012.
25. Zimmermann P, Gondan M, Fimm B. Testbatterie zur Aufmerksamkeitsprüfung für Kinder KiTAP. Herzogenrath: Psytest; 2003.
26. Földényi M, Imhof K, Steinhausen HC. Klinische Validität der computerunterstützten TAP bei Kindern mit Aufmerksamkeits-/Hyperaktivitätsstörungen. Zeitschrift für Neuropsychologie. 2000;11:154–67.
27. Drechsler R, Rizzo P, Steinhausen HC. Zur klinischen Validität einer computergestützten Aufmerksamkeitstestbatterie für Kinder (KITAP) bei 7-bis 10-jährigen Kindern mit ADHS. Kindheit und Entwicklung. 2009;18:153–61.
28. Renner G, Lessing T, Krampen G, Irblich D. Reliabilität und Retest-Stabilität der „Testbatterie zur Aufmerksamkeitsprüfung für Kinder"(KITAP) bei 6-bis 7-jährigen Kindern. Zeitschrift für Neuropsychologie. 2012;23:27–36.
29. Ulberstad F. QbTest technical manual. Stockholm: Qbtech AB; 2012.
30. QbTech A. QbTest plus technical manual. Sweden: Gothenburg; 2010.
31. Reh V, Schmidt M, Lam L, Schimmelmann BG, Hebebrand J, Rief W, et al. Behavioral assessment of core ADHD symptoms using the QbTest. J Atten Disord. 2015;19:1034–45.
32. Reh V, Schmidt M, Rief W, Christiansen H. Preliminary evidence for altered motion tracking-based hyperactivity in ADHD siblings. Behav Brain Funct. 2014;10:7.
33. Hult N, Kadesjo J, Kadesjo B, Gillberg C, Billstedt E. ADHD and the QbTest: diagnostic validity of QbTest. J Atten Disord. 2015. https://doi.org/10.1177/1087054715595697.
34. Soff C, Sotnikova A, Siniatchkin M, Christiansen H. Additiver Nutzen des QbTests in der Diagnostik der Aufmerksamkeitsdefizit-/Hyperaktivitätsstörung im Kindesalter; 2017 **(Manuscript in preparation)**.
35. Edebol H, Helldin L, Norlander T. Objective measures of behavior manifestations in adult ADHD and differentiation from participants with bipolar II disorder, borderline personality disorder, participants with disconfirmed ADHD as well as normative participants. Clin Pract Epidemiol Mental Health. 2012;8:134–43.
36. Edebol H, Helldin L, Norlander T. Measuring adult attention deficit hyperactivity disorder using the quantified behavior test plus. Psych J. 2013;2:48–62.
37. Hirsch O, Christiansen H. Factorial structure and validity of the quantified behavior test plus (Qb+®). Assessment. 2017;24:1037–49.
38. Soderstrom S, Pettersson R, Nilsson KW. Quantitative and subjective behavioural aspects in the assessment of attention-deficit hyperactivity disorder (ADHD) in adults. Nord J Psychiatry. 2014;68:30–7.
39. Lis S, Baer N, Stein-en-Nosse C, Gallhofer B, Sammer G, Kirsch P. Objective measurement of motor activity during cognitive performance in adults with attention-deficit/hyperactivity disorder. Acta Psychiatr Scand. 2010;122:285–94.

40. Berger I, Slobodin O, Cassuto H. Usefulness and validity of continuous performance tests in the diagnosis of attention-deficit hyperactivity disorder children. Arch Clin Neuropsychol. 2017;32:81–93.

41. Askland KD, Garnaat S, Sibrava NJ, Boisseau CL, Strong D, Mancebo M, et al. Prediction of remission in obsessive compulsive disorder using a novel machine learning strategy. Int J Methods Psychiatr Res. 2015;24:156–69.

42. Johnston BA, Mwangi B, Matthews K, Coghill D, Konrad K, Steele JD. Brainstem abnormalities in attention deficit hyperactivity disorder support high accuracy individual diagnostic classification. Hum Brain Mapp. 2014;35:5179–89.

43. Johnston BA, Mwangi B, Matthews K, Coghill D, Steele JD. Predictive classification of individual magnetic resonance imaging scans from children and adolescents. Eur Child Adolesc Psychiatry. 2013;22:733–44.

44. Orru G, Pettersson-Yeo W, Marquand AF, Sartori G, Mechelli A. Using support vector machine to identify imaging biomarkers of neurological and psychiatric disease: a critical review. Neurosci Biobehav Rev. 2012;36:1140–52.

45. APA. Diagnostic and statistical manual of mental disorders-fourth edition (DSM IV). Arlington: American Psychiatric Publishing, Inc.; 2000.

46. Wechsler D. Wechsler intelligence scale for children-fourth edition. 3rd ed. San Antonio: The Psychological Corporation; 2003.

47. Sattler JM. Assessment of children: cognitive foundations. 5th ed. San Diego: JM Sattler; 2008.

48. Döpfner M, Frölich J, Lehmkuhl G. Leitfaden Kinder- und Jugendpsychotherapie. Aufmerksamkeitsdefizit-/Hyperaktivitätsstörung. 2nd ed. Göttingen: Hogrefe; 2013.

49. Hodges K. Structured interviews for assessing children. J Child Psychol Psychiatry. 1993;34:49–68.

50. Renou S, Hergueta T, Flament M, Mouren-Simeoni MC, Lecrubier Y. Entretiens diagnostiques structures en psychiatrie de l'enfant et de l'adolescent (Diagnostic structured interviews in child and adolescent's psychiatry). L'Encephale. 2004;30:122–34.

51. Roelofs J, Muris P, Braet C, Arntz A, Beelen I. The structured clinical interview for DSM-IV childhood diagnoses (Kid-SCID): first psychometric evaluation in a Dutch sample of clinically referred youths. Child Psychiatry Hum Dev. 2015;46:367–75.

52. Kaufman J, Birmaher B, Brent D, Rao U, Ryan N. Kiddie-Sads-present and lifetime version (K-SADS-PL). Pittsburgh: University of Pittsburgh, School of Medicine; 1996.

53. Kaufman J, Birmaher B, Brent D, Rao U, Flynn C, Moreci P, et al. Schedule for affective disorders and schizophrenia for school-age children-present and lifetime version (K-SADS-PL): initial reliability and validity data. J Am Acad Child Adolesc Psychiatry. 1997;36:980–8.

54. Wender PH. Adult attention deficit hyperactivity disorder. Oxford: University Press; 1995.

55. Corbisiero S, Buchli-Kammermann J, Stieglitz RD. Reliabilität und Validität des Wender-Reimherr-Interviews (WRI). Zeitschrift für Psychiatrie Psychologie und Psychotherapie. 2010;58:323–31.

56. Mariani MA, Barkley RA. Neuropsychological and academic functioning in preschool boys with attention deficit hyperactivity disorder. Dev Neuropsychol. 1997;13:111–29.

57. Rucklidge JJ, Tannock R. Psychiatric, psychosocial, and cognitive functioning of female adolescents with ADHD. J Am Acad Child Adolesc Psychiatry. 2001;40:530–40.

58. Kuntsi J, Eley T, Taylor A, Hughes C, Asherson P, Caspi A, et al. Co-occurrence of ADHD and low IQ has genetic origins. Am J Med Genet Part B Neuropsychiatr Genet. 2004;124:41–7.

59. Bouchard TJ. The Wilson effect: the increase in heritability of IQ with age. Twin Res Hum Genet. 2013;16:923–30.

60. Brant AM, Munakata Y, Boomsma DI, Defries JC, Haworth CM, Keller MC, et al. The nature and nurture of high IQ: an extended sensitive period for intellectual development. Psychol Sci. 2013;24:1487–95.

61. Conners CK, Erhardt D, Sparrow E. Conner's adult ADHD rating scales: CAARS, technical manual. North Tonawande: MHS; 1999.

62. Christiansen H, Hirsch O, Philipsen A, Oades RD, Matthies S, Hebebrand J, et al. German validation of the conners adult ADHD rating scale-self-report: confirmation of factor structure in a large sample of participants with ADHD. J Atten Disord. 2013;17:690–8.

63. Christiansen H, Kis B, Hirsch O, Philipsen A, Henneck M, Panczuk A, et al. German validation of the Conners adult ADHD rating scales-self-report (CAARS-S) I: factor structure and normative data. Eur Psychiatry. 2011;26:100–7.

64. Christiansen H, Kis B, Hirsch O, Matthies S, Hebebrand J, Uekermann J, et al. German validation of the Conners adult ADHD rating scales (CAARS) II: reliability, validity, diagnostic sensitivity and specificity. Eur Psychiatry. 2012;27:321–8.

65. Christiansen H, Hirsch O, Abdel-Hamid M, Kis B. CAARS. Conners adult ADHD rating scales. German version. Bern: Huber; 2014.

66. Conners CK. Conners 3rd edition: manual. Toronto: Multi-Health Systems; 2008.

67. Christiansen H, Hirsch O, Drechsler R, Wanderer S, Knospe EL, Gunther T, et al. German validation of the Conners 3(R) rating scales for parents, teachers, and children. Z Kinder Jugendpsychiatr Psychother. 2016;44:139–47.

68. Schwaighofer A. SVM toolbox. 2.51 edition. 2001. https://pdollar.github.io/toolbox/. Accessed 16 May 2018.

69. Vapnik VN. The nature of statistical learning theory. New York: Springer; 1995.

70. Vapnik VN. Statistical learning theory. New York: Wiley; 1998.

71. Bishop CM. Pattern recognition and machine learning. New York: Springer; 2006.

72. Johnston BA, Coghill D, Matthews K, Steele JD. Predicting methylphenidate response in attention deficit hyperactivity disorder: a preliminary study. J Psychopharmacol. 2015;29:24–30.

73. Hervey AS, Epstein JN, Curry JF. Neuropsychology of adults with attention-deficit/hyperactivity disorder: a meta-analytic review. Neuropsychology. 2004;18:485–503.

74. Biedermann J, Mick E, Faraone SV. Age-dependent decline of symptoms of attention deficit hyperactivity disorder: impact of remission definition and symptom type. Am J Psychiatry. 2000;157:816–8.

75. Michielsen M, Comijs HC, Aartsen MJ, Semeijn EJ, Beekman AT, Deeg DJ, et al. The relationships between ADHD and social functioning and participation in older adults in a population-based study. J Atten Disord. 2015;19:368–79.

76. Novak SP, Kroutil LA, Williams RL, Van Brunt DL. The nonmedical use of prescription ADHD medications: results from a national Internet panel. Subst Abuse Treat Prev Policy. 2007;2:32.

77. Rabiner DL. Stimulant prescription cautions: addressing misuse, diversion and malingering. Curr Psychiatry Rep. 2013;15:375.

78. Hirsch O, Christiansen H. Faking ADHD? Symptom validity testing and its relation to self-reported, observer-reported symptoms, and neuropsychological measures of attention in adults with ADHD. J Atten Disord. 2015. https://doi.org/10.1177/1087054715596577.

79. Bijlenga D, Jasperse M, Gehlhaar SK, Sandra Kooij JJ. Objective QbTest and subjective evaluation of stimulant treatment in adult attention deficit-hyperactivity disorder. Eur Psychiatry. 2015;30:179–85.

80. Andreou P, Neale BM, Chen W, Christiansen H, Gabriels I, Heise A, et al. Reaction time performance in ADHD: improvement under fast-incentive condition and familial effects. Psychol Med. 2007;37:1703–15.

81. Slaats-Willemse D, Swaab-Barneveld H, de Sonneville L, van der Meulen E, Buitelaar J. Deficient response inhibition as a cognitive endophenotype of ADHD. J Am Acad Child Adolesc Psychiatry. 2003;42:1242–8.

82. Uebel H, Albrecht B, Asherson P, Borger NA, Butler L, Chen W, et al. Performance variability, impulsivity errors and the impact of incentives as gender-independent endophenotypes for ADHD. J Child Psychol Psychiatry. 2010;51:210–8.

83. Hinshaw SP, Owens EB, Sami N, Fargeon S. Prospective follow-up of girls with attention-deficit/hyperactivity disorder into adolescence: evidence for continuing cross-domain impairment. J Consult Clin Psychol. 2006;74:489–99.

84. Lahey BB, Willcutt EG. Predictive validity of a continuous alternative to nominal subtypes of attention-deficit/hyperactivity disorder for DSM-V. J Clin Child Adolesc Psychol. 2010;39:761–75.

Effects of social defeat stress on dopamine D2 receptor isoforms and proteins involved in intracellular trafficking

Vishwanath Vasudev Prabhu[1,2], Thong Ba Nguyen[1,2], Yin Cui[4], Young-Eun Oh[1,2], Keon-Hak Lee[3], Tarique R. Bagalkot[5] and Young-Chul Chung[1,2]*

Abstract

Background: Chronic social defeat stress induces depression and anxiety-like behaviors in rodents and also responsible for differentiating defeated animals into stress susceptible and resilient groups. The present study investigated the effects of social defeat stress on a variety of behavioral parameters like social behavior, spatial learning and memory and anxiety like behaviors. Additionally, the levels of various dopaminergic markers, including the long and short form of the D2 receptor, and total and phosphorylated dopamine and cyclic adenosine 3',5'-monophosphate regulated phosphoprotein-32, and proteins involved in intracellular trafficking were assessed in several key brain regions in young adult mice.

Methods: Mouse model of chronic social defeat was established by resident-intruder paradigm, and to evaluate the effect of chronic social defeat, mice were subjected to behavioral tests like spontaneous locomotor activity, elevated plus maze (EPM), social interaction and Morris water maze tests.

Results: Mice were divided into susceptible and unsusceptible groups after 10 days of social defeat stress. The susceptible group exhibited greater decreases in time spent in the open and closed arms compared to the control group on the EPM. In the social interaction test, the susceptible group showed greater increases in submissive and neutral behaviors and greater decreases in social behaviors relative to baseline compared to the control group. Furthermore, increased expression of D2L, D2S, Rab4, and G protein-coupled receptor associated sorting protein-1 was observed in the amygdala of the susceptible group compared to the control group.

Conclusion: These findings suggest that social defeat stress induce anxiety-like and altered social interacting behaviors, and changes in dopaminergic markers and intracellular trafficking-related proteins.

Keywords: Dopamine receptor isoforms, Elevated plus maze, GASP-1, Rab4, Social behaviors, Social defeat stress

Background

Social defeat is the result of a confrontation between male animals and is an ethologically relevant experimental paradigm that can be used to understand the physiological and behavioral adaptations to repeated social stress. The social defeat stress paradigm has been widely used as an animal model for depression, anxiety disorders, and drug abuse [1, 2]. This paradigm may also be useful for identifying the environmental factors associated with schizophrenia given that social defeat results in deficits in prepulse inhibition [3], an enhanced mesocorticolimbic dopamine response [4, 5], increased phasic activity in ventral tegmental area (VTA) dopaminergic neurons [6], reductions in striatal dopamine transporter (DAT) binding [7], and behavioral and neuronal cross-sensitization to amphetamine [8].

Social defeat stress also induces depression-like behaviors, such as a reduced sucrose preference, decreased social interaction and, and enhances anxiety-like

*Correspondence: chungyc@jbnu.ac.kr
[1] Department of Psychiatry, Chonbuk National University Medical School, Jeonju 561-756, South Korea
Full list of author information is available at the end of the article

behaviors [9, 10], such as more time spent in a dark box in the light/dark preference test [11] and an enhanced and prolonged response in the acoustic startle test [12]. For the present study, a particular focus was placed on changes in social behaviors, including dominant and submissive behaviors, and social avoidance because these symptoms are relatively commonly observed in patients with depressive disorder or schizophrenia. Several studies have addressed this issue but most have used rats [13] rather than mice [6, 14].

Two isoforms of the dopamine D2 receptor (D2R) have been identified; a long form (D2L) and a short form (D2S; [15]). The two isoforms are generated by alternative splicing of the same gene but show differential distributions [16] and functions [17, 18]. In the postmortem brains of patients with schizophrenia, there are changes in the mRNA levels of both D2S and D2L: increased expression of D2S in the dorsolateral prefrontal cortex (DLPFC) [19] and mixed results on D2L in the DLPFC and frontal cortex [19, 20]. However, to date, no studies have investigated the effects of social defeat stress on D2L or D2S except for one study from our research group [21], which found increased expression of D2S and D2L in the prefrontal cortex (PFC) of susceptible mice compared to controls. Dopamine and cyclic adenosine $3',5'$-monophosphate-regulated phosphoprotein-32 (DARPP-32) play central roles in mediating the effects of dopamine and glutamate [22, 23] and their expression can be altered by acute stress [24] and electroconvulsive stimulation [25]. Our research group reported significant increases in the expression of total DARPP-32 and phosphorylated DARPP-32 (p-DARPP-32) in the PFC and amygdala (AMY) of defeated mice [26]. However, those studies did not separate defeated mice into susceptible and unsusceptible groups, which is important for exploring the mechanisms that underlie the susceptibility to stress.

Schubert et al. [27] proposed that abnormalities in clathrin-mediated endocytosis and protein trafficking are core pathophysiological processes associated with schizophrenia and bipolar disorder. Of the various proteins involved in the trafficking of dopamine receptors, three are of particular interest: ADP-ribosylation factor 6 (ARF-6; [28]), Rab proteins [29] and G protein-coupled receptor (GPCR) associated sorting protein-1 (GASP-1; [30]) because they are involved in the regulation of vesicular traffic and organelle structure and associated with the degradation of D2Rs respectively.

Thus, the present study aimed to investigate the effects of chronic social defeat on a variety of behavioral parameters, including the social interaction, EPM, and MWM tests, and the levels of dopaminergic markers (D2L, D2S, and total and p-DARPP-32) and proteins involved in

intracellular trafficking in several brain regions of mice known to be affected in stress-related disorders such as anxiety and depressive disorders [31], and schizophrenia [32].

Methods

Animals
The social defeat procedure included male C57BL/6N mice and male CD1 (ICR) mice (Orient Company; Seongnam, South Korea) aged 6 and 15 weeks, respectively, and weighing 18–22 and 40–44 g, respectively, at the time of arrival. The C57BL/6N mice were group-housed while the CD1 mice were single-housed. The social interaction test included CD1 mice (4 weeks old) with similar weights that were matched to the C57BL/6N mice. All animals were housed in temperature-controlled rooms at 22 °C under a 12 h light/dark cycle with ad libitum food and water and were handled daily for 1 week to minimize stress during the behavioral experiments.

All the protocols in this experiment complied with the National Institutes of Health's Guide for the Care and Use of Laboratory Animals (NIH Pub. No. 85-23, revised 1996) [33]. The entire project was reviewed and approved by the Institutional Animal Care and Use Committee (cuh-IACUC-151027-32) of Chonbuk National University Medical School on the basis of 3Rs (replacement, refinement and reduction).

Study design
Following the 1-week habituation period, the behavioral tests were initiated in order of stress intensity (Fig. 1). Next, the C57BL/6N mice were subjected to the chronic social defeat procedure for 10 consecutive days; the defeated mice were categorized into susceptible and unsusceptible groups based on performance in the social avoidance test. Then, the behavioral tests were performed again. On day 39, the mice were sacrificed and brain tissues were obtained for the molecular studies.

Behavioral tests
All mice were habituated to the behavioral testing room for 30–60 min prior to all behavioral tests. After each behavioral test mice were rested for 1 day.

Spontaneous locomotor activity
Locomotor activity was measured in an open acrylic box ($30 \times 40 \times 50$ cm) using a video tracking system with SMART software (Panlab; Barcelona, Spain). The mice were placed into the testing apparatus and their activities, including distance traveled, locomotion time, and time spent in a central zone (defined as 25% or 50% of the total box area), were recorded for 30 min.

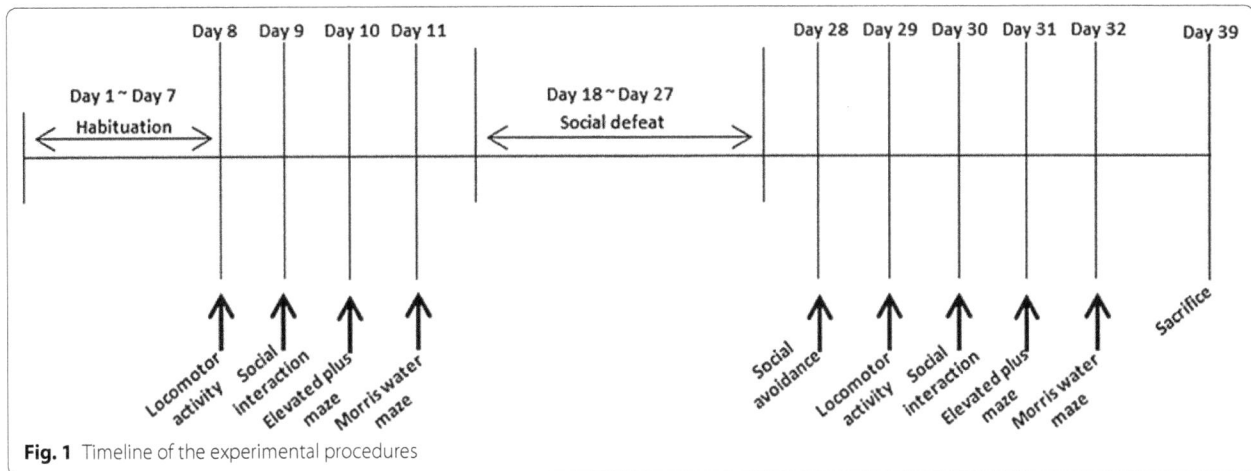

Fig. 1 Timeline of the experimental procedures

Social interaction test

The social interaction apparatus consisted of a standard polypropylene rectangular box (30 cm height × 40 cm width × 50 cm length) with an open top in which each C57BL/6N mouse was paired with an unfamiliar CD1 mouse with a similar weight. First, the C57BL/6N mice were habituated to the interaction box for 10 min and then returned to the home cage. Next, after the CD1 mouse was habituated for 10 min, the previously habituated C57BL/6N mouse was reintroduced into the box. Behaviors were recorded for 10 min with two video cameras under dimly lit conditions (40 lx) and the following behaviors were analyzed: (a) dominant behaviors, including upright/sideways offensive posture, attacks or bites, mounting/climbing, aggressive or violent grooming, and tail rattling; (b) submissive behaviors, including upright/sideways defensive posture, crouching, upright/sideways submissive posture, full submission posture, passive anogenital sniffing/being sniffed at the body part, avoidance, and curling up in the corner and remaining motionless; (c) neutral behaviors, including rearing/wall rearing, sniffing at the air or cage, and self-grooming; and (d) social behaviors, including approaching/following, nose sniffing, anogenital sniffing, and social grooming/sniffing. Total time spent and total numbers (frequency) of each behavior (counted when the duration was ≥ 1 s) were scored by an investigator blind to the conditions.

Elevated plus maze test

The test apparatus for the EPM was constructed from white plexiglas material and included two open arms (35 cm long × 5 cm wide) and two closed arms (35 cm long × 5 cm wide enclosed by 15 cm high walls) that extended from a central platform (5 × 5 cm). The maze was elevated 40 cm above the floor, illuminated at an intensity of 40 lx, and the edges of the open arms were

raised 0.25 cm to minimize the chance of a mouse falling. Each mouse was placed in the center facing an open arm and allowed to explore the apparatus for 5 min. Times spent in the open and closed arms and the numbers of open and closed arm entries were calculated; arm entries were defined as entry of all four paws into an arm [34]. If freezing occurred for more than 30% of the total test time (> 100 s), the mouse was excluded from data analysis [35].

Morris water maze test

The MWM consisted of a circular tank that was 100 cm in diameter and filled with opaque water (23 ± 1 °C) containing non-toxic white paint (Tempera, Dick Blick Holdings, Inc.; Galesburg, IL, USA). A circular escape platform (10 cm in diameter) was hidden 1 cm below the surface of the water. SMART software (Panlab) was used to calculate escape latency, distance traveled, and average swim speed. One day of pre-training (six trials to a fixed visible platform from a fixed start) was performed to assess motor and visual ability and then each animal participated in five trials per day for 5 consecutive days using the submerged platform and extra-maze cues. After end of the trial, wet body of the mouse was dried using towel and returned to its home cage and 1 min interval was given between trials.

When an animal failed to locate the platform within the 90-s time limit, an escape latency of 90 s was assigned. If a mouse floated, it was left alone. If a mouse floated the entire trial, it was removed and given a second trial at a later time. If the same mouse floated in the second trial, it was given up to two trials the next day. If a mouse never searched the maze, it was eliminated from the analyses [36]. Mice with repeated episodes of excessive floating (> 10 s/trial in ≥ 25% of trials) were also excluded from the analyses [37]. Floating was empirically determined as swimming at a speed < 4 cm/s. A different starting position was used for each trial performed on the same day with the sequence of starting positions varying from day to day. On the day after the acquisition training was completed (day 6), a probe test was performed in which the platform was removed and the animals were allowed to search for the maze for 90 s. Time spent and distance traveled in the target quadrant (where the platform had been located) were computed.

Chronic social defeat stress (CSDS)

The exact procedure for inducing social defeat stress has been described in previous articles from our research group [21, 38]. Briefly, C57BL/6N mice were introduced into the home cage of an unfamiliar CD1 aggressor mouse and they were allowed to interact for 10 min. We intervened to stop serious or prolonged confrontation [39]. During this exposure, all subject mice were defeated and showed signs of subordination (i.e., lying on their backs, freezing, or showing upright submissive postures). The social defeat procedure lasted for 10 consecutive days. We checked the wounds every time after social defeat bout. The mice with wound size greater than 1 cm were supposed to be removed based on the recommendation by Golden et al. [40] but we never saw mice with large wounds. The eight mice with small wounds were treated with betadine and excluded from the experiments. Control group experienced similar experimental conditions. During social defeat stress control mice were housed by pairs in equivalent cages with members of the same strain, one on each side of a perforated plexiglass partition and rotated on daily basis [40]. Based on the results of the social avoidance test, the animals were divided into susceptible and unsusceptible subgroups on day 11.

Social avoidance test

On 28th day mice were divided into the susceptible and unsusceptible group by performing social avoidance test. The defeated mouse was placed in interaction box (42×42 cm) with an empty wire mesh cage (10×45 cm) located at the one end. Interaction zone of 8 cm wide area surrounding the wire mesh cage was created. Test performed in two sessions. The first session without target i.e. wire mesh cage is empty and movement of the defeated animal tracked for 2.5 min. There was an interval of 1 min between 2 sessions. In the second session, novel CD1 mouse was introduced into wire mesh cage and the same defeated animal from first session was placed into the box and tracked for another 2.5 min. Mice activity near interaction zone was tracked by automated video tracking system based on the spontaneous motor activity recording tracking (SMART) software (Panlab, Barcelona, Spain). Social interaction (SI) ratio of 100

was set as the cut-off value. The interaction ratio is calculated as $100 \times$ (time spent in the interaction zone with an aggressor)/(time spent in the interaction zone without an aggressor). Mice which scores ≥ 100 were considered as unsusceptible group and mice which scores < 100 were considered as susceptible mice [40].

Preparation of brain tissue

Approximately 1–2 days after the completion of the behavioral experiments, all animals were killed by cervical dislocation. Brain tissues were collected from the PFC, striatum (ST), AMY, and hippocampus (HIP). An adult mouse brain slicer matrix cooled on ice (BSMAS001-01, Zivic Instruments; Pittsburgh, PA-15237, USA) was used to obtain coronal sections of brain tissues at 1.0 mm intervals. The targeted tissues (PFC, ST, and HIP) were removed from these brain sections on the ice cooled plate using single edge blades and preserved at -80 °C. The brain slices containing the AMY were immediately cryopreserved using liquid nitrogen and then punched at a later time using a 1.0-mm Harris Uni-Core micro-punch (Electron Microscopy Sciences; Hatfield, PA 19440, USA) in the microtome cryostat (Microm HM 525, Microm international GmbH, part of Thermos Fisher Scientific, Otto-han-str. 1A 69190 Wall Dorf/Germany).

Western blot analyses

Due to a sufficient number of samples, randomly selected tissues (approximately half) were processed for the Western blot analyses. The tissue samples were homogenized with a radio immunoprecipitation assay (RIPA) cell lysis buffer ($1\times$) containing 150 mM sodium chloride, 1% triton X-100, 1% sodium deoxycholate, 0.1% sodium dodecyl sulfate, 50 mM Tris–HCl, 2 mM EDTA, 1% protease (Sigma-Aldrich Korea Ltd.; Yongin, Korea), and phosphatase inhibitor cocktails (Sigma-Aldrich Korea Ltd.) at pH 7.5 using a Teflon pestle (Vintage Thomas; Philadelphia, PA, USA). The tissue homogenates were subjected to sonication for 5 min (amplitude 20%, on/off cycle as 10 s on and 5 s off) and then centrifuged for 15 min at 14,000 rpm at 4 °C. The resulting supernatant fractions were analyzed to estimate protein concentrations with Bio-Rad Protein assays (Bio-Rad Laboratories; Hercules, CA, USA).

The protein samples (20 μg/lane for ARF6, Rab4, Rab11, and p-DARPP-32 at Threonine 34 [p-DARPP-32 Thr34] and p-DARPP-32 at Threonine 75 [p-DARPP-32 Thr75] and 10 μg/lane for GASP-1 and total DARPP-32) were prepared with $2\times$ Laemmli sample buffer and lysis buffer (1:1 dilution) and boiled for 10 min. The protein samples were separated using either 12% or 10% sodium dodecyl sulfate–polyacrylamide gel electrophoresis (SDS-PAGE) for samples with 20 μg/lane and 10 μg/lane, respectively, and then transferred to a hydrophobic polyvinylidene difluoride (PVDF) membrane; prior to the transfer, the PVDF membranes were treated with methanol for 10 min. The membranes were then blocked with 5% skim milk or 5% bovine serum albumin (BSA) for 2 h at room temperature and incubated overnight at 4 °C with primary antibodies, including mouse monoclonal ARF6 (1:1000, Santa Cruz Biotechnology Inc.; Dallas, Texas, USA), mouse monoclonal Anti-Rab4 and Rab11 (1:1000, BD Transduction Laboratories; Erembodegem, Belgium), rabbit polyclonal GASP-1 (1:1000, Synaptic System; Gottingen, Germany), rabbit monoclonal total DARPP-32 (1:10,000, Epitomics, an Abcam Company; Cambridge, MA 02139-1517, USA), rabbit monoclonal p-DARPP-32 Thr34, and rabbit polyclonal p-DARPP-32 Thr75 (1:1000, Cell Signaling Technology; Denvers, MA, 01923, USA). After washing the membranes three times with Tris-buffered saline (TBS) containing 0.2% Tween 20 (TBST), the primary antibodies were detected using secondary goat anti-mouse IgG-HRP antibodies for ARF6, Rab4, and Rab11 (1:5000, Santa Cruz Biotechnology Inc.) and peroxidase-labeled goat anti-rabbit IgG(H+L) antibodies for GASP-1, total DARPP-32, p-DARPP-32 Thr34, and p-DARPP-32 Thr75 (1:5000, Vector Laboratories; Burlingame, CA, USA) for 2 h at room temperature (25 °C). The density of intracellular trafficking protein bands were normalized to β-actin.

The D2R isoforms (D2L and D2S) were analyzed using a procedure described by McDougall et al. [41] with a few modifications. The protein samples were prepared with 10 μg/lane and sample buffer and lysis buffer (1:1 dilution), kept at room temperature for 1 h, and then separated on 15% gel. The stacking gel was run at 60 V for 30 min during the initial phase, then at 60 V for 30 min until a good separation of the protein markers at 50 kDa was visible and, finally, at 140 V for 150 min. After transfer to the PVDF membranes, they were treated with 0.25% glutaraldehyde for 15 min [42] to improve the signal/noise ratio by decreasing the non-specific binding of secondary antibodies. Next, the glutaraldehyde-treated membrane were washed three times with TBST and blocked with 5% skim milk. The membrane was incubated in 5% skim milk overnight at 4 °C with the synthesized rabbit polyclonal antibodies for D2L (1:2000) and D2S (1:5000) (Abclon Inc. Seoul, Korea). After the membranes were washed three times, the primary antibodies were detected using peroxidase-labeled goat anti-rabbit IgG (H+L) (1:3000 for D2L and 1:5000 for D2S, Vector Laboratories) for 2 h at room temperature (25 °C). Western blot bands were developed using enhanced chemiluminescence reagents (GE Healthcare Inc.; Piscataway, NJ, USA), visualized using the Fusion Solo S imaging system (Vilber Lourmat; Marne-la-Vallee, France), and quantified with a densitometric measurement using Image J software a java based freeware by Wayne Rasband from National Institute of Health, USA. The density of the D2R isoform's protein bands were normalized to glyceraldehyde-3-phosphate dehydrogenase (GAPDH).

Synthesis and specificity of antibodies for *D2L and D2S*

Primary antibodies for D2L and D2S were ordered from Abclon Inc. (Seoul, Korea) to obtain subtype-specific staining against both the D2L and D2S isoforms using a procedure described by Khan et al. [43]. Briefly, the D2S peptide TPLKDAAR and the D2L peptide SNGSFPVNRRRM, which correspond to residues 238–245 and 259–270, respectively, were derived from the third cytoplasmic loop of the receptor. The D2S peptide was arranged by adopting four amino acids from each side of the insertion site to differentiate it from D2L. The peptides were coupled to the keyhole limpet hemocyanin (KLH) protein, the peptide/KLH conjugate (100 μg) was emulsified in complete Freund's adjuvant, and the solution was injected into rabbits for antibody development.

Specificity was tested using blocking peptides: SNGSFPVNRRRM-C (purity 94.86%) and TPLKDAAR-C (purity 92.78%) for D2L and D2S respectively (Abclon Inc. Seoul, Korea). The membranes incubated with blocked antibodies showed no band around 50 kDa markers whereas the membranes treated with control antibodies generated good signals near 50 kDa without non-specific bands surrounding the target protein bands. For the results of antibody specificity test, refer to the Additional file 1.

Statistical analysis

Outliers were defined as values outside a range of two standard deviations from the mean i.e., Mean ± 2SD of the respective group and were excluded from the analyses. The proportions of outliers were approximately 5–10% for the locomotion and social interaction tests and all Western blot analyses and 20% for the EPM test. For EPM outlier numbers were more than other behavioral tests because we applied one more criteria in which we excluded mice which shown freezing behavior for extended period of time on open arms (time spent on open arms is more than 30% of the total test time i.e., more than 100 s) due to noise or movement by experimenter during testing [35]. The behavioral and Western blot results are presented as a mean ± standard error of the mean (Mean ± S.E.M). For all the data except the frequency of social interacting behaviors, we performed one-way ANOVA. The social interacting behaviors were analyzed by Kruskal–Wallis H test because of skewed distribution. All data were analyzed using SPSS version 21.0 (SPSS Inc.; Chicago, USA). Pearson's correlation was performed to assess the correlation between SI ratio, and protein expression levels and behavioral data obtained after defeat stress. Correlation plots were constructed using PRISM version 6.0 (GraphPad software, California, USA). In all cases, p values < 0.05 were considered to indicate statistical significance.

Results
Social defeat stress
During the social defeat procedure (n = 69), eight mice were found to have small wounds. They were all removed from the experiments. The remaining defeated mice (n = 61) exhibited signs of subordination during the attack including fleeing, vocalizing, freezing, showing upright and sideway submissive postures, and lying on the back and exposing the belly to the attacker. Following this procedure, 65.6% of mice were classified as susceptible (n = 40) and 34.4% were classified as unsusceptible (n = 21).

Spontaneous locomotor activity
Following the social defeat procedure, the distances traveled and locomotion times significantly decreased compared to baseline (i.e., prior to social defeat) in both the unsusceptible ($p = 0.001$ and $p < 0.001$, respectively) and susceptible ($p = 0.018$ and $p = 0.026$, respectively) groups (Table 1). Times spent in the central zone also significantly decreased in all three groups but a group comparison of the change values revealed that only locomotion time significantly differed among the groups ($F_{[2, 70]} = 8.023$, $p = 0.001$). Post hoc analyses revealed significant differences between the unsusceptible and control groups ($p = 0.001$) and susceptible and unsusceptible groups ($p = 0.004$).

EPM test
Following the social defeat procedure, time spent in the open arms and number of entries into the open arms significantly decreased compared to baseline in all three groups (Table 2 and Fig. 2). Time spent in the closed arms increased in all three groups whereas the number of entries into the closed arms decreased in the unsusceptible and susceptible groups. A group comparison of the change values revealed that times spent in the open ($F_{[2, 59]} = 6.884$, $p = 0.002$) and closed ($F_{[2, 59]} = 7.252$, $p = 0.002$) arms and the number of entries into the closed arms ($F_{[2, 59]} = 6.866$, $p = 0.002$) significantly differed among the groups. The post hoc analyses revealed that the change in time spent in the open arms in the susceptible group was greater than those in the control ($p = 0.009$) and unsusceptible ($p = 0.017$) groups and that the change in time spent in the closed arms in the susceptible group was greater than that in the control group ($p = 0.003$). Additionally, the number of entries into the

closed arms in the susceptible ($p = 0.003$) and unsusceptible ($p = 0.013$) groups were greater than those of the control group.

Social interaction test
A group comparison of the change values revealed significant differences in submissive ($F_{[2, 68]} = 5.771$, $p = 0.005$), social ($F_{[2, 70]} = 5.509$, $p = 0.006$), and neutral ($F_{[2, 72]} = 19.830$, $p = <0.001$) behaviors among the groups (Fig. 3). The post hoc analyses revealed that the changes in submissive and neutral behaviors in the susceptible group were greater than those in the control ($p = 0.017$) and unsusceptible ($p = 0.026$) groups and that the change in social behaviors in the susceptible group was greater than in the control group ($p = 0.005$). In terms of time spent performing the behaviors, similar patterns of social and neutral behaviors were observed for all groups.

MWM test
Within- and between-group comparisons of the change values revealed that there were no significant differences in escape latency or path length.

Dopaminergic marker proteins
D2 isoforms
There were significant differences in the expression of D2L ($F_{[2, 32]} = 5.970$, $p = 0.006$) and D2S ($F_{[2, 33]} = 5.035$, $p = 0.009$] in the AMY among the three groups (Table 3, Fig. 4). The post hoc analyses revealed a significant increase in the expression of D2L in the susceptible group ($p = 0.008$) compared to the control group. The susceptible group also exhibited a significant increase in the expression of D2S compared to the control ($p = 0.030$) and unsusceptible ($p = 0.044$) groups.

Darpp-32
Of the DARPP-32 proteins, only the level of p-DARPP-32 Thr75 in the AMY significantly differed among the three groups [$F_{(2, 35)} = 7.406$, $p = 0.002$]. Post hoc analyses revealed a significant increase in the expression of p-DARPP-32 Thr75 in the unsusceptible ($p = 0.002$) and susceptible ($p = 0.008$) groups compared to the control group.

Intracellular trafficking-related proteins
A one-way ANOVA revealed significant differences in the levels of Rab4 ($F_{[2, 34]} = 6.126$, $p = 0.005$) and GASP-1 ($F_{[2, 37]} = 3.435$, $p = 0.043$) in the AMY among the three groups (Table 4 and Fig. 5). Post hoc analyses revealed that the expression of Rab4 ($p = 0.004$) and GASP-1 ($p = 0.048$) exhibited significant increases in the susceptible group compared to the control group.

Table 1 Comparison of locomotor activities obtained before and after social defeat stress among three groups

Parameters	Control group (n = 15)			p^a	Unsusceptible group (n = 20–21)			p^a	Susceptible group (n = 38–39)			p^a	p^b
	Before	After	Change		Before	After	Change		Before	After	Change		
Distance travelled (cm)	10,265.16 ± 813.84	9520.58 ± 635.32	−593.49 ± 812.32	0.401	9416.40 ± 565.47	7138.97 ± 483.44	−1457.57 ± 617.62	0.001	9082.38 ± 296.26	8313.24 ± 292.81	−629.96 ± 317.99	0.018	0.431
Time spent in central zone (25%)	83.87 ± 17.63	27.24 ± 4.96	−49.88 ± 9.92	0.004	104.49 ± 15.02	51.70 ± 7.66	−57.66 ± 13.48	0.002	103.65 ± 11.94	28.54 ± 5.23	−67.35 ± 7.88	<0.001	0.494
Time spent in central zone (50%)	357.77 ± 65.91	158.46 ± 31.14	−154.02 ± 33.75	0.008	335.34 ± 36.32	134.81 ± 24.06	−177.15 ± 33.68	<0.001	296.35 ± 30.94	152.84 ± 20.38	−125.55 ± 25.92	<0.001	0.449
Locomotion time (sec)	1205.35 ± 78.34	1121.15 ± 62.03	−41.86 ± 65.94	0.347	1138.77 ± 56.74	841.68 ± 65.19	−330.28 ± 59.17*†	<0.001	1123.74 ± 33.28	1038.77 ± 29.33	−116.99 ± 32.72	0.026	0.001

Data expressed as mean ± S.E.M

[a] Student's paired t test between the data obtained before and after social defeat stress

[b] One-way ANOVA for the change

* $p < 0.05$ versus susceptible group

† $p < 0.05$ versus control group

Table 2 Comparison of the results with elevated plus maze test obtained before and after social defeat stress among three groups

Parameters	Control group (n=12)			p^a	Unsusceptible group (n=16)			p^a	Susceptible group (n=34)			p^a	p^b
	Before	After	Change		Before	After	Change		Before	After	Change		
Time spent in arms (s)													
Open arm	39.90±6.36	18.89±4.90	−21.01±7.72	0.020	32.77±4.70	10.38±3.08	−22.38±5.83	0.003	53.12±4.95	5.93±1.66	−47.18±4.97*†	<0.001	0.002
Closed arm	212.43±8.54	249.29±9.48	36.85±12.04	0.011	221.55±6.68	270.98±4.72	49.42±8.79	<0.001	199.25±5.28	277.99±2.83	78.74±5.84*	<0.001	0.002
Number of entries													
Open arm	6.16±1.02	2.33±0.52	−3.83±1.19	0.008	7.09±1.54	1.54±0.65	−5.54±0.85	<0.001	7.00±0.55	1.03±0.24	−5.96±0.58	<0.001	0.275
Closed arm	14.91±1.00	16.25±1.23	1.33±2.11	0.541	16.90±1.58	11.0±1.09	−5.90±1.86*	0.010	15.5±0.61	9.25±0.78	−6.25±0.99*	<0.001	0.002

Data expressed as mean ± S.E.M

a Student's paired t test between the data obtained before and after social defeat stress

b One-way ANOVA for the change

* $p < 0.05$ versus control group

† $p < 0.05$ versus unsusceptible group

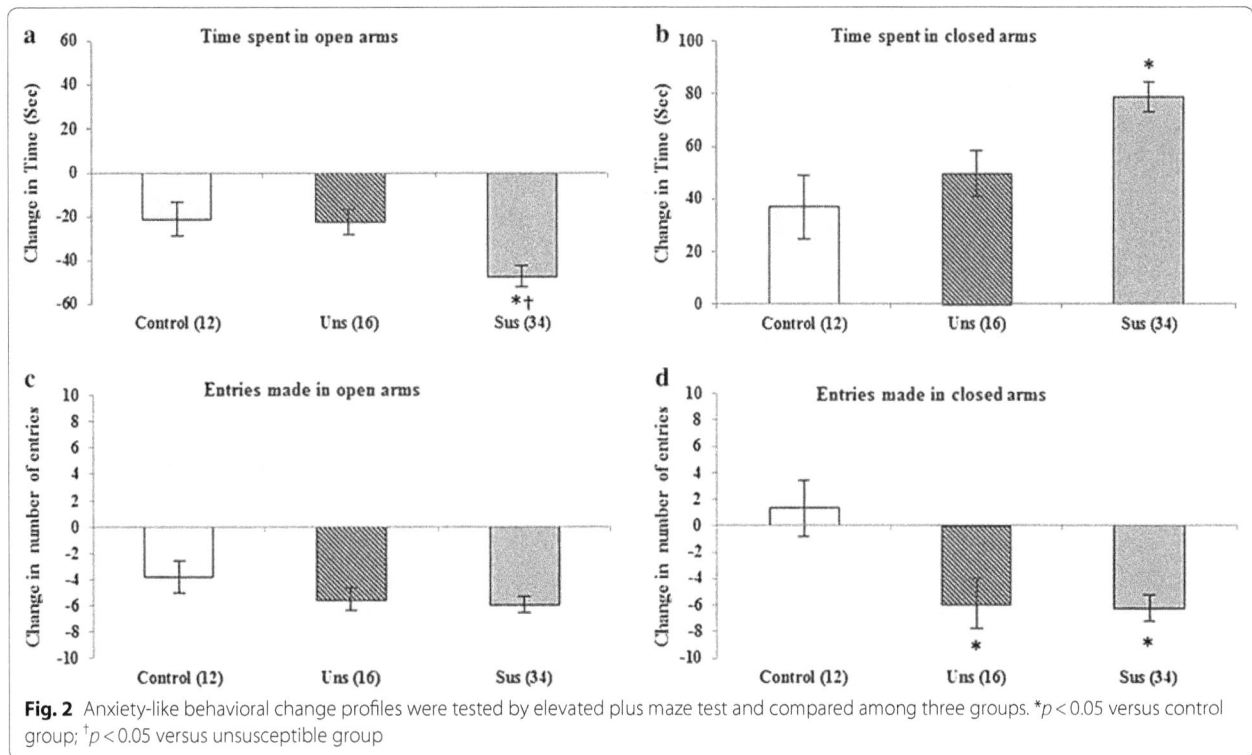

Fig. 2 Anxiety-like behavioral change profiles were tested by elevated plus maze test and compared among three groups. *$p < 0.05$ versus control group; †$p < 0.05$ versus unsusceptible group

Correlation analysis

Significant negative correlations were observed between SI score, and distance travelled ($r = -0.2615$; $p = 0.0418$), locomotion time ($r = -0.3608$; $p = 0.0043$), and submissive ($r = -0.2665$; $p = 0.0379$) and neutral ($r = -0.2918$; $p = 0.0225$) behaviors (Fig. 6a–c, e). Significant positive correlation was found with social ($r = 0.3107$; $p = 0.0148$) behavior (Fig. 6d).

As for D2 isoforms, we observed negative and positive correlation between SI ratio and D2L expression levels in the AMY ($r = -0.3751$; $p = 0.0492$) and HIP ($r = 0.3529$; $p = 0.0298$), respectively (Fig. 7a). On the other hand, no significant correlations were found between SI ratio and D2S in any of the brain regions (Fig. 7b). As for intracellular trafficking proteins, only p-DARPP-32 Thr34 ($r = 0.3428$; $p = 0.0472$) in the HIP was positively correlated with SI ratio (Fig. 8d).

Discussion

The present study investigated the effects of social defeat stress on a variety of behavioral parameters, including the social interaction, EPM, and MWM tests, and assessed the levels of various dopaminergic markers (D2L, D2S, and total and p-DARPP-32) and proteins involved in intracellular trafficking in several key brain regions of C57BL/6N mice. Following the social defeat procedure,

there were significant changes in behavior during the EPM and social interaction tests and significant alterations in the expression levels of D2L, D2S, p-DARPP-32 Thr75, Rab4, and GASP-1 in the AMY of the susceptible and/or unsusceptible groups compared to the control group.

Locomotor activity and anxiety-like behaviors in response to CSDS

In the spontaneous locomotor activity test, only the change in locomotion time after social defeat was greater in the unsusceptible group compared to the control and susceptible groups. These findings are consistent with those of previous reports [11, 44] but these studies did not classify the subjects into susceptible and unsusceptible subpopulations. On the other hand, Krishnan et al. [9] reported no change in locomotor activity in both susceptible and unsusceptible mice compared to controls. This discrepancy may be due to methodological differences between the studies. More specifically, the present study compared changes from baseline among three groups while Krishnan et al. [9] compared behavior among three groups only after social defeat. The present study found that locomotion time significantly decreased after social defeat in both the susceptible and unsusceptible groups but the degree of change was greater in the unsusceptible

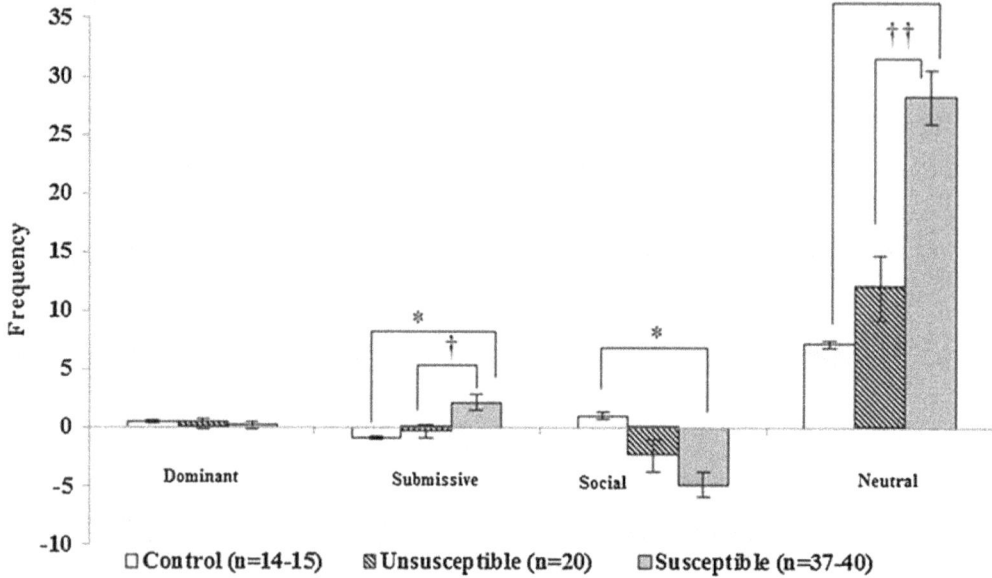

Fig. 3 Comparison of the changes in behavior frequencies obtained before and after social defeat stress in social interaction test among three groups. Data are total number (frequency) of each behavioral type and expressed as mean ± S.E.M, *$p < 0.05$, **$p < 0.001$ versus control group; [†]$p < 0.05$, [††]$p < 0.001$ versus unsusceptible group by Kruskal–Wallis test

Table 3 Western blot results of dopamine D2 receptor isoforms and total- and p-DARPP-32 among three groups

	Brain regions	Control group (n = 7–9)	Unsusceptible group (n = 8–11)	Susceptible group (n = 16–20)	p
D2L	PFC	1 ± 0.19	1.44 ± 0.24	1.29 ± 0.17	0.453
	ST	1 ± 0.16	1.18 ± 0.15	1.10 ± 0.09	0.695
	AMY	1 ± 0.17	1.17 ± 0.16	1.65 ± 0.16*	0.006
	HIP	1 ± 0.22	1.39 ± 0.32	0.96 ± 0.13	0.307
D2S	PFC	1 ± 0.16	1.04 ± 0.19	1.02 ± 0.14	0.988
	ST	1 ± 0.17	0.77 ± 0.10	0.91 ± 0.08	0.503
	AMY	1 ± 0.11	1.08 ± 0.23	1.77 ± 0.17*[†]	0.009
	HIP	1 ± 0.19	0.70 ± 0.09	1.14 ± 0.09	0.058
Total DARPP-32	PFC	1 ± 0.14	1.38 ± 0.16	1.16 ± 0.11	0.246
	ST	1 ± 0.15	0.81 ± 0.13	0.88 ± 0.11	0.719
	AMY	1 ± 0.18	1.23 ± 0.14	0.93 ± 0.08	0.191
	HIP	1 ± 0.28	1.02 ± 0.17	0.60 ± 0.06	0.071
p-DARPP-32 Thr34	PFC	1 ± 0.07	1.15 ± 0.12	1.33 ± 0.09	0.113
	ST	1 ± 0.11	1.15 ± 0.14	0.98 ± 0.07	0.475
	AMY	1 ± 0.14	1.31 ± 0.14	1.42 ± 0.13	0.185
	HIP	1 ± 0.23	0.93 ± 0.13	0.86 ± 0.07	0.781
p-DARPP-32 Thr75	PFC	1 ± 0.08	1.20 ± 0.11	1.09 ± 0.06	0.349
	ST	1 ± 0.14	0.97 ± 0.09	0.96 ± 0.07	0.976
	AMY	1 ± 0.02	0.70 ± 0.02*	0.77 ± 0.04*	0.002
	HIP	1 ± 0.13	1.11 ± 0.13	1.05 ± 0.13	0.899

Data were expressed in mean ± S.E.M

* $p < 0.05$ versus control group

[†] $p < 0.05$ versus unsusceptible group

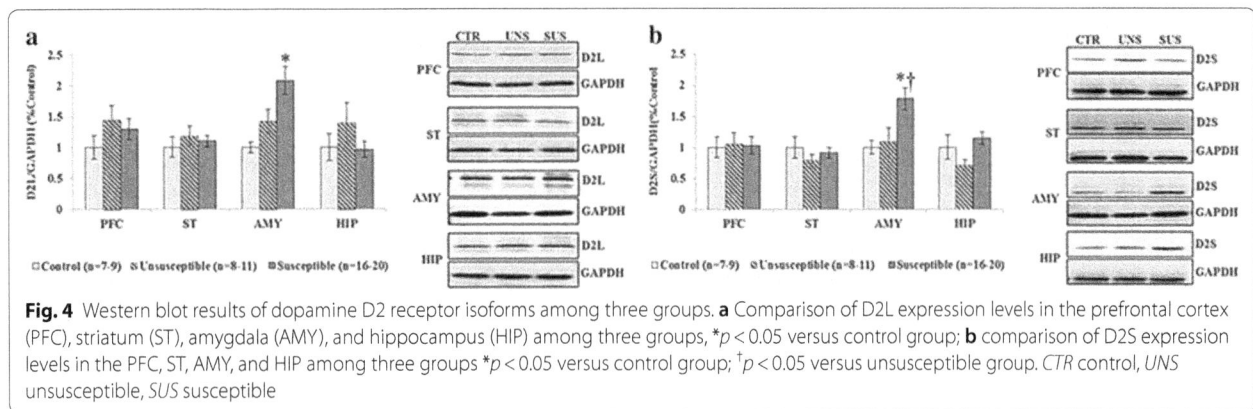

Fig. 4 Western blot results of dopamine D2 receptor isoforms among three groups. **a** Comparison of D2L expression levels in the prefrontal cortex (PFC), striatum (ST), amygdala (AMY), and hippocampus (HIP) among three groups, *$p < 0.05$ versus control group; **b** comparison of D2S expression levels in the PFC, ST, AMY, and HIP among three groups *$p < 0.05$ versus control group; $^{†}p < 0.05$ versus unsusceptible group. *CTR* control, *UNS* unsusceptible, *SUS* susceptible

Table 4 Western blot results of intracellular trafficking related proteins (ARF-6, GASP-1, Rab4 and Rab11) among three groups

	Brain regions	Control group (n = 7–9)	Unsusceptible group (n = 7–10)	Susceptible group (n = 16–19)	p
ARF-6	PFC	1 ± 0.13	0.87 ± 0.12	0.99 ± 0.04	0.552
	ST	1 ± 0.12	1.15 ± 0.03	0.95 ± 0.08	0.371
	AMY	1 ± 0.09	1.37 ± 0.09	1.20 ± 0.08	0.094
	HIP	1 ± 0.12	0.95 ± 0.11	1.06 ± 0.07	0.691
GASP-1	PFC	1 ± 0.13	1.31 ± 0.19	0.91 ± 0.06	0.054
	ST	1 ± 0.14	0.89 ± 0.07	0.94 ± 0.05	0.249
	AMY	1 ± 0.10	1.33 ± 0.12	1.32 ± 0.06*	0.043
	HIP	1 ± 0.10	1.24 ± 0.13	0.98 ± 0.06	0.123
Rab4	PFC	1 ± 0.07	1.20 ± 0.14	1.30 ± 1.10	0.276
	ST	1 ± 0.11	1.04 ± 0.16	1.08 ± 0.06	0.944
	AMY	1 ± 0.07	1.17 ± 0.06	1.27 ± 0.04*	0.005
	HIP	1 ± 0.11	1.04 ± 0.09	0.88 ± 0.04	0.303
Rab11	PFC	1 ± 0.06	1.17 ± 0.08	1.21 ± 0.04	0.097
	ST	1 ± 0.12	1.22 ± 0.05	1.17 ± 0.06	0.204
	AMY	1 ± 0.10	1.07 ± 0.09	1.07 ± 0.04	0.742
	HIP	1 ± 0.13	1.20 ± 0.09	1.21 ± 0.04	0.185

Data were expressed in mean ± S.E.M

ARF-6 ADP-ribosylation factor 6, *GASP-1* GPCR associated sorting protein-1

* $p < 0.05$ versus control group

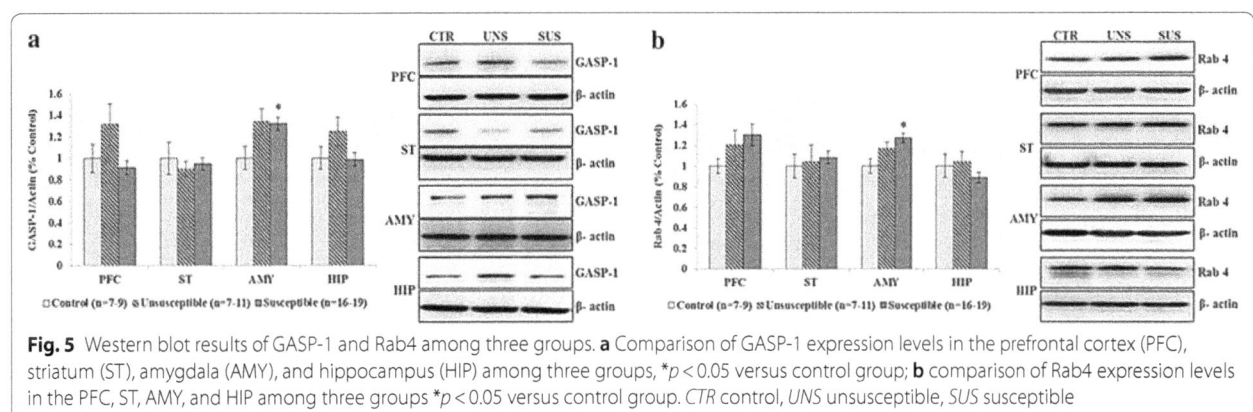

Fig. 5 Western blot results of GASP-1 and Rab4 among three groups. **a** Comparison of GASP-1 expression levels in the prefrontal cortex (PFC), striatum (ST), amygdala (AMY), and hippocampus (HIP) among three groups, *$p < 0.05$ versus control group; **b** comparison of Rab4 expression levels in the PFC, ST, AMY, and HIP among three groups *$p < 0.05$ versus control group. *CTR* control, *UNS* unsusceptible, *SUS* susceptible

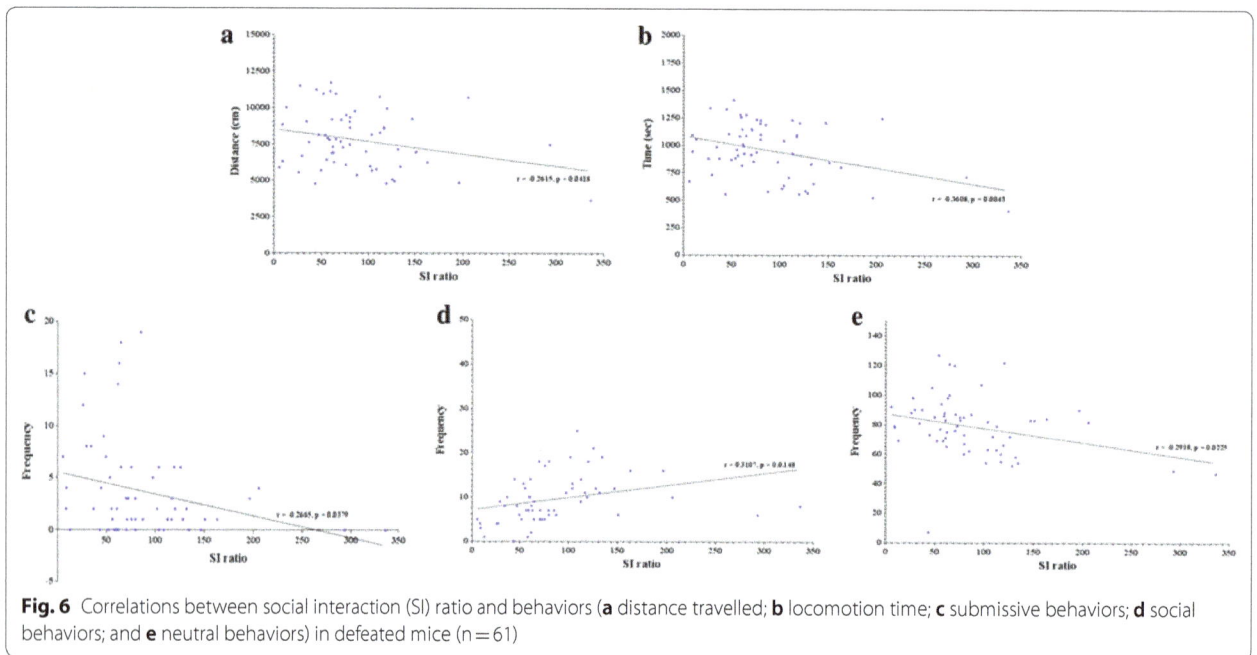

Fig. 6 Correlations between social interaction (SI) ratio and behaviors (**a** distance travelled; **b** locomotion time; **c** submissive behaviors; **d** social behaviors; and **e** neutral behaviors) in defeated mice (n = 61)

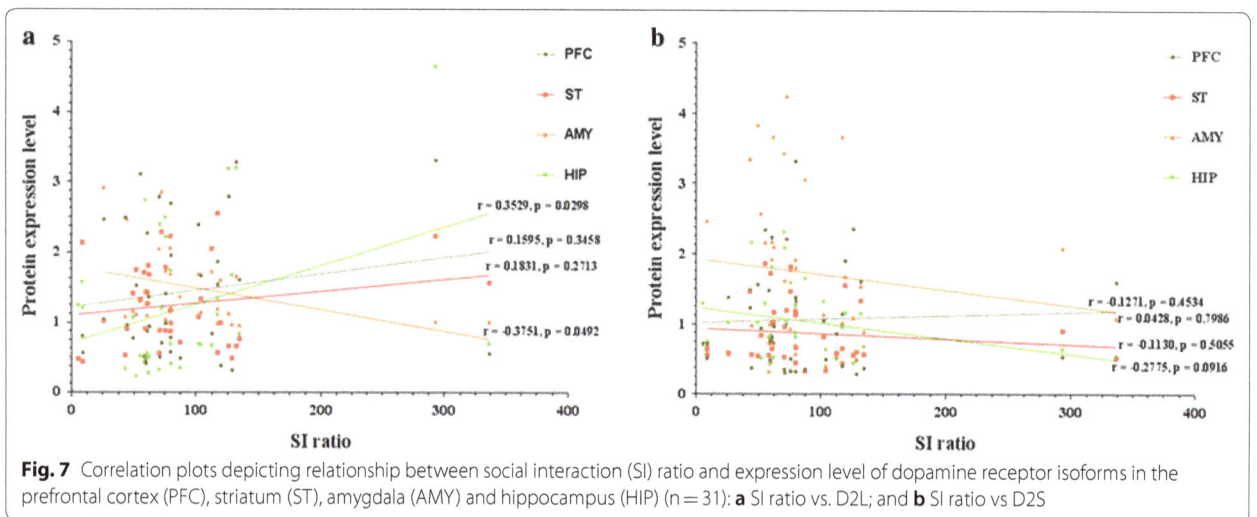

Fig. 7 Correlation plots depicting relationship between social interaction (SI) ratio and expression level of dopamine receptor isoforms in the prefrontal cortex (PFC), striatum (ST), amygdala (AMY) and hippocampus (HIP) (n = 31): **a** SI ratio vs. D2L; and **b** SI ratio vs D2S

group. The observed negative correlation results with SI ratio suggest that susceptible mice are more hyperactive compared to unsusceptible mice. This study also showed that there were greater decrease in time spent in the open arm and greater increase in time spent in the closed arm in the susceptible group compared to the control group and greater decreases in the number of entries into the closed arms in the susceptible and unsusceptible groups compared to the control group in the EPM test. These findings are consistent with those of Krishnan et al. [9] and a study showing that C57BL/6J male mice defeated by a conspecific display fewer open and total entries than controls [45]. Various environmental stressors, including prolonged isolation, foot shock, and forced swim, increase behavioral indices of anxiety in the EPM test [46, 47]. Therefore, the present EPM data indicate that social defeat stress increased anxiety-like behaviors in all defeated mice and that the degree of change was greater in the susceptible group. It was interesting to see decreases of the several parameters in control mice suggesting increased anxiety. This is in same line with Espezo study [48] that anxiety is enhanced after test repetition. Alternatively, it may be due to reduced novelty in the second test.

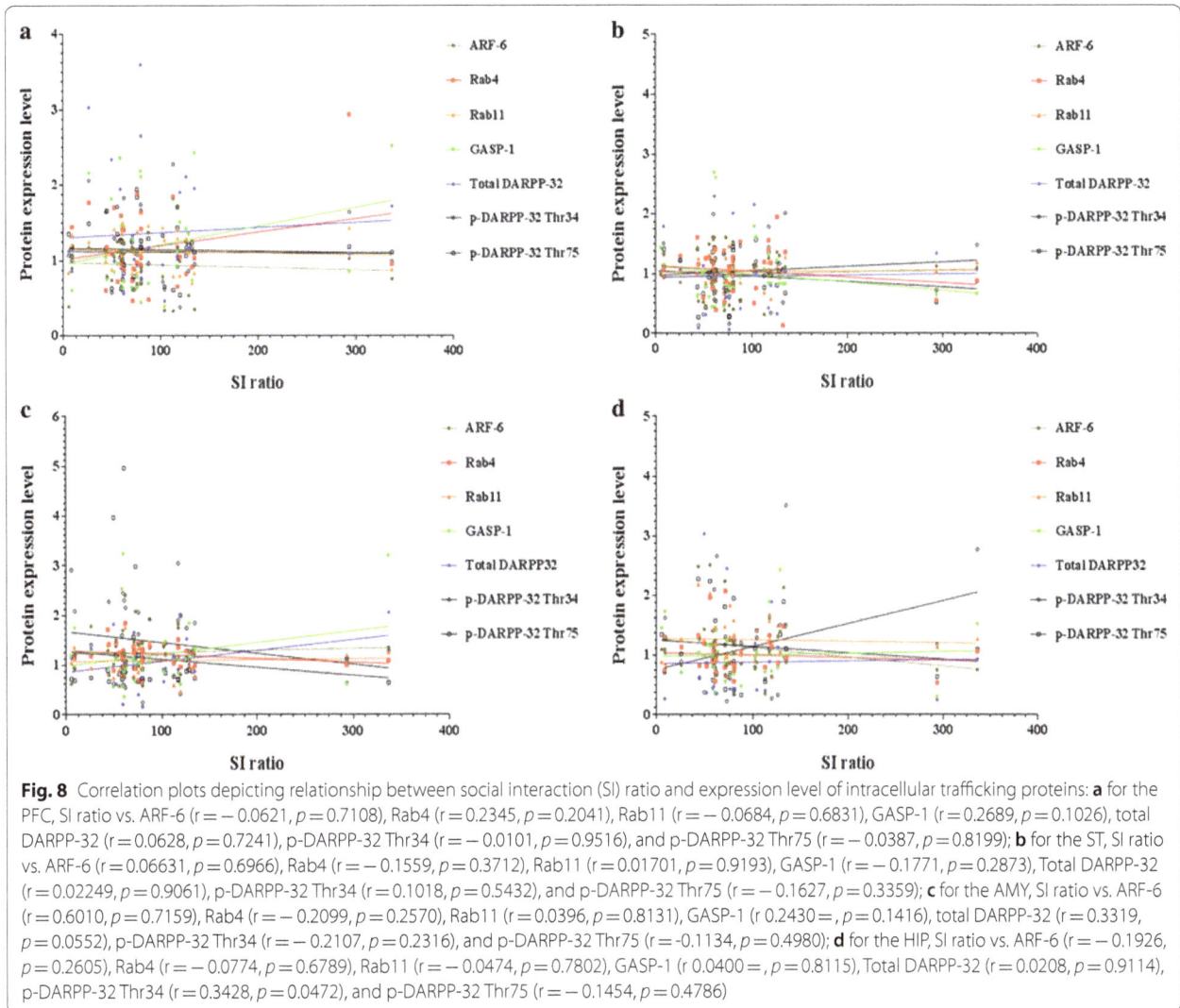

Fig. 8 Correlation plots depicting relationship between social interaction (SI) ratio and expression level of intracellular trafficking proteins: **a** for the PFC, SI ratio vs. ARF-6 ($r = -0.0621$, $p = 0.7108$), Rab4 ($r = 0.2345$, $p = 0.2041$), Rab11 ($r = -0.0684$, $p = 0.6831$), GASP-1 ($r = 0.2689$, $p = 0.1026$), total DARPP-32 ($r = 0.0628$, $p = 0.7241$), p-DARPP-32 Thr34 ($r = -0.0101$, $p = 0.9516$), and p-DARPP-32 Thr75 ($r = -0.0387$, $p = 0.8199$); **b** for the ST, SI ratio vs. ARF-6 ($r = 0.06631$, $p = 0.6966$), Rab4 ($r = -0.1559$, $p = 0.3712$), Rab11 ($r = 0.01701$, $p = 0.9193$), GASP-1 ($r = -0.1771$, $p = 0.2873$), Total DARPP-32 ($r = 0.02249$, $p = 0.9061$), p-DARPP-32 Thr34 ($r = 0.1018$, $p = 0.5432$), and p-DARPP-32 Thr75 ($r = -0.1627$, $p = 0.3359$); **c** for the AMY, SI ratio vs. ARF-6 ($r = 0.6010$, $p = 0.7159$), Rab4 ($r = -0.2099$, $p = 0.2570$), Rab11 ($r = 0.0396$, $p = 0.8131$), GASP-1 ($r 0.2430 =$, $p = 0.1416$), total DARPP-32 ($r = 0.3319$, $p = 0.0552$), p-DARPP-32 Thr34 ($r = -0.2107$, $p = 0.2316$), and p-DARPP-32 Thr75 ($r = -0.1134$, $p = 0.4980$); **d** for the HIP, SI ratio vs. ARF-6 ($r = -0.1926$, $p = 0.2605$), Rab4 ($r = -0.0774$, $p = 0.6789$), Rab11 ($r = -0.0474$, $p = 0.7802$), GASP-1 ($r 0.0400 =$, $p = 0.8115$), Total DARPP-32 ($r = 0.0208$, $p = 0.9114$), p-DARPP-32 Thr34 ($r = 0.3428$, $p = 0.0472$), and p-DARPP-32 Thr75 ($r = -0.1454$, $p = 0.4786$)

Social interaction in response to CSDS

In the social interaction test, there were greater increases in submissive and neutral behaviors and greater decreases in social behaviors from baseline in the susceptible group compared to the control group, which is similar with the findings of previous studies from our research group [38, 49]. However, the present results are unique in that the behavioral parameters were measured twice, before and after social defeat stress, in each group and interaction was performed with an unfamiliar CD1 mouse, not the same genetic background. The greater increase in submissive behaviors in the susceptible group compared to the control and unsusceptible groups was interesting as it could be regarded as an indicator of susceptibility. However, it is also possible that the development of subordinate behaviors is a more adaptive and flexible behavioral strategy [50]. This issue needs to be addressed in future studies. The correlation results reflect

the same profile, i.e., lesser social behaviors and greater neutral and submissive behaviors in susceptible mice. We performed the MWM test to evaluate whether CSDS affects spatial learning and memory in defeated mice. No significant findings in the MWM test are similar to the results of previous study [10].

Dopaminergic marker protein: D2 receptor isoforms

The present analyses of dopaminergic marker proteins showed that the expression of D2L and D2S increased in the AMY of the susceptible group compared to the control and unsusceptible groups. These findings are consistent with those of our previous report [21] except that the previous study also found significant changes in the PFC. The discrepancy may be due to delayed timing of sacrifice in the present study compared to the timing of the previous study in which animals were killed immediately after social avoidance test. The mechanisms underlying the increased expression of D2L and D2S in the AMY in susceptible mice remain unknown but it has been shown that conditioned fear stress enhances dopamine release in the AMY [51]. Because D2Rs are expressed at significant levels in the AMY [52] and the role of presynaptic D2S receptors is to inhibit dopamine release [53], the increased expression of D2S in the AMY of susceptible mice may be a compensatory mechanism that reduces dopamine release induced by social defeat stress. Assuming that released dopamine is more likely to bind to D1Rs, which are several times more abundant in the AMY than D2Rs [53], it could lead to the over activation of adenylyl cyclase. Subsequently, the increased expression of D2L may occur to cope with the over activation of adenylyl cyclase because D2R activation inhibits adenylyl cyclase. The AMY is usually maintained under the control of the medial prefrontal cortex but under the pressure of environmental threats, dopaminergic neurotransmission restores its activity allowing the development of anxiety responses [54, 55]. Accumulating evidence indicates that the mesoamygdaloid dopamine pathway modulates fear and anxiety by innervating preferentially GABAergic interfaces controlling the main input and output of the AMY [56]. More specifically, it has also been suggested that dopamine D1 receptor (D1R) may participate in danger recognition facilitating conditioned–unconditioned associations by retrieving the affective properties of the unconditioned environmental stimuli while D2R may instead participate in the modulation of reflex-like behaviors organized in the brain stem and in the setting up of adaptive responses to cope with aversive environmental situations [56]. Hence, our findings on D2S and D2L expressions in the AMY, and social interaction test indicate that susceptible mice are more likely to perceive defeat stress as threatening and in greater need to cope with aversive situations. The correlation analysis shows similar finding for D2L but different for D2S which should be compared cautiously to the results by one-way ANOVA because of no SI ratio for control group in the correlation.

Dopaminergic marker protein: p-DARPP-32 Thr75

In the present study, only p-DARPP-32 Thr75 expression was found to be significantly decreased in the AMY of defeated mice (susceptible and unsusceptible groups) compared to the control group. Enhanced dopamine states induced by amphetamine or cocaine increase the activity of protein kinase A (PKA) and lead to increases in p-DARPP-32 Thr34 but decreases in p-DARPP-32 Thr75 [57]. Assuming that social defeat stress may increase the release of dopamine in the AMY, the present results are partially consistent with earlier studies that used cocaine or amphetamine [57] suggesting defeated mice are under

high dopamine state. Despite the important potential role of DARPP-32 in neuropsychiatric disorders, few studies have investigated the roles of these proteins. In animal studies, increases in total DARPP-32 expression are induced by calorie restriction [58], electroconvulsive stimulation [25], and the inhibitory avoidance task [24]. On the other hand, the expression of DARPP-32 exhibits decreases in the post-mortem brain of patients with schizophrenia [59] and in the leukocytes of patients with schizophrenia and bipolar disorder [60]. Ours is the first report on the levels of p-DARPP-32 in relation to social defeat stress. The correlation analysis shows different findings which should be compared cautiously to the results by one-way ANOVA because of no SI ratio for control group in the correlation.

Intracellular trafficking protein measures (Rab4 and GASP-1)

The present study also assessed trafficking-related proteins and observed increased expression of Rab4 and GASP-1 in the AMY of the susceptible group compared to the control group. Li et al. [29] demonstrated that there are two D2R recycling pathways that play distinct roles in determining D2R function: the Rab4-sensitive constitutive D2R recycling pathway determines the steady-state surface expression levels of D2Rs whereas the Rab11-sensitive dopamine activity-dependent D2R recycling pathway is important for the functional resensitization of D2Rs. Moreover, acute stress increases the expression of Rab4 and subsequent trafficking processes in rats [61]. Therefore, the present findings that social defeat stress increased the expression of Rab4 in the AMY of susceptible mice may be associated with an increase in the recycling of internalized D2Rs induced by a high dopamine state, which, in turn, would lead to increased D2L levels in the cell membrane. However, this is pure speculation and needs to be confirmed in membrane proteins extracted from subcellular fractionation samples (post-synaptic density fraction) rather than total cell proteins, such as in the present study. GASP-1 is a recently discovered sorting protein for GPCRs that seems to be involved in directing internalized GPCRs to lysosomes for degradation [62]. Hence, the increased expression of GASP-1 observed in the present study may reflect an increased demand for the degradation of internalized D2Rs due to the high dopamine state. The physiological relevance of Rab4 and GASP-1 in terms of D2R expression in the cell membrane should be explored further.

Taken together of our findings, it may be inferred that defeated mice may be under high dopamine state especially in the AMY and increased expression of D2R isoforms seems compensatory mechanism. These changes may be associated with increased anxiety-like behaviors and decreased social behaviors of defeated mice. As negative symptoms including decreased social behaviors are known to be associated with hypo dopaminergic state in the limbic areas [63, 64], this speculation seems counterintuitive. However, considering the report that social withdrawal, a core feature of negative symptoms, is differentiated into passive social withdrawal (PSW) and active social avoidance (ASA) which are associated with negative and positive symptoms respectively [65], decreased social behaviors in the present study may reflect ASA rather than PSW. In light of the demonstrated role of inflammation in behavioral and neuronal phenotypes, it would be interesting to measure inflammatory markers and compare levels of inflammation between susceptible, unsusceptible and control mice in future studies.

Limitations

The present study has several limitations that should be mentioned. First, although two separated bands were consistently observed at about 48 and 52 kDa, using the protocol adopted from McDougall et al. [41] with subtype-specific antibodies synthesized from Abclon, Inc. (#1403, Ace Twin Tower1, 285 Digital-ro Guro-gu, Seoul 152-779, Korea) Western blot analyses of recombinant Sf9 cell lines expressing D2L and D2S should be carried out to test the specificity and selectivity of the antibodies to D2S and D2L. Second, the Western blot results may not reflect true changes induced by social defeat stress because the animals were exposed to another stressful test, MWM test and sacrificed 12 days after the social defeat stress; this issue should be considered when designing future studies. Third, to explore abnormalities in trafficking caused by social defeat stress, it is desirable to use subcellular fractionation samples rather than whole protein samples as in the present study. Despite these shortcomings, the present study assessed the behavioral parameters twice (before and after social defeat stress), identified D2R isoforms with subtype-specific antibodies, and included a relatively large number of mice in the susceptible and unsusceptible groups.

Conclusion

This study showed that (i) social defeat stress induces anxiety-like behaviors in spontaneous locomotor activity test or EPM test in defeated mice, (ii) altered submissive, social, and neutral behaviors in susceptible mice, and (iii) altered expression levels of D2 receptor isoforms (D2L and D2S) and intracellular trafficking proteins like Rab4 and GASP-1 in AMY brain region of susceptible mice. Taken together, these results suggest that social defeat stress induce changes in social behaviors and dopaminergic marker proteins which are closely related with pathogenesis of schizophrenia.

Abbreviations
EPM: elevated plus maze; MWM: Morris water maze; D1R: D1 receptor; D2R: D2 receptor; D2L: D2 long form; D2S: D2 short form; ARF-6: ADP ribosylation factor-6; GASP-1: G protein-coupled receptor (GPCR) associated sorting protein-1; DARPP-32: dopamine and cyclic adenosine 3′,5′-monophosphate-regulated phosphoprotein-32; p-DARPP-32 Thr34 and Thr75: phosphorylated DARPP-32 Thr34 and Thr75; GAPDH: glyceraldehyde-3-phosphate dehydrogenase; KLH: keyhole limpet hemocyanin; RIPA: radio immunoprecipitation assay cell lysis buffer; EDTA: ethylene diamine tetra acetic acid; PFC: pre frontal cortex; ST: striatum; AMY: amygdala; HIP: hippocampus; SDS-PAGE: sodium dodecyl sulfate–polyacrylamide gel electrophoresis; BSA: bovine serum albumin; PVDF: polyvinylidene difluoride; TBS: Tris-buffered saline; TBST: Tris buffered saline containing Tween 20; S.E.M: mean ± standard error of the mean; CTR: control; UNS: unsusceptible; SUS: susceptible; PSW: passive social withdrawal; ASA: active social avoidance.

Authors' contributions
C-YC planned experiments, interpreted data, and approved the version to be published. VVP performed most of the experiments and analyzed data. VVP and C-YC wrote the paper. TBN, YC, Y-EO, K-HK and TRB participated in the behavioral tests and discussion. All authors read and approved the final manuscript.

Author details
[1] Department of Psychiatry, Chonbuk National University Medical School, Jeonju 561-756, South Korea. [2] Research Institute of Clinical Medicine of Chonbuk National University-Biomedical Research Institute of Chonbuk National University Hospital, Jeonju 561-756, South Korea. [3] Department of Psychiatry, Maeumsarang Hospital, 465-23, Wanju, Jeollabuk-do, South Korea. [4] Shanghai Mental Health Center, Shanghai Jiao Tong University of Medicine, 600 Wan Ping Nan Road, Shanghai 200013, P. R. China. [5] Department of Cell Biology, University of Pittsburgh, 200 Lothrop Street, Biomedical Science Tower S372, Pittsburgh, PA 15213, USA.

Acknowledgements
I am grateful to Dr. Chung-Young Chul for guidance and insightful comments while preparing this manuscript and thanks to following lab mates (Tarique Rajasab Bagalkot, Thong Ba Nguyen, Yin Cui, Keon-Hak Lee and Young-Eun Oh) for their valuable contribution to complete this project.

Competing interests
The authors declare that they have no competing interests.

Funding
This research was supported by the Basic Science Research Program through the National Research Foundation (NRF) funded by the Ministry of Science, ICT and future Planning (NRF-2015R1A2A2A01003999).

References
1. Blanchard RJ, McKittrick CR, Blanchard DC. Animal models of social stress: effects on behavior and brain neurochemical systems. Physiol Behav. 2001;73:261–71.
2. Martinez M, Calvo-Torrent A, Pico-Alfonso MA. Social defeat and subordination as models of social stress in laboratory rodents: a review. Aggress Behav. 1998;24:241–56.
3. Adamcio B, Havemann-Reinecke U, Ehrenreich H. Chronic psychosocial stress in the absence of social support induces pathological pre-pulse inhibition in mice. Behav Brain Res. 2009;204:246–9.
4. Cabib S, D'Amato FR, Puglisi-Allegra S, Maestripieri D. Behavioral and mesocorticolimbic dopamine responses to non aggressive social interactions depend on previous social experiences and on the opponent's sex. Behav Brain Res. 2000;112:13–22.
5. Tidey JW, Miczek KA. Social defeat stress selectively alters mesocorticolimbic dopamine release: an in vivo microdialysis study. Brain Res. 1996;721:140–9.
6. Razzoli M, Andreoli M, Michielin F, Quarta D, Sokal DM. Increased phasic activity of VTA dopamine neurons in mice 3 weeks after repeated social defeat. Behav Brain Res. 2011;218:253–7.
7. Isovich E, Engelmann M, Landgraf R, Fuchs E. Social isolation after a single defeat reduces striatal dopamine transporter binding in rats. Eur J Neurosci. 2001;13:1254–6.

8. Nikulina E, Covington H, Ganschow L, Hammer R, Miczek K. Long-term behavioral and neuronal cross-sensitization to amphetamine induced by repeated brief social defeat stress: fos in the ventral tegmental area and amygdala. Neuroscience. 2004;123:857–65.

9. Krishnan V, Han M-H, Graham DL, Berton O, Renthal W, Russo SJ, LaPlant Q, Graham A, Lutter M, Lagace DC. Molecular adaptations underlying susceptibility and resistance to social defeat in brain reward regions. Cell. 2007;131:391–404.

10. Yu T, Guo M, Garza J, Rendon S, Sun X-L, Zhang W, Lu X-Y. Cognitive and neural correlates of depression-like behaviour in socially defeated mice: an animal model of depression with cognitive dysfunction. Int J Neuropsychopharmacol. 2011;14:303–17.

11. Kinsey SG, Bailey MT, Sheridan JF, Padgett DA, Avitsur R. Repeated social defeat causes increased anxiety-like behavior and alters splenocyte function in C57BL/6 and CD-1 mice. Brain Behav Immun. 2007;21:458–66.

12. Pulliam JV, Dawaghreh AM, Alema-Mensah E, Plotsky PM. Social defeat stress produces prolonged alterations in acoustic startle and body weight gain in male Long Evans rats. J Psychiatr Res. 2010;44:106–11.

13. Kabbaj M, Devine D, Savage V, Akil H. Neurobiological correlates of individual differences in novelty-seeking behavior in the rat: differential expression of stress-related molecules. J Neurosci. 2000;20:6983–8.

14. Berton O, McClung CA, Dileone RJ, Krishnan V, Renthal W, Russo SJ, Graham D, Tsankova NM, Bolanos CA, Rios M, et al. Essential role of BDNF in the mesolimbic dopamine pathway in social defeat stress. Science. 2006;311:864–8.

15. Giros B, Sokoloff P, Martres MP, Riou JF, Emorine LJ, Schwartz JC. Alternative splicing directs the expression of two D2 dopamine receptor isoforms. Nature. 1989;342:923–6.

16. McVittie LD, Ariano MA, Sibley DR. Characterization of anti-peptide antibodies for the localization of D2 dopamine receptors in rat striatum. Proc Natl Acad Sci. 1991;88:1441–5.

17. Usiello A, Baik JH, Rouge-Pont F, Picetti R, Dierich A, LeMeur M, Piazza PV, Borrelli E. Distinct functions of the two isoforms of dopamine D2 receptors. Nature. 2000;408:199–203.

18. Xu R, Hranilovic D, Fetsko LA, Bucan M, Wang Y. Dopamine D2S and D2L receptors may differentially contribute to the actions of antipsychotic and psychotic agents in mice. Mol Psychiatry. 1075;2002:7.

19. Kaalund S, Newburn E, Ye T, Tao R, Li C, Deep-Soboslay A, Herman M, Hyde T, Weinberger D, Lipska B. Contrasting changes in DRD1 and DRD2 splice variant expression in schizophrenia and affective disorders, and associations with SNPs in postmortem brain. Mol Psychiatry. 2014;19:1258.

20. Tallerico T, Novak G, Liu IS, Ulpian C, Seeman P. Schizophrenia: elevated mRNA for dopamine D2 Longer receptors in frontal cortex. Mol Brain Res. 2001;87:160–5.

21. Bagalkot TR, Jin HM, Prabhu VV, Muna SS, Cui Y, Yadav BK, Chae HJ, Chung YC. Chronic social defeat stress increases dopamine D2 receptor dimerization in the prefrontal cortex of adult mice. Neuroscience. 2015;311:444–52.

22. Fernandez É, Schiappa R, Girault J-A, Le Novère N. DARPP-32 is a robust integrator of dopamine and glutamate signals. PLoS Comput Biol. 2006;2:e176.

23. Svenningsson P, Tzavara ET, Witkin JM, Fienberg AA, Nomikos GG, Greengard P. Involvement of striatal and extrastriatal DARPP-32 in biochemical and behavioral effects of fluoxetine (Prozac). Proc Natl Acad Sci. 2002;99:3182–7.

24. Rosa DV, Souza RP, Souza BR, Guimarães MM, Carneiro DS, Valvassori SS, Gomez MV, Quevedo J, Romano-Silva MA. DARPP-32 expression in rat brain after an inhibitory avoidance task. Neurochem Res. 2008;33:2257–62.

25. Rosa DV, Souza RP, Souza BR, Motta BS, Caetano F, Jornada LK, Feier G, Gomez MV, Quevedo J, Romano-Silva MA. DARPP-32 expression in rat brain after electroconvulsive stimulation. Brain Res. 2007;1179:35–41.

26. Jin H-M, Muna SS, Bagalkot T, Cui Y, Yadav B, Chung Y-C. The effects of social defeat on behavior and dopaminergic markers in mice. Neuroscience. 2015;288:167–77.

27. Schubert KO, Focking M, Prehn JH, Cotter DR. Hypothesis review: are clathrin-mediated endocytosis and clathrin-dependent membrane and protein trafficking core pathophysiological processes in schizophrenia

28. Cho DI, Zheng M, Min C, Kwon KJ, Shin CY, Choi HK, Kim KM. ARF6 and GASP-1 are post-endocytic sorting proteins selectively involved in the intracellular trafficking of dopamine D2 receptors mediated by GRK and PKC in transfected cells. Br J Pharmacol. 2013;168:1355–74.

29. Li Y, Roy BD, Wang W, Zhang L, Zhang L, Sampson SB, Yang Y, Lin DT. Identification of two functionally distinct endosomal recycling pathways for dopamine D(2) receptor. J Neurosci. 2012;32:7178–90.

30. Bartlett SE, Enquist J, Hopf FW, Lee JH, Gladher F, Kharazia V, Waldhoer M, Mailliard WS, Armstrong R, Bonci A, Whistler JL. Dopamine responsiveness is regulated by targeted sorting of D2 receptors. Proc Natl Acad Sci USA. 2005;102:11521–6.

31. Myers Schulz B, Koenigs M. Functional anatomy of ventromedial prefrontal cortex: implications for mood and anxiety disorders. Mol Psychiatry. 2012;17:132–41.

32. Lawrie SM, Abukmeil S. Brain abnormality in schizophrenia. Br J Psychiatry. 1998;172:110–20.

33. Council NR. Guide for the care and use of laboratory animals. Institute of laboratory animal resources, commission on life sciences. Washington, D.C: National Academy of Sciences; 1996.

34. Pellow S, Chopin P, File SE, Briley M. Validation of open:closed arm entries in an elevated plus-maze as a measure of anxiety in the rat. J Neurosci Methods. 1985;14:149–67.

35. Walf AA, Frye CA. The use of the elevated plus maze as an assay of anxiety-related behavior in rodents. Nat Protoc. 2007;2:322–8.

36. Vorhees CV, Williams MT. Morris water maze: procedures for assessing spatial and related forms of learning and memory. Nat Protoc. 2006;1:848–58.

37. Wolf A, Bauer B, Abner EL, Ashkenazy-Frolinger T, Hartz AM. A comprehensive behavioral test battery to assess learning and memory in 129S6/Tg2576 mice. PLoS ONE. 2016;11:e0147733.

38. Huang GB, Zhao T, Muna SS, Bagalkot TR, Jin HM, Chae HJ, Chung YC. Effects of chronic social defeat stress on behaviour, endoplasmic reticulum proteins and choline acetyltransferase in adolescent mice. Int J Neuropsychopharmacol. 2013;16:1635–47.

39. Savignac H, Finger B, Pizzo R, O'leary O, Dinan T, Cryan J. Increased sensitivity to the effects of chronic social defeat stress in an innately anxious mouse strain. Neuroscience. 2011;192:524–36.

40. Golden SA, Covington HE 3rd, Berton O, Russo SJ. A standardized protocol for repeated social defeat stress in mice. Nat Protoc. 2011;6:1183–91.

41. McDougall SA, Der-Ghazarian T, Britt CE, Varela FA, Crawford CA. Postnatal manganese exposure alters the expression of D2L and D2S receptor isoforms: relationship to PKA activity and Akt levels. Synapse. 2011;65:583–91.

42. Ikegaki N, Kennett RH. Glutaraldehyde fixation of the primary antibody-antigen complex on nitrocellulose paper increases the overall sensitivity of immunoblot assay. J Immunol Methods. 1989;124:205–10.

43. Khan ZU, Mrzljak L, Gutierrez A, de la Calle A, Goldman-Rakic PS. Prominence of the dopamine D2 short isoform in dopaminergic pathways. Proc Natl Acad Sci USA. 1998;95:7731–6.

44. Razzoli M, Carboni L, Andreoli M, Ballottari A, Arban R. Different susceptibility to social defeat stress of BalbC and C57BL6/J mice. Behav Brain Res. 2011;216:100–8.

45. Avgustinovich DF, Gorbach OV, Kudryavtseva NN. Comparative analysis of anxiety-like behavior in partition and plus-maze tests after agonistic interactions in mice. Physiol Behav. 1997;61:37–43.

46. Jankowska E, Pucilowski O, Kostowski W. Chronic oral treatment with diltiazem or verapamil decreases isolation-induced activity impairment in elevated plus maze. Behav Brain Res. 1991;43:155–8.

47. Steenbergen HL, Heinsbroek RP, Van Hest A, Van de Poll NE. Sex-dependent effects of inescapable shock administration on shuttlebox-escape performance and elevated plus-maze behavior. Physiol Behav. 1990;48:571–6.

48. Espejo EF. Effects of weekly or daily exposure to the elevated plus-maze in male mice. Behav Brain Res. 1997;87:233–8.

49. Zhao T, Huang GB, Muna SS, Bagalkot TR, Jin HM, Chae HJ, Chung YC. Effects of chronic social defeat stress on behavior and choline acetyltransferase, 78-kDa glucose-regulated protein, and CCAAT/enhancer-

binding protein (C/EBP) homologous protein in adult mice. Psychopharmacology. 2013;228:217–30.

50. Koolhaas JM, Korte SM, De Boer SF, Van Der Vegt BJ, Van Reenen CG, Hopster H, De Jong IC, Ruis MA, Blokhuis HJ. Coping styles in animals: current status in behavior and stress-physiology. Neurosci Biobehav Rev. 1999;23:925–35.

51. Yokoyama M, Suzuki E, Sato T, Maruta S, Watanabe S, Miyaoka H. Amygdalic levels of dopamine and serotonin rise upon exposure to conditioned fear stress without elevation of glutamate. Neurosci Lett. 2005;379:37–41.

52. Beaulieu JM, Gainetdinov RR. The physiology, signaling, and pharmacology of dopamine receptors. Pharmacol Rev. 2011;63:182–217.

53. Rouge-Pont F, Usiello A, Benoit-Marand M, Gonon F, Piazza PV, Borrelli E. Changes in extracellular dopamine induced by morphine and cocaine: crucial control by D2 receptors. J Neurosci. 2002;22:3293–301.

54. Kröner S, Kröner S, Rosenkranz JA, Grace A, Barrionuevo G. Dopamine modulates excitability of basolateral amygdala neurons in vitro. J Neurophysiol. 2005;93:1598–610.

55. Marowsky A, Yanagawa Y, Obata K, Vogt KE. A specialized subclass of interneurons mediates dopaminergic facilitation of amygdala function. Neuron (Cambridge, Mass). 2005;48:1025–37.

56. de la Mora MP, Gallegos-Cari A, Arizmendi-García Y, Marcellino D, Fuxe K. Role of dopamine receptor mechanisms in the amygdaloid modulation of fear and anxiety: structural and functional analysis. Prog Neurobiol. 2010;90:198–216.

57. Greengard P. The neurobiology of slow synaptic transmission. Science. 2001;294:1024–30.

58. Yamamoto Y, Tanahashi T, Kawai T, Chikahisa S, Katsuura S, Nishida K, Teshima-Kondo S, Sei H, Rokutan K. Changes in behavior and gene expression induced by caloric restriction in C57BL/6 mice. Physiol Genomics. 2009;39:227–35.

59. Albert KA, Hemmings HC Jr, Adamo AI, Potkin SG, Akbarian S, Sandman CA, Cotman CW, Bunney WE Jr, Greengard P. Evidence for decreased DARPP-32 in the prefrontal cortex of patients with schizophrenia. Arch Gen Psychiatry. 2002;59:705–12.

60. Torres KC, Souza BR, Miranda DM, Nicolato R, Neves FS, Barros AG, Dutra WO, Gollob KJ, Correa H, Romano-Silva MA. The leukocytes expressing DARPP-32 are reduced in patients with schizophrenia and bipolar disorder. Prog Neuropsychopharmacol Biol Psychiatry. 2009;33:214–9.

61. Yuen EY, Liu W, Karatsoreos IN, Ren Y, Feng J, McEwen BS, Yan Z. Mechanisms for acute stress-induced enhancement of glutamatergic transmission and working memory. Mol Psychiatry. 2011;16:156–70.

62. Moser E, Kargl J, Whistler JL, Waldhoer M, Tschische P. G protein-coupled receptor-associated sorting protein 1 regulates the postendocytic sorting of seven-transmembrane-spanning G protein-coupled receptors. Pharmacology. 2010;86:22–9.

63. Brisch R, Saniotis A, Wolf R, Bielau H, Bernstein HG, Steiner J, Bogerts B, Braun K, Jankowski Z, Kumaratilake J, et al. The role of dopamine in schizophrenia from a neurobiological and evolutionary perspective: old fashioned, but still in vogue. Front Psychiatry. 2014;5:47.

64. O'donnell P, Grace AA. Dysfunctions in multiple interrelated systems as the neurobiological bases of schizophrenic symptom clusters. Schizophr Bull. 1998;24:267–83.

65. Hansen CF, Torgalsboen AK, Melle I, Bell MD. Passive/apathetic social withdrawal and active social avoidance in schizophrenia: difference in underlying psychological processes. J Nerv Ment Dis. 2009;197:274–7.

Frontal dysconnectivity in 22q11.2 deletion syndrome: an atlas-based functional connectivity analysis

Leah M. Mattiaccio[1], Ioana L. Coman[2], Carlie A. Thompson[1], Wanda P. Fremont[1], Kevin M. Antshel[3] and Wendy R. Kates[1]* (ORCID)

Abstract

Background: 22q11.2 deletion syndrome (22q11DS) is a neurodevelopmental syndrome associated with deficits in cognitive and emotional processing. This syndrome represents one of the highest risk factors for the development of schizophrenia. Previous studies of functional connectivity (FC) in 22q11DS report aberrant connectivity patterns in large-scale networks that are associated with the development of psychotic symptoms.

Methods: In this study, we performed a functional connectivity analysis using the CONN toolbox to test for differential connectivity patterns between 54 individuals with 22q11DS and 30 healthy controls, between the ages of 17–25 years old. We mapped resting-state fMRI data onto 68 atlas-based regions of interest (ROIs) generated by the Desikan-Killany atlas in FreeSurfer, resulting in 2278 ROI-to-ROI connections for which we determined total linear temporal associations between each. Within the group with 22q11DS only, we further tested the association between prodromal symptoms of psychosis and FC.

Results: We observed that relative to controls, individuals with 22q11DS displayed increased FC in lobar networks involving the frontal–frontal, frontal–parietal, and frontal–occipital ROIs. In contrast, FC between ROIs in the parietal–temporal and occipital lobes was reduced in the 22q11DS group relative to healthy controls. Moreover, positive psychotic symptoms were positively associated with increased functional connections between the left precuneus and right superior frontal gyrus, as well as reduced functional connectivity between the bilateral pericalcarine. Positive symptoms were negatively associated with increased functional connectivity between the right pericalcarine and right postcentral gyrus.

Conclusions: Our results suggest that functional organization may be altered in 22q11DS, leading to disruption in connectivity between frontal and other lobar substructures, and potentially increasing risk for prodromal psychosis.

Keywords: Functional connectivity, Connectives, Frontal lobe dysconnectivity, Velo-cardio-facial syndrome, 22q11.2 deletion syndrome, Schizophrenia

Background

Chromosome 22q11.2 deletion syndrome (22q11DS) is caused by a microdeletion of approximately 50 genes on one copy of the q11.2 band of chromosome 22. Youth with the syndrome typically present with physical anomalies, cognitive impairments, and behavioral disorders [1, 2]. During adolescence and young adulthood, approximately 30–40% of individuals with 22q11DS develop a psychotic illness, usually schizophrenia [3–5]. This represents a significant increase over the risk for schizophrenia in the general population [6]. The neurobiological mechanisms underlying this increased risk for schizophrenia in individuals with 22q11DS are not well-understood.

*Correspondence: katesw@upstate.edu
[1] Department of Psychiatry and Behavioral Sciences, State University of New York Upstate Medical University, 750 East Adams Street, Syracuse, NY, USA
Full list of author information is available at the end of the article

Converging evidence supports the notion that idiopathic (non-syndromal) schizophrenia is a disorder of functional and structural dysconnectivity [7–11]. Studies of functional connectivity point to a preponderance of anomalies in frontal–temporal connectivity [12, 13], although frontal–parietal and frontal–occipital connections have also been implicated [14, 15]. Moreover, abnormalities have been observed in several large-scale, functional networks, including the default mode network, the salience network and the central executive network [16–18].

Although studies examining functional dysconnectivity in 22q11DS are much fewer in number, the findings are consistent with studies of idiopathic schizophrenia [19]. Results of these studies indicate anomalous connectivity in frontal lobe connections [20] and parieto–occipital connections [20–22]. Decreases in functional connectivity have also been observed, in partially overlapping samples, in the default mode [23–26], salience [24] and frontal–parietal networks [22, 24]. In a modularity analysis of overall functional network organization, Scariati and colleagues [27] observed increased modular segregation across superior parietal, frontal and inferior temporal lobes in individuals with 22q11DS. Associations between anomalous functional connectivity in 22q11DS and increased symptoms of psychosis have been observed in most [20, 22, 24], but not all studies [25].

To our knowledge, two studies by Scariati and colleagues [20, 27] have conducted a functional connectivity analysis of atlas-based, ROI-to-ROI structural connections in 22q11DS. Scariati and colleagues first reported widespread functional connectivity in individuals with 22q11DS, primarily affecting frontal and temporal lobe regions. In a more recent study [27], they focused on age differences by examining connectivity in a sample of 9–30 year-old individuals with 22q11DS that were divided into two age groups (groups split at 18 years old) for subanalyses. In both age groups, alterations of modular communities were found to affect the anterior cingulate cortex and parieto-occipital processing regions. However, in adults with 22q11DS, they observed non-typical modularity partition of the dorsolateral prefrontal cortex.

Here, we conduct an atlas-based functional connectivity analysis of ROI-to-ROI connections in individuals with 22q11DS who are specifically between the ages of 18 and 24 years, a time-frame that poses the greatest risk for developing psychotic illness. In this ROI-to-ROI based approach, we sought to assess connectivity patterns by matching an anatomical atlas to each subject's own fMRI space. The methodological advantage of this approach is that data were not normalized to a standard template, thus obviating potentially problematic effects of warping

the brain. Conceptually, a subject-specific, atlas-based approach can yield additional data about the functional architecture and organization of the brain [28, 29]. Moreover, the use of atlas-based ROIs provides a common framework to increase reproducibility across studies, and can be incorporated for use in multimodal studies. In order to implement this approach, we applied the functional connectivity toolbox, CONN [28–30], which has shown a high degree of interscan reliability [28] and has demonstrated disease-relevant functional connections between anatomically defined regions of the brain [30]. We hypothesized that ROI-to-ROI connectivity between sublobar frontal–parietal gyri, and frontal–temporal gyri would be anomalous in individuals with 22q11DS relative to controls, and that aberrant connectivity would be associated with symptoms of psychosis.

Methods
Participants
Data were acquired from a large-scale longitudinal study of risk factors for psychosis in 22q11DS conducted at SUNY Upstate Medical University, Syracuse, NY. Our sample consisted of 84 participants: 54 with 22q11DS (30 males; mean age 20.98, SD 2.35) and 30 controls (16 males; mean age 20.97, SD 1.46). The control sample consisted of 12 healthy siblings of individuals with 22q11DS, and 18 community controls. Since siblings and community controls did not differ in either demographic variables or measures of functional connectivity (Additional file 1), they were combined into one control group. A previous publication included 39 of the 54 (72.2%) participants with 22q11DS in the current report, which tested differential connectivity in resting-state networks utilizing independent component analysis and associations with psychiatric and neurocognitive functioning [22]. Additionally, a recent publication including a partially overlapping sample of the 22q11DS group in this report demonstrated hypoconnectivity as a classifier in the identification of 22q11DS versus control groups [24].

Diagnosis of 22q11DS was confirmed by fluorescence in situ hybridization (FISH). Recruitment details have been described previously [31]. Briefly, exclusion criteria included seizure disorder, fetal exposure to alcohol or drugs, parent-reported elevated lead levels or birth weight under 2500 g, loss of consciousness lasting longer than 15 min, paramagnetic implants, or orthodontic braces. Potential controls with a personal or family history of schizophrenia or bipolar disorder were also excluded [31]. Since data for the current report were taken from a longitudinal study, control participants who had presented with an anxiety disorder and/or depression at the first timepoint were excluded. However, the current report depicts data from the last (fourth) timepoint, and controls that subsequently developed an anxiety disorder or depression in the longitudinal study were included. Controls with ADHD or a learning disability were not excluded at any timepoint in the study to maximize comparability to higher functioning participants in the 22q11DS group. Of the 54 participants, 22 were being treated with one or more antidepressant, antianxiety, antipsychotic, or stimulant medications at the time of their scan. Three controls were being treated with either a stimulant and/or antidepressant/antianxiety medication. Details of the samples can be found in Table 1.

Within the 22q11DS group, 10 participants were currently experiencing positive prodromal symptoms of psychosis (based on a frequency of symptoms > 1 week, and a score of equal or greater than 3 on the positive symptoms subscale of the Structured Interview for Prodromal Symptoms [SIPS; [32]]). An additional 5 participants were diagnosed with overt psychosis. Additional details regarding these subgroups can be found in Table 2. The institutional review board of SUNY Upstate Medical University approved all study procedures, and each participant provided written informed consent or assent.

Psychiatric assessment

Participants had psychiatric evaluations administered by two doctoral-level clinicians (WF and KMA). To determine the presence of DSM-IV psychiatric diagnoses in both the 22q11DS and control group, the Structured Clinical Interview for DSM-IV Axis I disorders (SCID; [33]) was administered. Inter-rater reliability was calculated based on 5 consecutive, audio-recorded interviews

Table 1 Demographic and psychiatric data

	22q11DS N = 54	Controls N = 30	p value
Age[a]	20.98 (2.35)	20.97 (1.46)	0.990
Gender (male, %)	30 (55.6%)	16 (53.3%)	0.847
Full scale IQ[a]	74.41 (12.0)	109.47 (16.02)	< 0.001
Psychiatric diagnosis, n (%)			
Psychotic disorder	5 (9.26%)	0 (0%)	0.024
ADHD	8 (14.81%)	5 (16.67%)	0.825
Anxiety disorder	11 (20.37%)	4 (13.33%)	0.426
Mood disorder	7 (12.96%)	1 (6.25%)	0.094
Current medication, n (%)			
Antipsychotic/mood stabilizer	8 (14.81%)	0 (0%)	0.004
Antidepressant/anti-anxiety	16 (29.63%)	2 (6.67%)	0.004
Stimulant	9 (16.67%)	2 (6.67%)	0.151

Demographic and psychiatric data for participants in our group analyses; from our initial sample of 85, one proband was excluded due to image quality

[a] Mean and standard deviation are provided for age and full scale IQ. Independent t tests were conducted to determine differences between 22q11DS and control samples

Table 2 Demographic data for prodromal and nonprodromal subgroups

	Prodromal N = 10	Overt N = 5	Nonpro-dromal N = 39	p value
Age[a]	22.60 (2.50)	19.43 (1.54)	20.76 (2.21)	0.320
Gender (male, %)	5 (50.0%)	2 (40.0%)	23 (58.97%)	0.436
Full scale IQ[a]	71.0 (6.65)	61.6 (4.62)	76.92 (12.53)	0.002

Demographic and psychiatric data for prodromal, nonprodromal, and participants with overt psychosis from our initial sample of 55; 1 proband was excluded due to image quality

[a] Mean and standard deviation are provided for age and full scale IQ. Independent t tests were conducted to determine differences between prodromal and nonprodromal subgroups; participants with overt psychosis were combined with the prodromal group for subsequent analyses

resulting in an interclass correlation coefficient of 0.91. The presence of prodromal, positive symptoms of psychosis was determined utilizing the Structured Interview for Prodromal Syndromes (SIPS; [32]), conducted within the context of the psychiatric evaluation. Additional details regarding psychiatric diagnoses can be found in Table 1.

Image acquisition

Both anatomical and functional resting-state imaging data were acquired with a Siemens Tim Trio, 3 Tesla scanner with an 8-channel head coil receiver (Siemens Medical Solutions, Erlangen, Germany) during the same scanning session. T1-weighted images were acquired in the sagittal plane utilizing a MPRAGE pulse sequence with the following parameters: TR/TE = 2530/3.31 ms, voxel size = $1.0 \times 1.0 \times 1.0$, flip angle = 7°, field of view = 256 mm, and 256×256 acquisition matrix. Blood oxygen level dependent (BOLD) images were acquired during a 5-minute resting-state scan, which included 152 images (34 axial slices, 4 mm thickness, no gap) utilizing an ep2d_bold sequence: TR/TE = 2000/30 ms, voxel size $4.0 \times 4.0 \times 4.0$, flip angle = 90°, field of view = 256, acquisition matrix = 64×64. Participants were instructed to keep their eyes open and not to fall asleep during the scanning session.

Image processing

Raw structural data were imported into the FreeSurfer image analysis suite (v5.1.0, https://surfer.nmr.mgh.harvard.edu/ [34]) for removal of non-brain tissue. The generated brain mask was then manually edited in 3DSlicer 4 (https://www.slicer.org/ [35]). Edited brain masks were then aligned in 3DSlicer along the anterior and posterior commissure using a cubic spline transformation. Resolution was maintained at 1 mm cubic isotropic voxels. Preprocessed data were then introduced into FreeSurfer's automated surface-based reconstruction and volume-based subcortical processing streams to segment, and parcellate the brain into 68 regions based on the Desikan-Killiany atlas [36]. To briefly summarize, this processing pipeline includes motion correction, intensity normalization, registration to Talairach space, removal of non-brain matter, cortical reconstruction, and segmentation of subcortical structures and white matter. Before final reconstruction was run, manual intervention using control points were placed to minimize motion and hyperintensities that were not corrected by the automated pipeline. Details of manual intervention protocols can be found in McCarthy and colleagues [37]. Second reconstruction was then conducted considering any manual intervention. Final reconstruction steps were then run to complete the processing pipeline.

Functional data were preprocessed using statistical parametric mapping (SPM5; Wellcome Trust Centre for Neuroimaging, 2005, London, UK, http://www.fil.ion.ucl.ac.uk/spm/ [38]). Images were visually inspected for the presence of significant signal dropout, ghosting, excessive noise, and any other artifact that would impact the ability to analyze the images. Visual inspection was repeated throughout different stages of preprocessing. Images were first motion corrected using INRIalign [39], an algorithm that is unbiased by local signal changes. Motion adjustment, an algorithm that suppresses residual fluctuations due to errors in interpolation from large motions was subsequently conducted using ArtRepair [40]. A despiking function was then applied to remove any spikes caused by motion. No participants were excluded due to motion based on the following criteria: > 2 mm across the entire run and rotation greater than 2°. One proband was excluded due to a significant signal dropout in the raw BOLD images, and no other participants were excluded for any other artifacts mentioned above.

Anatomical T1-weighted images from FreeSurfer, (including each ROI for both hemispheres) were then coregistered to the mean functional EPI image in SPM for each participant.

Functional connectivity analysis
Functional connectivity analyses were conducted utilizing the CONN toolbox (https://www.nitrc.org/projects/conn [28]). This toolbox implements a CompCor method, which reduces physiological and movement effects: CSF and white matter effects, task-related effects, and realignment parameter noise without removing the global signal [29]. A band-pass filter of 0.008–0.09 was applied to the data. Realignment parameters from preprocessing were entered as confounds in the first-level analysis. Using the Desikan-Killany atlas in FreeSurfer [36], which generates 34 bilateral, or 68 ROI's, we conducted a seed-based ROI-to-ROI analysis to create a 68 × 68 functional connectivity map. A bivariate correlation was used to determine total linear temporal associations between each of the resulting 2278 ROI-to-ROI functional connections. Second-level analyses of group differences in functional connectivity between 22q11DS and controls was conducted through the CONN toolbox and FDR-corrected, $p < 0.05$, two-tailed.

We then repeated the aforementioned ROI-to-ROI analysis to compare functional connectivity between prodromal and nonprodromal participants with 22q11DS based on positive symptoms that were present at a frequency of greater than once per week, and that obtained summed scores of ≥ 3 (reflecting intensity of the symptom) on the Structured Interview for Prodromal Symptoms (SIPS; [32]) positive symptoms subscale. These criteria have been applied in previous studies of individuals with 22q11DS [20, 24].

Associations with positive symptoms
We then tested associations between positive symptom scores in 22q11DS (taken from summed scores of the SIPS Positive Symptoms subscale) and functional connectivity values for ROI-to-ROI connections that were significantly different between individuals with 22q11DS and the control group. Functional connectivity values were taken from Fisher-transformed correlation coefficients from the first-level analysis conducted in the CONN toolbox. Since many participants with 22q11DS scored 0 on the SIPS Positive Symptoms Scale (29 participants, 53.7%), and since the SIPS produces a count variable, we conducted a zero-inflated Poisson (ZIP) regression analysis to examine these associations. Results were then FDR-corrected, *p < 0.05.*

Results
Second-level analyses of the functional connectome analysis revealed significant differences in functional connectivity between 22q11DS and controls ($p_{FDR} < 0.05$). (Table 3 and Fig. 1) At the lobar level, we observed differential connectivity between ROIs within frontal–frontal, frontal–occipital, frontal–parietal, occipital–occipital, and parietal–temporal regions.

Increased functional connectivity in 22Q11DS vs. controls
Within frontal–frontal connections, we observed increased functional connectivity in individuals with 22q11DS relative to controls between the right precentral gyrus and right posterior cingulate, right superior frontal gyrus to left posterior cingulate, and right superior frontal gyrus to right posterior cingulate. Table 3 displays differential functional connections between 22q11DS and controls at both the lobar and sublobar level as well as t values, corrected p values, and averaged functional connectivity values.

Table 3 Differential functional connectivity between 22q11DS and controls

Functional connection (ROI–ROI) 22q11DS vs controls	Lobar-level connections	t value	p value, corr	22q11DS[a]	controls[a]
Right precentral–right posterior cingulate	Frontal–frontal	3.59	0.038	0.232	0.067
Right superior frontal–left posterior cingulate	Frontal–frontal	3.22	0.025	0.230	0.036
Right superior frontal–right posterior cingulate	Frontal–frontal	3.23	0.025	0.411	0.212
Right pars orbitalis–left cuneus	Frontal–occipital	3.79	0.019	0.011	− 0.187
Right pars orbitalis––right cuneus	Frontal–occipital	3.44	0.022	0.021	− 0.146
Right pericalcarine–left paracentral	Frontal–occipital	3.42	0.033	− 0.013	− 0.173
Right pericalcarine–right postcentral	Frontal–occipital	3.27	0.035	− 0.013	− 0.159
Right precuneus–right caudal middle frontal	Frontal–parietal	4.04	0.008	0.281	0.054
Left Precuneus–right pars orbitalis	Frontal–parietal	3.42	0.033	− 0.109	− 0.313
Right precuneus–right pars orbitalis	Frontal–parietal	3.23	0.04	0.014	− 0.174
Left precuneus–right superior frontal	Frontal–parietal	4.06	0.008	0.110	− 0.113
Right precuneus–right superior frontal	Frontal–parietal	3.30	0.04	0.289	0.092
Right superior frontal–right lateral orbito frontal gyrus	Frontal–frontal	− 3.37	0.025	0.102	0.312
Right pericalcarine–left pericalcarine	Occipital–occipital	− 3.98	0.01	1.254	1.488
Left superior parietal–left fusiform	Parietal–temporal	− 3.55	0.021	0.208	0.382
Left superior parietal–left inferior temporal gyrus	Parietal–temporal	− 3.63	0.021	0.156	0.379

Functional connections displayed within this table represent connections that were significantly different between 22q11DS and controls, FDR-corrected, $p < 0.05$

[a] Mean functional connectivity values reported for each study group

Increased functional connectivity was also observed in frontal–occipital connections: between the right pars orbitalis and left cuneus, right pars orbitalis and right cuneus, right pericalcarine and left paracentral gyri, and right pericalcarine and right postcentral gyri. Relative to controls, increased functional connectivity was again displayed within frontal-parietal connections: between the right precuneus to the right caudal middle frontal gyrus, left precuneus and right pars orbitalis, right precuneus and right pars orbitalis, left precuneus and right superior frontal gyrus, right precuneus and right superior frontal gyrus.

Reduced functional connectivity in 22Q11DS vs. controls

Reduced functional connectivity was observed between the right superior frontal gyrus and right lateral orbitofrontal cortex. We also observed reduced functional connectivity in 22q11DS in parietal-temporal connections: between the left superior parietal lobule and left fusiform gyrus and left superior parietal lobule and left inferior temporal lobe.

Functional connectivity within 22Q11DS

Between the nonprodromal and prodromal 22q11DS groups, we observed only one significant difference between groups: increased functional connectivity between the left inferior temporal and right pericalcarine gyri (t = 3.68, p_{FDR} = 0.038) (Fig. 2).

Associations with psychosis in 22q11DS

After correction for multiple comparisons, ($p_{FDR} < 0.05$) a ZIP regression analysis reported increased functional connectivity between the left precuneus and right superior frontal was positively associated with positive symptoms (z = 5.72, p = 0.008). Reduced functional connectivity between the right pericalcarine and left pericalcarine was positively associated with positive symptoms (z = 4.39, p = 0.008). Increased functional connectivity between the right pericalcarine and right postcentral were found to be negatively associated with positive psychotic symptoms (z = − 2.95, p = 0.016) (see Fig. 3).

Heterogeneity effects in controls

Since seven of our controls in the current report were diagnosed with an anxiety disorder, depression, or ADHD, we conducted a separate functional connectivity analysis in CONN excluding those seven participants to account for any potential confounding effects in our FC results. Our findings remained significant after FDR correction, $p < 0.05$, and we continued to observe the same patterns of increased/decreased functional connectivity between the frontal–occipital, frontal–parietal, occipital–occipital, and superior parietal-inferior temporal connections. However, we did observe that once these controls were excluded, functional connectivity between frontal–frontal regions (superior frontal lobe–posterior cingulum; precentral gyrus–posterior cingulum) and one

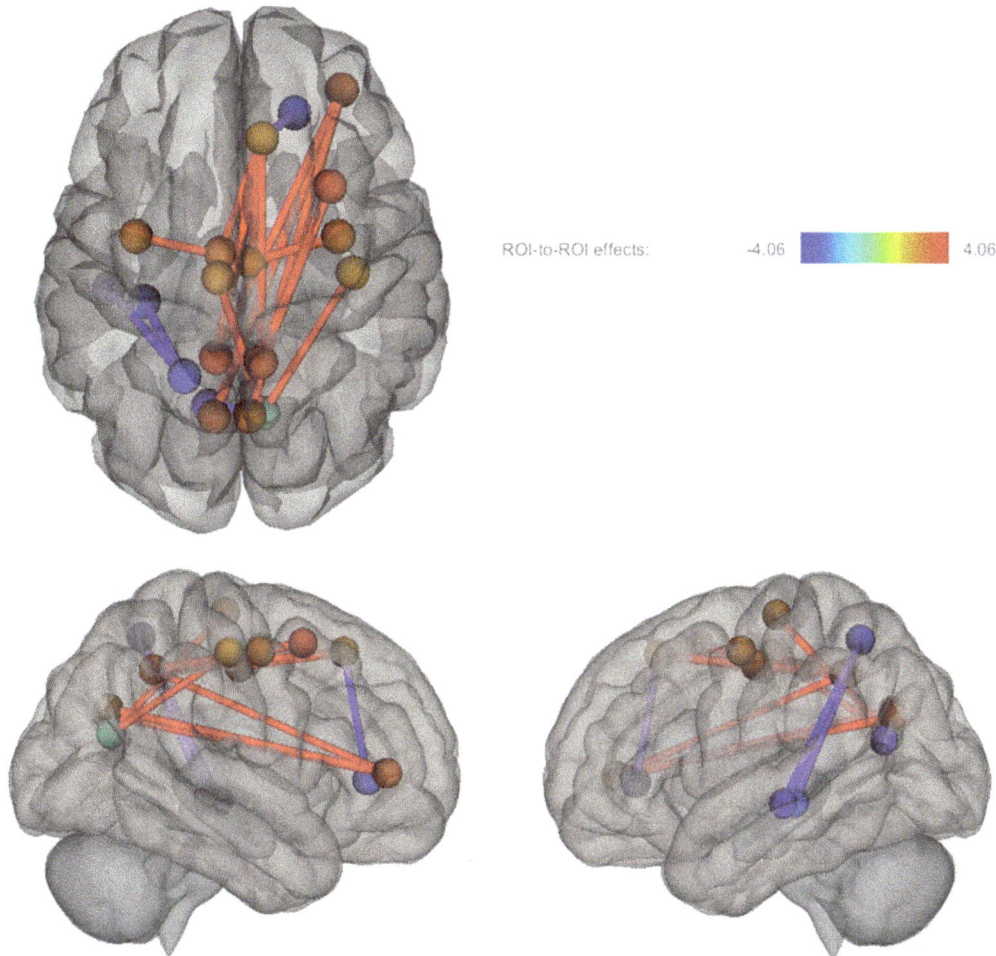

Fig. 1 This figure depicts significant differences in functional connectivity between 22q11DS and control samples. The color bar represents t values of results in axial (top) and left and right sagittal views. Red indicates increased FC in 22q11DS and blue indicates reduced FC in 22q11DS

frontal–parietal connection (pars orbitalis–precuneus) no longer met threshold for significance.

Discussion

Using a seed-based connectivity analysis of 2278 ROI-to-ROI connections, we observed both hyper- and hypo-connectivity in frontal–frontal gyri, frontal–parietal gyri, frontal–occipital gyri, parietal–temporal gyri and occipital–occipital gyri in young adults with 22q11DS relative to controls. Notable findings included (1) increased functional connectivity between frontal (superior frontal, caudal middle frontal and pars orbitalis) gyri and the precuneus, and (2) increased functional connectivity between posterior cingulate gyrus and both superior frontal and precentral gyri. Anomalies in frontal–parietal and occipital–occipital gyral connectivity were significantly associated with positive symptoms of psychosis.

The precuneus, caudal middle frontal and pars orbitalis (i.e., medial inferior frontal) regions constitute part

of the default mode network (DMN), which as noted above, is reported to be anomalous in both schizophrenia and 22q11DS. Studies have demonstrated that the DMN is active not only during rest but also during activities involving self-referential [41] and social-interpersonal processing [42]. Evidence suggests that the DMN may be involved in auditory hallucinations in individuals with schizophrenia [43–45], although other networks have been implicated as well [46, 47]. In individuals with 22q11DS, the DMN has been associated with prodromal symptoms [21], sustained attention [21] and reciprocal social behaviors [23]. It is not clear why we observed increased functional connectivity between these DMN regions, while several other studies [23–26] of 22q11DS have observed decreased functional connectivity between these regions. This may be attributable, in part, to our implementation of measurements within each subject's native brain space. In light of the anatomic differences that have been reported in brains of individuals

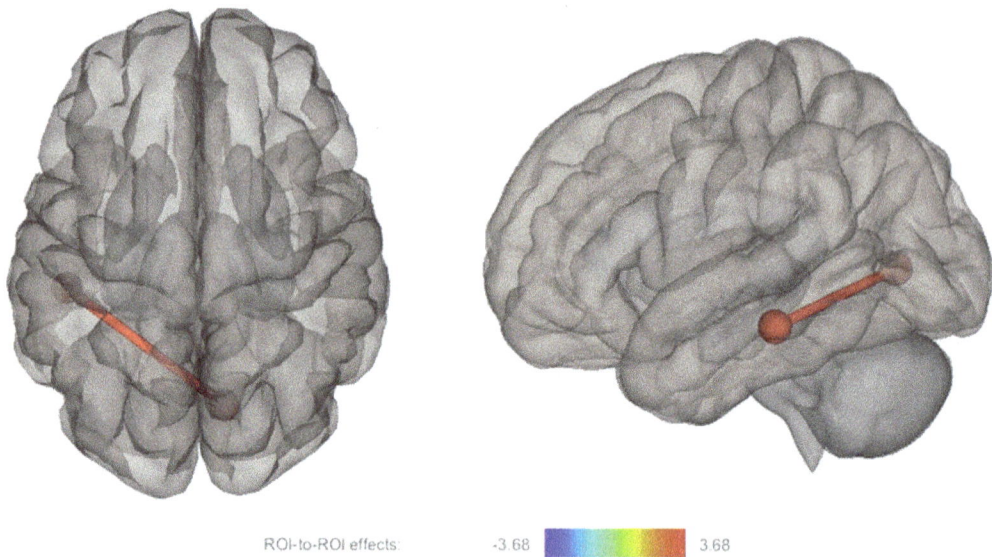

Fig. 2 This figure depicts differential functional connectivity between prodromal and nonprodromal (prodromal > nonprodromal) 22q11DS samples represented by left sagittal and superior axial views

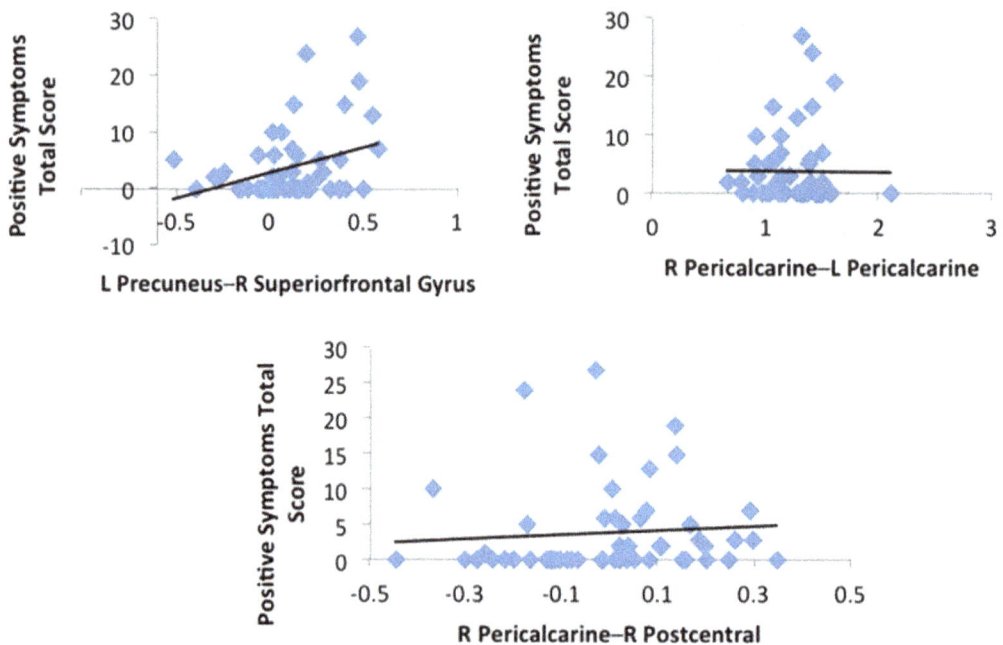

Fig. 3 This figure depicts plots representing associations between total positive symptoms scores measured by the SIPS and functional connectivity in connections that were significantly different between 22q11DS and controls

with 22q11Ds, retaining each subject's native brain space may have produced results that are not totally (anatomically) comparable to studies in which brains are warped to a standard template. Moreover, potential differences in sample characteristics (e.g. IQ levels; medication usage) between studies may also be contributing to differences in the direction of these results (see review by Scariati and colleagues [19]). Additional insight into why our finding of increased functional connectivity in the DMN differs from several (but not all [21, 22]) studies of 22q11DS is suggested by the results of two previously-published papers [22, 24] that included samples that overlapped with the sample of the current. In our two previously-published papers, we pooled samples from two research sites, and applied Independent Components Analyses to the pooled data. However, preprocessing methods differed somewhat between the two papers. In the first paper, by Mattiaccio and colleagues [22], for which data were preprocessed and analyzed at our site, increased functional connectivity in the DMN was observed. In the second paper, by Schreiner and colleagues [24], the data were preprocessed and analyzed by our collaborating site, and decreases in functional connectivity in the DMN were observed. Interestingly, our respective sites' preprocessing methods differed in motion correction and noise reduction strategies, potentially accounting for the discrepancies in results. This supports the notion that differences in image processing methods and in sample characteristics may be contributing to between-study differences in results.

The posterior cingulate gyrus (PCG) is also part of the default mode network, and we found anomalies in connectivity between PCG and superior frontal and precentral gyri. The extent to which PCG—superior frontal connections in our study reflects the DMN is not completely clear, since we utilized a predefined, atlas-based approach that maps onto regions that subsume, but are not synonymous with the DMN. Nonetheless, primate (and more recently, human imaging) studies indicate that the PCG has strong, reciprocal connections to the dorsolateral prefrontal cortex (DLPFC) [48–50], which overlaps with the superior frontal region included in the Desikan-Killany atlas. It has been suggested that PCG-DLPFC connections may be part of both the dorsal attention network and the frontal-parietal control network [51] both of which contribute to efficient cognitive function. Functional connectivity of the PCG and the superior aspect of the DLPFC has been linked to goal-directed thought processes [52], suggesting that this reciprocal connection may subserve executive planning [53, 54] and cognitive control [53, 55], both of which are impaired in individuals with 22q11DS [56–59]. Moreover, these functional brain networks have been shown to be impaired in schizophrenia [14, 60, 61] and 22q11DS [22, 24, 62].

Of the 16 ROI-to-ROI connections that significantly differentiated individuals with 22q11DS from controls, 13 (81%) of them included at least one ROI in the frontal lobe. These findings are consistent with other functional connectivity studies of both idiopathic schizophrenia [7, 12, 13, 63] and 22q11DS [20, 23] and suggest that both short-range and long-range connectivity of the frontal lobe is anomalous in individuals with this syndrome. To the extent that the frontal lobe subserves a myriad of cognitive and social-affective functions, functional dysconnectivity of networks that include the frontal lobe could underlie many of the cognitive and psychiatric impairments that are associated with 22q11DS [20, 23]. For example, in addition to schizophrenia, frontal dysconnectivity has been implicated in both autism spectrum disorders and in ADHD, both of which are elevated in 22q11DS [5, 57, 64–68].

In our sample, positive prodromal symptoms of psychosis were associated with increased connectivity between the superior frontal gyrus and the precuneus, and with decreased connectivity between the right and left pericalcarine gyri of the occipital lobe, and between pericalcarine and postcentral gyri. As noted above, the precuneus and aspects of the superior frontal gyrus are included in the DMN, which previous studies of 22q11DS have associated prodromal symptoms as well [21]. Associations between parietal–occipital and occipital–occipital functional connections and prodromal symptoms of psychosis have not been reported. However, anatomic connections between parietal and occipital lobes, via the superior longitudinal fasciculus (SLF), have been reported to be aberrant in 22q11DS [69–72]. Moreover, in an overlapping sample, our group [73] recently reported associations between anatomic anomalies in the SLF and prodromal symptoms.

When we divided the group of individuals with 22q11DS into prodromal and nonprodromal subgroups, we observed a significant difference in connectivity between the left inferior temporal and right pericalcarine gyri. Interestingly, we recently reported (in the same patient sample) significant associations between white matter microstructural anomalies in the temporal-occipital aspect of the inferior longitudinal fasciculus and symptoms of psychosis [74]. Temporal-occipital alterations in functional connectivity have also been reported in patients experiencing their first episode of psychosis [75], further supporting the validity of these observations.

Limitations and conclusions

Our study utilized an atlas-based approach to investigate functional connectivity in 22q11DS, which permitted us to examine, within each individual's own fMRI space, more than 2000 functional connections throughout the cortex. A potential limitation to our method is that the acquisition time of 5 min that we used to acquire our fMRI data, while minimally acceptable for an fcMRI study, may not be optimal in order to minimize the effects of noise and ensure the detection of small correlations that might otherwise go unobserved [76]. A second potential limitation is that the connections we examined do not necessarily map specifically onto the networks that are traditionally examined in resting state fcMRI studies, thus limiting comparisons to other studies to some extent, and rendering conclusions regarding these comparisons somewhat speculative. Nonetheless, our results concur generally with previous studies that have observed DMN anomalies in 22q11DS and associations between DMN anomalies and prodromal symptoms of psychosis. However, we observed increased functional connectivity in DMN regions, in contrast to several previous studies that have observed reduced connectivity. As noted above, this may be due in part to the potential impact of current medication usage in our sample, and to study differences in image preprocessing. In addition, it should be noted that when we removed the subset of controls with ADHD and anxiety, study group differences in the connections between the PCG and both the superior frontal and precentral gyri did not survive correction for multiple comparisons. This may suggest that the presence of psychiatric disorders in our sample may be influencing our observation of study group differences in connectivity between PCG and other frontal-based regions; however, the removal of the control subgroup also reduced power to detect differences. Accordingly, future studies would benefit from larger samples to elucidate the potential interplay between the presence of psychiatric disorders in 22q11DS and functional connectivity. To the extent that sampling and image preprocessing differences account for discrepancies across studies, it would be useful, in general, to apply different preprocessing methods to identical samples in order to elucidate the extent to which these methods account for differences in results of functional connectivity studies. Within the area of neurofunction in 22q11DS, future studies should examine the associations between functional and structural connectivity in 22q11DS, in order to elucidate the extent to which neuroanatomic structure underlies functional anomalies and leads to the psychiatric impairments for which individuals with this disorder are at great risk.

Abbreviations

22q11DS: 22q11.2 deletion syndrome; FC: functional connectivity; ROI: region of interest; SCID: Structured Clinical Interview for DSM-IV Axis I disorders; SIPS: Structured Interview for Prodromal Symptoms; SPM: statistical parametric mapping; DMN: default mode network; PCG: posterior cingulate gyrus; DLPFC: dorsolateral prefrontal cortex; ADHD: attention deficit hyperactivity disorder; SLF: superior longitudinal fasciculus; corr: corrected.

Authors' contributions

LM participated in data processing and analysis, and wrote the Methods and Results sections of the manuscript. WK conceived of the study design, wrote the Introduction and Discussion sections of the manuscript, and edited the remainder of the manuscript. KA and WF conducted neuropsychological and psychiatric assessments. CT participated in the processing of structural data. IC participated in study design, data analysis, and contributed to the manuscript. All authors read and approved the final manuscript.

Author details

[1] Department of Psychiatry and Behavioral Sciences, State University of New York Upstate Medical University, 750 East Adams Street, Syracuse, NY, USA. [2] Department of Computer Science, State University of New York at Oswego, Oswego, NY, USA. [3] Department of Psychology, Syracuse University, Syracuse, NY 13210, USA.

Acknowledgements

Not applicable.

Competing interests

The authors declare that they have no competing interests.

Funding

Support for this study was provided by the National Institutes of Health, MH064824, to Wendy R. Kates.

References

1. Shprintzen RJ, Goldberg RB, Lewin ML, Sidoti EJ, Berkman MD, Argamaso RV, Young D. A new syndrome involving cleft palate, cardiac anomalies, typical facies, and learning disabilities: velo-cardio-facial syndrome. Cleft Palate J. 1978;15:56–62.
2. Jonas RK, Montojo CA, Bearden CE. The 22q11.2 deletion syndrome as a window into complex neuropsychiatric disorders over the lifespan. Biol Psychiatry. 2014;75:351–60.
3. Murphy KC, Jones LA, Owen MJ. High rates of schizophrenia in adults with velo-cardio-facial syndrome. Arch Gen Psychiatry. 1999;56:940–5.
4. Monks S, Niarchou M, Davies AR, Walters JT, Williams N, Owen MJ, van den Bree MB, Murphy KC. Further evidence for high rates of schizophrenia in 22q11.2 deletion syndrome. Schizophr Res. 2014;153:231–6.
5. Schneider M, Debbane M, Bassett AS, Chow EW, Fung WL, van den Bree M, Owen M, Murphy KC, Niarchou M, Kates WR, Antshel KM, Fremont W, McDonald-McGinn DM, Gur RE, Zackai EH, Vorstman J, Duijff SN, Klaassen PW, Swillen A, Gothelf D, Green T, Weizman A, Van Amelsvoort T, Evers L, Boot E, Shashi V, Hooper SR, Bearden CE, Jalbrzikowski M, Armando M, Vicari S, Murphy DG, Ousley O, Campbell LE, Simon TJ, Eliez S. International consortium on brain and behavior in 22q11.2 deletion syndrome. Psychiatric disorders from childhood to adulthood in 22q11.2 deletion syndrome: results from the International consortium on brain and behavior in 22q11.2 deletion syndrome. Am J Psychiatry. 2014;171:627–39.
6. McGrath J, Saha S, Chant D, Welham J. Schizophrenia: a concise overview of incidence, prevalence, and mortality. Epidemiol Rev. 2008;30:67–76.
7. Fornito A, Zalesky A, Pantelis C, Bullmore ET. Schizophrenia, neuroimaging and connectomics. Neuroimage. 2012;62:2296–314.
8. Stephan KE, Friston KJ, Frith CD. Dysconnection in schizophrenia: from abnormal synaptic plasticity to failures of self-monitoring. Schizophr Bull. 2009;35:509–27.
9. Friston KJ, Frith CD. Schizophrenia: a disconnection syndrome? Clin Neurosci. 1995;3:89–97.
10. Lynall ME, Bassett DS, Kerwin R, McKenna PJ, Kitzbichler M, Muller U, Bullmore E. Functional connectivity and brain networks in schizophrenia. J Neurosci. 2010;30:9477–87.
11. Cole MW, Anticevic A, Repovs G, Barch D. Variable global dysconnectivity and individual differences in schizophrenia. Biol Psychiatry. 2011;70:43–50.
12. Fornito A, Yoon J, Zalesky A, Bullmore ET, Carter CS. General and specific functional connectivity disturbances in first-episode schizophrenia during cognitive control performance. Biol Psychiatry. 2011;70:64–72.
13. Liu Y, Liang M, Zhou Y, He Y, Hao Y, Song M, Yu C, Liu H, Liu Z, Jiang T. Disrupted small-world networks in schizophrenia. Brain. 2008;131:945–61.
14. Repovs G, Csernansky JG, Barch DM. Brain network connectivity in individuals with schizophrenia and their siblings. Biol Psychiatry. 2011;69:967–73.
15. Deserno L, Sterzer P, Wustenberg T, Heinz A, Schlagenhauf F. Reduced prefrontal-parietal effective connectivity and working memory deficits in schizophrenia. J Neurosci. 2012;32:12–20.
16. Manoliu A, Riedl V, Zherdin A, Muhlau M, Schwerthoffer D, Scherr M, Peters H, Zimmer C, Forstl H, Bauml J, Wohlschlager AM, Sorg C. Aberrant dependence of default mode/central executive network interactions on anterior insular salience network activity in schizophrenia. Schizophr Bull. 2014;40:428–37.
17. Orliac F, Naveau M, Joliot M, Delcroix N, Razafimandimby A, Brazo P, Dollfus S, Delamillieure P. Links among resting-state default-mode network, salience network, and symptomatology in schizophrenia. Schizophr Res. 2013;148:74–80.
18. Narr KL, Leaver AM. Connectome and schizophrenia. Curr Opin Psychiatry. 2015;28:229–35.

19. Scariati E, Padula MC, Schaer M, Eliez S. Long-range dysconnectivity in frontal and midline structures is associated to psychosis in 22q11.2 deletion syndrome. J Neural Transm. 2016;123:823–39.

20. Scariati E, Schaer M, Richiardi J, Schneider M, Debbane M, De Van, Ville D, Eliez S. Identifying 22q11.2 deletion syndrome and psychosis using resting-state connectivity patterns. Brain Topogr. 2014;27:808–21.

21. Debbane M, Lazouret M, Lagioia A, Schneider M, De Van, Ville D, Eliez S. Resting-state networks in adolescents with 22q11.2 deletion syndrome: associations with prodromal symptoms and executive functions. Schizophr Res. 2012;139:33–9.

22. Mattiaccio LM, Coman IL, Schreiner MJ, Antshel KM, Fremont WP, Bearden CE, Kates WR. Atypical functional connectivity in resting-state networks of individuals with 22q11. 2 deletion syndrome: associations with neurocognitive and psychiatric functioning. J Neurodev Disord. 2016;8(1):2.

23. Schreiner MJ, Karlsgodt KH, Uddin LQ, Chow C, Congdon E, Jalbrzikowski M, Bearden CE. Default mode network connectivity and reciprocal social behavior in 22q11.2 deletion syndrome. Soc Cogn Affect Neurosci. 2014;9:1261–7.

24. Schreiner M, Forsyth JK, Karlsgodt KH, Anderson AE, Hirsh N, Kushan L, Uddin LQ, Mattiacio L, Coman IL, Kates WR, Bearden CE. Intrinsic connectivity network-based classification and detection of psychotic symptoms in youth with 22q11.2 deletions. Cereb Cortex. 2017;27:3294–306.

25. Padula MC, Schaer M, Scariati E, Schneider M, Van De Ville D, Debbane M, Eliez S. Structural and functional connectivity in the default mode network in 22q11.2 deletion syndrome. J Neurodev Disord. 2015;7:23.

26. Padula MC, Schaer M, Scariati E, Maeder J, Schneider M, Eliez S. Multimodal investigation of triple network connectivity in patients with 22q11DS and association with executive functions. Hum Brain Mapp. 2017;38:2177–89.

27. Scariati E, Schaer M, Karahanoglu I, Schneider M, Richiardi J, Debbane M, De Van, Ville D, Eliez S. Large-scale functional network reorganization in 22q11.2 deletion syndrome revealed by modularity analysis. Cortex. 2016;82:86–99.

28. Whitfield-Gabrieli S, Nieto-Castanon A. Conn: a functional connectivity toolbox for correlated and anticorrelated brain networks. Brain Connect. 2012;2:125–41.

29. Chai XJ, Castanon AN, Ongur D, Whitfield-Gabrieli S. Anticorrelations in resting state networks without global signal regression. Neuroimage. 2012;59:1420–8.

30. McKenna F, Koo BB, Killiany R, Alzheimer's Disease Neuroimaging Initiative. Comparison of ApoE-related brain connectivity differences in early MCI and normal aging populations: an fMRI study. Brain Imaging Behav. 2016;10:970–83.

31. Kates WR, Miller AM, Abdulsabur N, Antshel KM, Conchelos J, Fremont W, Roizen N. Temporal lobe anatomy and psychiatric symptoms in velocardiofacial syndrome (22q11.2 deletion syndrome). J Am Acad Child Adolesc Psychiatry. 2006;45:587–95.

32. Miller TJ, McGlashan TH, Rosen JL, Cadenhead K, Cannon T, Ventura J, McFarlane W, Perkins DO, Pearlson GD, Woods SW. Prodromal assessment with the structured interview for prodromal syndromes and the scale of prodromal symptoms: predictive validity, interrater reliability, and training to reliability. Schizophr Bull. 2003;29:703–15.

33. First MB, Spitzer RL, Gibbon M, Williams JBW. Structured Clinical Interview for DSM-IV-TR Axis I Disorders, Research Version, Patient Edition (SCID-I/P). New York: Biometrics Research, New York State Psychiatric Institute; 2002.

34. Dale AM, Fischl B, Sereno MI. Cortical surface-based analysis. I. Segmentation and surface reconstruction. Neuroimage. 1999;9:179–94.

35. Fedorov A, Beichel R, Kalpathy-Cramer J, Finet J, Fillion-Robin J-C, Pujol S, Bauer C, Jennings D, Fennessy FM, Sonka M, Buatti J, Aylward SR, Miller JV, Pieper S, Kikinis R. 3D Slicer as an image computing platform for the Quantitative Imaging Network. Magn Reson Imaging. 2012;30:1323–41.

36. Desikan RS, Segonne F, Fischl B, Quinn BT, Dickerson BC, Blacker D. An automated labeling system for subdividing the human cerebral cortex on MRI scans into gyral based regions of interest. Neuroimage. 2006;31:968–80.

37. McCarthy CS, Ramprashad A, Thompson C, Botti JA, Coman IL, Kates WR. A comparison of FreeSurfer-generated data with and without manual intervention. Front Neurosci. 2015;9:379.

38. Friston KJ, Penny WD, Ashburner JK, Stefan J, Nichols TE. Statistical parametric mapping: the analysis of functional brain images. London: Academic Press; 2006.

39. Freire L, Mangin JF. Motion correction algorithms may create spurious brain activations in the absence of subject motion. Neuroimage. 2001;14:709–22.

40. Mazaika P, Hoeft F, Glover GH, Reiss AL. Methods and software for fMRI analysis for clinical subjects. Human Brain Mapp. 2009;47:S58.

41. Buckner RL, Andrews-Hanna JR, Schacter DL. The brain's default network: anatomy, function, and relevance to disease. Ann N Y Acad Sci. 2008;1124:1–38.

42. Li W, Mai X, Liu C. The default mode network and social understanding of others: what do brain connectivity studies tell us. Front Hum Neurosci. 2014;8:74.

43. Alderson-Day B, McCarthy-Jones S, Fernyhough C. Hearing voices in the resting brain: a review of intrinsic functional connectivity research on auditory verbal hallucinations. Neurosci Biobehav Rev. 2015;55:78–87.

44. Garrity AG, Pearlson GD, McKiernan K, Lloyd D, Kiehl KA, Calhoun VD. Aberrant "default mode" functional connectivity in schizophrenia. Am J Psychiatry. 2007;164:450–7.

45. Wolf ND, Sambataro F, Vasic N, Frasch K, Schmid M, Schonfeldt-Lecuona C, Thomann PA, Wolf RC. Dysconnectivity of multiple resting-state networks in patients with schizophrenia who have persistent auditory verbal hallucinations. J Psychiatry Neurosci. 2011;36:366–74.

46. Lavigne KM, Rapin LA, Metzak PD, Whitman JC, Jung K, Dohen M, Loevenbruck H, Woodward TS. Left-dominant temporal-frontal hypercoupling in schizophrenia patients with hallucinations during speech perception. Schizophr Bull. 2015;41:259–67.

47. Vercammen A, Knegtering H, den Boer JA, Liemburg EJ, Aleman A. Auditory hallucinations in schizophrenia are associated with reduced functional connectivity of the temporo-parietal area. Biol Psychiatry. 2010;67:912–8.

48. Mufson EJ, Pandya DN. Some observations on the course and composition of the cingulum bundle in the rhesus monkey. J Comp Neurol. 1984;225:31–43.

49. Vogt BA, Pandya DN. Cingulate cortex of the rhesus monkey: II. Cortical afferents. J Comp Neurol. 1987;262:271–89.

50. Greicius MD, Supekar K, Menon V, Dougherty RF. Resting-state functional connectivity reflects structural connectivity in the default mode network. Cereb Cortex. 2009;19:72–8.

51. Leech R, Sharp DJ. The role of the posterior cingulate cortex in cognition and disease. Brain. 2014;137:12–32.

52. Gerlach KD, Spreng RN, Madore KP, Schacter DL. Future planning: default network activity couples with frontoparietal control network and reward-processing regions during process and outcome simulations. Soc Cogn Affect Neurosci. 2014;9:1942–51.

53. Leech R, Kamourieh S, Beckmann CF, Sharp DJ. Fractionating the default mode network: distinct contributions of the ventral and dorsal posterior cingulate cortex to cognitive control. J Neurosci. 2011;31:3217–24.

54. Leech R, Braga R, Sharp DJ. Echoes of the brain within the posterior cingulate cortex. J Neurosci. 2012;32:215–22.

55. Vincent JL, Kahn I, Snyder AZ, Raichle ME, Buckner RL. Evidence for a frontoparietal control system revealed by intrinsic functional connectivity. J Neurophysiol. 2008;100:3328–42.

56. Maeder J, Schneider M, Bostelmann M, Debbane M, Glaser B, Menghetti S. Developmental trajectories of executive functions in 22q11.2 deletion syndrome. J Neurodev Disord. 2016;8:10.

57. Antshel KM, Faraone SV, Fremont W, Monuteaux MC, Kates WR, Doyle A, Mick E, Biederman J. Comparing ADHD in velocardiofacial syndrome to idiopathic ADHD: a preliminary study. J Atten Disord. 2007;11:64–73.

58. Campbell LE, Azuma R, Ambery F, Stevens A, Smith A, Morris RG, Murphy DG, Murphy KC. Executive functions and memory abilities in children with 22q11.2 deletion syndrome. Aust N Z J Psychiatry. 2010;44:364–71.

59. Shapiro HM, Tassone F, Choudhary NS, Simon TJ. The development of cognitive control in children with chromosome 22q11.2 deletion syndrome. Front Psychol. 2014;5:566.

60. Zhou Y, Liang M, Jiang T, Tian L, Liu Y, Liu Z, Liu H, Kuang F. Functional dysconnectivity of the dorsolateral prefrontal cortex in first-episode schizophrenia using resting-state fMRI. Neurosci Lett. 2007;417:297–302.

61. Woodward ND, Rogers B, Heckers S. Functional resting-state networks are differentially affected in schizophrenia. Schizophr Res. 2011;130:86–93.

62. Zoller D, Schaer M, Scariati E, Padula MC, Eliez S, De Van, Ville D. Disentangling resting-state BOLD variability and PCC functional connectivity in 22q11.2 deletion syndrome. Neuroimage. 2017;149:85–97.

63. Skudlarski P, Jagannathan K, Anderson K, Stevens MC, Calhoun VD, Skud-larska BA, Pearlson G. Brain connectivity is not only lower but different in schizophrenia: a combined anatomical and functional approach. Biol Psychiatry. 2010;68:61–9.

64. Antshel KM, Fremont W, Roizen NJ, Shprintzen R, Higgins AM, Dhamoon A, Kates WR. ADHD, major depressive disorder, and simple phobias are prevalent psychiatric conditions in youth with velocardiofacial syndrome. J Am Acad Child Adolesc Psychiatry. 2006;45:596–603.

65. Antshel KM, Hendricks K, Shprintzen R, Fremont W, Higgins AM, Faraone SV, Kates WR. The longitudinal course of attention deficit/hyperactivity disorder in velo-cardio-facial syndrome. J Pediatr. 2013;163:187–93.

66. Jalbrzikowski M, Ahmed KH, Patel A, Jonas R, Kushan L, Chow C, Bearden CE. Categorical versus dimensional approaches to autism-associated intermediate phenotypes in 22q11.2 microdeletion syndrome. Biol Psychiatry Cogn Neurosci Neuroimaging. 2017;2:53–65.

67. Niarchou M, Martin J, Thapar A, Owen MJ, van den Bree MB. The clinical presentation of attention deficit-hyperactivity disorder (ADHD) in children with 22q11.2 deletion syndrome. Am J Med Genet B Neuropsychiatr Genet. 2015;168:730–8.

68. Vorstman JA, Morcus ME, Duijff SN, Klaassen PW, Heineman-de Boer JA, Beemer FA, Swaab H, Kahn RS, van Engeland H. The 22q11.2 deletion in children: high rate of autistic disorders and early onset of psychotic symptoms. J Am Acad Child Adolesc Psychiatry. 2006;45:1104–13.

69. Jalbrzikowski M, Villalon-Reina JE, Karlsgodt KH, Senturk D, Chow C, Thompson PM, Bearden CE. Altered white matter microstructure is associated with social cognition and psychotic symptoms in 22q11.2 microdeletion syndrome. Front Behav Neurosci. 2014;8:393.

70. Radoeva PD, Coman IL, Antshel KM, Fremont W, McCarthy CS, Kotkar A, Wang D, Shprintzen RJ, Kates WR. Atlas-based white matter analysis in individuals with velo-cardio-facial syndrome (22q11.2 deletion syndrome) and unaffected siblings. Behav Brain Funct. 2012;8:38.

71. Villalon-Reina J, Jahanshad N, Beaton E, Toga AW, Thompson PM, Simon TJ. White matter microstructural abnormalities in girls with chromosome 22q11.2 deletion syndrome, Fragile X or Turner syndrome as evidenced by diffusion tensor imaging. Neuroimage. 2013;81:441–54.

72. Kikinis Z, Asami T, Bouix S, Finn CT, Ballinger T, Tworog-Dube E, Kucher-lapati R, Kikinis R, Shenton ME, Kubicki M. Reduced fractional anisotropy and axial diffusivity in white matter in 22q11.2 deletion syndrome: a pilot study. Schizophr Res. 2012;141:35–9.

73. Kikinis Z, Cho KI, Coman IL, Radoeva PD, Bouix S, Tang Y, Eckbo R, Makris N, Kwon JS, Kubicki M, Antshel KM, Fremont W, Shenton ME, Kates WR. Abnormalities in brain white matter in adolescents with 22q11.2 deletion syndrome and psychotic symptoms. Brain Imaging Behav. 2016. https://doi.org/10.1007/s11682-016-9602-x.

74. Tylee D, Kikinis Z, Quinn TP, Antshel KM, Fremont W, Tahir MA, Zhu A, Gong X, Glatt SJ, Coman IL, Shenton ME, Kates WR, Makris N. Machine learning classification of 22q11.2 deletion syndrome: A diffusion tensor imaging study. NeuroImage Clin. 2017;15:832–42.

75. Alonso-Solis A, Corripio I, de Castro-Manglano P, Duran-Sindreu S, Garcia-Garcia M, Proal E, Nunez-Marin F, Soutullo C, Alvarez E, Gomez-Anson B, Kelly C, Castellanos FX. Altered default network resting state functional connectivity in patients with a first episode of psychosis. Schizophr Res. 2012;139:13–8.

76. Van Dijk KR, Hedden T, Venkataraman A, Evans KC, Lazar SW, Buckner RL. Intrinsic functional connectivity as a tool for human connectomics: theory, properties and optimization. J Neurophysiol. 2010;103:297–321.

Permissions

All chapters in this book were first published in B&BF, by BioMed Central; hereby published with permission under the Creative Commons Attribution License or equivalent. Every chapter published in this book has been scrutinized by our experts. Their significance has been extensively debated. The topics covered herein carry significant findings which will fuel the growth of the discipline. They may even be implemented as practical applications or may be referred to as a beginning point for another development.

The contributors of this book come from diverse backgrounds, making this book a truly international effort. This book will bring forth new frontiers with its revolutionizing research information and detailed analysis of the nascent developments around the world.

We would like to thank all the contributing authors for lending their expertise to make the book truly unique. They have played a crucial role in the development of this book. Without their invaluable contributions this book wouldn't have been possible. They have made vital efforts to compile up to date information on the varied aspects of this subject to make this book a valuable addition to the collection of many professionals and students.

This book was conceptualized with the vision of imparting up-to-date information and advanced data in this field. To ensure the same, a matchless editorial board was set up. Every individual on the board went through rigorous rounds of assessment to prove their worth. After which they invested a large part of their time researching and compiling the most relevant data for our readers.

The editorial board has been involved in producing this book since its inception. They have spent rigorous hours researching and exploring the diverse topics which have resulted in the successful publishing of this book. They have passed on their knowledge of decades through this book. To expedite this challenging task, the publisher supported the team at every step. A small team of assistant editors was also appointed to further simplify the editing procedure and attain best results for the readers.

Apart from the editorial board, the designing team has also invested a significant amount of their time in understanding the subject and creating the most relevant covers. They scrutinized every image to scout for the most suitable representation of the subject and create an appropriate cover for the book.

The publishing team has been an ardent support to the editorial, designing and production team. Their endless efforts to recruit the best for this project, has resulted in the accomplishment of this book. They are a veteran in the field of academics and their pool of knowledge is as vast as their experience in printing. Their expertise and guidance has proved useful at every step. Their uncompromising quality standards have made this book an exceptional effort. Their encouragement from time to time has been an inspiration for everyone.

The publisher and the editorial board hope that this book will prove to be a valuable piece of knowledge for researchers, students, practitioners and scholars across the globe.

List of Contributors

Yuqin Deng, Xiaochun Wang and Chenglin Zhou
Department of Sport Psychology, School of Kinesiology, Shanghai University of Sport, 399 Chang Hai Road, Shanghai 200438, People's Republic of China

Yan Wang
Interdisciplinary Center for Social and Behavioral Studies, Dongbei University of Finance and Economics, Dalian 116025, Liaoning Province, People's Republic of China.

Santeri Yrttiaho and Jukka M. Leppänen
Tampere Center for Child Health Research, School of Medicine, University of Tampere, Lääkärinkatu 1, 33520 Tampere, Finland

Dana Niehaus and Eileen Thomas
Department of Psychiatry, Faculty of Health Sciences, Stellenbosch University, Stellenbosch, South Africa

Chanyoung Ko
College of Medicine, Yonsei University, 50 Yonsei-ro, Seodaemun-Gu, Seoul 120-752, South Korea

Namwook Kim and Dong Ho Song and Keun-Ah Cheon
Division of Child and Adolescent Psychiatry, Department of Psychiatry, College of Medicine, Severance Hospital, Yonsei University, Seoul, South Korea
Institute of Behavioral Science in Medicine, College of Medicine, Yonsei University, 50 Yonsei-ro, Seodaemun-Gu, Seoul 120-752, South Korea

Eunjoo Kim
Department of Psychiatry, Institute of Behavioral Science in Medicine, College of Medicine, Gangnam Severance Hospital, Yonsei University, 211 Eonju-ro, Gangnam-gu, Seoul 06273, South Korea

Marcus Augusto de Oliveira, Camila Mendes de Lima, César Augusto Raiol Fôro, Marcia Consentino Kronka Sosthenes and João Bento-Torres
Laboratório de Investigações Em Neurodegeneração e Infecção, Instituto de Ciências Biológicas, Universidade Federal do Pará, Hospital Universitário João de Barros Barreto, Rua dos Mundurucus 4487, Guamá, Belém, Pará CEP 66073-000, Brazil

Daniel Guerreiro Diniz and Cristovam Wanderley Picanço Diniz
Laboratório de Investigações Em Neurodegeneração e Infecção, Instituto de Ciências Biológicas, Universidade Federal do Pará, Hospital Universitário João de Barros Barreto, Rua dos Mundurucus 4487, Guamá, Belém, Pará CEP 66073-000, Brazil
Laboratory of Experimental Neuropathology, Department of Pharmacology, University of Oxford, Oxford, England, UK

Pedro Fernando da Costa Vasconcelos
Departamento de Arbovirologia e Febres Hemorrágicas, Instituto Evandro Chagas, Ananindeua, Pará, Brazil

Daniel Clive Anthony
Laboratory of Experimental Neuropathology, Department of Pharmacology, University of Oxford, Oxford, England, UK

Ole Bernt Fasmer
Department of Clinical Medicine, Section for Psychiatry, Faculty of Medicine and Dentistry, University of Bergen, Bergen, Norway
Division of Psychiatry, Haukeland University Hospital, Bergen, Norway.
K.G. Jebsen Centre for Research on Neuropsychiatric Disorders, Bergen, Norway

Espen Borgå Johansen
Oslo and Akershus University College, Stensberggata 26, 0170 Oslo, Norway

Qin-qin He, Xiang He, Yu Zou, Qing-jie Xia, Liu-Lin Xiong and Chao-zhi Luo
Department of Anesthesia and Critical Care Medicine Translational Neuroscience Center, West China Hospital, Sichuan University, Chengdu 610041, Sichuan, China

Ting-hua Wang
Department of Anesthesia and Critical Care Medicine Translational Neuroscience Center, West China Hospital, Sichuan University, Chengdu 610041, Sichuan, China
Institute of Neuroscience and Experiment Animal Center, Kunming Medical University, Kunming 650031, China

Yan-ping Wang and Jia Liu
Institute of Neuroscience and Experiment Animal Center, Kunming Medical University, Kunming 650031, China

Xiao-song Hu
Center for Experimental Technology for Preclinical Medicine, Chengdu Medical College, Chengdu 610083, Sichuan, China

Amy K. Olszewski, Ioana L. Coman, Wanda Fremont and Wendy R. Kates
Department of Psychiatry, SUNY Upstate Medical University, 750 E. Adams St., Syracuse, NY 13210, USA

Zora Kikinis, Xue Gong, Yogesh Rathi, Anni Zhu and Sylvain Bouix
Department of Psychiatry, Brigham and Women's Hospital, Harvard Medical School, Boston, MA, USA

Nikolaos Makris
Department of Psychiatry, Brigham and Women's Hospital, Harvard Medical School, Boston, MA, USA
Departments of Psychiatry and Neurology, Massachusetts General Hospital, Harvard Medical School, Boston, MA, USA

Marek R. Kubicki
Department of Psychiatry, Brigham and Women's Hospital, Harvard Medical School, Boston, MA, USA

Department of Radiology, Brigham and Women's Hospital, Harvard Medical School, Boston, MA, USA

Christie S. Gonzalez and Kevin M. Antshel
Syracuse University, Syracuse, NY, USA

Martha E. Shenton
Department of Radiology, Brigham and Women's Hospital, Harvard Medical School, Boston, MA, USA. VA Boston Healthcare System, Harvard Medical School, Brockton, MA, USA

Chang-Hong Wang, Jing-Yang Gu, Xiao-Li Zhang, Jiao Dong, Ying-Li Zhang, Qiu-Fen Ning and Xiao-Wen Shan
Department of Psychiatry, The Second Affiliated Hospital of Xinxiang Medical University, Xinxiang 453002, Henan, China

Jun Yang
Standard Technological Co. Ltd. (Xinxiang Institute for New Medicine), Xinxiang 453003, Henan, China. Xinjiang Hongda Food and Beverage Co. Ltd., Xinjiang 043102, Shanxi, China

Yan Li
Department of Child and Adolescent, Public Health College, Zhengzhou University, 100 Kexue Road, Zhengzhou 450001, Henan, China

Radu Ionita, Paula Alexandra Postu, Marius Mihasan and Lucian Hritcu
Department of Biology, Alexandru Ioan Cuza University of Iasi, Bd. Carol I, No. 11, 700506 Iasi, Romania

Galba Jean Beppe
Laboratory of Animal Physiology, Faculty of Science, University of Yaoundé I, Yaoundé, Cameroon.
Department of Biological Sciences, Faculty of Science, University of Maroua, Maroua, Cameroon

Brindusa Alina Petre
Department of Chemistry, Alexandru Ioan Cuza University of Iasi, Bd. Carol I, No. 11, 700506 Iasi, Romania

Monica Hancianu and Oana Cioanca
Faculty of Pharmacy, University of Medicine and Pharmacy "Gr. T. Popa", 16 University Str., 700115 Iasi, Romania

Lian Shien Lee
Integrative Pharmacogenomics Institute (iPROMISE), Level 7, FF3, Universiti Teknologi MARA Selangor, Puncak Alam Campus, 42300 Bandar Puncak Alam, Selangor, Malaysia

Mohd Zaki Farah Naquiah Richard Johari James, Mohd Zaki Salleh and Lay Kek Teh
Integrative Pharmacogenomics Institute (iPROMISE), Level 7, FF3, Universiti Teknologi MARA Selangor, Puncak Alam Campus, 42300 Bandar Puncak Alam, Selangor, Malaysia
Faculty of Pharmacy, Universiti Teknologi MARA Selangor, Puncak Alam Campus, 42300 Bandar Puncak Alam, Selangor, Malaysia

Suraya Suratman
Faculty of Pharmacy, Universiti Teknologi MARA Selangor, Puncak Alam Campus, 42300 Bandar Puncak Alam, Selangor, Malaysia

Mohd Izhar Mohd Hafidz
Comparative Medicine and Technology Unit, Institute Bioscience, Universiti Putra Malaysia, 43400 Serdang, Selangor, Malaysia

Akemi Uwaya, Hyunjin Lee and Shigeo Ohta
Department of Biochemistry and Cell Biology, Institute for Advanced Medical Sciences, Nippon Medical School, 1-396 Kosugi-cho, Nakahara-ku, Kawasaki, Kanagawa 211-8533, Japan

Jonghyuk Park
Department of Laboratory Medicine, The Jikei University School of Medicine, 3-25-8, Nishi-Shimbashi, Minato-ku, Tokyo 105-8641, Japan

Hosung Lee
Department of Cell Biology and Neuroscience, Juntendo Medical School, 2-1, Hongo, Bunkyo-ku, Tokyo 113-8421, Japan

Junko Muto
Graduate School of Health and Sport Science, Nippon Sport Science University, 7-1-1 Fukasawa, Setagaya-ku, Tokyo 158-8508, Japan

Sanae Nakajima
Kyoritsu Women's Junior College, 2-2-1 Hitotsubashi, Chiyoda-ku, Tokyo 101-8437, Japan

Toshio Mikami
Department of Health and Sport Science, Nippon Medical School, 1-7-1, Sakaiminami machi, Mushasino-shi, Tokyo 180-0023, Japan

Sayaka Yokota, Keigo Hamami and Akiko Harada
Graduate School of Biological Sciences, Nara Institute of Science and Technology, 8916-5 Keihanna Science City, Nara 630-0192, Japan

Shoji Komai
Graduate School of Biological Sciences, Nara Institute of Science and Technology, 8916-5 Keihanna Science City, Nara 630-0192, Japan
JST, PRESTO, Saitama, Japan

Yusuke Suzuki
Graduate School of Medicine, Kyoto University, Kyoto, Japan

Takahiro Yoshikawa and Yoko Yamano
Department of Sports Medicine, Osaka City University Graduate School of Medicine, 1-4-3 Asahi-machi, Abeno-ku, Osaka, Osaka 545-8585, Japan

Masaaki Tanaka and Akira Ishii
Department of Physiology, Osaka City University Graduate School of Medicine, 1-4-3 Asahi-machi, Abeno-ku, Osaka, Osaka 545-8585, Japan

Yasuyoshi Watanabe
Department of Physiology, Osaka City University Graduate School of Medicine, 1-4-3 Asahi-machi, Abeno-ku, Osaka, Osaka 545-8585, Japan
RIKEN Center for Life Science Technologies, 6-7-3 Minatojima-minamimachi, Chuo-ku, Hyogo 650-0047, Japan

Shu Ping Chen, Yu Kan, Jian Liang Zhang, Jun Ying Wang, Yong Hui Gao, Xiu Mei Feng, Ya Xia Yan and Jun Ling Liu
Department of Physiology, Institute of Acupuncture and Moxibustion, China Academy of Chinese Medical Sciences, 16 Nanxiaojie Street, Dongzhimennei, Beijing 100700, China

Li Na Qiao
Department of Biochemistry and Molecular Biology, Institute of Acu-Moxibustion, China Academy of Chinese Medical Sciences, Beijing, China

Xiao G. Wu, Hong Miao, Jian J. Cheng, Shu F. Zhang and Ya Z. Shang
Hebei Province Key Research Office of Traditional Chinese Medicine Against Dementia/Institute of Traditional Chinese Medicine, Chengde Medical College/Hebei Province Key Laboratory of Traditional Chinese Medicine Research and Development, Chengde, Hebei 067000, China

Shu S. Wang
Hebei Research Institute for Family Planning, Shijiazhuang, Hebei 050000, China

Hao Cao and Helgi B. Schiöth
Department of Neuroscience, Uppsala University, Husargatan 3, BMC, 75124 Uppsala, Sweden

Galina Y. Zheleznyakova
Department of Neuroscience, Uppsala University, Husargatan 3, BMC, 75124 Uppsala, Sweden
Department of Clinical Neuroscience, Karolinska Institute, Karolinska University Hospital, CMM L8:04, 17176 Stockholm, Sweden

Wei-Chih Ou, Chen-Nu Liu, Mei-Chih Chen and Pei-Lain Chen
Department of Medical Laboratory Science and Biotechnology, Central Taiwan University of Science and Technology, No. 666 Buzih Road, Beitun District, Taichung City 40601, Taiwan

Chih-Ling Huang
Department of Nursing, Chang Jung Christian University, Tainan, Taiwan

Min-Hsuan Lin, Yi-Chun Chen and Ching-Shan Huang
Administration Center for Research and Education, Changhua Christian Hospital, Changhua, Taiwan

Yi-Ju Chen
Company Limited of Ditech Enterprise, Taipei, Taiwan

Yi-Chin Huang
Division of Infectious Diseases, Jen-Ai Hospital, Taichung, Taiwan

Morteza Zangeneh Soroush and Keivan Maghooli
Department of Biomedical Engineering, Science and Research Branch, Islamic Azad University, Tehran, Iran

Seyed Kamaledin Setarehdan
Control and Intelligent Processing Centre of Excellence, School of Electrical and Computer Engineering, College of Engineering, University of Tehran, Tehran, Iran

Ali Motie Nasrabadi
Department of Biomedical Engineering, Faculty of Engineering, Shahed University, Tehran, Iran

Chu-Chu Qi, Xue-zhu Ma and Jie Yin
Institute of Anatomy and Histology and Embryology, Neuroscience, School of Basic Medical Sciences, Lanzhou University, No. 199 of Donggang West Road, Lanzhou 730000, Gansu, People's Republic of China

Yu-Hong Jing
Institute of Anatomy and Histology and Embryology, Neuroscience, School of Basic Medical Sciences, Lanzhou University, No. 199 of Donggang West Road, Lanzhou 730000, Gansu, People's Republic of China
Key Laboratory of Preclinical Study for New Drugs of Gansu Province, Lanzhou University, No. 199 of Donggang West Road, Lanzhou 730000, Gansu, People's Republic of China

Qing-Jun Wang, Hai-Chao Chen and Li-Ping Gao
Institute of Biochemistry and Molecular Biology, School of Basic Medical Sciences, Lanzhou University, No. 199 of Donggang West Road, Lanzhou 730000, Gansu, People's Republic of China

Hanna Christiansen
Clinical Child and Adolescent Psychology, Department of Psychology, Philipps University Marburg, Gutenbergstr. 18, 35037 Marburg, Germany

Theresa S. Emser
Clinical Child and Adolescent Psychology, Department of Psychology, Philipps University Marburg, Gutenbergstr. 18, 35037 Marburg, Germany
Clinic for Child and Adolescent Psychiatry, University Clinic Würzburg, Margarete-Höppel-Platz 1, 97080 Würzburg, Germany

Blair A. Johnston
Division of Neuroscience, Medical Research Institute, Ninewells Hospital and Medical School, University of Dundee, Dundee DD1 9SY, UK

J. Douglas Steele
School of Medicine (Neuroscience), University of Dundee, Dundee DD1 9SY, UK

Sandra Kooij
PsyQ, Psycho-medical Programs, Expertise Center Adult ADHD, Jan van Nassaustraat 125, 2596 BS The Hague, The Netherlands

Lisa Thorell
Department of Clinical Neuroscience, Karolinska Institutet, Tomtebodavägen 18A, 5th floor, 171 77 Stockholm, Sweden

Vishwanath Vasudev Prabhu, Thong Ba Nguyen, Young-Eun Oh and Young-Chul Chung
Department of Psychiatry, Chonbuk National University Medical School, Jeonju 561-756, South Korea
Research Institute of Clinical Medicine of Chonbuk National University-Biomedical Research Institute of Chonbuk National University Hospital, Jeonju 561-756, South Korea

Keon-Hak Lee
Department of Psychiatry, Maeumsarang Hospital, 465-23, Wanju, Jeollabuk-do, South Korea

Yin Cui
Shanghai Mental Health Center, Shanghai Jiao Tong University of Medicine, 600 Wan Ping Nan Road, Shanghai 200013, P. R. China

Tarique R. Bagalkot
Department of Cell Biology, University of Pittsburgh, 200 Lothrop Street, Biomedical Science Tower S372, Pittsburgh, PA 15213, USA

Leah M. Mattiaccio, Carlie A. Thompson, Wanda P. Fremont and Wendy R. Kates
Department of Psychiatry and Behavioral Sciences, State University of New York Upstate Medical University, 750 East Adams Street, Syracuse, NY, USA

Ioana L. Coman
Department of Computer Science, State University of New York at Oswego, Oswego, NY, USA

Kevin M. Antshel
Department of Psychology, Syracuse University, Syracuse, NY 13210, USA

Index

A

Acetylcholinesterase, 102, 105, 112-114, 147

Acute Immobilization Stress, 125, 129-130, 134-136

Acute Lung Injury, 61, 65, 70-71, 73

Adhd, 2, 7-8, 24, 26, 28, 49-50, 56-60, 75, 77, 89, 230-242, 262, 264, 267-270

Alcl3, 103, 113, 169-170, 174, 177

Alzheimer's Disease, 46-47, 102, 112-113, 122, 169, 177-178, 190, 269

Astrocytes Morphology, 30, 37

Autism Spectrum Disorder, 21, 28, 90-91, 231

Autistic Symptom Severity, 21, 24, 26, 28

Autonomic Nervous System, 10, 16, 19

B

Basolateral Amygdala, 97, 137, 217-218, 228, 259

Bone Marrow Mesenchymal Stem Cell, 61-63

Bovine Serum Albumin, 219, 247, 257

Brain Ischemia, 61-62, 64-72

Brain-derived Neurotrophic Factor, 125, 179, 190-192

C

Catechol-o-methyltransferase, 193-194

Cerebral Artery Occlusion, 61, 73

Cingulate-frontal-striatum Network, 1

Complex Partial Seizure, 21

Cotinine, 193-196, 198-201

Cytochrome P450 2a6,, 193

D

Dempster Shafer Theory, 202

Dentate Gyrus, 30-31, 33-34, 37-48, 167

Diffusion Tensor Imaging, 75-76, 78, 80, 90-91, 270

Dna Methylation, 122, 179-184, 186-192

Dorsolateral Prefrontal Cortex, 148, 153-154, 157, 244, 267-269

E

Elevated Plus Maze, 115-116, 118, 145, 243, 245, 250-251, 257-258

Epilepsy, 21-29, 122, 158, 216, 233

F

Functional Magnetic Resonance Imaging, 1, 89, 158

G

Gasp-1, 244, 246-248, 251, 253, 256-257

Glial Cells, 43, 47, 92-93, 98-100, 172, 188

H

Hippocampal-dependent Task, 37

Hippocampus, 31, 33, 42-43, 46-48, 92-93, 97-103, 105, 112-113, 125-137, 159-169, 173-174, 177, 182, 192, 217-218, 225, 228, 246, 253-254, 257

Histone Acetylation, 122, 125-126, 134-135, 137

I

Infant Face Stimuli, 11, 16, 19

Inferior Frontal Gyrus, 1, 5, 7

Interference Resolution, 1, 7

L

Luminance-matched Non-face Stimuli, 9-10, 16

M

M1 Machr, 159, 161-163, 165-167

M2 Machr, 159, 161-163, 165, 167

Magnetoencephalography, 148-149, 157-158

Markhamia Tomentosa, 102-103, 106-108, 110, 113

Medial Prefrontal Cortex, 1, 5, 137, 217-218, 228, 256

Meta-analysis, 1-8, 90, 93, 97, 241

Motor Activity, 49-60, 145, 241

Multi-source Interference Task, 1-2, 5, 7-8

N

Nachr, 159-167

Neuropathic Pain, 159-160, 162-165, 167

O

Orbitofrontal Cortex, 76, 148, 152-153, 155, 157-158

Oxidative Stress, 101-103, 112-114

P

Passive Avoidance Test, 139-143, 145

Psychiatric Disorders, 24, 77, 89, 124, 179-180, 182, 184, 188, 190-191, 268

Psychosis, 24, 26, 75, 77, 85-86, 88-90, 191, 260-262, 264-265, 267-270

Pulmonary Edema, 61-62, 69, 73

Pulmonary Injury, 61-62, 69
Pupil Dilation, 9-10, 12-18, 20

R
Rab4, 243, 246-248, 251, 253, 255-257
Resting Brain Activity, 148, 156

S
S100b Protein, 92-93, 95, 97-100
Schizophrenic, 58, 182, 259
Scopolamine, 102-104, 106-108, 110-114
Scutellaria Barbata Flavonoids, 169-170, 177-178
Shr, 49-60
Social Brain Network, 75, 88, 90
Social Responsiveness Scale, 21-22, 28-29, 75, 78, 82-84, 89-90
Spatial Memory, 37, 42-43, 46, 48, 102, 113, 137, 170-171, 174

Sucrose Preference Test, 94, 96
Superior Longitudinal Fasciculus, 76, 80-81, 89, 267-268

T
Tail Suspension Test, 140, 144, 147
Transgenerational Effects, 115, 122-123
Two-tensor Tractography, 75, 78-79, 89 142

V
Velo-cardio-facial Syndrome, 75, 77, 89, 260, 268, 270
Venlafaxine, 92-101

W
Wais-iii, 77-78, 89
Western Blot Analysis, 62, 65, 125, 162, 220
White Matter Tracts, 75-76, 78, 80, 87-88, 91
Whole Brain Tractography, 78-79, 87